Ultrasonography Examination

Notice

Medicine is an ever-changing science. As new research and clinical experience broaden our knowledge, changes in treatment and drug therapy are required. The authors and the publisher of this work have checked with sources believed to be reliable in their efforts to provide information that is complete and generally in accord with the standards accepted at the time of publication. However, in view of the possibility of human error or changes in medical sciences, neither the authors nor the publisher nor any other party who has been involved in the preparation or publication of this work warrants that the information contained herein is in every respect accurate or complete, and they disclaim all responsibility for any errors or omissions or for the results obtained from use of the information contained in this work. Readers are encouraged to confirm the information contained herein with other sources. For example and in particular, readers are advised to check the product information sheet included in the package of each drug they plan to administer to be certain that the information contained in this work is accurate and that changes have not been made in the recommended dose or in the contraindications for administration. This recommendation is of particular importance in connection with new or infrequently used drugs.

Ultrasonography Examination

Fifth Edition

Charles S. Odwin, BS, PA-C, RDMS
Senior GYN Physician Assistant
Women's Health NCB Hospital
Director of PA GYN Ultrasound
Department of Obstetrics and Gynecology
North Central Bronx Hospital
Clinical Assistant Professor, College of Health Professions
Pace University, New York, New York

Arthur C. Fleischer, MD
Cornelius Vanderbilt Professor
Departments of Radiology and Radiological Sciences
and Obstetrics and Gynecology
Medical Director, Sonography
Medical Director, Sonographer Training Program
Vanderbilt University Medical Center
Nashville, Tennessee

George L. Berdejo, BA, RVT, FSVU
Director, Vascular Ultrasound Services
White Plains Physician Associates
White Plains Hospital
White Plains, New York

McGraw Hill

New York   Chicago   San Francisco   Athens   London   Madrid   Mexico City
Milan   New Delhi   Singapore   Sydney   Toronto

LANGE REVIEW: Ultrasonography Examination, Fifth Edition

Copyright © 2021, 2012, 2004 by McGraw Hill. All rights reserved. Printed in China. Except as permitted under the United States Copyright Act of 1976, no part of this publication may be reproduced or distributed in any form or by any means, or stored in a data base or retrieval system, without the prior written permission of the publisher.

Previous editions copyright © 1993, 1987 by Appleton & Lange.

2 3 4 5 6 7 8 9   MER   28 27 26 25 24

ISBN 978-1-260-44135-2
MHID 1-260-44135-0

This book was set in Minion Pro by KnowledgeWorks Global Ltd.
The editors were Susan Oldenburg and Christie Naglieri.
The production supervisor was Catherine Saggese.
Project management was provided by Sarika Gupta, KnowledgeWorks Global Ltd.

This book is printed on acid-free paper.

Library of Congress Cataloging-in-Publication Data
Names: Odwin, Charles S., editor. | Fleischer, Arthur C., editor. |
  Berdejo, George L., editor.
Title: Lange review : ultrasonography examination / [edited by] Charles S.
  Odwin, Arthur C. Fleischer, George L. Berdejo.
Other titles: Ultrasonography examination
Description: Fifth edition. | New York : McGraw Hill, 2021. | Includes
  bibliographical references and index. | Summary: ""Since the publication
  of the 4th edition of Appleton and Lange"s Review for the
  Ultrasonography Examination, there have been many additional refinements
  in the applications of sonography. This new and updated 5th edition has
  been extensively revised to include more comprehensive material and
  instrumentation and contains chapters including 3D OB/GYN sonography,
  pediatric sonography, and breast sonography. In addition, the physics
  and instrumentation and vascular sonography chapters have been revised
  to current knowledge in order to better prepare candidates for the ARDMS
  board examinations. Hundreds of ultrasound images, including color
  Doppler is now included to assist the sonographer in visualizing
  pathologic conditions. This text contains 16 chapters with new enhanced
  color illustrations relevant anatomic information. The rapid expansion
  and evolution of sonographic techniques and their clinical applications
  requires that sonographers continually update, expand and enhance their
  clinical skills. Sonographers now routinely perform 3D sonography,
  duplex and color Doppler studies, and detailed examinations of the fetus
  and pelvic organs, and they provide vitally important guidance for
  interventional procedures using sonography. This rapid pace of
  innovation makes our field exciting and rewarding and, at the same time,
  demands that sonographers constantly improve their scanning skills. It
  is the intention of this book to enable both students as well as ""young""
  and experienced sonographers to enhance their knowledge base.
  Accordingly, it is much more than a study guide directed solely at
  passing a one-time test. It also provides a basis for the continuous
  study of diagnostic sonography"— Provided by publisher.
Identifiers: LCCN 2020029638 (print) | LCCN 2020029639 (ebook) | ISBN
  9781260441352 (paperback ; alk. paper) | ISBN 9781260441369 (ebook)
Subjects: MESH: Ultrasonography | Examination Questions
Classification: LCC RC78.7.U4 (print) | LCC RC78.7.U4 (ebook) | NLM WN
  18.2 | DDC 616.07/543—dc23
LC record available at https://lccn.loc.gov/2020029638
LC ebook record available at https://lccn.loc.gov/2020029639

McGraw Hill books are available at special quantity discounts to use as premiums and sales promotions, or for use in corporate training programs. To contact a representative, please visit the Contact Us pages at www.mhprofessional.com.

Dedication

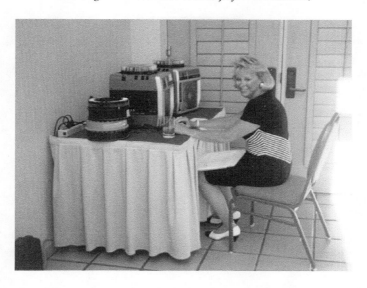

(Donna preparing for her lecture in the Mid-1990s in Florida. The little square objects that she is handling are slides. Photo courtesy of A.C. Fleischer.)

I would like to acknowledge the pride, professionalism, and enthusiasm of the late Donna Kepple, RT, RDMS, by dedicating this 5th edition of *Lange Review: Ultrasonography Examination* in her memory. Ms. Kepple was a prime example of how a caring and compassionate professional could combine technical expertise in sonography to enhance a patient's life and those that worked and interacted with her. Beginning in the early 1980s, Donna was one of the first students to graduate from our first Sonographer Training Program and then continue to excel at the local and national meetings. She touched not only her patients' lives, but those residents, medical students, and fellow sonographers nationwide that she came in contact with. She was a superb teacher, acting not only as Chief Sonographer for 18 years but was Program Director of our first "Era" of our sonography training program in 1982–1986. She was also involved in many sonographic societies, serving as an officer and in the American Registry of Diagnostic Medical Sonographers (ARDMS) and American Institute of Ultrasound in Medicine (AIUM), being recognized as "Sonographer of the Year" by AIUM 1996.

She exemplifies the impact of a dedicated, caring, and compassionate professional. On a lighter note she always insisted on being referred to as "sonographer" rather than "ultrasound technician." She leaves pleasant thoughts to those that knew her and an example of the impact that a committed medical professional can impart both to her patients and fellow professionals every day.

Acknowledgments

The author/editors would like to express their gratitude to Susan Barnes of McGraw Hill Publishers and her staff who guided and enabled the completion of this edition. Their commitment and guidance in this process is gratefully acknowledged. We would also like to express appreciation to Vera Merriweather, senior administrative assistant to Dr. Fleischer for her assistance with revisions of this edition.

We would also like to thank Michael Zinaman, MD, Chinyere Anyaogu, MD, and Tisha Brizz PA-C, from the North Central Bronx Hospital who were so kind to allow for a flexible work schedule for PA Odwin, which enable him to work on this edition and Lennox Tate for his help with the images.

We also want to acknowledge previous contributors and new ones for their expertise and assistance to the completion of this review. Finally, we cannot thank enough all of our sonographers and sonography students for providing the help, feedback, and inspiration for this project.

Sonography: Principles, Techniques, and Instrumentation

Mary Ann Keenan, Charles S. Odwin, and Arthur C. Fleischer

Study Guide

Diagnostic medical sonography, or diagnostic ultrasound imaging, is an imaging method that uses ultrasound waves to generate images of structures in the body for diagnosis of physical or medical conditions. It is typically performed by a sonographer, who is a medical professional specially trained in the use of ultrasound devices for acquiring medically diagnostic images. Other medical professionals, such as physicians, physician assistants, and nurses, may use ultrasound devices for imaging or special procedures. In this chapter, we will discuss the physical science behind ultrasound imaging. We will discuss the physical characteristics of ultrasound and how sound travels through different mediums. Additionally, this chapter will cover the mechanisms associated with the ultrasound transducer and how it generates and receives ultrasound waves. We will also explain the ultrasound imaging chain from formation to display and the basic functions of the ultrasound machine. We will end the discussion with methods for evaluation of the ultrasound system and the biological effects that are associated with ultrasound usage on human tissue.

PHYSICAL SCIENCE OF ULTRASOUND

Ultrasound is a wave that is comparable to the familiar water wave with its peaks and troughs. Ultrasound waves travel in a longitudinal format and are considered mechanical in nature. This means that an ultrasound wave has movement, force, and is measurable. We measure an ultrasound wave the same way one would measure any wave, by the number of times the wave repeats itself in a given time period, or by its cycles per unit time. Ultrasound is defined as a wave that repeats itself at a frequency greater than 20,000 times per second (or 20,000 Hz). The unit hertz (Hz) simply means cycles per second and is an internationally accepted term. Humans cannot hear sound generated at this high frequency.

Ultrasound must have a medium in which it travels. This is because it travels, or propagates by passing energy, from one particle to another in a rolling, or oscillatory motion. Oscillatory motion creates areas in the wave cycle where particles are compressed together (compression) and areas where particles are farther apart, (rarefaction). In areas of compression, the pressure, or force of the wave is highest. In areas of rarefaction, the pressure and force are lowest.

Ultrasound waves can be created with continuous motion (continuous wave) or from the pulsing of sound (pulsed-wave ultrasound). In continuous-wave ultrasound, the oscillatory vibrations are constant. For pulsed-wave ultrasound, pulses of sound are sent out to create the oscillatory wave motion. During periods between pulses, the system is "listening" for reflected sound waves to return. Most modern-day ultrasound units use pulsed ultrasound for normal imaging.

The following terms are commonly used in diagnostic medical sonography and help to describe how sound interactions with different medium:

Longitudinal wave is a wave in which the particles of the medium travel in a direction parallel to the direction of the wave propagation. This is opposite of a *transverse wave* (shear wave), in which particles are moving perpendicular to the direction of wave propagation.

Mechanical wave is a wave that requires a medium in which to travel. It cannot propagate through a vacuum (a space that has no medium or matter). The wave travels by transferring energy from one particle to another as it propagates in an oscillatory motion through the medium in.

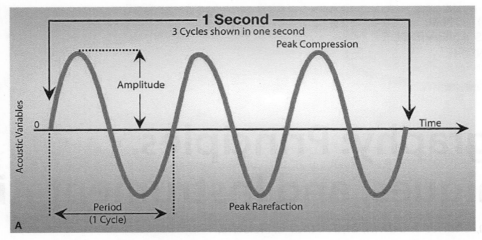

FIGURE 1–1A. The parameters of a wave. The frequency of the wave variable is 3 Hz (or three complete cycles per second). A period is one complete cycle. This wave consists of three periods. *Note*: In the vertical direction, a positive (upward) variable change represents compression and a negative (downward) variable change represents rarefaction. Both represent pressure and density.

Acoustic variable. *Pressure, temperature, density, particle motion (distance)* are all acoustic variables. Variable means that they change with time as the acoustic wave propagates through the medium.

Parameters of a wave (Fig. 1–1A). The following terms are common to all waves:

Cycle. A cycle is composed of one compression and one rarefaction, or one complete positive and negative change.

Frequency (f) in general is the number of times something happens per unit time. For ultrasound waves, it is the number of cycles per second. Ultrasound wave frequency describes how many times the acoustic variable (pressure, temperature, density, particle motion) goes through a complete cycle in one second. Mathematically, we represent frequency as follows and in units of hertz (Hz), megahertz (MHz), or kilohertz (kHz):

$$\text{frequency } (f) = \frac{\text{propagation speed}}{\text{wavelength}}, \quad f = \frac{c}{\lambda} \quad (1\text{--}1)$$

Period is the time it takes for 1 cycle to occur. It is the inverse of frequency. It is mathematically expressed as follows and typically in units of seconds (s) or microseconds (μs):

$$\text{period } (p) = \frac{1}{\text{frequency}}, \quad p = \frac{1}{f} \quad (1\text{--}2)$$

As the frequency increases, the period decreases. Conversely, as the frequency decreases, the period increases.

Wavelength (λ) is the distance the wave must travel in 1 cycle. Wavelength is determined by both the source of the wave and the medium in which it is propagating (Fig. 1–1B). It is

represented mathematically by the following and typically in units of meters (m) or millimeters (mm):

$$\text{wavelength } (\lambda) = \frac{\text{propagation speed}}{\text{frequency}}, \quad \lambda = \frac{c}{f} \quad (1\text{--}3)$$

The velocity or propagation speed of sound in soft tissue is 1540 m/s, which results in a wavelength of 1.54 mm for 1 MHz, 0.77 mm for 2 MHz, and 0.51 mm for 3 MHz.

Propagation speed is the maximum speed with which an acoustic wave can move through a medium and is determined by the density and stiffness of the medium. Propagation speed increases proportionally with the stiffness (ie, the stiffer the medium, the faster the variable will travel). Density is the

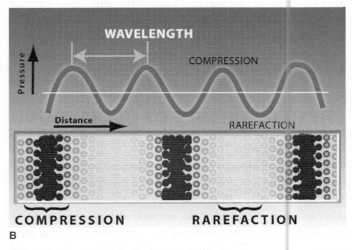

FIGURE 1–1B. A longitudinal sound wave demonstrating areas of compression corresponding to the peak positive amplitudes and areas of rarefaction corresponding to the negative amplitude peaks. This also demonstrates a wavelength, the distance between a point on one wave to the same point on the adjacent wave. In this example the points are adjacent positive peaks.

concentration of mass per unit volume, and propagation speed is inversely proportional to density. Propagation speed is mathematically represented by the following equations and in units of distance per second. Typically, meters per second (m/s) or millimeters per second (mm/s).

$$propagation\ speed\ (c) = \sqrt{\frac{elasticity\ (stiffness)}{density}},$$

$$c(m/s) = \sqrt{\frac{E(kg/m \cdot s^2)}{\rho(kg/m \cdot s^3)}} \qquad (1\text{-}4)$$

Compressibility is the opposite of stiffness. If a medium is more compressible, it is less rigid or stiff and the propagation speed in that medium will be less. Propagation speed is greater in solids > liquids > gases.

$$propagation\ speed\ (c) = wavelength \times frequency,$$

$$c\ (m/s) = \lambda(m) \times f(1/s) \qquad (1\text{-}5)$$

Note: Propagation speed is constant for a given medium. In other words, the propagation speed will always be the same in that specific medium. If the frequency increases, the wavelength will decrease. Conversely, if the frequency decreases, the wavelength will increase.

Example

An ultrasound wave traveling through soft tissue is increased from 2 to 4 MHz. What happens to the wavelength after this increase?

Step 1: Start with the equation. propagation speed (c) = wavelength (λ) × frequency (1/s).

Solve for the wavelength.

$\lambda = c_{soft\ tissue}$/frequency, where propagation speed in tissue = 1540 m/s or 1.54 mm/μs, frequency$_1$ is 2 MHz or 2/μs and frequency$_2$ is 4 MHz or 4/μs.

Step 2: Calculate the two wavelengths.

$$\lambda_1 = \frac{1.54\ mm/\mu s}{2/\mu s} = 0.77\ mm$$

$$\lambda_2 = \frac{1.54\ mm/\mu s}{4/\mu s} = 0.385\ mm$$

As you can see, doubling the frequency will halve the wavelength in a given medium. *Note:* the wavelength got smaller as the frequency increased.

PULSED-WAVE ULTRASOUND

Pulsed-wave ultrasound functions as an ultrasound wave with the same variables and characteristics described in the previous section. The formation of the pulsed ultrasound wave is different such that time between the production of one sound pulse and the next pulse is delayed. This allows time for returning echoes or "reflections" of the wave.

The following parameters are used to describe the characteristics associated with pulsed-wave ultrasound:

Pulse repetition frequency (PRF) is the number of pulses per second. It is typically represented with the units of hertz (Hz) or kilohertz (kHz). Imaging depth will determine the timing of the PRF. As imaging depth increases, PRF will decrease due to the increase in time needed for the echoes to return from a reflecting surface. The deeper the reflector, the more spacing required between pulses. The sonographer does not typically control the PRF. It is automatically adjusted by the system as the depth of penetration is changed.

Pulse repetition period (PRP) is the time from the beginning of one pulse to the beginning of the next. The units for PRP are usually represented in seconds (s) or milliseconds (ms).

$$PRP = \frac{1}{PRF}$$

The PRP increases as imaging depth increases. When depth decreases, the PRP decreases.

Pulse duration (PD) is the time it takes for a pulse to occur. Mathematically, PRP is the *period* of the pulse multiplied by the number of cycles in the pulse (Fig. 1–2A). The units for PD are typically represented in a form of seconds (s), milliseconds (ms), or microseconds (μs).

$$PD = period \times number\ of\ cycles = p \times n \qquad (1\text{-}6)$$

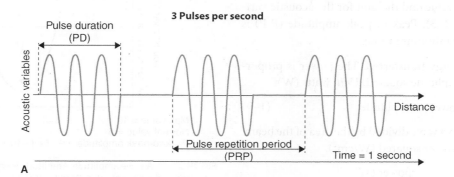

FIGURE 1–2A. Pulse repetition period (PRP).

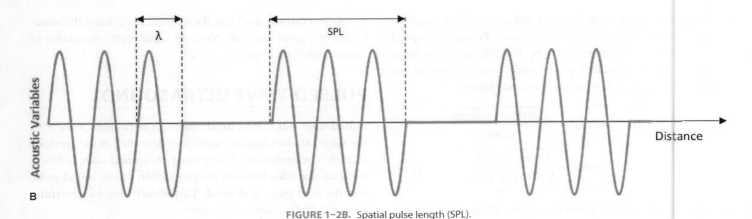

FIGURE 1–2B. Spatial pulse length (SPL).

Duty factor (DF) is the fraction of time that the transducer is generating a pulse.

Maximum value: 1.0. In continuous-wave ultrasound, the transducer is **always** generating a pulse. For reception, a second transducer acts as the listening device.

Minimum value: 0.0. The transducer is **not** being excited or activated, and no pulse will be generated. In clinical imaging, using pulse-echo systems, the DF ranges from 0.001 to 0.01. *Units:* unitless.

$$DF = \frac{PD(\mu s)}{PRP(ms) \times 1000} = \frac{PD(\mu s) \times PRF(1/ms)}{1000} \quad (1-7)$$

Note: DF is unitless. It may be necessary to use a conversion factor if PD units of time do not match with the PRP units of time. These must match to cancel each other out. In this example PD is in units of microseconds. It is necessary to divide by 1000 for the units to cancel out the units of PRP which are in milliseconds.

Spatial pulse length (SPL) is the distance over which a pulse occurs (Fig. 1–2B). *Units:* Typically represented in units of millimeters (mm). Mathematically, SPL = wavelength (λ) × number of cycles in the pulse (n).

$$SPL = \lambda \times n \quad (1-8)$$

Amplitude is the maximum variation that occurs in an acoustic variable. It indicates the strength of the sound wave. To arrive at this variation, the undisturbed value is subtracted from the maximum value and the unit for the acoustic variable is applied (Fig. 1–3). Peak-to-peak amplitude (P-P) is the maximum to the minimum value.

Power is the rate of energy transferred. The power is proportional to the wave amplitude squared. *Unit:* watts (W).

$$power \propto amplitude^2 \quad (1-9)$$

Intensity is the power in a wave divided by the area of the beam. *Unit:* watts per centimeter squared (W/cm^2).

$$intensity = \frac{power\ (W)}{area\ (cm^2)} \quad (1-10)$$

Note: For a given area, the intensity is proportional to the wave amplitude squared. Therefore, if the amplitude doubles, the intensity quadruples.

ULTRASOUND POWER AND INTENSITY

As noted above, the power and intensity of the ultrasound beam are not identical, although the two terms are sometimes used interchangeably. *Ultrasound power* is the rate at which work is done or energy is transferred from one medium or system to another. Mathematically, power is the amount of energy transferred divided by the time it takes to transfer the energy. For the purposes of this discussion, the units are simply represented in watts. Intensity is the power distributed over a certain area, or power divided by the area (W/cm^2). The value represents the strength of the ultrasound beam. Typically, for diagnostic ultrasound imaging, intensities range from 10 to 50 mW/cm^2. Later in this chapter, we will discuss the important relationship between intensity and biological effects.

Intensities are represented in both peak and average values. The intensity of the sound beam as it travels through a medium

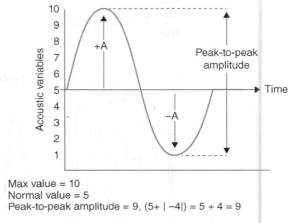

Max value = 10
Normal value = 5
Peak-to-peak amplitude = 9, (5+ | −4|) = 5 + 4 = 9

FIGURE 1–3. A wave amplitude. Amplitude is equal to the maximum value minus the normal value. Peak-to-peak (P-P) amplitude is equal to the maximum plus the absolute value of the minimum.

will vary with time (*temporal intensity*) and vary across the volume of the beam (*spatial intensity*).

Spatial peak (SP) is intensity at the center of the beam.

Spatial average (SA) is intensity averaged throughout the beam.

Temporal peak (TP) is the maximum intensity in the pulse (measured when the pulse is on).

Temporal average (TA) is intensity averaged over one on-off beam cycle (it includes the intensity from the beginning of one pulse to the beginning of the next).

Pulse average (PA) is intensity averaged over the duration of a single pulse.

The above descriptors can be combined to describe effects from both spatial and temporal intensities:

Spatial peak-temporal peak	SPTP Highest
Spatial Peak-pulse average	SPPA
Spatial average-pulse average	SAPA
Spatial average-temporal peak	SATP
Spatial peak-temporal average	SPTA (Tissue heating)
Spatial average-temporal average	SATA Lowest

In pulsed ultrasound, the TP is greater than the PA, which is greater than the TA (TP > PA > TA). When using continuous-wave ultrasound, TP and TA intensities are the same.

Spatial peak intensity is related to SA by the **beam non-uniformity ratio (BNR)**, sometimes called the beam uniformity ratio (BUR). BNR is a unitless coefficient that describes how uniform the sound beam intensity is distributed. The higher the SP, the more concentrated the intensity. The higher the SA, the less concentrated. A low BNR represents a more uniform beam.

$$\text{BNR} = \frac{\text{spatial peak intensity (W/cm}^2)}{\text{spatial average}}, \text{BNR} = \frac{\text{SP}}{\text{SA}} \quad (1\text{--}11)$$

Temporal average intensity is related to TP by the DF. *Units:* unitless.

$$\text{duty factor} = \frac{\text{temporal average}}{\text{temporal peak}}, \text{DF} = \frac{\text{TA}}{\text{TP}} \quad (1\text{--}12)$$

Attenuation

Attenuation describes the fading, or reduction of the sound beam's amplitude and intensity as it travels through a medium. It explains why echoes from deep structures are weak compared with those from superficial or shallow structures. The following factors, terms, and formulas are used to describe and assess attenuation and its components:

Absorption is the conversion of sound energy into heat energy. It is the major source of attenuation in soft tissue.

Scattering. *Diffuse scattering* is the redirection of the sound beam after it strikes rough boundaries or boundaries that are smaller than the wavelength of the sound wave. Liver parenchyma and red blood cells often cause diffuse scattering.

Reflection is the return of a portion of the ultrasound beam back toward the transducer (an echo). A special type of reflection, *specular reflection*, occurs when the wavelength of the pulse is much smaller than the boundary it is striking, and the boundary is smooth. Good examples of specular reflecting surfaces are the diaphragm, liver capsule, and gallbladder wall. Reflection of the ultrasound beam depends on the *acoustic impedance mismatch* at the boundary between two media. We will discuss impedance differences later in this chapter.

The decibel is the unit of intensity or power ratios. Mathematically, it is as expressed as ten times the log of the intensity or power ratio.

$$\text{decibels (dB)} = 10 \log \frac{\text{final intensity}}{\text{initial intensity}}, \text{dB} = 10 \log \frac{\text{I}_f}{\text{I}_i} \quad (1\text{--}13)$$

Attenuation coefficient is the attenuation per unit length the sound wave travels through a medium and is expressed in units of dB/cm. This value is dependent on the frequency of sound from the transducer and the medium through which it is traveling. For soft tissue, it is approximately one-half of the operating frequency of the transducer ($ac_{\text{soft tissue}} = 0.5 \text{dB/cm·MHz}$). In other words, there is about 0.5 dB of attenuation per MHz and per centimeter traveled by the sound wave.

$$\text{attenuation (dB)} = \text{attenuation coefficient (dB/cm)}$$
$$\times \text{ path length} \quad (1\text{--}14)$$

Note: For the sake of this discussion the sonographer need not know the complexities that derive the different attenuation coefficients. It should be understood that decibels are derived from exponents. Therefore, small changes in decibels can mean a large change in resulting values. The best technique for learning attenuation with respect to decibels is to memorize commonly encountered values (Table 1–1). In the first line of the table, the attenuation or loss of 3 dB (shown as −3 dB) means the intensities was reduced by half. A loss of 10 dB (or −10 dB) means the intensity was reduced to one-tenth of the initial intensity.

TABLE 1-1 • Decibel Values of Attenuation

Decibels (dB)	Value
−3	(1/2) 0.5
−6	(1/4) 0.25
−9	(1/8) 0.13
−10	(1/10) 0.10
−20	(1/100) 0.01
−30	(1/1,000) 0.001

Half-intensity depth is the distance at which the intensity will be one-half of the original. Also stated as, the distance the sound beam will travel through a medium before its intensity is reduced by 50%. It is calculated by the following formula:

$$\text{half-intensity depth} = \frac{3\ \text{dB}}{\text{attenuation coefficient (dB/cm)}} \quad (1\text{-}15)$$

For soft tissue, the half-intensity depth can be calculated from the frequency, using the following equation:

$$\text{half-intensity depth} = \frac{6\ \text{cm} \cdot \text{MHz}}{\text{frequency (MHz)}} \quad (1\text{-}16)$$

The half-intensity depth is a good indicator of the frequency that should be selected to view different structures in the body. For example, if 50% of the intensity is gone before one reaches a certain depth, then it is obvious that the deeper structures will receive less of the sound beam, generating weaker echoes. To visualize deep structures, it is necessary to use a lower frequency.

Example 1

The ultrasound beam produced by a 4 MHz had an original intensity of 20 mW/cm² with a pathlength of 3 cm. Assume an attenuation coefficient of soft tissue ($ac_{\text{soft tissue}} = 0.5$ dB/cm · MHz). Find the final intensity value.

Step 1: Find the attenuation coefficient with respect to the transducer frequency.

$$ac_{\text{soft tissue}} = \frac{0.5\,\text{dB}}{(\text{cm} \cdot \text{MHz})} \times 4\,\text{MHz} = 2\,\text{dB/cm}$$

Step 2: Apply to the given attenuation equation to find the dB loss.

attenuation = 2 dB/cm × 3 cm = 6 dB of attenuation or −6 dB

Step 3: From the table, we can see that a loss of 6 dB means the intensity was reduced to 1/4th (or 25%) its original intensity. The original intensity was 20 mW/cm².

$$\frac{20\ \text{mW/cm}^2}{4} = 5\ \text{mW/cm}^2$$

The final intensity could also have been predicted another way. We know that for every 3 dB loss, the intensity is reduced by half or 50%, thus 3dB plus 3dB is a 6dB loss. You can calculate this in your head often. For the first 3 dB loss, the beam was reduced to 10 mW/cm² (half of the 20). For the second 3 dB, the beam was reduced again by half, yielding 5 mW/cm² (half of the 10).

Example 2

An ultrasound beam with an initial intensity of 100 mW/cm² passes through soft-tissue media which results in a final intensity of 0.01 mW/cm². How much attenuation occurred?

Step 1: Know your givens. $I_{\text{final}} = 0.01$ mW/cm²; $I_{\text{initial}} = 100$ mW/cm²

and Knowns: attenuation (dB) = 10 log ($I_{\text{final}}/I_{\text{initial}}$)

Step 2: Calculate based on the original attenuation formula.

$$\text{attenuation (dB)} = 10 \log \frac{0.01}{100} = 10 \log 0.0001$$
$$= 10\,(-4) = -40\ \text{dB or a loss of 40 dB}$$

Note: It is not uncommon for attenuation to be given without the negative sign. Strictly mathematically speaking, the negative value denotes loss or attenuation. A positive value mathematically represents gain. When the negative value is not given, the value should be stated as "a loss" or "attenuation" of *x* number of decibels.

The ultrasound system allows for electronic adjustments to improve visualization due to loss of echo strength from attenuation effects. Terms used to describe this mechanism are as follows:

Time gain compensation (TGC) is an electronic compensation for tissue attenuation.

TGC near gain increases or decreases the echo brightness in the near field.

TGC far gain increases or decreases the echo brightness in the far field.

Overall gain increases or decreases the overall brightness in the image.

Echoes

Echoes are the reflections of the sound beam as it travels through the media. An echo is generated each time the beam encounters an acoustic impedance mismatch, but its strength depends on several factors. One very important factor is the *angle of incidence*. This is the angle at which the incident beam strikes a boundary. The angle of incidence (θ_i) is equal to the angle of reflection (θ_R) (Fig. 1–4A).

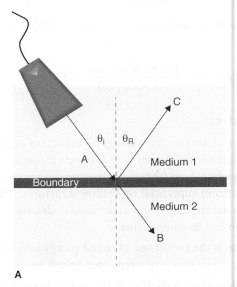

A

FIGURE 1–4A. (A) An oblique incidence striking a boundary; **(B)** refraction of the sound beam; **(C)** reflection of the sound beam. *Note:* There are only two approaches for the incident angle. *Oblique* and *normal* incidence (Normal means perpendicular to or at a 90° angle). Any incidence angle that is not a normal incidence is considered an oblique incidence.

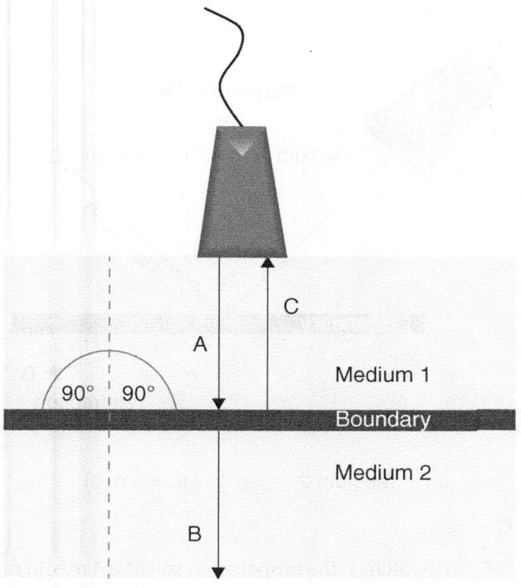

FIGURE 1–4B. The transmission of the perpendicular incidence sound beam, also called normal incidence. (**A**) Normal incidence striking a boundary perpendicularly; (**B**) the intensity transmitted; (**C**) reflection of energy at the boundary of medium 1 and medium 2. *Note:* Beam C travels back along the same beam path as (**A**), although shown here as separate.

Perpendicular incidence is a beam traveling through a medium perpendicular to a boundary and encountering the boundary at a 90° angle (Fig. 1–4B). Perpendicular incidence is also known as *normal incidence.*[1] The portion of the beam that is not reflected continues in a straight line. This continuation is called *transmission.*

Perpendicular incidence will produce a reflection when the acoustic impedance of the medium changes at the boundary. *Acoustic impedance (Z) is the product of the density of a medium and the velocity of sound in that medium.*

$$\text{Acoustic impedance (rayls)} = \text{density (kg/m)}$$
$$\times \text{propagation speed(m/s)}, Z = \rho \times c \quad (1\text{--}17)$$

At an acoustic impedance mismatch, the sound beam will proceed (transmission), be reflected, or both. The relationship between perpendicular incidence and the intensity of the echoes can be characterized by the following formulas:

$$\text{intensity reflection coefficient (IRC)} = \left(\frac{z_2 - z_1}{z_2 + z_1}\right)^2 \quad (1\text{--}18a)$$

$$\text{intensity reflection coefficient (IRC)} = \frac{\text{reflected intensity}}{\text{incident intensity}}$$
$$= \frac{I_r(W/cm^2)}{I_i(W/cm^2)} \quad (1\text{--}18b)$$

$$\text{intensity transmission coefficient (ITC)} = \frac{\text{transmitted intensity}}{\text{incident intensity}}$$
$$= \frac{I_t(W/cm^2)}{I_r(W/cm^2)}$$

$$(1\text{--}19a)$$

The intensity transmission coefficient (ITC) represents the part of sound that is not reflected. It can also be calculated from the intensity reflection coefficient by the following formula:

$$\text{ITC} = 1 - \text{IRC} \quad (1\text{--}19b)$$

As you can see, if the IRC increases, the ITC decreases. If the IRC decreases, the ITC will increase. The incident intensity is reflected and transmitted. The sum of these two parts represents one hundred percent of the incident intensity of the beam.

Example

Given two media, one with an acoustic impedance of 20 rayls and the other with an acoustic impedance of 40 rayls, calculate the intensity reflection coefficient (IRC), the intensity transmission coefficient (TC), the reflected intensity, and the transmitted intensity. (Assume that the incident intensity is 10 mW/cm².)

Step 1: You are given Z_1 = 20 rayls, Z_2 = 40 rayls, from this you can calculate IRC.

$$\text{IRC} = \left(\frac{Z_2 - Z_1}{Z_2 + Z_1}\right)^2 = \left(\frac{40-20}{40+20}\right)^2 = \left(\frac{20}{60}\right)^2 = \left(\frac{1}{3}\right)^2 = 0.11$$

Step 2: Calculate the ITC from the above IRC of 0.11.

$$\text{ITC} = 1 - \text{IRC} = 1 - 0.11 = 0.89$$

Step 3: You are given the incident intensity as I_i = 10 mW/cm². Solve for the reflected intensity by rearranging the IRC *equation 1-18b*. Note the units are given in mW/cm², so the answer will also be in these units. Also note that the IRC is unitless, because it is a ratio of values with the same units. The units are cancelled out.

reflected intensity (I_r (mW/cm²))
= IRC × I_i (mW/cm²)
= 0.11 × 10 mW/cm² = 1.1 mW/cm²

Step 4: The transmitted intensity is equal to the ITC (calculated in Step 2) times the original intensity. Rearranging the ITC **equation 1-19a**, just as above.

transmitted intensity (I_t (mW/cm²))
= ITC × I_i (mW/cm²)
= 0.89 × 10 mW/cm² = 8.9 mW/cm²

Oblique incidence is used to describe the angle of incidence that is not 90° or perpendicular to the boundary it approaches. When oblique incidence occurs, the angle of transmission will equal the angle of incidence only if the propagation speeds of the media on each side of the boundary are equal. If the propagation speeds are different, the transmission angle will not be equal to the incident angle. The beam will change direction. This change in direction or change between incident and transmission angles is called refraction (Snell's law). Figs. 1–5A–C illustrates the changes that occur based on the propagation speed differences of the media on either side of the boundary.

the characters appeared to be moving in a jerky fashion. In order for the motion to appear smooth to the perceiving eye, a presentation of images must be at least 30 per second. A 2D ultrasound image is a single frame consisting of a number of lines of data across the FOV or width of the sector. Each line of data consists of the echo information received back into the transducer from along the trajectory of the line. Factors affecting temporal resolution are the following:

- Frame rate
- Sector width (width of the FOV)
- Number of pulses or lines
- Line density (spacing of lines distributed evenly across the FOV)

The best temporal resolution will have a high frame rate, a narrow sector width, fewer pulses, and a low line density. However, adjusting each of these factors has a cost. This will be discussed later in the image quality section.

IMAGING PRODUCTION

The basic components that make up the pulsed-echo ultrasound system are the beam former (pulse generator and receiver), signal processor, image processor, and the display. Along with the transducer, each component is required to generate, display, and store ultrasound images. *Fig. 1–22 is a simplified block diagram of the main and subcomponents of the system. The order of function can be slightly different, depending on the system, but the general operations are consistent. Operations of very modern systems may vary from this discussion, but at present we will present the traditional operations.*

Beam Former

Pulser. The *pulser* produces an electric voltage that activates the piezoelectric element. This causes the element to contract and expand to produce the longitudinal compression wave (sound beam), as discussed in the section on Transducers. A second function of the pulser is to signal the receiver and scan converter that the transducer has been activated.

Each electric pulse generates an ultrasonic pulse. The number of ultrasonic pulses per second is defined as the *pulse repetition frequency* (PRF). As discussed earlier in the chapter, the PRF is determined by the imaging depth. If the sonographer chooses to image at a deeper depth, more time is required to "listen" for the return echoes and the system will automatically reduce the PRF. For diagnostic ultrasound imaging the PRF typically ranges from approximately 1 to 10 kHz, and for Doppler ultrasound, it is from approximately 5 to 30 kHz. *Remember, PRF is referring to the number of pulses generated per second. The definition of frequency is: how often something occurs in a sample, or the number of times something occurs in a specific window of time. When we discuss the frequency of the sound wave generated, we are discussing the number of cycles in the pulse (Fig. 1–1A). These are two different distinctions.*

With multielement array transducers, the pulser is responsible for the delay and variations in pulse amplitude needed for electronic control of beam scanning, steering, and shaping. Part of this control serves to reduce off axis (grating lobe) energy, which could interfere with image quality. The term used for the process of reducing off axis energy is *dynamic apodization*. Dynamic apodization improves the dynamic range of multielement transducers. A more detailed discussion of off axis energy can be found in the Attenuation Artifacts section.

The pulser controls the intensity of the beam by way of the voltage amplitude (height). If you recall from earlier in the chapter, *power* is proportional to the wave amplitude squared and *intensity* is the power in a wave divided by the area of the beam. By increasing the output (transmit) power, the pulser is signaled to generate increased voltage amplitudes. Remember the rule: If the amplitude doubles, the intensity quadruples. Increasing the strength of the output signal will increase the strength of the returned echo, while reducing noise and

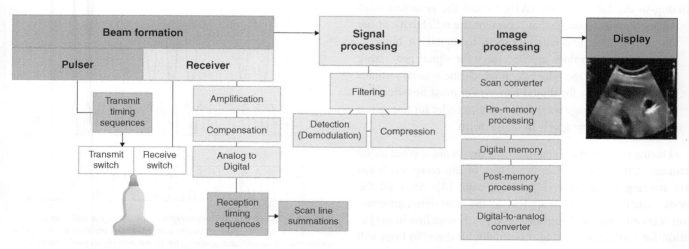

FIGURE 1–22. Simplified block diagram of the main and subcomponents of the system.

improving SNR ratio. But there is a cost, increased intensity could result in harmful biological effects. (Bioeffects are discussed later in the chapter.)

Receiver. When an echo returns from a reflector, its mechanical force generates an electrical, or voltage signal in the transducer. The *receiver* not only captures all of the returned electric echo signals, but it must process the signals in order for them to be usable for the creation of the image. Processing involves **amplification, compensation,** conversion of the **analog signal to digital, filtering (rejection), compression,** and **detection (demodulation).**

Amplification. Voltages from the transducer, or return echo signals, are extremely weak compared with the transmitted signal, which is controlled by the output (transmit) power. The returned signals must be enhanced to be acceptable for further processing and storage. Amplifiers enhance the signals by increasing the returned voltage amplitudes. This process is sometimes described as, increasing the "overall gain" because all signals are increased, including the noise, proportionately. The SNR ratio remains the same. Receiver gain is mathematically defined as the ratio of the amplifier output electric power to the input electric power and is expressed in units of decibels (dB).

Compensation is another mechanism that improves echo information that is lost due to attenuation at depth. When simultaneous pulses produce echoes from two objects with equal reflective properties, but located at different depths, the echo traveling from the deeper object will be weaker, due to attenuation (see Attenuation, page 5). It will arrive at a later time than the echo from the shallower reflector. The weaker echo will have a decreased amplitude signal, which must be enhanced to match the brightness of the earlier echo. Compensation at depth is often referred to as "time-gain-compensation" or TGC. Attenuation increases with depth and with transducer frequency. For soft tissue, 0.5 dB of attenuation per centimeter of travel, per MHz of frequency.

Analog-to-digital converter (ADC) takes the returned echo voltage signals (analog) that represent the reflectivity of the tissue structures, and converts them to digital, or numeric values. Numeric values are necessary for signal processing and memory storage. The rate at which the system samples the voltage signals for digital conversion must be twice that of the highest voltage wave frequency, in order for the values to be represented properly in digital form.

During the reception chain, timing delays are applied to the returned echo signals for optimization of the reception focus and steering (*recall Receive focusing*, page 13). After all the receive functions have been applied, all the echo signal information is coordinated and summed along each scan line in preparation for further processing. Eventually, all the scan lines will make up the completed image.

Signal Processing

Signal processing takes the digital echo information from each scan line and prepares it for the image processing operation. The information must be filtered, smoothed, and compressed to a usable range.

Filtering. Filtering is primarily a means for reducing electronic noise. Although this is a step of signal processing, it is also a function of the amplifier. Amplifiers are adjusted such that they only allow signals within a certain range to pass through for amplification, thus eliminating (rejecting) frequencies above and below the set range. This mechanism helps to reduce signals that do not provide meaningful information in the image.

Detection (Demodulation). Demodulation is another method for transforming the signal information into a more useful form. Recall the amplitude descriptor of Fig. 1–3, which shows the peaks of the waves as peak amplitudes. Note there is a positive amplitude and a negative amplitude to the waveform. Demodulation uses a process called rectification, which inverts the negative values of the voltage signals, making them positive values. The strength of the voltage amplitude is maintained, yet the negative values now become positive (Figs. 1–23A and B). Additionally, the pulse information is smoothed, allowing for one mean signal per pulse to be recorded (Fig. 1–23C).

Compression. *Dynamic range* is the range between the smallest amplitude, or power that the system can process to the largest. This ratio is expressed in decibels (dB). The human eye is capable of discerning about 20 dB of gray levels in an image. Additionally, most image displays are limited to a range of about 30 dB of gray level. Although the system can produce a much wider dynamic range, more range means more information to be stored in the computer memory. Compression narrows the difference between the largest echo signals and the smallest signals, compressing them to a useful range and reducing the amount of stored information. The system can do this in many ways, for

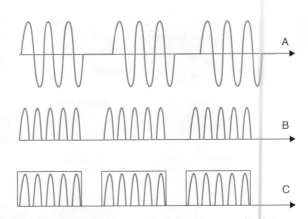

FIGURE 1–23. (A and B) The strength of the voltage amplitude is maintained, yet the negative values now becomes positive. **(C)** The pulse information is smoothed, allowing for one mean signal per pulse to be recorded.

example normalizing smaller signals to a zero value, limiting the largest signals to a maximum value, or manipulating both ends of the range at the same time. Compression, or dynamic range is typically adjustable by the sonographer.

Image Processing

After the signal information is neatly processed, it must again be processed in a form capable of being displayed on the ultrasound monitor as an image. There are processing steps that occur before the information is stored in the memory, because once information is stored in the memory it is irreversible. Further steps are performed with the memory data.

Prememory processing. Preprocessing of the acquired image data typically refers to advance image processing. These steps are done before the information is stored in the memory. Some preprocessing operations include the following:

- write magnification
  - allows selection of a specific region in the image and discards the remainder to create a new image with better resolution
- edge enhancement
  - sharpens edges by increasing the brightness or darkness at boundaries
- temporal and spatial compounding (persistence)
  - averages information from several frames to improve image quality
- Pixel interpolation
  - a way of filling in the missing gaps
- Volume imaging
  - information from multiple 2D scans are combined to render 3D image information

Scan Converter. The scan converter takes each scan-line of processed data and stores it to the memory.

Modern ultrasound units use *digital scan converters*. Previously, we discussed the role of the ADC, which takes the analog voltage amplitude signals and converts them to numerical

values representing echo strength. Here, the scan converter takes the numeric values and stores them in the computer's digital memory. Each unit of memory is correlated with a circuit that corresponds to each element in the transducer. A complex computational system correlates the direction and location of the outgoing pulse, with the timing and strength of the returned echo, sending that information through the circuitry to the memory unit. Eventually, all of this information is converted back to analog voltage to activate the individual units of the presentation monitor which will correspond with the location and strength (in the form of brightness) of the echo signal, creating the displayed image. This conversion starts with numeric values being stored in the digital memory.

Digital Scan Converter memory. A single scan consists of one or more frames, made up of many scanned lines of numeric data. Memory stores the numeric data so it can be organized, processed, and converted to a form acceptable to be displayed on the monitor. Computers use physical hardware, often referred to as "memory chips" that temporarily store all of this data. Each memory chip consists of many cells that are part of an integrated computer circuitry. The more memory units the system's computer has, the more data it can handle at one time. This is an important factor as many frames are acquired each second of scanning. Even with all of the data being processed, the memory continually stores the last few frames it has acquired. If the user chooses to freeze an image, they can typically view a **cine loop**, meaning they can review the last few image frames acquired.

As complex as this seems, the memory cells only have two states, on or off, which the computer recognizes as 0 or 1. This two-state counting system is called a **binary system**. We are accustomed to a decimal system, which represents numeric values in increasing powers of ten, or ten to the nth power (10^n). The binary system uses increasing powers of two (2^n), which can represent any number possible in the decimal system. In the decimal system, the digit farthest to the right represents the single unit position, moving to the left the next position represent tens, then hundreds, then thousands, etc (Fig. 1–24A). In a

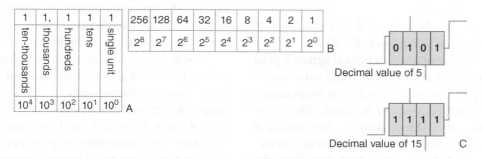

FIGURE 1–24. (A) In the decimal system, the digit farthest to the right represents the single unit position, moving to the left the next position represent tens, then hundreds, then thousands. **(B)** The binary system uses increasing powers of two (2^n), which can represent any number possible in the decimal system. In a binary system, the binary digit (bit) farthest to the right represents one, next on the left represents two, then four, then eight, and so on. **(C)** If all the cells are turned "on" or assigned a one (1) designation, the highest gray-level value of 15 is represented.

TABLE 1-2 • Conversion of Decimal Values to Binary For a 4-bit System

Decimal Value	Activated Binary Switch	Summation of Binary Switch Values	Decimal Value	Activated Binary Switch	Summation of Binary Switch Values
0	0000	0+0+0+0 = 0	8	1000	8+0+0+0 = 8
1	0001	0+0+0+1 = 1	9	1001	8+0+0+1 = 9
2	0010	0+0+2+0 = 2	10	1010	8+0+2+0 = 10
3	0011	0+0+2+1 = 3	11	1011	8+0+2+1 = 11
4	0100	0+4+0+0 = 4	12	1100	8+4+0+0 = 12
5	0101	0+4+0+1 = 5	13	1101	8+4+0+1 = 13
6	0110	0+4+2+0 = 6	14	1110	8+4+2+0 = 14
7	0111	0+4+2+1 = 7	15	1111	8+4+2+1 = 15

binary system, the binary digit (bit) farthest to the right represents one, next on the left represents two, then four, then eight, and so on (Fig. 1–24B and Table 1–2).

A light switch also has two states, on or off. However, if you replace it with a dimmer switch, you are able to vary the level of brightness. Similarly, the ultrasound digital memory has levels or bit depth, that allow it to display many gray-level values. Each level of bit depth represents an increasing power of two. *In the simplest of terms*, imagine four cells in a memory data chip. In that chip, up to 15 decimal values can be displayed simply by turning each cell "on" or "off" in a specific sequence. If all the cells are turned "on" or assigned a one (1) designation, the highest gray-level value of 15 is represented (Fig. 1–24C). If none of the cells are activated, the lowest level, or zero is represented. Typically, the highest level is assigned a gray value of white and the lowest level black, with all the intermediate shades assigned in between. Table 1–2 demonstrates the conversion of decimal values to binary for a 4-bit system.

Mathematically, the number of gray shades possible = 2^n and the largest value that can be represented = $2^n - 1$.

For the system to display an image, it must assign each pixel in the image matrix with a numeric gray-scale value corresponding to the strength of the returned echo. An image matrix is similar to checkerboard. Each box in the checkerboard correlates to the position of the 2D slice anatomy. The squares of the image matrix are called pixels, which is short for picture elements. Fig. 1–25B is divided into a 10×10 matrix. Typically, ultrasound images are divided into a 512×512 matrix of pixels. Dividing the matrix into many, very tiny squares allows the viewer to see a smooth whole image, rather than seeing each individual square (Fig. 1–26).

Each pixel must have enough bit depth such that each can represent enough shades of gray to accurately describe the anatomical information. The human eye can distinguish approximately 100 levels of gray. Most modern ultrasound units have up to 8 bits of memory depth and can display approximately 256 levels of gray, representing gray values of 0 up to 255. A specific pixel cell must have 8 bits of depth to display these 256 levels of gray. This is accomplished by layering the matrices (see Fig. 1–25A).

If a sensor receives a signal indicating a specific amplitude strength, it will activate the circuit to turn "on" cells such that their binary value adds up to the value of the signal at their location. For instance, a processed signal assigned a value of 25 will cause cells at depths $2^0 + 2^3 + 2^4$, or $1 + 8 + 16$ to be activated, adding up to 25 and all other cells at that location turned off. The subsequent shade of gray corresponding to that numeric value will be represented at that location. In Fig. 1–25B, cell A3 should have a gray-scale value of 96. The cells in green of Fig. 1–25A demonstrate activation with respect to the memory location in this 8-bit system. Of course, the actual memory circuits in the ultrasound systems look much different (Fig. 1–27).

As stated previously, most ultrasound units generate images with up to 8 bits of gray scale (up to 256 shades of gray). Color-flow Doppler machines need more bits to represent the various colors. The machine cannot make the distinction of color; it can only represent an array of numbers. Colors are stored as number values representing the three primary colors, which are typically red, yellow, and blue. Various combinations of these colors will generate almost any color in the color spectrum.

To calculate the number of bits per image, calculate the number of pixels. Multiply the number of rows with the number of columns.

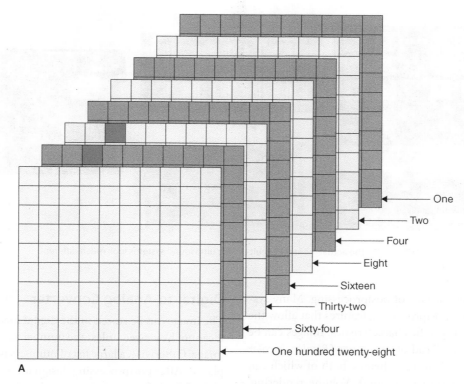

FIGURE 1–25A. Demonstrate activation with respect to the memory location in this 8-bit system.

Example: a matrix of 512 rows × 512 columns = 262,144 pixels

Multiply the number of pixels with the bit depth.

Example: 262,144 pixels × 8 bits/pixel = 2,097,152 bits per image

In computer language, eight binary digits or 8-bits is equal to 1 *byte*. To determine the number of bytes of memory in an image, divide the number of bits per image by eight.

Example:

$$\frac{2,097,152 \text{ bits/image}}{8 \text{ bits/byte}} = 262,144 \text{ bytes}$$

As you can see, a single image can typically contain over 2 million bits, or more than a quarter of a million bytes. Because of the vast amount of information that must be stored, multipliers are applied to reduce the number of digits required. Typical multipliers are kilo-, mega-, and giga-. These multipliers do not represent the same values as we see in the metric system. For example, a kilobyte is not 1000 bits. Instead it is 1024 bits or 2 to the 10th power (2^{10}). For convenience, large numbers may be rounded. For example, 262,144 bytes may be rounded to 260 kilobytes. Table 1–3 describes the typical multipliers.

Postprocessing. In a nutshell, postprocessing is anything done to echo data after it has been stored in the digital memory and while it is being prepared for display. For instance,

	1	2	3	4	5	6	7	8	9	10
A			96							
B				96						
C				45	45					
D					75					
E						15				
F						15	15			
G										
H										
I										
J										

B

FIGURE 1–25B. Cell A3 should have a gray-scale value of 96.

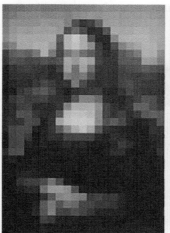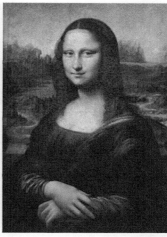

FIGURE 1–26. Too few pixels and the image loses detail.

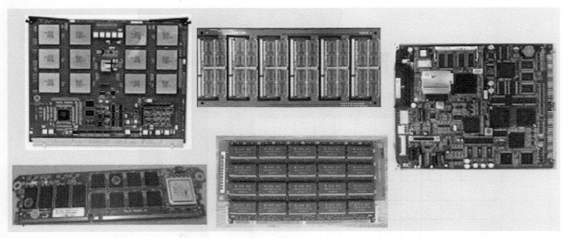

FIGURE 1–27. The actual memory circuits in the ultrasound systems look much different.

assigning echo brightness is part of postprocessing. Many systems have preprogramed postprocessing features that allow the user to display data with specific characteristics. Images can be displayed with color tint instead of gray tones (*B color or color scale*), or with different brightness schemes, both of which can often improve image contrast perception. Volume rendering, which provides 3D image information from data of several 2D images, is another postprocessing function of some systems. Surface renderings, transparent visualization, or 2D slices are typical options for volume imaging display.

Other Forms of Processing

Coded Excitation. Conventional ultrasound transducers are based on the principle that high-frequency ultrasound has difficulty penetrating deep into the body. A processing method used with digital technology called *coded excitation* allows the use of high frequency while providing good penetration and high resolution at the same time. When applied, this technique improves axial resolution, contrast resolution, SNR, and depth of penetration. There are several methods used for coded excitation, which primarily apply coding sequences during transmit and reception steps. *Harmonic imaging and strain imaging* use coded excitation.

Digital-to-Analog Converter

The image can be stored in the digital memory as numbers, but it cannot be viewed unless the numbers are converted back to an image. Otherwise, a large list of numbers is all that would be displayed. After postprocessing designations have been made, display of the information requires that the number values stored in memory are changed back into an analog voltage. To generate different levels of brightness in the image, the voltage is applied to a cathode ray tube or light-emitting diode, depending on the type of display monitor. The hardware that performs this function is the digital-to-analog converter (DAC).

Display

The display monitor takes data from many vertical scan lines and displays it with many horizontal lines across the screen. A *frame* is a single image composed of multiple scan lines. To produce a dynamic or moving image, numerous frames are required. To freeze a frame, or stop the image to record or view it, the memory of the system is activated. The *frame rate* (FR) is the number of image frames displayed or scanned per second. Typically, most diagnostic medical sonography or echocardiography systems have frame rates of 10–60 frames per second. If the FR is below 20 frames per second, the human eye can resolve the frames separately and the image will appear to flicker.

The PRF is the number of pulses produced by the transducer in a given time period. It is related to the number of lines per frame (LPF) and the FR as follows:

$$\text{pulse repetition frequency (PRF)} = n \times \text{LPF} \times \text{FR}$$

where n is the number of focal zones. A separate scan line is required for each focal zone.

The PRF, LPF, and FR are directly related to the propagation speed. Recall, propagation speed is the maximum speed with which an acoustic wave can move through a medium and is determined by the density and stiffness of the medium. The

TABLE 1–3 • Unit of Measurement in Computer Terminology			
Unit	Prefix	Symbol	Quantity
byte[a]	kilo-	K	1,000
byte	mega-	M	1,000,000
byte	giga-	G	1,000,000,000

[a]1 kilobyte equals 1024 characters but can be rounded off to 1,000.

maximum effective velocity is 77,000 cm/s, or ½ the propagation speed of ultrasound in soft tissue (1540 m/s or 154,000 cm/s). Why ½ the propagation speed? The pulse must have time to travel to the reflector and then back to the receiver, or to make a "round-trip."

Mathematically, for a single focus scan the following holds true:

$$\text{penetration depth (cm)} \times \text{LPF} \times \text{FR (Hz)} \leq 77{,}000 \text{ cm/s}$$

Since the PRF for a single focus is equal to LPF × FR, the above equation can also be defined as:

$$\text{penetration depth (cm)} \times \text{PRF} \leq 77{,}000 \text{ cm/s}$$

If imaging depth remains constant, improving image quality by increasing the lines per frame will cause a decrease in frame rate. Increasing the penetration depth, while maintaining the same LPF will also cause a decrease in frame rate. In order for the above equations to be true, the product of the components on the left must remain less than or equal to 77,000 cm/s. A change in one component requires a change of one or more of the others.

The *display format* refers to how the image appears on the screen. Typical formats are either *rectangular* or a type of *sector display*. The width of the display is typically given in centimeters; the *line density* is express as the number of lines per centimeter. To determine the line density for a rectangular display, the lines per frame are divided by the display width in centimeters.

$$\text{line density}_{\text{rectangular}} \text{ (lines/cm)} = \frac{\text{lines per frame (LPF)}}{\text{display width (cm)}}$$

A sector display appears as a pie-shaped image. The scans lines are formed at angles so that the line density is expressed as lines per degree.

$$\text{line density}_{\text{sector}} \text{ (lines/degree)} = \frac{\text{lines per frame (LPF)}}{\text{sector angle (degrees)}}$$

Information from the rectangular or sector image scan lines is read out row by row from the image memory. The information is then written or transposed to the video frame in horizontal lines (Fig. 1–28). The computer electronics also add the text and graphic information (such as depth markers) to the displayed image.

Modes of Display

The *A-mode*, or amplitude mode, is a one-dimensional graphic display with vertical deflections of the baseline. The height of the deflection represents the amplitude, or strength, of the echo (*y*-axis); the distance in time is a function of where on the horizontal baseline the deflection occurs (*x*-axis). All ultrasound images contain this information. However, it is the *B-mode*, or brightness mode that displays the A-mode information as variations in brightness on an image. Each spot on an image represents the position of the reflector and its brightness is

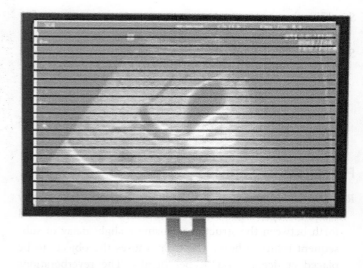

FIGURE 1–28. The information is then written or transposed to the video frame in horizontal lines.

proportional to the strength of the echoed pulse. In B-mode, the *x*-axis represents depth and the *z*-axis represents brightness. There is no *y*-axis in B-mode.

M-mode, or motion mode, is a two-dimensional recording of the reflector's change in position, or its motion with respect to time. It can be a moving B-mode image, or a changing A-mode graph, or both. The vertical axis represents depth and the horizontal axis represents time. Most M-modes display the brightness of the signal in proportion to the strength of the echo. This mode is most commonly used for the study of dynamic structures, such as the heart.

ARTIFACTS

We are accustomed to using the term "artifact" when describing things such as historical remnants. However, for medical imaging the term describes something seen on an image that is not really in the anatomy we are viewing. Sometimes, an artifact is beneficial and tells us specific characteristics of the anatomy being imaged. Other times the artifact can interfere with the viewer's ability to interpret the anatomical information or can falsely mimic anatomical structures. For ultrasound, we typically distinguish artifacts based on the physical principles that produce them. We generally recognize four categories of artifacts: resolution, propagation, attenuation, and miscellaneous artifacts.

Resolution Artifacts

When an ultrasound system cannot resolve two objects laying parallel to the beam as separate, we describe it has having limited *axial resolution* (see Fig. 1–21B). If the two objects are laying perpendicular to the beam's axis, and cannot be resolved as separate, we describe the system as having poor *lateral resolution* (see Fig. 1–20B).

Speckle is the scatter of echo signals in tissues, causing interference effects referred to as *noise*.

Section thickness artifact appears due to the finite thickness of the sound beam (see Fig. 1–15). Echoes from objects or tissue next to the center of the beam appear in structures that normally are echo free (anechoic). This makes the echo-free structure appear as though it has 'debris' or echo producing structures within in it, when in actuality it does not.

Propagation Artifacts

Reverberation is repetitive reflections between two highly reflective layers or structures. The sound bounces back and forth between the structures causing a slight delay of subsequent return echoes. The delay causes the objects to be placed at deeper and deeper depths. The reverberations appear on the image as equally spaced bands of diminishing brightness or amplitude.

Refraction is the change in direction of the sound beam as it passes from one medium to another medium with a different propagation speed. If the refracted sound wave encounters a reflector, its return echo signal will be improperly positioned on the image.

Multipath artifact is a form of refraction occurring when the primary sound beam gets reflected from an object at a different angle. The echo returning along the original path places the reflector in the correct position, while the refracted signal returns the echo along a different path, placing the object at a different location. The refracted signal will typically place the object slightly deeper, due to the slight delay of the return signal.

Mirror Image artifacts typically occur at large smooth boundaries, such as at the diaphragm. The transmitted signal reflects off an object placing it correctly before the smooth boundary. When a signal first reflects off the smooth boundary and then strikes the object, the object will be placed on the other side of the boundary, positioned along the path of the signal before it was reflected. The mirrored object appears the same, only inverted.

Propagation Artifacts

Shadowing is the loss of signal or reduction of echo strength for signals returning from behind a strong reflector or attenuating structure. Shadows are typically seen behind gallstones, renal calculi, and bone, but can occur behind other highly attenuating structures. Shadowing is unrelated to the propagation speed of the medium.

Enhancement is an increase in the amplitude of echoes returning from behind weakly attenuating structures. The increase pertains to the relative strength of the signals when compared with neighboring signals, which pass through more attenuating media. It is common to see strong reflections behind fluid-filled structures (such as a urine-filled bladder) as opposed to solid structures, like tumors.

Edge shadowing occurs when the beam loses intensity as it is refracted or bent at the edges of a curved reflector. The loss of intensity causes shadows to occur at the edges of the curved object. The loss of intensity could be caused by redirection and loss of the echo information, or due to destructive phase interferences caused from changes in propagation speeds of the associated mediums.

Miscellaneous Artifacts

Comet tail artifact is produced by a strong reflector. It is a form of reverberation. The comet tail is composed of thin lines of closely spaced discrete echoes. Comet tail artifacts frequently occur with the presence of gas bubbles, surgical clips, biopsy needles, or bullet fragments.

Ring down is *associated with imaging of gas bubbles*. Its appearance is similar to reverberation artifact, but it originates from resonance energy, caused by the vibrations of air bubbles, rather than reverberations between highly attenuating objects. It can appear as multiple descending parallel echoes or may have more of a continuous streak appearance, typically emanating posterior to the gaseous structure or as the result of gas bubbles.

Propagation speed error. Ultrasound systems typically assume the speed of sound in the tissue is 1540 m/s. However, this does not always hold true. Different tissues have different propagation speeds. When the ultrasound beam passes from one tissue type to another with a higher (faster) propagation speed, the calculated distance will place the echo closer to the transducer because it returned more quickly. The opposite also holds true. If the ultrasound beam passes to another tissue medium with a lower (slower) propagation speed, the return echo takes longer, and the system places the echo farther away. The displacement is termed *propagation speed error*.

Side-lobe artifacts are due to off-axis energy emanating away from the primary ultrasound beam. The off-axis energy can generate reflections outside the main beam which interfere with image quality. Side-lobe artifacts are associated with single element transducers and are uncommon in modern diagnostic ultrasound imaging.

Grating lobe artifacts are similar to side-lobe interferences except that their production is associated with multielement transducers. The structure of multielement arrays inherently pushes the off-axis energy farther away from center compared with the side-lobe energy of the single-element transducer. As discussed previously, dynamic apodization greatly reduces the effects of grating lobe artifacts by systematic activation of specific elements to focus the energy of the beam to its center, reducing the energy at the outside.

Range ambiguity. As noted earlier, the range equation relates the depth of a reflector to the propagation speed and the pulse round-trip time. The maximum depth (d_{max}) of a reflector that can be unambiguously recorded is:

$$d_{max} = \frac{1}{2} \times \text{propagation speed} \times \text{PRP} = \frac{\text{propagation speed}}{2 \times \text{PRF}}$$

Thus, the PRP that controls the FOV also determines the maximum depth of a reflector that can be unmistakably recorded. The PRP is the timing window that includes the pulse and the listening time (see Fig. 1–2A). Echoes received by the transducer after the PRP timing window will arrive after the second pulse has been transmitted and the system will assume it is associated with the second pulse. The system will mistakenly place the echo closer to the transducer.

QUALITY OF PERFORMANCE

All ultrasound equipment is tested and maintained under a quality management (QM) program. Quality management ensures the system is operating correctly, consistently, and safely. A good QM program includes the following:

1. Assessment of imaging performance
2. Assessment of equipment conditions, performance, and safety
3. Assessment of acoustic output
4. Routine preventive maintenance
5. Assessment of primary interpretation display performance
6. Oversight of routine quality control (QC)
7. Oversight of operator credentials and continuing education

Image Performance

Test Objects (Phantoms).
To ensure ultrasound systems are providing accurate information and acceptable image quality, a qualified service engineer, physicist, or trained sonographer will utilize test objects or image quality phantoms to measure the characteristics of the image information. There are many phantoms available, and their selection will depend on the types of transducers and imaging performed by the ultrasound unit. For routine imaging, an ideal image quality phantom will be made of a material with a propagation speed similar to tissue (such as graphite-filled aqueous gel or urethane rubber) and will contain objects for the assessment of the following:

- System sensitivity (Gray Scale Contrast Resolution)
- Anechoic Mass Resolution
- Limiting Axial Resolution
- Limiting Lateral Resolution
- Dead Zone depth (ring down)

- Horizontal and Vertical Distance Accuracy
- Uniformity
- Gray-Scale Performance (Dynamic Range)

System sensitivity measures the weakest signal the system will display correctly within the noise of the background. Test objects in the phantom can vary in scatter strength from strong (hyperechoic) to weak (anechoic), will typically range in size, and may be embedded at increasing depths to give the tester quantitative measurements for comparison.

Anechoic mass resolution is a specific form of system sensitivity testing that looks at the system's ability to discern objects with low scattering qualities from the noise background. Test phantoms will typically imbed the objects at increasing depths and typically use objects of varying sizes for a quantitative comparison.

Limiting axial resolution describes the smallest distance a system (transducer) can resolve for two reflectors positioned along (vertically) the beam axis (see Figs. 1–21A and B). The phantom will contain objects of decreasing spacing, sometimes at different depths that provide a quantitative measurement (Fig. 1–29).

Limiting lateral resolution describes the smallest distance a system (transducer) can resolve for two reflectors positioned perpendicular (horizontally) to the beam axis (see Figs. 1–20A and B). The phantom will contain objects of decreasing spacing, sometimes at different depths that provide a quantitative measurement (see Fig. 1–29).

Dead zone (near field) is the distance between the front surface of the transducer and the first identifiable echo at the patient skin or phantom interface. It is a test that measures the ability of the transducer to image surface structures. Reflecting objects are placed toward the surface of the phantom at known distances of depth. The tester will image the objects and determine the shallowest distance that is discernable. Fig. 1–30 shows a CIRS phantom diagram with a dead zone (near field) target group containing six targets ranging from 6 mm to 1 mm deep. Dead zone measurement is particularly important for determining a transducer's usefulness for shallow imaging such as dermatological or breast imaging. To improve dead zone imaging, "stand-off" pads or other materials can be used to create additional transmission depth or surface uniformity between the transducer face and the shallow reflector.

Horizontal and vertical distance accuracy measures the system's ability to place reflectors at their actual location and measures the system's accuracy of the internal measuring calipers. Reflecting targets are spaced with known distances, allowing the tester to use the system calipers to measure those distances. Physicians rely on distance calipers for making accurate anatomical measurements.

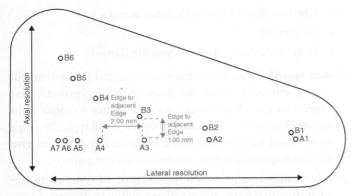

FIGURE 1–29. The axial-lateral resolution targets in the CIRS phantom (Fig. 1–30). The phantom will contain objects of decreasing spacing, sometimes at different depths that provide a quantitative measurement. *(Reproduced with permission from Computerized Imaging Reference Systems, Inc (CIRS), Norfolk, VA.)*

Uniformity measurements are used to determine the presence of artifacts due to the transducer or ultrasound system malfunction. Measurements will be made in a phantom with tissue mimicking material of uniform or equal reflective properties. There will be no other test objects in that area. The resulting image should appear with equal echogenicity across the FOV. Fig. 1–31 demonstrates non-uniformity due to element "drop-out" or defective elements. This test is sometimes performed with "in air" measurements with similar results. This test will often discern issues early on, before they become problematic with patient imaging.[11]

Gray-scale performance (dynamic range) assessment determines the system's ability to display reflectors with many varying levels of echo intensities, specifically displaying the smallest to the largest measured intensity, and as many of the intermediate intensities in between. Recall that the system may be capable of measuring a very wide range of echo intensities. The final information stored in the memory has a smaller dynamic range due to various processing steps, for example steps to reduce noise and to facilitate storage. If the system has limited dynamic range, or if too much compression processing is applied by the user, a smaller range of echo intensity information is stored in the memory. This will result in an image that displays mostly black and white, losing gray-level detail that may be imperative for diagnostic interpretation (Fig. 1–32). The ability to store a large dynamic range allows the image interpreter access to a wider range of echo information, and the ability to display that gray-scale information with a narrower range of brightness assignments if desired. Because the observer differentiates echo intensities based on the gray-scale values in comparison with the surrounding background gray-level values, image quality phantoms are designed with inserts that allow visual and quantitative measurements for this assessment (see Fig. 1–30, gray scale targets). Other phantoms may have

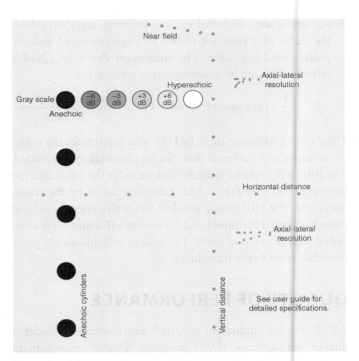

FIGURE 1–30. A CIRS phantom diagram showing measurable targets for assessing image quality of the system. *(Reproduced with permission from Computerized Imaging Reference Systems, Inc (CIRS), Norfolk, VA.)*

several gray-scale group targets that also vary by depth and/or size. Currently, the two most common tissue mimicking materials used in QC phantom design are Urethane Rubber and solid elastic water-based polymers with a form of plastic membrane that allows for scanning.

Specialty Testing Phantoms or Devices. Many ultrasound units perform specialty imaging, such as elasticity measurements, Doppler ultrasound, or 3D imaging. These usages require special equipment to assess performance. An ultrasound

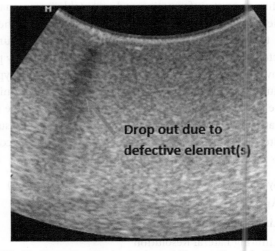

FIGURE 1–31. Nonuniformity due to element "drop-out" or defective elements.

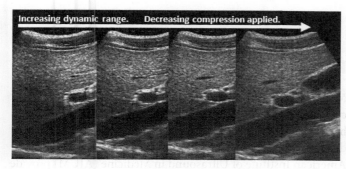

FIGURE 1–32. The dynamic range determines the system's ability to display reflectors with varying levels of echo intensities. If the system has limited dynamic range, or if too much compression processing is applied, the image will have limited echo intensity information. If it is limited too much, the image will appear mostly black or white and will lose gray-level detail.

unit performing Doppler ultrasound may be tested for sensitivity, waveform, and velocity accuracy using a Doppler Flow Simulator device. Special phantoms are designed for ensuring the accuracy of tissue elasticity measurements as well as phantoms designed with embedded 3D structures to ensure 3D imaging performance and measurement accuracy.

The first **hydrophone** was invented during World War I[4] and used for underwater echo detection. Hydrophones used in diagnostic ultrasound are used by engineers and physicists to measure or calculate: pressure amplitude, intensities, period and wavelength, pulse duration, and PRP.

BIOEFFECTS OF ULTRASOUND

For ultrasound, *bioeffects* describe the potential consequences to tissues or biological structures exposed to ultrasound energy. Up to the present time, no definitive evidence has been presented to substantiate any detrimental biological effects associated with the use of routine diagnostic ultrasound imaging. Cautionary statements and reports have been published regarding safe use of diagnostic ultrasound for pre- and postnatal subjects as well as for the use of ultrasound contrast agents.[5] Continued research is essential in ascertaining potential bioeffects associated with newer technologies and modern ultrasound imaging techniques. As a general rule, most scientists and physicians agree that a risk versus benefit approach should be made when utilizing ultrasound for imaging procedures. In the latest 2014 AIUM statement, As Low As Reasonably Achievable (ALARA) Principle, AIUM reiterates that a conservative approach, while maintaining adequate image information, is best *when adjusting system controls that affect the acoustical output and when considering transducer dwell times.* The potential for bioeffects are typically separated into two categories: Thermal effects and Mechanical effects. Ultrasound systems are designed to present index values associated with these affects,

allowing the user to monitor and adjust to avoid bioeffects while imaging.

Thermal index (TI). Sound waves are energy. The absorption, or attenuation of energy in tissue can cause heating to occur. Permanent damage can occur in tissues when heated beyond critical limits. Thermal index is defined as the ratio of total acoustic power that is required to cause a rise in temperature of 1°C anywhere in the beam. If focusing remains constant in a given tissue type, the TI is directly related to the output power of the system.

Some tissues absorb ultrasound energy at different rates. Because of this, thermal index values are reported according to tissue type.

TIS. Thermal index for soft tissue

TIB. Thermal index for bone (important for fetal imaging)

TIC. Thermal index for cranial bone (important for fetal imaging)

Experts agree, for adults a rise of less than 2°C beyond the normal temperature of a tissue, will not cause harm to the tissue, this correlates to a TI < 2.[1] The fetus is more sensitive to heating effects, with sensitivity changing with the age of the fetus. Experts recommend TI ≤ 0.7 and limiting exposure time, particularly for Doppler imaging.[6]

Mechanical Index (MI) is a measure of pressure amplitude that occurs in tissue. It is an indicator of potential cavitation. FDA limits general diagnostic ultrasound imaging systems to a MI ≤1.9.[7] Studies suggest that under certain conditions, such as fetal imaging, contrast imaging, or imaging of structures containing naturally occurring gas bodies, the MI should be limited further (MI ≤0.3 to <0.7 for most fetal imaging).[8, 9]

Cavitation is the result of rapid pressure changes in a medium causing gas bubbles to form, and can cause gas bubbles already present to rapidly increase and decrease in size (oscillate.) Ultrasound waves propagating through tissues can cause cavitation. There are two types of cavitation:

Stable cavitation, the bubbles oscillate in size in response to the changing pressure of the sound wave. These oscillations can cause increases in temperature and pressure within the bubbles, which in turn can create mechanical stress on the tissues or fluids surrounding them.

Transient cavitation occurs when pressure changes are great, causing the net change in bubble size to increase, eventually causing implosion of the bubbles. Animal research has shown that cavitation can occur in tissues containing gas bodies at MI levels of less than 1.9.[8] Caution should be used when imaging tissues of this description, such as lung/pulmonary, cardiac, intestinal, or fetal imaging involving exposure around the lungs, etc.

Both forms of cavitation can cause damage to surrounding tissues or vessels, with transient cavitation having a higher potential to do harm. However, cavitation is also utilized to form the gas bubbles used for contrast imaging, and sometimes for the purpose of rupturing the micro bubbles during therapeutic use, such as for the delivery of a therapeutic agent encapsulated in the bubble.

ALARA

ALARA (As Low As Reasonably Achievable) is a principle recommended to minimize patient ultrasound exposure by the following:

- Using a high receiver gain setting and a low power output setting
- Avoiding high TI and MI values
- Minimizing scanning time
- Using a higher frequency transducer when possible
- Using a focused transducer
- Avoiding temperature elevation
- Avoiding the use of spectral Doppler for early embryo imaging when possible

The following guidelines are adapted from official AIUM statements. The reader is encouraged to read the full AIUM texts:[10, 11, 12, 13]

Intensity: There are no independently confirmed significant biological effects in mammalian tissues exposed *in vivo* with unfocused transducers with SPTA intensities below 100 mW/cm^2 and below 1 W/cm^2 for focused transducers, or for temperature increases less than 1.5°C.

Exposure: Exposure times can be greater than 1 second and less than 500 seconds for an unfocused transducer; and less than 50 seconds per pulse for a focused transducer. With these exposure times, no significant bioeffects have been observed even at higher intensities than those noted above, as long as the (intensity x time) is <50 J/cm^2.

Thermal: A maximum temperature rise of 1.5°C above normal for exposure durations of up to 50 hours is acceptable for general adult imaging. For fetal imaging, temperature increases are progressively greater for color and spectral Doppler applications compared with normal B-mode imaging. Additionally, animal studies have shown that the first trimester is the most sensitive period for adverse thermal exposure outcomes. Exposures during this period should be limited to the lowest outputs required to obtain sufficient imaging detail. In general, for current diagnostic medical ultrasound units, limiting TI values to 2.5 or below for exposure times of less than 4 minutes will not result in adverse thermal heating of fetal tissue.

Mechanical (cavitation): For diagnostic medical ultrasound units, no adverse effects have been observed in tissues containing naturally occurring gas bodies at MI values less than 0.4. For contrast-enhanced diagnostic ultrasound imaging, no adverse effects have been confirmed for MI values below 0.4. For imaging of tissue that does not contain well-defined gas bodies, no adverse mechanical bioeffects have been confirmed for MI values below 1.9.

PATIENT CARE AND SAFETY

Medical errors are preventable adverse effects involving patient care and treatment. Patient safety experts at Johns Hopkins have estimated that medical errors are the third leading cause of death in the United States.[14] National organizations, such as the American Institute of Ultrasound in Medicine (AIUM) provide guidelines and resources to educate the sonographer about the many aspects of patient safety and care. Education and training are the key to minimizing or eliminating medical errors. Common causes for medical errors include the following:

- Wrong patient
- Wrong site
- Wrong procedure
- Missed diagnosis
- Missed pathology
- Improper hygiene
- Poor patient monitoring (patient injuries from falls)

Preprocedure Safety Check

Preventing wrong patient, wrong site, and wrong procedure errors can be accomplished with the establishment and compliance of standard clinical procedures. A typical procedure scenario might be the following:

1. Identify yourself and your role in the patients care. Ensure your employee identification badge is visible.
2. With the appropriate orders or scheduling document, confirm you have the correct patient by confirming name, date of birth, medical record number, checking the patient's ID bracelet, or by scanning the ID bracelet.
3. Does the patient's clinical history correspond to the requested examination?
4. Confirm the examination and site of the exam with the patient and the examination orders.
5. Check for latex allergies.
6. Ensure the patient is stable when positioning and exiting the examination table.

Postprocedure Safety Check

To ensure patient safety and that proper diagnoses can be made by the radiologist or physician, the following steps are recommended prior to releasing the images:

1. Verify the appropriate anatomical features were captured in the image.
2. Verify the images are of diagnostic quality for interpretation.
3. Ensure the patient is stable when exiting the examination table.

4. Before sending the image information to the physician or Picture Archiving System (PACS), confirm the images correspond to the correct patient.

5. Confirm the side markers on the postprocedure images are correct.

INFORMED CONSENT

Informed consent is a means for obtaining permission from the patient to perform specific medical procedures under the full disclosure of possible side effects or limitations of the procedure. A patient has the right to revoke informed consent at any time. The sonographer has the obligation to assess and ensure the patient's or caregiver's ability to understand the informed consent. A proper informed consent document should be easily understood and include the following:[15]

- A thorough description of what the procedure involves.
- A description of the risks and benefits associated with the procedure.
- A statement describing the patient's right to refuse the procedure.
- A statement providing a reasonable alternative(s) to the procedure.
- Witness to the consent.
- A Certified Language line for patients with limited English proficiency (LEP).*

UNIVERSAL PRECAUTIONS

Universal precautions are a set of precautions designed to prevent HIV, hepatitis B virus, and other blood-borne pathogens when providing health care. For the sonographer, these precautions involve the utilization of protective barriers such as gloves, gowns, and masks. The following are applicable for implementation of universal precautions:

- Vaginal secretions
- Semen
- Amniotic fluid
- Cerebrospinal fluid
- Pleural fluid
- Peritoneal fluid

Feces, sweat, urine, nasal secretions, tears, vomit, and sputum do not apply to the universal precautions unless they contain visible blood. The Centers for Disease Control and Prevention (CDC) recommend hand washing before and after procedures to reduce the spread of microorganisms. Hand washing should be done for at least 20 seconds with water and soap. For hand sanitizer use, apply the correct gel amount according to the label and rub the gel over all surfaces of your hands and fingers until your hands are dry, approximately 20 seconds. Either should be done even if gloves will be worn during the procedure. [16, 17]

DISINFECTION OF INTERNAL TRANSDUCERS

Internal transducers, such as vaginal, rectal, and transesophageal transducers, are reusable medical instruments. Cross-contamination is possible with these devices if cautionary methods are not employed. Internal transducers should undergo high-level disinfection (HLD) between patients to prevent transmission of infection. The FDA provides details regarding available high-level disinfectants. The AIUM recommends the following steps:[18, 19]

1. Remove and dispose of used probe cover and clean probe with running water and soap
2. Disinfect with HLD-cold chemical disinfectants
3. Cover again using a disposable probe cover, its sterility appropriate for the upcoming procedure

Although the disposable probe covers provide a barrier, nonvisible microscopic tears in the covers could expose the transducer to bacteria or viruses from mucosal tissue secretions. Therefore, the above steps are required to prevent cross-infection from the transducer.

The use of cold chemical disinfectants is preferred over heating methods for disinfecting. The piezoelectric crystal arrays of the transducer are heat-sensitive. Mechanisms that use heat for disinfection, such as steam autoclaves, could damage the sensitive crystals rendering them useless.

DOPPLER AND DOPPLER COLOR-FLOW IMAGING INSTRUMENTATION

Color Doppler—Brief Historical Overview

Color Doppler imaging (CDI) began with the development of multigate Doppler systems, which first appeared around 1975.[20] Although this early technology only used color Doppler inside an M-mode display, it started the advancement of the multigate approach combined with the color encoding of motion. In 1983, the first real-time echocardiography color-flow system became commercially available.[21] The first commercial color-flow vascular imaging device followed in 1986. Today, most current clinical ultrasound systems have color-flow imaging capabilities.

The Federal Food and Drug Administration (FDA) (21 CFR 50.25 and 21 CFR 50.27) and US Department of Health and Humans Services (DHHS) (45 CFR 46.116 and 45 CFR 46.117) require that Informed Consent documents be translated for all LEP medical research patients. The regulations state that informed consent information should be given in writing and must be given in a language that is understood by the patient or their authorized representative.

There are many descriptors for CDI, for example, Doppler color-flow imaging and color-flow Doppler. Today, there are multiple applications that utilize CDI, such as for the depiction of myocardial motion along with blood flow,[22] fetal heart and placenta perfusion evaluations, vascular imaging, and general echocardiography to name a few. There are new and emerging applications on the horizon continuously. Recent advances include the ability to noninvasively image vasculature and blood flow in the head,[23] improved frame rate acquisition for enhanced dynamic flow with 4-D echocardiography, and vector flow mapping (VFM) for quantification of blood flow abnormalities in the heart and vascular structures.[24]

No matter the application, the main advantage of CDI is its ability to simultaneously display gray-scale (B-mode) information of the stationary tissue along with the color-encoded information of the Doppler-shifted frequencies, and flow velocity information of the moving tissue or blood flow. However, the information is not perfect. Any moving echo source within, and often outside the scan field, can produce color in the image. Setting up the system correctly can limit the color-flow information to that of the moving blood.[21]

Modern-day ultrasound systems use signal-handling techniques which keep the image frame rate as high as possible allowing the following fundamental pieces of information to be displayed in the color-flow presentation:

1. existence of flow
2. flow location in the image
3. flow location in the anatomy
4. direction of flow relative to the transducer
5. direction of flow relative to the anatomy
6. the flow pattern over space and time

Due to the system's ability to show color-encoded flow over space and time, the image can be used to locate specific characteristics within the flow pattern. For example, one would be able to see high-velocity flow segments within the heart and larger vessels as well as complex or chaotic flow patterns. Changes in flow patterns may be due to anatomy or could be related to disease states, such as stenosis.[25] Characteristics of blood flow are described in the following section entitled *Hemodynamics* and in more detail in Chapter 13.

Hemodynamics

The circulatory system is one of ten organ systems in the human body and is responsible for blood flow throughout the body. Its components consist of the heart, blood vessels (arteries, veins, and capillaries), and blood components. The circulatory system uses blood to deliver nutrients, oxygen, hormones, and blood cells to the different parts of the body. After metabolism of these deliveries, the cardiovascular system removes the metabolic waste products from the body. The circulatory system helps stabilize the body's temperature and pH balance, helps the body fight illness and disease, and in general helps the body maintain an essential equilibrium of all its organ systems. *Hemodynamics* describes the blood flow characteristics of the circulatory system. Perturbations or disruptions in the human body's hemodynamic function can lead to serious health consequences and death. The ability to image flow characteristics of the circulatory system are imperative for proper diagnosis. Today's ultrasound systems provide technology that helps us gain invaluable information of flow patterns as well as cardiac motion in the displayed image and in the image's correlating measured data.

Blood flow in the circulatory system is measured by the volume of blood moving between two points in a specified unit of time. This measurement is called the *volumetric flow rate* and is commonly displayed in liters per unit time (eg, mL/min). For imaging of the circulatory system, we are also concerned with how fast blood flows, or the blood velocity, measured as a unit of distance per time (eg, cm/s). One primary way blood moves through the body is by the pumping action of the heart which causes a pulsatile motion, or a varying of the blood velocity. Breathing can also cause variations in blood velocity and is usually associated with movement through the venous system. This form of flow is referred to as phasic flow. However, when breathing stops a steady flow is observed in the venous system. Flow characteristics are also influenced by properties of the blood fluid, such as density and viscosity, anatomical characteristics, such as vessel diameter and elasticity, the amount of blood volume in the body, and peripheral vascular resistance, also referred to as vascular compliance. *A detailed discussion of hemodynamics can be found in Chapter 13.* For the purposes of this Doppler discussion, it is important to understand the correlation between Doppler ultrasound and hemodynamics. It is therefore advised that the reader include Chapter 13 as part of their preparation for the physics portion of the exam.

Color Doppler Basics

Doppler Ultrasound imaging uses the Doppler effect for measuring the change in frequency that occurs as sound is reflected from moving reflectors, such as moving blood cells. Your ears measure changes in the sound frequency of an ambulance's siren wail. The frequency sounds higher when the ambulance is approaching you and lower as it moves away from you (Fig. 1–33). The ultrasound instrument similarly measures this change or shift in frequency as echoes from moving reflectors (ie, flowing blood cells) move toward the transmit/receive transducer, or away. This change of frequency is called the Doppler shift.

Several factors determine the measured Doppler shift: The speed of the reflector, the direction of the flow path, the angle between the path direction and the sound source direction, and the frequency of the emitted sound wave source. These factors can be quantitatively described with the Doppler shift equation.

$$f_D(\text{kHz}) = f_R(\text{kHz}) - f_o(\text{kHz}) = f_o(\text{kHz}) \times \frac{[2 \times v(\text{cm/s})]}{c(\text{cm/s})}$$

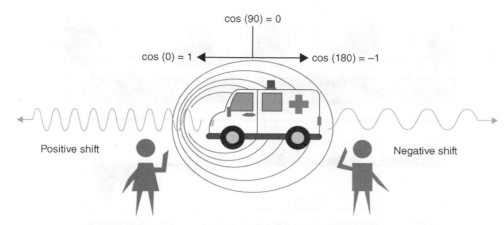

FIGURE 1–33. Doppler shift principle as the sound moves toward the receiver and away from the receiver. The receiver is stationary, the source direction is changing.

where f_D is the **Doppler shift** frequency, v is the velocity or speed of the reflector, c is the propagation speed of the medium, f_R is the received frequency of the reflected sound wave, and f_o is the source frequency of the initial sound wave.

If the moving reflector is approaching the sound source, the Doppler shift is positive, because the received frequency f_R will be greater than the source frequency f_o. If the reflector is moving away from the sound source, the Doppler shift will be negative, as the received frequency will be less than the source frequency.

Doppler color-flow imaging was developed out of a necessity for imaging cardiovascular blood flow noninvasively. You can intuitively understand that the blood flow direction cannot move directly toward or away from the direction of the sound beam if the transducer is placed at the surface of the skin. Instead, the sound approaches the moving reflectors at an angle (Fig. 1–34). The imaging angle, or *angle of insonation* is very important. The Doppler shift is dependent on the cosine of the angle of insonation (Doppler angle, θ), and the above equation is better defined by including this angle:

$$f_D(kHz) = f_o(kHz) \times \frac{[2 \times v(cm/s) \times \cos\theta]}{c(cm/s)}$$

The ultrasound system typically assigns a color value for Doppler shifts that are positive, or moving toward the transducer (typically red) and for those that are negative, moving away from the transducer (typically blue). Depending on the system's bit color capabilities, these depictions can be reassigned by the user. The most common graphic for display is a color bar (Fig. 1–35A) with the positive signals represented by the color on top and negative on bottom. However, other color schematics can apply (Figs. 1–35B–D).

The system measures and could just present the Doppler shift information (flow direction), as indicated for the first color map (see Fig. 1–35A) using the Doppler shift equation $f_D = f_R - f_o$ (measuring the difference between the frequency emitted and the frequency received for the moving reflector(s)). However, for most applications the desired measurement is ultimately for motion or blood flow velocity or speed, as well as direction. The Doppler shift is proportional to the blood flow velocity or speed. The above equation can be rearranged to solve for the

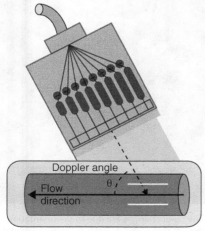

FIGURE 1–34. Instead, the sound approaches the moving reflectors at an angle.

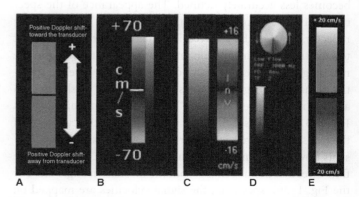

FIGURE 1–35. (**A**) Doppler shift color map, no velocity information. (**B**) This color variance map shows direction and velocity intensity, along with a gray-scale intensity map. (**C**) This color map is reversed. The color on top always represents flow toward the transducer. This is a good trick question for reviewers, as most sonographers are accustomed to the A and B map schematic with red representing flow toward the transducer. (**D**) Another type of color map using a color wheel to display direction and velocity information. (**E**) Color saturation map.

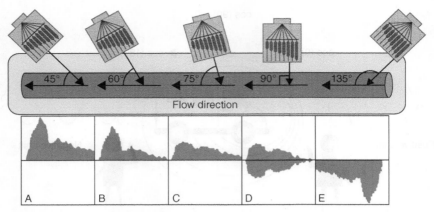

FIGURE 1–36. Possible spectral images based on differences with the Doppler angle.

speed, or velocity of the moving reflector, and simplified assuming the propagation speed of sound in tissue.

$$v(\text{cm/s}) = \frac{[77(\text{cm/ms}) \times f_D(\text{kHz})]}{[f_o(\text{MHz}) \times \cos\theta]}$$

As stated previously, it is mostly impossible for the insonation angle to be placed at zero degrees, or directly in line with the blood flow, which should produce the maximum Doppler shift signal. Instead, the system will correct its calculation to maximize the signal based on the angle assigned by the sonographer. Artifacts and inaccurate velocity flow measurements result when the sonographer poorly defines flow direction. The general "Rule of Thumb" for the ideal angle is less than 60 degrees (60°) for accuracy and greater than 30 degrees (30°) to reduce reflections at the vessel surface.

Fig. 1–36 shows possible spectral images based on differences with the Doppler angle. Beginning with an appropriate angle of 45° up to the 60° angle, the spectral velocity information (A & B) appears as good representations of the flow velocities in the vessel. As the angle increases, the spectral information becomes less accurately defined. The appearance of the spectrum for the 90° insonation angle is the result of the moving reflectors. Part of the received information is from movement toward the line of insonation and part is away, resulting in the mapping of the spectrum on both sides of the baseline (positive signals and negative signals). This can also be shown with a color map image (Fig. 1–37). In the anatomical image of Fig. 1–37, you can see the angle changes due to the curvature of the transducer as well as the curvature of the vessel. Blue represents flow away from the transducer, red toward. Obviously, the flow direction did not change, but the insonation angle did. For the Fig. 1–36E spectrum, the signal velocities are mapped on the opposite side of the baseline, as negative signals. The movement is away from the receiver.

Producing an Image

Doppler color-flow imaging begins by making a multigate image for both the gray scale and the Doppler segments of the image. Multigate means the system purposefully divides each sound beam location in the scanning field into a series of small volume sampling sites. Each site translates into a specific location in the digital scan converter image.[26] Fig. 1–38 is an example of this division using a linear array. The ultrasound unit's digital scan converter design determines the size and spacing of these sampling sites.[27]

The amount of time between sampling pulses, the *sampling interval*, must be long enough for the pulse to travel to and from the reflector, or sample site (recall Figs. 1–21A and B). The sampling interval requirement is different for the gray-scale information than it is for the color Doppler information. The gray-scale image depends on detection of echo signal amplitudes, which are then converted into gray-scale intensities by the signal processor. If the sampling interval is greater than one wavelength, there will not be enough information to display appropriate variations in tissue texture in the gray-scale image.

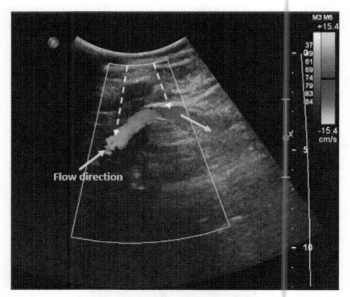

FIGURE 1–37. The color changes are due to the orientation of the Doppler angle. Flow on the left side of the vessel is traveling toward the direction of the sound source. Because the probe is curvilinear, the sound direction changes and flow is moving away from the sound beam on the right.

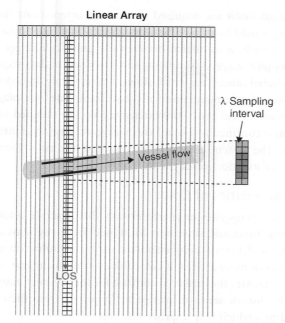

Linear Array

λ Sampling interval

Vessel flow

LOS

FIGURE 1–38. In a multi-gate system, the sound beam is purposefully divided into a series of small volume sampling sites.

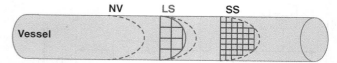

NV LS SS

Vessel

FIGURE 1–39. Image resolution of flow and sampling intervals. The dashed blue line NV, is the normal velocity profile, LS is the large-interval sampling profile, and SS is the small-interval sampling profile. The smaller the sampling interval, the more accurate the depiction of flow patterns.

More time is required to sample the color Doppler signal information than for sampling amplitude signal information. A single pulse-listen cycle can provide enough information for a single gray-scale image line of site (LOS). CDI requires anywhere from 4 to 100 pulse-listen cycles to build a single Doppler image LOS.[28] We refer to the number of pulse-listen cycles per LOS as the *ensemble length, package length,* or *dwell time.* Each Doppler pulse-listen cycle is gathering information. After an appropriate amount of *dwell time,* the system will have enough information to accurately depict the frequency shifts in each sampling interval containing reflector motion. It is important to remember that the reflectors are tiny red blood cells which produce very small frequency shifts. To increase sensitivity to these small shift signals and improve SNR, the more cycles the better. However, more cycles equate to longer dwell times. Using too many cycles slows image formation (reduces the frame rate). For the system to produce timely image information most limit the dwell time range to around 4–32 cycles, with 10–20 on average.[1]

The smallest Doppler sampling interval sites are about one-wavelength (λ). However, to reduce frame rates, enabling combined gray-scale and real-time color Doppler images, these sampling sites may increase to several wavelengths. There is a caution here—just as sampling intervals greater than one wavelength produce poor variations in tissue texture for gray-scale imaging, sampling sites larger than 1 mm produce poor representations of vascular flow patterns. Fig. 1–39 demonstrates how sampling interval size from each line of site (LOS) can affect the depiction of flow patterns in a vessel.

The information in the vessel is singled out by applying a range gate at the position of the Doppler sampling site. Within

this gate a range, or spectrum of Doppler shift frequencies exists. It is not possible for the system to display a spectrum of frequencies in each colored pixel. To represent the color-flow information within the vessel, the system will determine a representative frequency for each sample site or sampling interval, and will encode that sample with a corresponding color intensity. The representative frequency is typically an averaged value within the sampled site. By choosing an averaged value to represent the Doppler shift frequency, noise is reduced in the sampled volume. Depending on the system, different methods are used to determine the representative frequency such as autocorrelation, online spectral analysis, or various signal averaging techniques.[27] Additionally, each system will define the color intensity or quality associated with that value, depending on the color bit depth and color combination characteristics of the system.

As discussed previously, CDI displays color information asynchronously with the gray-scale anatomical information. Using the Doppler effect, it measures the changing frequency of moving reflectors. Unfortunately, mathematically the calculation cannot distinguish between a moving sound beam versus a stationary object, or a moving object (blood cells) versus a stationary sound beam. This means the system may pick up low-frequency measurements from the moving sound beams reflecting off stationary objects and encode those areas with color. This was problematic for mechanically scanned transducers. To remedy this, modern-day ultrasound imaging systems with multielement phased array, linear, and curvilinear transducers use electronic scanning beams (discussed earlier in the chapter). Electronic manipulation of the beams allows for a stationary reference beam for every line of site so that a differentiation can be made between the reference beam and the multiple samples being sent out to capture the moving Doppler information.

Color Doppler Signal Processing

Processing the echoed signals of the Doppler information involves complicated analysis. As discussed, CDI uses asynchronous signal processing. Using separate signal data for each, the system maps the anatomical gray-scale information along with the Doppler shift information. This is done using separate transmitters, an image transmitter and a coherent transmitter. Typically, beam steering is used to acquire the signals used for the Doppler information, while perpendicular beams are used

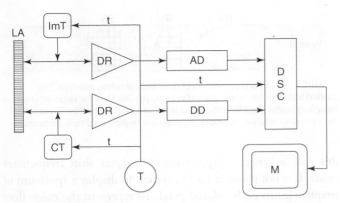

FIGURE 1–40. Asynchronous signal processing. LA is the linear array, ImT is the image transmitter, CT is the coherent transmitter, DR is a receiver, AD represents amplitude detection, DD represents Doppler detection, DSC is the digital scan converter, M is the color monitor, T is a common timer with control signals (t), and DR is the Doppler receiver. Asynchronous signal processing uses different signals for the gray-scale and color portions of the image.

for the gray-scale information. As discussed above, the Doppler sampled frequency information can be different from the main imaging frequency allow the main frequency to work as a reference. An example might be a Doppler sampling frequency of 3 MHz and a gray-scale image sampling frequency of 5 MHz. Fig. 1–40 is a simplified schematic of asynchronous signal processing.

As discussed earlier, extremely fast and sophisticated timing delays can be manipulated to sample information from the gray-scale lines of site and then interweave it with information from the Doppler sampled sites (Fig. 1–41). However, because the information is obtained separately, it must be stored in the system memory separately. The digital scan converter retrieves the separated information and overlays it for the composite image.

Despite extremely fast timing for modern systems, there is still a delay between the two acquisitions. Additionally, the

two acquisitions are acquired at different orientations (beam steering is used to acquire the Doppler information). These differences cause a mismatch between the gray-scale image and the Doppler image. Assimilating these two sets of data requires complicated processing which slows the frame rate. In order for the acquisition to maintain an adequate frame rate to display the information "real time," the extensive Doppler sampled information is confined to a small area within the region of interest (ROI). The system computes and displays the color-Doppler image information inside the ROI only.

Characteristics of Color

The main properties or characteristics that describe color are hue, brightness, and saturation. Most modern-day systems allow the user to define the color characteristics. The human observer can discern more shades of color than variations in gray scale. Color increases the observed contrast for the reviewer allowing hard to discern areas of interest to "pop out" from their surroundings, which may improve diagnosis.

Hue represents variation of the main colors in the color spectrum. Red, blue, and yellow are different hues of color. Even greater nuances of hue can ensue from these main colors. For instance, a pink hue is a variation of red, gold is a variation of yellow, and aqua is a variation of blue. As stated previously in this chapter, by varying the combinations of three main colors, such as red, blue, and yellow, the system can produce almost any color hue in the color spectrum.

Brightness is the perceived luminance of an object. Roughly speaking, in our case it's how much light is emanating from a pixel. For ultrasound, brightness typically represents strength, intensity, or energy of a signal. For example, a very bright white pixel represents a strong reflector compared with a gray pixel. For color imaging, increased brightness typically represents increasing velocity. Brightness for CDI is usually represented

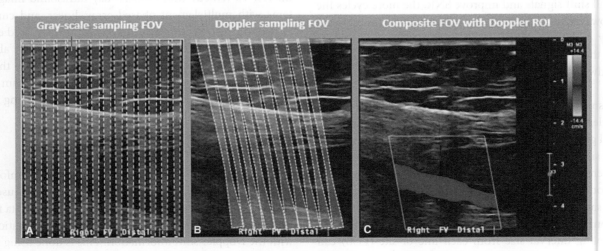

FIGURE 1–41. (A) Simplified graphic of gray-scale sampling of the linear array. (B) Simplified orientation of the Doppler sampling, steering the beam to optimize the Doppler angle and to differentiate from the gray-scale information. (C) The composite image. Information for the color-Doppler sampling and display is confined to a smaller region of interest (ROI).

with variations in hue, for instance dark red up to gold, or dark blue up to aqua (see Figs. 1–35B and C).

Saturation describes the purity of a color at a constant luminance level. A 100% pure red will appear on the image as a deep red. To reduce the purity of a color, white light is added making the color appear faded. Saturation color maps are another method for representing Doppler signals (see Fig. 1–35E).

Power Doppler Imaging-Amplitude Signal Processing

For color flow imaging, processing a Doppler signal requires the ability to separate the frequency components that make up the returning echo signal. To do this, the composite waveform is analyzed often using Fast Fourier transform (FFT) analysis which separates the waveform into a range of its distinct frequency parts. More specifically, FFT analysis provides the Doppler signal amplitudes and the Doppler signal frequencies. The information is used to color encode the Doppler shift information for both direction of blood flow and speed of flow. What if we were not concerned with flow speed and direction and were only concerned with the presence of flow. *Power Doppler* is an alternate method of CDI that measures the strength or power of the Doppler signal, independent of angle and frequency. It has the advantage of being more sensitive to very low or weak blood flow in the body as well as flow in microvascular environments. This makes it ideal for three-dimensional depictions of perfusion into organs and masses.[29] Power Doppler is also less prone to aliasing and angle dependent image artifacts.

Disadvantages of power Doppler are its lack of detail for flow information. It is also very sensitive to soft-tissue motion which produces an artifact commonly called "flash artifact." Modern systems do a good job of reducing flash artifact while maintaining sensitivity, yet it can still be an issue.

Color-Doppler Echocardiography

When imaging the heart, it is not necessary to see the same detailed flow patterns used for vascular imaging. Because of this, color Doppler of the heart or *color-Doppler echocardiography* is able to use larger sampling intervals and fewer LOS,[28] thus reducing the time to acquire the colored portion of an image.[21] As with color-flow imaging, both the gray-scale image and the color-flow image are presented asynchronously (Fig. 1–42). Because the color-flow echocardiography time requirement has decreased, the combined frame rate can be accelerated allowing for detailed cardiac motion imaging, which is particularly important for capturing details during pediatric cardiac imaging.

Imaging of the heart has an added complication regarding the ability to image between intercostal and subcostal spacing with low-frequency pulses.[21] Parasternal CFI places the ultrasound beam at about 90° to the flow pattern. To place flow patterns parallel to the beam, apical and subcostal views are

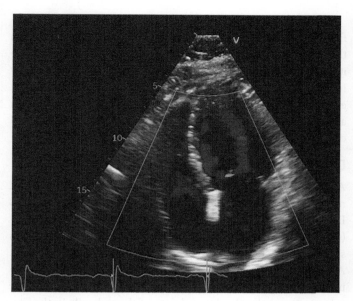

FIGURE 1–42. Color Doppler imaging of the heart.

required. To this end, phased-array transducers with short-radius curved arrays are the best transducer for imaging under these conditions. Their sector angles typically range from 30° to 180°.

Because blood is a low attenuator (0.15 dB/cm per MHz), using ultrasound to view the heart does not require the same pulse/receive timing design that is required for vascular imaging. Instead cardiac imaging uses high frame rates, a large FOV, large sampling intervals, and uses a sector format. The use of these parameters for vascular imaging would be impossible.

A disadvantage for the use of large sampling intervals for echocardiography is difficulty in detection of regional turbulences. To help locate flow disorganization (or spectral broadening) within a sampling location, most cardiac systems determine not only the mean frequency at a sample site, but the signal variance as well.[21] In many cardiac devices, color-coding for an increasing variance introduces a green tint to the primary color.

Vascular Imaging Requirements

Vascular CFI involves all accessible peripheral vessels, the large, upper thoracic vessels, and the deeper vessels in the abdomen. A linear array is typically used to view the peripheral vessels. This linear scanning geometry sets the stage for using changes in color to show changes in the direction of flow. In contrast, a sector scan of a linear vessel produces a continuously changing Doppler angle similar to example shown in Fig. 1–37 and, thus, continuously changing color. Instead, sector-scanning transducers, such as the phased array and the curved linear array, are used to view abdominal vasculature rather than peripheral vessels. As stated above, these transducers permit both subcostal and intercostal scanning to visualize the deeper abdominal vessels that may be within the rib cage.

However, sector fields make reading the images more difficult. Identifying arteries and veins requires knowing both the direction and the pulsatility, variability of the blood velocity. Large FOVs and longer processing times for the color-flow image often make the effective frame rates too low to permit easy determination of pulsatility. Using a single-point spectrum and a color-flow image together, along with decreasing the ROI can yield information about vascular pulsatility.

Displays of Frequency and Velocity

All current color-flow images using Doppler are two-dimensional maps of the Doppler shift frequencies. After all, color flow uses Doppler, too. Many systems show the color values in velocity (centimeters per second) rather than frequency (hertz). This sort of display suggests a direct measurement of velocity in color. As in all color-flow Doppler determinations of velocity, the values represent a solution to the Doppler equation. However, the velocity is not the absolute velocity of the red cells in the vessel. Instead, the image values represent the sampled velocity, or the component of motion along the ultrasound beam. Absolute velocities would require a continuous correction of all angles to the flow patterns throughout the image. Fig. 1–43 shows this sampled velocity relationship.

Color Flow Imaging Artifacts

Color flow imaging uses gray-scale imaging and therefore is susceptible to the same artifacts. This section will discuss artifacts with respect to the color-Doppler contribution. The three primary artifacts of concern are (1) range ambiguity artifacts, (2) Doppler high-frequency artifacts, and (3) soft-tissue vibration artifacts.

The definition for the *Range ambiguity artifact* was discussed previously on page 25. The high power and faster frame rates typical of Doppler CFI offer ample opportunities for this artifact.[31] In Doppler CFI, the artifact appears as diffuse, nonpulsatile colors, suggesting flow that may not actually exist where it appears in the image. As discussed, range ambiguity occurs when the PRF is set improperly. The PRP is the time from the beginning of one pulse to the beginning of another, PRP = 1/PRF. Just as for gray-scale imaging, time is required between pulses

to "listen" for the return echo signals or these signals get crossed and misinterpreted.

Range ambiguity occurs with Pulsed Wave (PW) Doppler imaging only. Continuous-wave (CW) Doppler will not produce this artifact. Remember that for continuous-wave ultrasound, the transducer is **always** generating an oscillating pulse. For reception, a second transducer (separate elements) acts as the listening or receiving device. The side by side transmit/receive beams overlap. The overlapped area is the sample volume. The sample volume for CW Doppler is larger than PW Doppler. Because the Doppler shift frequency, or velocity never exceeds the PRF, range ambiguity aliasing does not occur.

For PW Doppler imaging, the Doppler shift frequencies are being sampled at the PRF of the system. *High-frequency aliasing* occurs when the Doppler shift frequency exceeds the system's PRF sampling frequency. To accurately sample the Doppler shift frequency of the moving reflector, there is a limit to the number of samples that can be acquired while maintaining the appropriate delay between these samples. That limit is called the *Nyquist limit (NL)* or *Nyquist frequency*, and is equal to ½ PRF. In Fig. 1–1A, recall that we measure sound wave frequencies in cycles. For sampling the maximum Doppler shift frequency (f_{Dmax}), the system must sample at least twice for every Doppler shift cycle. Therefore, the PRF must be greater than or at least equal to two times the Doppler shift frequency (PRF $\geq 2f_{Dmax}$) of the moving reflector or aliasing will occur.

Recall the system is measuring the Doppler shift to display the velocity of the moving blood along with the direction. It is helpful to envision the Doppler shift frequency as a wave (see Fig. 1–44). Each sampling pulse is used to form the interpreted characteristics of the Doppler shift frequency wave. In a given amount of time, there must be enough samples to accurately define the wave. If it is not accurately defined, the system will display the velocity incorrectly and define the direction incorrectly.

$$f_D(kHz) = f_R(kHz) - f_o(kHz)$$
$$v(cm/s) = \frac{[77(cm/ms) \times f_D(kHz)]}{[f_o(MHz) \times \cos\theta]}$$

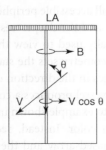

FIGURE 1–43. The "closing" or average velocity geometry. LA is the linear array, B is the ultrasound beam, V is the target velocity, and V cos θ is the sampled velocity. Sampled velocity is the component of motion along the ultrasound beam.

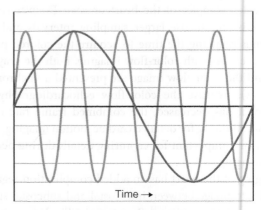

FIGURE 1–44. Orange line is the actual frequency. The gray line shows the misinterpreted frequency due to slow sampling.

For CFI, range artifacts can appear misrepresented on the spectrum or in the color shown on the image. The spectrum and the color will appear to "wrap around" if the sampling frequency is too low. This is due to the system mapping a lower frequency than the actual Doppler shift frequency. When the Doppler shift frequency is lower than actual or negative, the velocity appears less, and could be shown as negative.

The sonographer will not typically have a control knob for adjustment of the PRF. However, as we discussed, decreasing the focal depth or shortening the FOV increases the PRF. The sonographer can control the Doppler shift frequency by adjusting the transducer position or Doppler angle toward the 90° angle (This is not an optimum choice. Recall, Doppler angles greater than 60° are prone to error) to reduce the Doppler frequency. Another option to control the Doppler shift frequency is by reducing the Doppler carrier frequency, also called transmit or initial frequency (f_o). These techniques all aid in controlling high-frequency aliasing artifacts.

Another common source of artifacts associated with Doppler imaging and CFI arises from mechanical vibrations of moving soft tissues. These vibrations create low frequency signals, or noise, and can occur when patients talk, around an area of turbulent blood flow (*bruit*),[32] or from pulsative motion of the heart. This artifact appears as unusual brightness or color variation where it normally would not appear, such as outside vessel walls or within abdominal images. As discussed earlier, Power Doppler is particularly sensitive to this artifact.

Applications of Color Doppler Imaging

Color Doppler imaging is a mainstay of clinical ultrasound. In this section, we will explore nuances of the different imaging types. Fig. 1–45 is an example of color flow imaging of a carotid artery with corresponding Doppler spectral waveform. On the right of this image is transverse view of the carotid bifurcation. The blue area connotes the internal jugular vein overlying the carotid vessels. The color blue in the color bar on the right represents flow moving toward the transducer.

Fig. 1–46A shows a cardiac continuous wave Doppler image with spectral display. This image also shows significant turbulent flow and elevated velocities distal to a stenosis related to atherosclerotic plaque at the carotid bulb. The mosaic colors distal to the plaque indicate turbulent flow. Fig. 1–46B color image clearly shows multiple velocities related to flow turbulence. Fig. 1–47A shows a diagram depicting the multiple lines of sight that can be used to examine the carotid artery and its major branches. This is a Matrix array transducer/probe. Recent enhancements in computational abilities and transducer design have resulted in development of matrix array probes. These transducer/probes afford real time 3D depiction of anatomy and simultaneous depiction of multiple scan planes. Fig. 1–47B shows a 3D representation of the common, internal and external carotid arteries and the adjacent internal jugular vein. Fig. 1–47C shows a 3D sonogram depicting an extensive plaque at the carotid bulb.

Doppler color-flow Imaging is a combination of gray-scale anatomical information and colored depiction of flow events. It is

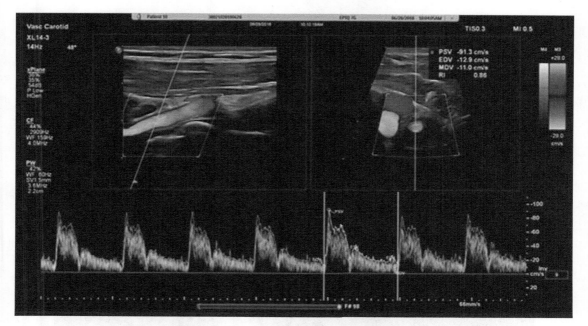

FIGURE 1–45. A color and spectral Doppler sonogram of a normal internal carotid artery as depicted in simultaneous long and short axis with a Matrix array transducer/probe. The top-left image shows the long axis, the top right in short axis. The spectral waveform shows laminar flow. This probe affords simultaneous depiction of long and orthogonal (at 90°) short axis. The lighter shade of red in the center of the vessel implies higher velocity, indicative of laminar flow.

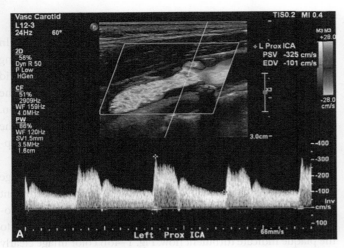
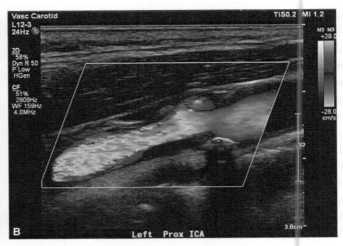

FIGURE 1–46. **(A)** Significant turbulent flow and elevated velocities distal to a stenosis related to atherosclerotic plaque at the carotid bulb. The mosaic colors distal to the plaque indicates turbulent flow. **(B)** The spectral waveforms resulting in turbulent flow and markedly elevated systolic and diastolic velocities. Instead of the waveform being a clear line, there is "filling in" resulting from multiple velocities related to flow turbulence.

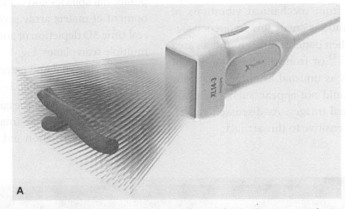

FIGURE 1–47A. Diagram depicting the multiple lines of sight that can be used to examine the carotid artery and its major branches. This is a Matrix array transducer/probe. Recent enhancements in computational abilities and transducer design have resulted in development of matrix array probes. These transducer/probes afford real time 3-D depiction of anatomy and simultaneous depiction of multiple scan planes.

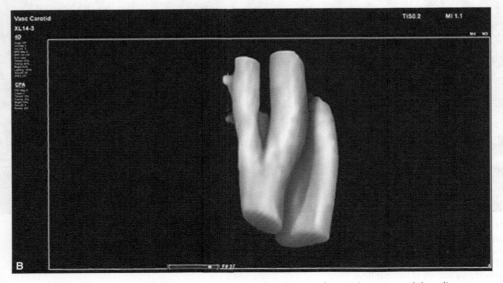

FIGURE 1–47B. 3D representation of the common, internal, and external carotid arteries and the adjacent internal jugular vein.

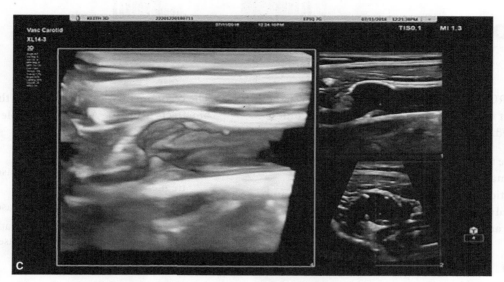

FIGURE 1–47C. Diagram depicting the multiple lines of sight that can be used to examine the carotid artery and its major branches.

an integrated image of form with function, anatomy, and physiology. The color portion of the image is not an image of blood; rather, it is an image of motion. Using power Doppler, the color can depict the presence of flow with great sensitivity, but without some flow details. Within each Doppler color-flow system, the amplitudes of echo signals become gray-scale intensities, while the frequency information of the signals becomes color. The echo signals for both may be the same or different, even in carrier frequency. This imaging modality depends on the sophistication and speed of contemporary digital signal processing. It also is an imaging modality that is ever changing and will continue to improve the clinical diagnostic value of ultrasound in medicine.

Questions

GENERAL INSTRUCTIONS: For each question, select the best answer. Select only one answer for each question unless otherwise specified.

1. Which of the following is the standard protocol for digital imaging that allows compatibility and communication between computers, workstations, and network hardware provided by various manufacturers of CT, MRI, and ultrasound equipment?

   (A) PACS
   (B) DICOM
   (C) AIUM
   (D) ALARA

2. The spatial pulse length

   (A) determines the speed of ultrasound in tissue
   (B) usually increases with higher frequency
   (C) is improved with rectification
   (D) usually decreases with higher frequency

3. Axial resolution is improved by

   (A) focusing
   (B) acoustic mirrors
   (C) damping
   (D) beam diameter

4. Lateral resolution is improved by

   (A) ring-down
   (B) decreased beam diameter
   (C) spatial pulse length
   (D) imaging in the far zone

5. The beam of an unfocused transducer diverges

   (A) because of inadequate damping
   (B) in the Fresnel zone
   (C) in the Fraunhofer zone
   (D) when the pulse length is long

6. Reverberation artifacts are a result of

   (A) electronic noise
   (B) improper time gain compensation (TGC) settings
   (C) the presence of two or more strong reflecting surfaces
   (D) duplication of a true reflector

7. The recommendations for reducing the potential for bioeffects using the ALARA principle is to

   (A) increase receiver gain and decrease the power output
   (B) increase power output and decrease transducer frequency
   (C) decrease power output and increase scanning time
   (D) decrease scanning time when a patient has a maternal temperature and decrease overall gain and increase power output

8. What technique can be employed to reduce grating side lobes?

   (A) depolarization
   (B) apodization
   (C) subsonic beam tapering
   (D) magnification

9. A technique that uses an ensemble of pulses to improve penetration and contrast resolution is

   (A) coded excitation
   (B) harmonic imaging
   (C) apodization
   (D) subdicing

10. A 75-year-old patient suffering from Alzheimer's disease arrived in the ultrasound department from the surgical ward for ultrasound of the right legs to rule out deep venous thrombosis. The patient has no name band. What is the most appropriate next step?

   (A) Retrieve the name and medical record number from the chart that accompanied the patient.
   (B) Return the patient to the ward for appropriate identification and tagging.
   (C) Scan the patient now and retrieve identification later.
   (D) Call the nurse on the floor by telephone to identify the patient.

Questions 11–15:   Match the following group of wires with its function for the AIUM test object (Fig. 1–48).

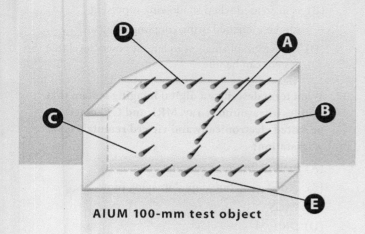

AIUM 100-mm test object

FIGURE 1–48.

11. registration or B-mode alignment _____

12. axial resolution _____

13. lateral resolution _____

14. dead zone _____

15. depth calibration _____

16. **Decreasing the spatial pulse length**

   (A) reduces the field of view (FOV)
   (B) reduces lateral resolution
   (C) improves axial resolution
   (D) improves lateral resolution

17. **How much will a 3.5-MHz pulse be attenuated after passing through 2 cm of soft tissue?**

   (A) 7 dB
   (B) 3.5 dB
   (C) 17 dB
   (D) 1.75 dB

18. **Which of the following is the role of the pulse?**

   (A) voltage generation to drive the transducer
   (B) gain adjustment for the receiver
   (C) beam focusing
   (D) beam steering

19. **Enhancement is caused by**

   (A) reduction in echo amplitude distally
   (B) propagation speed errors
   (C) Snell's law
   (D) weakly attenuating structures

20. **The Doppler shift frequency is**

   (A) directly proportional to the velocity of the reflector
   (B) greater in pulsed Doppler systems
   (C) greater at high-intensity levels
   (D) dependent on the number of transducer elements being used

21. **The number of frames per second necessary for a real-time image to be flicker free is**

   (A) more than 15
   (B) less than 1
   (C) between 5 and 10
   (D) between 2 and 5

22. **A non–English-speaking patient presented for an ultrasound-guided breast biopsy in which an informed consent is required. What is the most appropriate step to take?**

   (A) get a family member who speaks the patient's language to be an interpreter.
   (B) use a sign-language interpreter licensed for the deaf and hearing impaired.
   (C) use any full-time employee who speaks that language as an interpreter.
   (D) use a certified language line.

23. **The intensity of the ultrasound beam is usually greater at the focal zone because of**

   (A) decreased attenuation
   (B) smaller beam diameter
   (C) diffraction effects
   (D) a shorter duty factor

24. **If the amplitude is doubled, the intensity is**

   (A) doubled
   (B) cut in half
   (C) increased by four times
   (D) unchanged

25. The attenuation for soft tissue is

(A) increased with tissue thickness

(B) determined by the slope of the TGC curve

(C) increased with decreasing wavelength

(D) unimportant when using digital scan converters

26. The acoustic impedance of the matching layer

(A) can be chosen to improve transmission into the body

(B) must be much larger than the transducer material to reduce attenuation

(C) is not necessary with real-time scanners

(D) must be made with the same material as the damping material

27. Which of the following is necessary additional confirmation required to ensure that the patient you are about to scan is the correct patient?

(A) which ward the patient is from

(B) documented ultrasound request

(C) what part to scan

(D) date of birth

28. If a patient's body fluids (blood or vaginal secretions) come into contact with the ultrasound machine, what would be the most appropriate action?

(A) cancel the cases for the day and wait for the blood to dry before cleaning the machine.

(B) document the date and time and call the biomedical department.

(C) call the manufacturer of the ultrasound for advice.

(D) use approved disinfectant solution to clean the machine.

29. The operating frequency

(A) depends on the transducer's ring-down time

(B) depends on the thickness of the crystal

(C) is increased as the crystal diameter is decreased

(D) depends on the strength of the pulsar

30. The period of an ultrasound wave is

(A) the time at which it is no longer detectable

(B) the number of times the wave is repeated per second

(C) the time to complete one cycle

(D) the speed of the wave

31. The dynamic range of a system

(A) is increased when specular reflectors are scanned

(B) is decreased when shadowing is present

(C) can be increased using coupling gel

(D) is the ratio of smallest to largest power level that the system can handle

32. What term describes a digital imaging system that enables ultrasound, x-ray, MRI, and CT images to be stored electronically and viewed remotely on a workstation?

(A) high-definition harmonic imaging

(B) coded excitation digital imaging protocol

(C) PACS

(D) DICOM

33. Increasing the pulse repetition period (PRP)

(A) improves resolution

(B) increases the maximum depth that can be imaged

(C) decreases the maximum depth that can be imaged

(D) increases refraction

34. Ultrasound bioeffects with an unfocused beam

(A) do not occur

(B) cannot occur with diagnostic instruments

(C) are not confirmed below 100 mW/cm^2 spatial peak temporal average (SPTA)

(D) are not confirmed above 1 W/cm^2 SPTA

35. When can an informed consent be revoked?

(A) after 72 hours for an adult older than 21 years

(B) at any time

(C) only by a court order

(D) cannot be revoked after signing, because it is a legally binding document

36. What is the first thing you should do when a patient enters the ultrasound room?

(A) introduce yourself with name and title

(B) disinfect the transducer

(C) turn on the ultrasound machine

(D) check the ultrasound machine for electrical safety

37. How often should you disinfect the transvaginal transducer?

(A) before and after each use

(B) every day at the end of the work shift

(C) only when the transducer probe cover is broken

(D) if the patient has a vaginal infection or bleeding

38. Which of the following should be minimized in order to comply with the ALARA principle?

    (A) TGC
    (B) overall gain
    (C) frequency
    (D) transmit power

39. Which of the following *best* describes autocorrelation?

    (A) mathematical process in which a waveform is multiplied by a time-shifted version of itself
    (B) the automatic correlation between the transmitted echo and the reflected echo
    (C) the repositioning of the incident acoustic energy scattered back toward the source
    (D) the continuously repeated display of a recorded image from memory

40. What is the name of the mechanism of ultrasound bioeffects in which microbubbles oscillate without collapsing?

    (A) stable
    (B) ionization
    (C) thermal effect
    (D) fluid streaming

41. Which of the following would *not* typically be related to ultrasound bioeffects?

    (A) power output
    (B) thermal index (TI)
    (C) examination time
    (D) high-frequency transducer

42. Harmonic frequencies are derived from

    (A) nonlinear wave propagation
    (B) perpendicular wave propagation
    (C) symmetrical wave propagation
    (D) proportional behavior

43. Which of the following has an effect on the propagation speed of the ultrasound?

    (A) high-frequency transducers
    (B) output power
    (C) angle of the ultrasound beam
    (D) tissue type

44. Which of the following is equivalent to the prefix giga?

    (A) 10^6
    (B) 10^{-6}
    (C) 10^9
    (D) 10^3

45. What percentage of intensity of an ultrasound pulse incident on an interface of 0.25 and 0.75 rayls is reflected?

    (A) 50%
    (B) 100%
    (C) 25%
    (D) 75%

46. Axial resolution can be improved by

    (A) higher-frequency transducers
    (B) lower-frequency transducers
    (C) larger transducers
    (D) poorly damped transducers

47. When particle motion of a medium is parallel to the direction of a wave propagation, what is the wave being transmitted called?

    (A) longitudinal wave
    (B) shear wave
    (C) surface wave
    (D) electromagnetic wave

48. The wavelength in a material having a wave velocity of 1500 m/s employing a transducer frequency of 5 MHz is

    (A) 0.3 mm
    (B) 0.3 cm
    (C) 0.6 mm
    (D) 0.6 cm

49. Which of the following determines the amount of reflection at the interface of two dissimilar materials?

    (A) the index of refraction
    (B) the frequency of the ultrasonic wave
    (C) Young's modulus
    (D) the difference in specific acoustic impedances

50. Which equation describes the relationship among wave propagation speed, wavelength, and frequency?

    (A) $V = f\lambda$
    (B) wavelength = 2(frequency × velocity)
    (C) $Z = pV$
    (D) wavelength = frequency + velocity

51. When a sound wave strikes a tissue interface at an oblique angle of incidence, what other condition must be present in order for refraction to occur?

   (A) a change in the angle of reflection
   (B) a difference in propagation speeds
   (C) a strong specular reflector
   (D) the presence of several small reflectors

52. The range of the pulse repetition frequency (PRF) used in diagnostic ultrasound is

   (A) 4–15 kHz
   (B) 2.5–10 MHz
   (C) 2.5–3.5 MHz
   (D) 10–15 MHz

53. What is the average velocity of ultrasonic waves in soft tissue?

   (A) 1540 m/s
   (B) 154,000 cm/s
   (C) 0.154 cm/μs
   (D) all of the above

54. A soft-tissue mass is measured to be 80 mm in diameter; what is the diameter in centimeters?

   (A) 80.00 cm
   (B) 8.0 cm
   (C) 4.0 cm
   (D) 0.8 cm

55. When a sound wave strikes a boundary between two tissues with a normal incidence, what other condition must be present in order for reflection to occur?

   (A) an oblique incidence
   (B) a difference in acoustical impedance
   (C) a weak nonspecular reflector
   (D) a thick boundary

56. Ultrasound transducers convert

   (A) mechanical to thermal energy and vice versa
   (B) thermal to cavitation energy and vice versa
   (C) electromagnetic to kinetic energy and vice versa
   (D) mechanical to electrical energy and vice versa

57. The velocity of sound waves is primarily dependent on

   (A) angulation
   (B) reflection
   (C) the medium and the mode of vibration
   (D) frequency

58. Increasing the frequency of an ultrasonic longitudinal wave will result in which of the following changes in the velocity of the wave?

   (A) an increase
   (B) a decrease
   (C) no change
   (D) a reversal

59. Which of the following terms describes the change in direction of an ultrasonic beam when it passes from one medium to another in which elasticity and density differ from those of the first medium?

   (A) refraction
   (B) rarefaction
   (C) angulation
   (D) reflection

60. A long near zone can be obtained by

   (A) using a higher-frequency transducer
   (B) adding a convex lens to the transducer
   (C) decreasing the diameter of the transducer
   (D) increasing the damping

61. If a 2-MHz frequency is used in human soft tissue, what is the approximate wavelength?

   (A) 0.75 mm
   (B) 0.15 mm
   (C) 0.21 mm
   (D) 0.44 mm

62. What is the ratio of particle pressure to particle velocity at a given point within the ultrasonic field?

   (A) interference
   (B) impedance
   (C) incidence
   (D) interface

63. What is the following formula used to determine?

$$\frac{2 \times \text{velocity of reflector} \times \text{original frequency}}{\text{velocity of sound}}$$

   (A) shift in frequency caused by the Doppler effect
   (B) degree of attenuation
   (C) distance a wave front travel
   (D) amount of amplification necessary to produce diagnostic ultrasound

244. The term *bit* in computer science denotes

    (A) binary digit
    (B) pixel
    (C) baud rate
    (D) matrix

245. An 8-bit binary number is referred to as a

    (A) byte
    (B) baud
    (C) pixel
    (D) voxel

246. What is the purpose of employing an acoustic lens on transducers?

    (A) decrease the spatial pulse length
    (B) increase the frequency bandwidth
    (C) steer the beam
    (D) narrowing of the ultrasound beam

247. A needle or membrane hydrophone is used to measure

    (A) pressure amplitude
    (B) MI
    (C) TI
    (D) dead zone

248. Viscosity is measured in units of

    (A) megahertz
    (B) millimeters
    (C) poise
    (D) pascal

249. Which one of the following will increase the speed of ultrasound?

    (A) increased frequency
    (B) decreased frequency
    (C) increased tissue stiffness
    (D) decreased tissue stiffness

250. The resistance to flow offered by a fluid in motion is called

    (A) turbulence
    (B) eddies
    (C) variance
    (D) viscosity

251. Autocorrelation is the mathematical process commonly used to detect

    (A) aliasing
    (B) spectral dispersion
    (C) Doppler shifts
    (D) inertia

252. A decrease in dynamic aperture results in

    (A) increased temporal resolution
    (B) decreased lateral resolution
    (C) decreased the near-zone length
    (D) increased near-zone length

253. Which one of the following would normally have the lowest viscosity?

    (A) molasses
    (B) coupling gel
    (C) blood
    (D) water

254. An 8-bit word microcomputer with 128K words of memory can store how many bits of data?

    (A) 128
    (B) 1000
    (C) 1024
    (D) 128,000

255. Harmonics are created

    (A) when the focal length is changed
    (B) when nonlinear oscillations occur in tissues
    (C) when acoustic lens are used
    (D) when the TGC is increased

256. Frequency compounding improves

    (A) contrast resolution
    (B) penetration depth
    (C) temporal resolution
    (D) lateral resolution

257. What is the unit for acoustic pressure?

    (A) pascal
    (B) poise
    (C) torr
    (D) pag

258. What does the horizontal axis (*x*-axis) on an M-mode display represent?

(A) time

(B) brightness

(C) depth

(D) strength

259. Which ultrasound frequency is commonly used in the clinical setting?

(A) 3.5 kHz

(B) 5 kHz

(C) 7 MHz

(D) 2.5 kHz

260. The ratio of the minimum to maximum signal amplitude that can be applied to a device without producing distortion is called

(A) Nyquist ratio

(B) dynamic range

(C) spectral range

(D) harmonic ratio

261. What does the vertical axis (*y*-axis) on an M-mode display represent?

(A) amplitude

(B) brightness

(C) depth

(D) strength

262. Each binary digit can represent how many different digital memory states?

(A) 1

(B) 2

(C) 4

(D) 8

263. How many digits are utilized in a binary number?

(A) 1

(B) 2

(C) 4

(D) 10

264. What is the binary equivalent of the decimal number 30?

(A) 0110

(B) 1110

(C) 1001

(D) none of the above

265. How many gray levels (echo amplitude levels) can a 4-bit deep digital scan converter store?

(A) 2

(B) 4

(C) 8

(D) 16

266. An ultrasound instrument that could represent 64 shades of gray would require how many bits memory?

(A) 8

(B) 6

(C) 4

(D) 16

267. What are the two categories of cavitation?

(A) turbulent and laminar

(B) stable and transient

(C) compression and rarefaction

(D) analog and digital

268. Which of the following functions are performed by the receiver in the ultrasound machine?

(A) inspection, detection, correction, rejection, depression

(B) randomization, amplification, modulation, rectification, limitation

(C) amplification, compensation, compression, rejection

(D) demodulation, contraction, band limitation, depolarization

269. A large amplitude voltage pulse from the pulser applied to the transducer results in

(A) a long duration pulse from the transducer

(B) a short duration pulse from the transducer

(C) a small amplitude pressure pulse from the transducer

(D) a large amplitude pressure pulse from the transducer

270. Voltage pulses from the pulser to the transducer are also used to

(A) automatically adjust receiver gain

(B) synchronize the receiver for the arrival time determination

(C) adjust the gray-scale display dynamic range

(D) determine FOV

271. The five major components of a pulse-echo ultrasound system are

   (A) flux capacitor, image memory, transducer, scan arm, amplifier

   (B) synchronizer, pulser, receiver, display, power supply

   (C) image memory, display, scan arm, TGC control, foot switch

   (D) transducer, receiver, image memory, pulser, display

272. Transducers may be focused by internal focusing and external focusing. These are accomplished by

   (A) crystal thickness and/or by adding water path offset

   (B) concave transducer elements and/or by using an acoustic lens

   (C) "doping" the crystal with metal ions and/or by added damping

   (D) adjustment of frequency and/or crystal diameter

273. Which unit is used to specify the Q factor (quality factor)?

   (A) pascal

   (B) poise

   (C) Nyquist

   (D) none of the above

Questions 274–282:   Match each term in Column A with the correct definition in Column B.

COLUMN A

274. acoustic shadow _____

275. acoustic enhancement _____

276. anechoic _____

277. artifact _____

278. echogenic _____

279. hyperechoic _____

280. hypoechoic _____

281. interface _____

282. sonolucent _____

COLUMN B

   (A) without echoes

   (B) echoes of lower amplitude than surrounding tissues

   (C) the boundary between two media having different acoustic impedances

   (D) an echo that does not correspond to a real structure

   (E) reduction in echo amplitudes within a region distal to a strongly attenuating structure

   (F) the property of a medium allowing easy passage of sound: low attenuation (echo-free)

   (G) an increase in echo amplitudes within a region distal to a weakly attenuating structure

   (H) echoes of higher amplitude than the normal surrounding tissues

   (I) a structure that produces echoes

283. Which of the following is a commonly used backing material for CW Doppler transducers?

   (A) epoxy resin

   (B) cork

   (C) metal powder

   (D) no backing material

284. Which one of the following is *not* associated with CW Doppler?

   (A) no backing material

   (B) no Nyquist limit

   (C) aliasing

   (D) no TGC

285. The strength of the echo in B-mode ultrasound is displayed as

   (A) y-axis deflection

   (B) x-axis position

   (C) pixel brightness

   (D) decibels

286. Ultrasound cannot travel in which one of the following?

   (A) intravenous pyelogram (IVP) contrast

   (B) solid tissue

   (C) vacuum

   (D) blood

287. Lambda (λ) represents

   (A) period

   (B) wavelength

   (C) frequency

   (D) velocity

288. The time it takes to complete a single cycle is called

   (A) period

   (B) wavelength

   (C) frequency

   (D) velocity

289. A wave vibration at 20 cycles per second has a frequency of

   (A) 20 MHz

   (B) 20 Hz

   (C) 20 kHz

   (D) 120 kHz

290. A wave vibrating at 1 million cycles per second has a frequency of

    (A) 1 GHz
    (B) 1 kHz
    (C) 1 MHz
    (D) 100 MHz

291. A damaged active element in a mechanical transducer may result in

    (A) a horizontal band of signal dropout at a particular depth
    (B) the loss of an entire image
    (C) a reduced frame rate
    (D) a vertical line of dropout extending from the top to the bottom of the image

Questions 292–294:   Match the question in Column A with the correct answer in Column B.

COLUMN A

292. Which statement best describes A-mode? _____

293. Which statement best describes B-mode? _____

294. Which statement best describes M-mode? _____

COLUMN B

(A) a graphic presentation with vertical spikes arising from a horizontal baseline; the height of the vertical spikes represents the amplitude of the deflected echo

(B) a two-dimensional image of internal body structures displayed as dots; the brightness of the dots is proportional to the amplitude of the echo; the image is applicable to both real-time and static scanners

(C) one-dimensional presentation of moving structures displayed in a pie-shaped or rectangular image; the image is applicable only to real-time scanners

(D) a graphic presentation of moving structures in a waveform; the display is presented as a group of lines representing the motion of moving interfaces versus time

295. A long dead zone may indicate

    (A) a fluid-filled mass
    (B) a short spatial pulse length
    (C) high tissue temperature
    (D) detached backing material

296. The frame rate in ultrasound is strongly affected by

    (A) transducer frequency
    (B) focal method
    (C) cavitation
    (D) imaging depth

297. Doppler signals and velocities cannot be measured at what Doppler angle?

    (A) 90°
    (B) 30°
    (C) 40°
    (D) 50°

298. A device used to visualize the dead zone.

    (A) radiation force balance
    (B) analog-digital converter
    (C) acoustic standoff
    (D) Schlieren camera

299. The intensity of the ultrasound beam from a pulsed-echo system

    (A) is measured in watts
    (B) is constant at all depths
    (C) will depend upon the beam diameter
    (D) is constant in time

300. Whose principle states that all points on an ultrasound waveform can be considered as point sources for the production of secondary spherical wavelets?

    (A) Doppler
    (B) Curie
    (C) Huygens
    (D) Nyquist

301. The fraction of time that a pulsed ultrasound system is actually producing ultrasound is called the

    (A) duty factor
    (B) Curie factor
    (C) frame rate
    (D) transmission factor

302. Real-time ultrasound transducers can be classified as

    (A) annular, sector, linear, and static scanners
    (B) sector scanners, vector, and annular
    (C) phased, linear, annular, and vector
    (D) linear sequenced array and vector

303. The speed at which ultrasound propagates within a medium depends primarily on

(A) its frequency
(B) the compressibility of the medium
(C) its intensity
(D) the thickness of the medium

304. An artifact that results from a pulse that has traveled two or more round-trip distances between the transducer and the interface is called

(A) a multipath
(B) a side lobe
(C) reverberation
(D) scattering

305. The ratio of output of electric power to input electric power is termed

(A) power
(B) intensity
(C) gain
(D) voltage

306. Multipath artifacts result from

(A) echoes that return directly to the transducer
(B) shotgun pellets
(C) echoes that take an indirect path back to the transducer
(D) sound wave propagates through a medium at a speed other than soft tissue

307. What type of noise is associated with Doppler shift?

(A) clutter
(B) speckle
(C) flash
(D) harmonics

308. To achieve the best possible digital representation of an analog system, the echo signals should undergo

(A) postprocessing
(B) preprocessing
(C) rectification
(D) amplification

309. Near-zone length may be increased by increasing

(A) wavelength
(B) wavelength and bandwidth
(C) small transducer aperture
(D) high frequency and large diameter transducer

Questions 310–319:   Match each term in Column A with the correct definition in Column B.

COLUMN A

310. density _____
311. propagation _____
312. frequency _____
313. power _____
314. duty factor _____
315. bandwidth _____
316. acoustic impedance _____
317. absorption _____
318. quality factor _____
319. intensity _____

COLUMN B

(A) rate at which work is done
(B) mass divided by volume
(C) conversion of sound to heat
(D) number of cycles per unit time
(E) density multiplied by sound propagation speed
(F) range of frequencies contained in the ultrasound pulse
(G) the fraction of time that the ultrasound pulse is on
(H) progression or travel
(I) operating frequency divided by bandwidth
(J) power divided by area

320. Which of the following is a true definition for a highly damped transducer?

(A) increased efficiency, sensitivity, and spatial pulse length
(B) decreased efficiency, sensitivity, and spatial pulse length
(C) increased efficiency and sensitivity, but decreased spatial pulse length
(D) decreased efficiency, but increased sensitivity and spatial pulse length

321. Gain compensation is necessary due to

(A) reflector motion
(B) gray scale
(C) attenuation
(D) resolution

322. The frequency bandwidth may be determined by which of the following?

(A) spectral analysis
(B) Schlieren system
(C) hydrophone analysis
(D) cathode analysis

323. Which of the following is *not* true of power output?

(A) bioeffects concerns
(B) does not affect signal-to-noise ratio
(C) can be used to change the brightness of the entire image
(D) alters patient exposure

491. What increases the acoustic energy that a patient receives?

(A) high frequency
(B) wavelength
(C) gain
(D) examination time

492. Frequency is a significant factor in

(A) propagation speed
(B) tissue compressibility
(C) tissue attenuation
(D) transducer diameter

493. In a pulse-echo system, a 3.5 MHz beam of 2 cm of tissue will be attenuated by

(A) 3.5 dB/cm
(B) 7.0 dB/cm
(C) 3.5 dB
(D) 7.0 dB

494. The characteristic acoustic impedance of a material is equal to the product of the material density and

(A) path length
(B) wavelength
(C) frequency
(D) propagation speed

495. In what area of a stenotic blood vessel does the maximum velocity of blood occur?

(A) within the stenosis
(B) before the stenosis
(C) after the stenosis
(D) before and after the stenosis

496. For normal incidence, if the intensity reflection coefficient is 30%, the intensity transmission coefficient will be

(A) 15%
(B) 30%
(C) 60%
(D) 70%

497. Turbulent flow is possible when blood flow exceeds what Reynolds number?

(A) 100
(B) 200
(C) 1500
(D) 2000

498. The range equation relates

(A) frequency, velocity, and wavelength
(B) frequency, velocity, and time
(C) distance, velocity, and time
(D) distance, frequency, and time

499. Which of the following predicts the onset of turbulent flow?

(A) dosimetry
(B) acoustic pressure
(C) Reynolds number
(D) wall thump

500. The Doppler shift frequency is zero when the angle between the receiving transducer and the flow direction is

(A) 0°
(B) 45°
(C) 90°
(D) 180°

501. Turbulence flow occurs at what area of a stenotic blood vessel?

(A) within the stenosis
(B) before the stenosis
(C) after the stenosis
(D) all of the above

502. The dynamic range of a pulse-echo ultrasound system is defined as

(A) the ratio of the maximum to the minimum intensity that can be processed
(B) the range of propagation speeds
(C) the range of gain settings allowed
(D) the difference between the transmitted and the received ultrasound frequency

503. The thermal paper printer is not working, what is the first step?

(A) call the manufacturer for service
(B) check for a paper jam
(C) call biomedical services
(D) call the ultrasound supervisor

504. The time gain or depth gain compensation control

(A) compensates for attenuation effects
(B) compensates for increased patient scan time
(C) compensates for machine malfunctions
(D) compensates for video-image drifts

505. A digital scan converter is essentially a

   (A) radio receiver

   (B) video monitor

   (C) television set

   (D) computer memory

506. An increase in peak rarefactional pressure could result in which of the following?

   (A) increased TI

   (B) hypothermia of biological tissue

   (C) necrotic tissue

   (D) inertial cavitation

507. Acoustic enhancement can be observed when scanning

   (A) highly attenuating structures

   (B) weakly attenuating structures

   (C) highly reflective structures

   (D) structures with large speed differences

508. Ultrasound depth penetration is inversely related to

   (A) period

   (B) propagation speed

   (C) magnification

   (D) frequency

509. Lateral resolution

   (A) is affected by the beam diameter

   (B) is affected by aperture size and acoustic lens

   (C) is improved at the focal zone

   (D) all of the above

510. If the lines per degree in a mechanical sector scanner remain constant, a decreased sector angle can result in

   (A) decreased resolution

   (B) increased frame rate

   (C) decreased frame rate

   (D) increased resolution

511. What letter represents a group of nylon lines used to evaluate horizontal distance accuracy in this tissue-equivalent phantom (Fig. 1–62)?

   (A) line A

   (B) line B

   (C) line C

   (D) line D

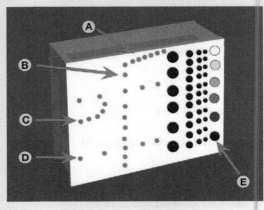

FIGURE 1–62.

512. What letter represents a group of nylon lines used to evaluate range accuracy in this tissue-equivalent phantom (Fig. 1–62)?

   (A) line A

   (B) line B

   (C) line C

   (D) line D

513. The advantages of CW include all of the following *except*

   (A) ability to measure very high velocities

   (B) ability to use high frequencies

   (C) no aliasing

   (D) range ambiguity

514. If the gain of an amplifier is 18 dB, what will the new gain setting be if the gain setting is reduced by one-half?

   (A) 9 dB

   (B) 36 dB

   (C) 15 dB

   (D) 0.5 dB

515. Decreasing the PRP

   (A) decreases spatial resolution

   (B) decreases axial resolution

   (C) decreases the maximum depth imaged

   (D) increases the maximum depth imaged

516. The AIUM 100-mm test object is used to evaluate all of the following except

   (A) registration

   (B) attenuation

   (C) range accuracy

   (D) azimuthal resolution

517. **A 3.5-MHz transducer is used on a patient with the ultrasound wave propagating the various tissues listed below. Which one will have the longest wavelength?**

    (A) muscle
    (B) blood
    (C) water
    (D) fat

518. **What type of resolution is degraded in the presence of grating lobes and side lobes?**

    (A) lateral
    (B) axial
    (C) temporal
    (D) range

519. **Spatial compounding improves the quality of the image in several ways *except***

    (A) reducing the amount of reverberation and shadowing in the image
    (B) reduced clutter artifacts
    (C) structures previously hidden beneath distal acoustic shadow can be visualized
    (D) creating multiple images in a single angle

520. **A 7.5-MHz transducer is used on a patient with the ultrasound wave propagating various tissues listed below. Which one will have the shortest wavelength?**

    (A) lungs
    (B) blood
    (C) water
    (D) fat

521. **The ability of a system to detect low-amplitude echoes accurately is referred to as**

    (A) resolution
    (B) sensitivity
    (C) accuracy
    (D) dynamic accuracy

522. **The primary mechanisms whereby ultrasound can produce biologic effects are**

    (A) thermal and cavitation
    (B) absorption and reflection
    (C) reflection and transmission
    (D) photon energies and ultraviolet

523. **The near-zone length of a transducer depends on**

    (A) propagation speed and frequency
    (B) frequency and transducer diameter
    (C) FOV and transducer diameter
    (D) magnification

524. **The AIUM Committee on Biological Effects in 2019 stated what biologic effects with the use of ultrasound intensities below SPTA 100 mW/cm^2?**

    (A) has small amount reported cases of cancer of the fetal kidneys
    (B) has no confirmed effects in mammalian
    (C) result in maternal leukemia in mothers who had multiple sonograms during pregnancy
    (D) minimal amount of neurological and musculoskeletal biologic injury to sonographers

525. **The intensity of a focused beam is generally**

    (A) constant
    (B) highest at the transducer surface
    (C) highest at the focal zone
    (D) lowest at the transducer surface

526. **The wavelength of a 5-MHz wave passing through soft tissue is approximately**

    (A) 0.1 mm
    (B) 0.3 mm
    (C) 0.5 mm
    (D) 1.0 mm

527. **An echo that has undergone an attenuation of 3 dB will have an intensity that is _____ than its initial intensity.**

    (A) three times smaller
    (B) three times larger
    (C) two times smaller
    (D) two times larger

528. **Linear array transducers are commonly called**

    (A) vector
    (B) phased
    (C) convex
    (D) annular

529. A 5-MHz transducer used in a pulse-echo system will generally produce

(A) a wide band of frequencies centered at 5 MHz

(B) frequencies only at 5 MHz

(C) frequencies only at 5 MHz or multiples of 5 MHz

(D) a wide band of frequencies above 5 MHz

530. The transducer _____ determines its _____.

(A) diameter; intensity

(B) damping; lateral resolution

(C) thickness; sensitivity

(D) thickness; resonance frequency

531. The axial resolution of a transducer can be improved with _____ but at the expense of _____.

(A) increased damping; sensitivity

(B) frequency; lateral resolution

(C) focusing; sensitivity

(D) focusing; lateral resolution

532. A material that changes its dimensions when an electric field is applied is called which of the following?

(A) piezoelectric

(B) acoustic-optics

(C) RAID

533. The process of making the impedance values on either side of a boundary as close as possible to reduce reflections is known as which of the following?

(A) damping

(B) refracting

(C) matching

(D) compensating

534. Which of the following data medium has the largest storage capacity used in diagnostic ultrasound?

(A) flash drive

(B) CD

(C) magneto-optical

(D) RAID

535. Shadowing occurs with

(A) highly attenuating structures

(B) large changes in propagation speed

(C) low frequencies more often than with high frequencies

(D) weak reflectors

536. Reverberation artifacts

(A) occur most often at high frequencies

(B) occur with multiple strong reflecting structures

(C) occur only with real-time arrays

(D) cannot occur in color Doppler systems

537. A transducer with a large bandwidth is likely to have

(A) good axial resolution

(B) a large ring-down time

(C) poor resolution

(D) a high Q factor

538. The region of the ultrasound beam from the focus to beam diversion is called which of the following?

(A) Fraunhofer zone

(B) Fresnel zone

(C) focal zone

(D) divergence zone

539. Refraction will not occur at an interface

(A) when high frequencies are used

(B) if the acoustic impedances are equal

(C) if the propagation speeds are significantly different

(D) with normal incidence of the ultrasound beam

540. Acoustic power output is determined primarily by

(A) the diameter of the transducer

(B) the thickness of the transducer

(C) the pulser voltage spike

(D) focusing

541. Specular reflections occur when

(A) the reflecting object is small with respect to the wavelength

(B) the reflecting surface is large and smooth with respect to the wavelength

(C) the reflecting objects are moving

(D) the angle of incidence and angle of reflection are unequal

542. The angle at which an ultrasound beam is bent as it passes through a boundary between two different materials is described mathematically by which of the following?

(A) Huygens-Fresnel principle

(B) Curie's principle

(C) Snell's law

(D) Nyquist limit

543. **What type of transducer is composed of multiple ring-shaped elements?**

    (A) annular

    (B) linear sequential arrays

    (C) trapezoidal

    (D) phased array

544. **The percentage of an ultrasound beam reflected at an interface between gas and soft tissue is approximately**

    (A) 90–100%

    (B) 70–80%

    (C) 45–55%

    (D) 10–25%

545. **The percentage of an ultrasound beam reflected at an interface between fat and muscle is approximately**

    (A) 90–100%

    (B) 70–80%

    (C) 45–55%

    (D) 1–10%

546. **Which of the following is a reason to use an acoustic standoff?**

    (A) to reduce tissue attenuation

    (B) to move the focal zone closer to the skin surface

    (C) to allow a lower frequency transducer to be used

    (D) to move the focal zone deeper in the body structure

547. **Ultrasound waves in tissue are referred to as**

    (A) shear waves

    (B) transverse waves

    (C) vibrational waves

    (D) longitudinal compression waves

548. **High-frequency transducers have**

    (A) shorter wavelengths and less penetration

    (B) longer wavelengths and greater penetration

    (C) shorter wavelengths and greater penetration

    (D) longer wavelengths and less penetration

549. **When the piezoelectric crystal continues to vibrate after the initial voltage pulse, this is referred to as**

    (A) ring-down time

    (B) pulse delay

    (C) pulse retardation

    (D) overdamping

550. **Annular phased arrays, unlike linear phased arrays,**

    (A) can be dynamically focused

    (B) electronically focus in two dimensions rather than one

    (C) can be used in Doppler systems

    (D) can achieve high frame rates

551. **Which group is arranged in the correct order of increasing propagation speed?**

    (A) gas, bone, muscle

    (B) bone, muscle, gas

    (C) gas, muscle, bone

    (D) muscle, bone, gas

552. **The lower useful range of diagnostic ultrasound is determined primarily by _____, whereas the upper useful range is determined by _____.**

    (A) resolution; penetration

    (B) scattering; propagation speed

    (C) cost; resolution

    (D) scattering; resolution

553. **Convert the number 125,000,000,000 to engineering notation.**

    (A) 125×10^{-11}

    (B) 1.25×10^{11}

    (C) 1.25×10^{-11}

    (D) 125×10^{9}

554. **Which of the following is true?**

    (A) SPTA is always equal to or greater than SPTP.

    (B) SPTP is always equal to or greater than SPTA.

    (C) SATA is always equal to or greater than SATP.

    (D) SPTA is always equal to or greater than SATP.

555. **A beam-intensity profile is often mapped with**

    (A) dosimetry

    (B) acousto-optics

    (C) a hydrophone

    (D) AIUM test object

556. **If the direction of flow is perpendicular to the sound beam, what is the velocity and cosine?**

    (A) Velocity is 1 and the cosine is 1.

    (B) Velocity is 0.87 and the cosine is 0.87.

    (C) Velocity is 0.5 and the cosine is 0.5.

    (D) Velocity is zero and the cosine is zero.

166. **(D)** SATA has the lowest intensity because the intensity is averaged over the whole beam profile (SA), and over the whole duration of exposure (TA).

167. **(B)** The beam uniformity ratio is defined as the spatial peak intensity (measured at the beam center) divided by the spatial average intensity (the average intensity across the beam).

168. **(C)** The duty factor is the fraction of time the transducer is emitting sound. In a pulsed echo system, it is normally less than 1%.

169. **(D)** Axial resolution is defined as one-half the SPL. Therefore, the shorter the SPL, the better the axial resolution.

170. **(C)** Propagation speed (mm/μs); f = frequency (cycle/s) and λ wavelength (mm).

171. **(D)** Attenuation of an ultrasound beam can occur by divergence of a beam, scattering, and reflection. It can also occur by absorption.

172. **(A)** Attenuation coefficient of sound is determined by knowing dB/cm/MHz and then multiplying that quantity by the frequency expressed in MHz.

173. **(B)** Transducer Q factor (quality factor) is equal to the operating frequency divided by the bandwidth. Therefore, if the transducer Q factor is low, the bandwidth is wide.

174. **(A)** Axial resolution can be improved by shortening pulse length, increasing damping, and a higher-frequency transducer.

175. **(B)** Axial resolution is primarily affected by SPL. Because the SPL is the product of wavelength, reducing the wavelength or increasing the frequency will affect axial resolution.

176. **(D)** Increasing transducer frequency will improve both lateral and axial resolution but decrease depth of penetration.

177. **(C)** Range resolution is another name for *axial* resolution.

178. **(B)** The duty factor is the fraction of time that sound is being emitted from the transducer. In continuous wave, the sound is being emitted 100% of the time.

179. **(A)** The arrow (B) points to blood cells moving toward the transducer.

180. **(D)** Acoustic impedance is calculated as $Z = p \times c$ and measured with units of rayls. The average soft-tissue impedance is 1,630,000 rayls.

181. **(C)** Constant depth mode (C-mode). Its application is PW Doppler.

182. **(A)** The height of the vertical spike corresponds to the strength of the echo received by the transducer (y-axes).

183. **(B)** The arrow (C) points to blood cells moving away from the transducer.

184. **(A)** The correct equation for calculating reflection percentage is

$$R = \left(\frac{Z_2 - Z_1}{Z_2 + Z_1} \right)^2 \times 100$$

185. **(D)** The reflection coefficient between water and air interface is 100%. Air prevents the sound from entering the body. It is for this reason that a coupling gel is necessary.

186. **(B)** Beyond the critical angle, 100% of the sound beam is reflected and 0% is transmitted.

187. **(A)** Rayleigh scattering occurs when the particle size is smaller than a wavelength (for ultrasound typically in the 1-mm range).

188. **(D)** The least likely way to decrease the dead zone (main bang) is to increase pulse length. The dead zone is decreased with high frequency, short pulse length, and increasing the output power and acoustic standoff pad.

189. **(C)** Power is defined as the rate at which work is done or energy is transferred (energy per unit time).

190. **(A)** Lateral resolution is the minimum separation between two reflectors perpendicular to the sound path.

191. **(D)** In most soft tissues, the attenuation coefficient increases directly with frequency. As frequency is increased, the attenuation coefficient increases, thereby limiting depth of perception.

192. **(A)** Absorption is the conversion of ultrasound energy into heat. Absorption, scattering, and reflection are all factors of attenuation.

193. **(D)** The rule of thumb for attenuation in soft tissue is 0.5 dB/cm/MHz. Therefore, an ultrasound beam of 1 MHz frequency will lose 0.5 dB of amplitude for every centimeter traveled.

194. **(C)** Reverberation produces false echoes.

195. **(D)** The acoustic impedance mismatch between fat and muscle is small; therefore, approximately 90% of the sound beam is transmitted.

196. **(D)** Huygens's principle states that all points on a wavefront can be considered as a source for secondary spherical wavelets.

197. **(B)** Enhancement is the "burst of sound" visualized posterior to weak attenuations.

198. **(A)** Half-value layer (HVL—sometimes called half-intensity depth) is defined as the thickness of tissue that reduces the beam intensity by one-half.

199. **(D)** Propagation speed error. The ultrasound machine assumes a speed of 1540 m/s. If the sound passes through a medium of a different velocity, the result is an error in the range equation.

200. **(B)** The range equation explains the distance to the reflector, which is equal to one-half of the propagation speed × the pulse round-trip time.

201. **(A)** For a specular reflector, the angle of incidence is equal to the angle of reflection. This type of reflection occurs from a surface, which is larger than the wavelength.

202. **(C)** Propagation speed is determined by the medium. The transducer determines amplitude, period, intensity, and frequency.

203. **(D)** Acoustic variables include density, pressure, temperature, particle motion, and distance.

204. **(D)** Acoustic parameters include frequency, power, intensity, period, amplitude, wavelength, and propagation speed.

205. **(C)** CW Doppler requires two active elements mounted side by side. One element transmits and the other receives the echoes.

206. **(D)** Reynold's number is a dimensionless index that indicates the likelihood of turbulence to occur.

207. **(A)** A is correct, with the propagation velocity in this order, respectively: 331 m/s, 1450 m/s, 1585 m/s, and 4080 m/s.

208. **(C)** Backscatter is increased by increasing frequency and increasing heterogeneous media.

209. **(A)** Critical angle is the angle at which sound is totally reflected and none is transmitted.

210. **(D)** The PRF is the number of pulses occurring per second. The PRF is inversely proportional to the PRP. The PRF and depth of view are inversely related and the PRF is equal to the number of scan lines per second.

211. **(D)** The duty factor is the fraction of time that the transducer is emitting a pulse. It is unitless.

212. **(A)** The attenuation coefficient is the attenuation per unit length of sound travel. It's typical value is 3 dB/cm, for 6 MHz sound in soft tissue (0.5 dB/cm/MHz × 6 MHz = 3 dB/cm).

213. **(B)** Normal incidence is also known as orthogonal, perpendicular, right angle, or 90°. At normal incidence, sound may be reflected or transmitted in various degrees.

214. **(A)** The difference (mismatch) of acoustic impedance between two media is what determines how much energy will be transmitted or reflected.

215. **(A)** Acoustic impedance is equal to the product of the density of a substance and the velocity of sound. The propagation speed in solids is higher than that in liquids, and the propagation speed in gas is low. The increase in propagation speed is caused by increasing stiffness of the media, not by the density.

216. **(A)** According to Snell's law,

$$\frac{\sin i}{\sin r} = \frac{V_1}{V_2}$$

the transmission angle is proportional to the incidence angle times the medium 2 propagation speed divided by the medium 1 propagation speed.

217. **(C)** The depth of the interface is 3 cm. Ultrasound equipment is programmed at 1.54 mm/µs, and because the average speed in soft tissue is known, the depth and time can be calculated using the following equation:

$$\text{depth (mm)} = \frac{1.54 \text{ mm/µs} \times \text{transmitted and reflected time (µs)}}{2}$$

This equation is called range equation.

Another method is using the 13-µs rule. This rule states that for every 13 µs of transmitted time, the reflected interface is 1 cm depth; therefore, 26 µs is 2 cm depth and 39 µs is 3 cm depth.

218. **(D)** The mirror image artifact duplicates a structure on the other side of a strong curved reflector, eg, the diaphragm and pleura.

219. **(C)** The comet tail is a bright tapering trail of echoes just distal to a strongly reflecting structure. The greater the acoustic impedance mismatch, the greater the possibility of this artifact to occur.

220. **(C)** The acoustic impedance mismatch between tissue and gas is very great; therefore, it may produce the comet tail artifact.

221. **(C)** Aliasing occurs when the Doppler shift frequency exceeds one-half of the PRF. This is known as Nyquist limit.

222. **(D)** By increasing damping, one also increases the bandwidth. Bandwidth is the range of frequency involved in a pulse.

223. **(D)** All of the above

224. **(C)** Using the range equation 13-µs rule, 4 × 13 = 52 µs. Therefore, the depth is 4 cm for 52 µs.

225. **(A)** An ultrasound transducer generally can resolve reflectors along the sound path better than it can resolve those perpendicular to it.

226. **(D)** The number of electrical pulses produced per second is typically 1000 Hz.

227. **(B)** The most common artifact in Doppler ultrasound is aliasing.

228. **(B)** With a typical PRF of 1000 Hz, each pulse–receive interval is 1 ms (1000 µs) long. Because an average pulse is 1 µs long, this leaves 999 µs for receiving. 999/1000 is 99.9%.

229. **(C)** Frequency equals velocity divided by wavelength. Because velocity is standard at 1540 m/s, doubling the frequency will result in decreasing the wavelength by one-half.

230. **(A)** Real-time transducers display two formats: sector and rectangular. The linear-sequenced array transducer displays a rectangular format.

231. **(C)** Z is the acoustic impedance; p is the material density; and c is the propagation speed. Z (rayls) = p (kg/m^3) × c (m/s). *(25:28)*

232. **(A)** Lead zirconate titanate (PZT) is a ceramic material with piezoelectric properties. It is most commonly used in transducers because of its greater efficiency and sensitivity. *(20:236)*

233. **(D)** The pulse travels to the interface and back to the transducer, the total time for the distance travel is 39 μs. Using the 13 μs rule, 3 × 13 = 39 μs; therefore, the depth of the reflector is 3 cm. The total distance traveled is 2 × 3 = 6 cm.

234. **(C)** The total round-trip time in human tissue for reflected echo at a depth of 2 cm is 26 μs.

235. **(A)** PRF is the number of pulses emitted per second.

236. **(D)** The pulser produces the electric voltage pulses; this, in turn, drives the transducer to emit ultrasound pulses. It also tells both the memory and the receiver when the ultrasound pulses were produced.

237. **(C)** Shadowing is a useful artifact that helps with diagnosis. The ultrasound beam striking a highly reflective or highly attenuating structure causes this artifact.

238. **(D)** PRF 18 kHz = 9 Nyquist limit

239. **(A)** Lateral resolution is dependent on beam diameter, which varies with distance from the transducer.

240. **(C)** A period is the time it takes for one full cycle to occur.

241. **(B)** Half-intensity depth decreases with increasing frequency. As frequency increases, the wavelength decreases both axial and lateral resolution.

242. **(C)** Redirection of a portion of the sound beam from a boundary

243. **(C)** 7 MHz. The transmitted frequency is called the fundamental frequency. The second harmonic frequency is twice the fundamental frequency.

244. **(A)** Bit is an acronym for binary digit and represents the basic digital unit for storing data in the main computer memory.

245. **(A)** Eight bits equal 1 byte. A bit is a unit of data in binary notation and assumes one of two states: "on" representing the number 1, or "off" representing the number 0.

246. **(D)** The purpose of using an acoustic lens on transducers is to narrow the ultrasound beam, which improves lateral resolution.

247. **(A)** The needle or membrane hydrophone is used to measure pressure amplitude, wavelength, intensity, and PRF

248. **(C)** Viscosity is measured in units of *poise* or *kilograms per meter-second* (kg/m-s).

249. **(C)** The speed of ultrasound is dependent on bone, muscle, soft tissue, and fat, which make up the medium. The speed is not dependent on the range of frequency or output power. If stiffness increases, speed increases, and if density increases, speed decreases.

250. **(D)** The resistance to flow offered by a fluid in motion is called viscosity.

251. **(C)** Autocorrelation is the mathematical process commonly used to detect Doppler shifts in color Doppler instruments.

252. **(C)** A decrease in frequency or transducer aperture size will decrease the near-zone length (Fresnel zone).

253. **(D)** Water has the lowest viscosity.

254. **(C)** While the symbol k represents kilo or 1000 in metric, in computer terminology K = 1024. Then, the amount that can be stored in memory is 128 × 1024 × 8 bits = 1,048,576 bits, referred to as 1 megabit.

255. **(B)** Harmonics frequencies are created when structures undergo nonlinear oscillations. These nonlinear vibrations can occur both in tissue as well as with microbubbles used as contrast agents. Harmonics frequencies are multiples of the fundamental frequency, eg, twice that of the fundamental frequency.

256. **(A)** Frequency compounding reduces speckle and as a result, improves image contrast.

257. **(A)** The unit for acoustic pressure is pascal (Pa).

258. **(A)** The horizontal (or x-axis) on the M-mode display represents time.

259. **(C)** 7 MHz. Diagnostic ultrasound transducers used in the clinical setting range from 2.5 to 10 MHz. Ultrasound frequencies in the kilohertz range are not useful in diagnostic range.

260. **(B)** The ratio of the minimum to maximum signal amplitude that can be applied to a device without producing distortion is called dynamic range.

261. **(C)** The vertical (y-axis) on the M-mode display represents depth of the reflector.

262. **(B)** Two: off or on. "Off" represented by the number 0. "On" represented by the number 1. *(20:62)*

263. **(B)** Two (0 or 1). *(20:62)*

264. **(D)** The number 30 is represented by 011110. To convert from decimal to binary, repeatedly divide by two and note the remainder.

30 ÷ 2 = 15 remainder 0	3 ÷ 2 = 1 remainder 1
15 ÷ 2 = 7 remainder 1	1 ÷ 2 = 0 remainder 1
7 ÷ 2 = 3 remainder 1	0 ÷ 2 = 0 remainder 0

265. **(D)** The binary system, which is used in digital scan converter memory, is based on the powers of two. For four bits, 2^4 ($2 \times 2 \times 2 \times 2$) or 16 different gray levels can be represented. Another way of looking at this is to list all possible states:

0000	0100	1000	1100
0001	0101	1001	1101
0010	0110	1010	1110
0011	0111	1011	1111

There are 16 possible unique states.

266. **(B)** Digital memory, where the electronic components are either on (1) or off (0), is based on the binary number system. We can say that the number of discrete levels possible, N, is equal to 2 raised to the power of that number of bits. $N = 2^n$. Therefore, to make 64 shades of gray would require 2^6 bit memory.

$$(2 \times 2 \quad 4 \times 2 \quad 8 \times 2 \quad 16 \times 2 \quad 32 \times 2 = 64)$$
$$2 \quad 3 \quad 4 \quad 5 \quad 6$$

267. **(B)** The acoustic output with potential for producing cavitational effects in tissue is characterized by the MI. Cavitation is classified as either stable or transient.

268. **(C)** The receiver processes echoes detected by the transducer. These echoes may be amplified (gain), compensated for depth (TGC), compressed (to fit into the dynamic range of the system), and rejected (eliminating low-level signals).

269. **(D)** The greater the pulse amplitude (electronic voltage applied to the transducer), the greater the amplitude of the ultrasound pulse provided by the transducer.

270. **(B)** The pulser produces electric voltage pulses that drive the transducer and serve to synchronize the receiver so that the arrival time of returning echoes can be accurately determined.

271. **(D)** Components of a pulse-echo system include the *pulser* that produces the electrical pulse, which drives the *transducer*. For each reflection received from the tissue by the transducer, an electrical voltage is produced that goes to the *receiver*, where it is processed for display. Information on transducer position and orientation is delivered to the *image memory*. Electric information from the memory drives the *display*.

272. **(B)** Transducers may be focused by using a curved piezo-electric transducer element (internal focusing) or by using an acoustic lens.

273. **(D)** Quality factor (Q factor) is equal to the operating frequency divided by the bandwidth and is unitless.

274. **(E)** Reduction in echoes from a region distal to an attenuating structure

275. **(G)** An increase in echoes from a region distal to a weakly attenuating structure or tissue

276. **(A)** A structure that is echo-free; not necessarily cystic unless there is good through transmission. A solid mass can be anechoic but will not have good through transmission.

277. **(D)** An echo that does not correspond to the real target.

278. **(I)** A structure that possesses echoes.

279. **(H)** Echoes of higher amplitude than the normal surrounding tissues.

280. **(B)** Echoes of lower amplitude than the normal surrounding tissues.

281. **(C)** The surface forming the boundary between two media having different acoustic impedances.

282. **(A and F)** A structure without echoes and with low absorption; not necessarily cystic unless there is good through transmission. *Sonolucent* is a misnomer for *anechoic*.

283. **(D)** Air. There are numerable backing materials used for damping. Pulse-echo transducer backing materials are (1) epoxy resin, (2) tungsten, (3) cork, and (4) rubber. CW Doppler transducers have little or no backing materials.

284. **(C)** Aliasing.

285. **(C)** Brightness of pixel.

286. **(C)** For ultrasound to propagate a medium, it must be composed of particles of matter. A vacuum is a space empty of matter; therefore, ultrasound cannot travel in a vacuum.

287. **(B)** Wavelength.

288. **(A)** Period.

289. **(B)** Hertz (Hz) represents cycles per second (cps). Therefore, 20 cps = 20 Hz.

290. **(C)** 1 MHz.

291. **(B)** Mechanical transducers have only one crystal, so this will result in total image loss.

292. **(A)** A-mode is a shortened form of amplitude mode. This mode is presented graphically with vertical spikes arising from a horizontal baseline. The height of the vertical spikes represents the amplitude of the deflected echo.

293. **(B)** B-mode is a shortened form of brightness modulation. This mode presents a two-dimensional image of internal body structures displayed as dots. The brightness of the dots is proportional to the amplitude of the echo. B-mode display is employed in all two-dimensional images, static or real-time.

294. **(D)** M-mode is short for time-motion modulation. This mode is a graphic display of movement of reflecting structures related to time. M-mode is used almost exclusively in echocardiography.

295. **(D)** A long dead zone may indicate a detached backing material. The use of a high-frequency transducer or a short PD will typically decrease the dead zone.

296. **(D)** The frame rate in ultrasound is determined by image depth and the speed of sound in the medium.

297. **(A)** Doppler signals and velocities cannot be measured with perpendicular incidence (90°).

298. **(C)** The technique used to visualize the dead zone is acoustic standoff.

299. **(C)** The intensity of the ultrasound beam depends on the beam diameter. Intensity is defined as the beam power divided by the beam cross-sectional area.

300. **(C)** Huygens principle

301. **(A)** The fraction of time that a pulsed ultrasound is actually producing ultrasound is called the duty factor.

$$\text{duty factor (DF)} = \frac{\text{pulse duration (PD)}}{\text{pulse repetition period (PRP)}}$$

302. **(C)** Real-time ultrasound instrumentation is classified as phased, linear, annular, and vector.

303. **(B)** The speed at which ultrasound propagates within a medium depends primarily on the compressibility of the medium.

304. **(C)** The reverberation artifact occurs when two or more reflections are present along the path of the beam. This gives rise to multiple reflections, which will appear behind one another at intervals equal to the separation of the real reflectors.

305. **(C)** Gain is the ratio of electric power. Gain governs the electric compensation for tissue attenuation and is expressed in decibels (dB).

306. **(C)** Multipath reverberation artifacts result from sound reflected from a highly curved specular surface when the echo takes an indirect path back to the transducer.

307. **(A)** Doppler shift artifacts are called clutter. Clutter is eliminated by wall filters.

308. **(B)** Echo signals that are in analog format as they emerge from the receiver are transferred to a digital format by an analog-to-digital (A–D) converter. Preprocessing then produces the best possible digital representation of the analog signal.

309. **(D)** By increasing frequency (MHz) (f) and/or transducer diameter (mm), the near-zone length (mm) is increased, as shown in the equation:

$$\text{near zone length} = \frac{(\text{transducer diameter})^2\, f}{6}$$

310. **(B)** Mass divided by volume.

311. **(H)** Progression or travel.

312. **(D)** Number of cycles per unit time.

313. **(A)** Rate at which work is done.

314. **(G)** The percentage of time the system is transmitting a pulse.

315. **(F)** Range of frequencies contained in the ultrasound pulse.

316. **(E)** Density multiplied by sound propagation speed.

317. **(C)** Conversion of sound to heat.

318. **(I)** Operating frequency divided by bandwidth.

319. **(J)** Power divided by area.

320. **(B)** The damping material reduces SPL, efficiency, and sensitivity.

321. **(C)** Gain is electric compensation for tissue attenuation.

322. **(A)** Spectral analysis allows the determination of the frequency spectrum of a signal.

323. **(B)** The output power is a knob on the ultrasound equipment that is used to increase or decrease the brightness of the entire image; increasing the power output improves the signal-to-noise ratio, and increasing this output also increases patient exposure with potential bioeffect concerns.

324. **(C)** Gray-scale resolution is the ability of a gray-scale display to distinguish between echoes of slightly different amplitudes or intensities. The first step in this problem is to figure out how many shades of gray are contained in a 5-bit digital system. The total number of shades of gray is 32 ($2^5 = 32$). The next step is to divide the dynamic range (42 dB) by the number of levels. This will give the number of decibels per level. 42 dB ÷ 32 gray levels = 1.3 dB/gray level.

325. **(B)**

$$\begin{aligned} \text{Distance} &= \text{velocity} \times \text{time} \\ &= 1540 \text{ m/s} \times 0.01 \text{ s} \\ &= 15.4 \text{ m} \end{aligned}$$

However, 0.1 seconds is only the time to reach the echo source. The time of the round-trip must be calculated by multiplying by 2. Round-trip distance = 15.4 m × 2 = 30.8 m. *(4:2)*

326. **(B)** An edge artifact. Edge shadowing results from refraction and reflection of the ultrasound beam on a rounded surface, for example, the fetal skull.

327. **(A)** A split image artifact (ghost artifact) may produce duplication or triplication of an image, resulting in ultrasound beam refraction at a muscle–fat interface.

328. **(A)** Multipath, mirror image, and side lobe artifacts are most likely to produce a pseudomass. A comet tail artifact is least likely.

329. **(A)** Split image artifact is more noticeable in athletic and mesomorphic habitus patients.

330. **(C)** Split image artifact (ghost artifact) is *not* caused by a gas bubble. The most likely cause is refraction of the sound beam at a muscle–fat interface. The artifact is more evident at an interface between subcutaneous fat and abdominal muscle or between rectus muscles and fat in the pelvis. The artifact can also be produced by an abdominal scar or superficial abdominal skin keloids.

331. **(C)** The most likely cause of beam thickness artifact is partial volume effect. This type of artifact occurs most often when the ultrasound beam interacts with a cyst or other fluid-filled structures.

332. **(C)** Beam thickness artifacts depend on beam angulation, not gravity. Therefore, if an image of the gallbladder has what appears to be sludge, a change in the patient's position relative to the beam could differentiate pseudosludge caused by artifact from layering of biliary sludge.

333. **(D)** Side lobe artifacts are weaker than the primary beam.

334. **(B)** Shotgun pellets and metallic surgical clips produce a trail of dense continuous echoes. Bone, gas, calcifications, and gallstones produce a distal acoustic shadow.

335. **(A)** The most common type of artifact observed in patients with shotgun pellets or metallic surgical clips are comet tail artifacts. This type of reverberation artifact is characterized by a trail of dense continuous echoes distal to a strongly reflecting structure.

336. **(D)** A ring-down artifact is characterized sonographically as high-amplitude parallel lines occurring at regular intervals distal to a reflecting interface. This type of artifact is commonly associated with bowel gas.

337. **(A)** It is possible to calculate the displacement in split images by using Snell's law.

338. **(C)** The first large vertical reflection at the start of the A-mode is called "main bang," or transducer artifact.

339. **(C)** Annular-array real-time uses a combination of mechanical and electronic devices. The annular array is used for dynamic focusing; the mechanical part for beam steering.

340. **(A)** A decrease in the amplitude of the returning echo and also a decrease in the amount of transmitted sound: these result in a fade-away picture. The combination of the coupling medium and matching layers enables passage and return of echoes from the body to the transducer.

341. **(A)** Spatial compounding.

342. **(C)** M-mode stands for time-motion modulation. This mode displays a graphic representation of motion of reflecting surfaces. It is used primarily in echocardiography.

343. **(A)** B-mode stands for brightness modulation. This mode displays a two-dimensional view of internal body structures in cross section or sagittal section. The images, displayed as dots on the monitor, result from interaction between ultrasound and tissues. The brightness of the dots is proportional to the amplitude of the echo. Real-time equipment uses B-mode.

344. **(B)** A-mode stands for amplitude modulation. This mode displays a graphic representation of vertically reflected echoes arising from a horizontal baseline. The height of the vertical reflection is proportional to the amplitude of the echo, and the distance from one vertical reflection to the next represents the distance from one interface to another. A-mode is one-dimensional. The horizontal baseline is the x-axis and the vertical reflection represents the y-axis.

345. **(B)** The effects of ultrasound on human soft tissue are called bioeffects, or biologic effects.

346. **(E)** The speed of ultrasound in soft tissue is 1540 m/s, 1.54 mm/μs, 0.154 cm/μs, or 1 mile/s.

347. **(C)** Slope.

348. **(B)** Delay.

349. **(D)** Far gain.

350. **(A)** Near gain.

351. **(C)** Progressive weakening of the sound beam as it travels through a medium. *(2:30)*

352. **(F)** A new imaging technique used to assess tissue stiffness. This is based on a well-established principle that malignant tissue is stiffer than benign tissue.

353. **(G)** Binary digit.

354. **(B)** The production and behavior of microbubbles within a medium.

355. **(D)** A liquid placed between the transducer and the skin.

356. **(H)** A method of reducing PD by mechanical or electrical means.

357. **(E)** The number of intensity levels between black and white.

TABLE 2-1 • Ischemic Cascade

Imbalance in supply and demand	Myocardial perfusion is decreased by obstructed coronary vessel
Decreases in LV compliance	Changes in diastolic function occur such as slowed relaxation, increased L stiffness and increased end-diastolic pressure (LVEDP)
Decreased or changes in systolic function	Segmental or regional wall motion abnormalities develop
ECG changes develop	Significant changes in ST segment (elevation or depression)
Patient symptoms	Chest pain

impaired myocardial function. Coronary artery stenoses may have little or no effect in the resting state but become manifested during stress or exercise. Therefore, evaluation of patients with exercise has become a standard part of the echocardiographic examination.

Exercise echocardiography has evolved as a test ideally suited for the evaluation of patients with coronary artery disease (CAD) or valvular heart disease. It is a cost-effective, reliable tool for detecting the presence, extent, and distribution of coronary stenosis. Echocardiography rapidly detects regional wall motion at rest and after exercise, which allows highly accurate predictions of the extent and distribution of CAD.[1] Other capabilities of stress echocardiography include the following:

- Assessment of LV size and ejection fraction
- Identification of thrombus or aneurysm that may have resulted from previous MI
- Identification of other causes of chest pain unrelated to vascular obstruction, such as hypertrophic cardiomyopathy, aortic dissection, or pericardial disease
- The evaluation of valvular heart lesions, especially if used in conjunction with Doppler echocardiography

Indications for stress echocardiography include: (1) screening of new patients for CAD, (2) assessing states before and after intervention, (3) determining prognosis after MI, and (4) evaluating hemodynamic significance of valvular heart disease.[1]

Contraindications include: (1) recent MI, (2) unstable angina, (3) potentially life threatening dysrhythmias, (4) acute pericarditis, (5) severe hypertension, (6) acute pulmonary embolism, and (7) critical aortic valve stenosis. Interpretation of the test includes the evaluation of the patient's blood pressure, ECG, symptoms, and the echocardiographic response to exercise. The LV myocardial segments are divided into three perfusion zones, each dictated by coronary artery anatomy. The left

anterior descending artery (LAD) supplies the anterior, septal, and apex. The left circumflex coronary artery supplies the posterolateral segments but may also supply the inferior segments depending on dominance. The right coronary artery, or posterior descending artery (PDA), supplies the inferior segments.

An exercise echocardiogram is considered positive if any of these three findings are present: (1) there is an exercise-induced wall motion abnormality, (2) there is an increase in LV volume, or (3) there is a decrease in global LV ejection fraction. The greater the wall motion abnormality, the more severe the disease. There are many factors that affect wall motion abnormalities. Perhaps the most important of these include the duration of exercise; the less exercise the patient does, the less likely the patient will achieve an adequate heart rate. False positives and false negatives are listed in Table 2–2.

Contrast Echocardiography

The use of contrast agents has gained widespread use in the field of echocardiography. Their uses range from the evaluation of left and right heart structures and function, enhancements of regurgitant and stenotic lesions, enhanced assessment of pulmonary artery pressures, presence of various shunts such as patent foramen, ASD and VSDs and other shunts, and patency coronary artery perfusion.[1]

Contrast agents come in many forms from the simplest, such as agitated saline solution, to complex agents composed of perfluorocarbon shells (or other substances) filled with gases. These later forms of contrast agents hold special promise not only in aiding in the identification of cardiac structures and function, but more recently in the evaluation of myocardial perfusion imaging. Currently (at the time of this writing), contrast agents are only approved by the Food and Drug Administration (FDA) in the evaluation of LV opacification and not for the evaluation of myocardial perfusion imaging. Still, research continues in the use of microbubbles to help identify coronary distribution.

TABLE 2-2 • False Positives and Negatives

False-Negative Exams	False-Positive Exams
Mild coronary artery disease	Cardiomyopathies
Inability to reach maximal heart rate	Inadequate exercise
Presence of extensive collateral vessels (improves flow to diseased area)	Preexisting myocardial dysfunction Left ventricular hypertrophy Left ventricular fibrosis Aging of the heart High blood pressure (220/110 mm Hg) Severe hypertension

Internal contrast or spontaneous echo contrast (SEC) is the discrete reflections in the blood within the cardiac chambers or vessels without the injection of contrast media. SEC is observed when blood becomes echogenic in a region of decreased flow. It is not seen with shear rates greater than 40 seconds. SEC may be seen in normal states as well as abnormal conditions. SEC has the potential to induce embolic events caused by thrombus formation.[1] As technology and equipment improve, visualization of SEC may become more prevalent, even in totally healthy patients.

Contrast agents in the form of microbubbles range in size from 0.1 to 8.0 μm. These tiny spheres are strong reflectors of ultrasound but are small enough to pass through the capillary bed. The microbubbles must be small to avoid harmful effects, must remain tiny after injection, and must stay in the circulation long enough to be detected by ultrasound. The reflective property of the microbubbles comes from the material within the bubbles or spheres, which is usually gas or air bodies. Because of the acoustic impedance of the air or gas versus blood, there is a strong signal. Other factors that affect reflective properties are:

- Transmitted frequency
- Microbubble diameter
- Microbubble concentration
- Microbubble survival rate

The microbubble eventually disappears through natural processes of the body. Table 2–3 lists the currently available agents in the United States and their potential uses.

Transesophageal Examination

Transesophageal echocardiography (TEE) is another echocardiographic technique routinely used to evaluate cardiac structure and function. It is performed by a physician with specialized training in TEE performance and interpretation.[1] TEE examinations provide complete evaluation of all regions of the heart, including the great vessels. Although it is considered more invasive than a transthoracic or surface echocardiogram, it is a relatively simple procedure tolerated by most patients.

Atrial paced TEE is performed by attaching a flexible silicone-coated pacing catheter to the TEE probe. Pacing is increased incrementally to 85% of patient age predicted maximum heart scale. LV function is monitored by TEE examination at baseline, as well as during and immediately after maximal pacing. This technique has a high sensitivity and specificity for detection of CAD and a high success rate of 90–100% of patients.[1]

TEE plus pharmacologic agents is used to assess CAD and has proved to be feasible and accurate. At each stage of dobutamine infusion, it is important to use longitudinal and transverse planes to optimize visualization of all wall segments.

There are several advantages of using TEE, which include the following:

- TEE provides higher resolution than the transthoracic echocardiographic (TTE) exam because of the use of the transesophageal window that allows the use of higher frequencies. The transducer is mounted on a flexible gastroscope that is sufficient in length to be advanced down the esophagus. It is positioned behind the posterior wall of the left ventricle.
- TEE provides additional viewing of structures that are often not seen well on the TTE exam in technically difficult studies. These structures include the posterior cardiac structures such as the aorta, atria, left atrial appendage, and cardiac valves.
- TEE provides "off-axis planes" in addition to the standard planes, which often provides a clearer view of the anatomy or anomalies.

There are contraindications to performing the TEE examination. These include: esophageal tumors or tumors of the mouth, esophageal stenosis or strictures, diverticulum, esophageal varices, perforated viscus, gastric volvulus or perforation, active gastrointestinal tract bleeding, and patient refusal or unwillingness to cooperate.[1] Occasionally, the TEE probe cannot be easily passed and should never be forced.

Table 2–4 lists the indications for TEE.

CARDIAC ANATOMY

To become proficient in the techniques of echocardiography, a thorough understanding of cardiac anatomy is essential. One must know the normal structures and be able to recognize normal variants from pathologic states. One must also understand the anatomic orientation of the heart within the chest cavity.

The heart is a cone-shaped, hollow, fibromuscular organ located in the middle mediastinum between the lungs and the pleurae. It has a base, apex, and multiple surfaces and borders. It is enclosed within the pericardium. The pericardium is made of fibrous and serosal components. The fibrous pericardium is the tough outer sac that completely surrounds the heart but does not adhere to it. The serosal component is the inner layer, which has two components. The visceral, or epicardial, layer adheres to the surface of the heart and makes up the epicardium and the serosal pericardium, which is the outer or parietal layer. The serosal pericardium lines the inside surface of the fibrous

TABLE 2–3 • Microbubble Agents

Available Agents	Manufacturer	Uses (FDA approved)
Optison	Amersham	• LV opacification
Definity	Bristol-Myers Squibb	• LV opacification

TABLE 2–4 • Indications for TEE

Left ventricular function	• Regional wall motion abnormalities • Global LV function
Endocarditis	• Valvular vegetations • Valvular strands
Valvular disorders/ pathology	• Mitral valve prolapse • Mitral, aortic, pulmonic, tricuspid stenosis • Mitral, aortic, pulmonic, tricuspid regurgitation • Flail leaflets • Torn chordal structures
Pericardial disease	• Pericarditis • Pericardial fluid • Tamponade
Aortic abnormalities	• Presence and extent of arteriosclerotic disease • Traumatic aortic rupture • Aortic dissection • Nondissecting aneurysms
Shunts (atrial, ventricular, other)	• Atrial septal defects • Ventricular septal defects • Patent foramen ovale • Atrial septal aneurysms
Source of embolus	• Can help identify patients at risk for stroke • Used to screen patients for cardioversion • Allows interrogation of left atrial appendage
Right heart function	• Monitoring during and after open heart surgery

ventricles and contains the main trunk of the coronary arteries and coronary sinus. The interventricular groove separates the right and left ventricles. The anterior interventricular groove runs on the anterior surface and contains the descending branch of the left coronary artery. The posterior interventricular groove lies on the diaphragmatic surface of the heart and contains the posterior interventricular descending coronary artery and the middle cardiac vein. The interatrial grooves separate the atria. The interatrial grooves are shallow and less prominent than the other grooves. The interatrial, atrioventricular, and posterior interventricular grooves meet and form the crux of the heart. The terminal groove or sulcus terminalis demarcates the true atrium and the venous component of the right atrium. These external grooves are filled with fatty tissue that varies with overall body fat and increases with age.[1]

There are basically two important types of heart valves: the semilunar and the atrioventricular. Semilunar valves are the aortic and the pulmonary. AV valves are the tricuspid and the mitral.

Numerous pathologies can affect the heart in the adult. These disease states can cause a variety of primary as well as secondary anatomical changes in the heart. Knowing what these changes are greatly enhances the echocardiographic examination. Once the student has an understanding of the heart anatomy, the echocardiographic images are better understood. The basic two-dimensional echocardiographic views are illustrated in Figs. 2–1 to 2–8. These figures are from the ASE and are the accepted nomenclature for two-dimensional imaging.

Left Ventricle

Anatomy. The left ventricle is the largest cardiac chamber, accounting for 75% of the heart mass. It consists of two papillary muscles, has trabeculations in the apex, and a

pericardium. Within the serosal layers is a thin film of pericardial fluid. The purpose of the pericardium is to (1) reduce friction with cardiac movement; (2) allow the heart to move freely with each beat, facilitating ejection and volume changes; (3) contain the heart within the mediastinum, especially during trauma; and (4) serve as a barrier to infection.[1]

The average adult heart measures approximately 12 cm from the apex to the base, 8–9 cm transversely in the broadest diameter, and 6 cm anterior–posterior. The weight varies in males ranging from 280 to 340 g and in females from 230 to 280 g. Cardiac weight is approximately 0.45% of total body weight in men and 0.40% of total body weight in women.[1,2]

The heart is divided into four chambers: two atria and two ventricles. The external surface contains numerous grooves and sulci. The coronary or AV groove separates the atria from the

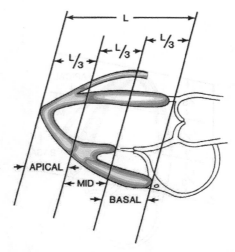

FIGURE 2–1. Parasternal long-axis view of the heart demonstrating the method of subdividing the myocardial walls along the long axis (L) into three regions of equal length using the left ventricular papillary muscles as landmarks.

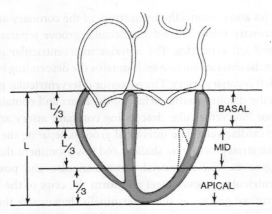

FIGURE 2–2. Apical four-chamber view of the heart demonstrating the method of subdividing the myocardial walls into three regions using the left ventricular papillary muscles as landmarks.

smooth-walled basal area. Its end-diastolic diameter is 3.6–5.6 cm, and its end-systolic diameter is 2.3–4.0 cm. Normal fractional shortening (difference between diastolic and systolic diameters) is:

$$FS = (LVEDD - LVESD)/LVEDD \times 100$$

Normal LV wall thickness in diastole ranges from 0.6 to 1.1 cm.

Hemodynamics. The ventricle receives oxygenated blood from the left atrium and pumps it through the aortic valve to the body by way of arteries, arterioles, and capillaries. Its systolic pressure is 100–120 mm Hg.

Echocardiographic Views. Almost all the standard views allow visualization of at least part of the left ventricle. The apical views allow examination of the apex, which can be difficult to

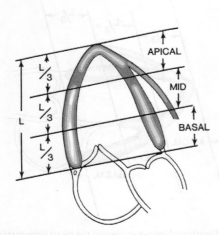

FIGURE 2–3. Apical long-axis view of the heart demonstrating the method of subdividing the myocardial walls into three regions of equal length.

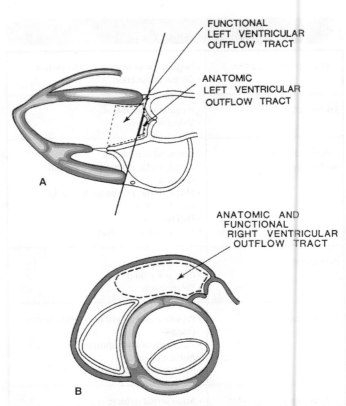

FIGURE 2–4. The functional and anatomic left ventricular outflow tracts of the heart are diagrammed in the upper panel (**A**), whereas the functional and anatomic right ventricular outflow tract is illustrated in the bottom panel (**B**).

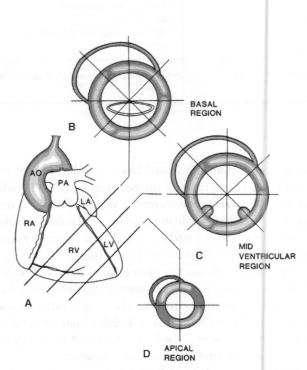

FIGURE 2–5. Diagram of the heart (**A**) and the short-axis views of the basal region (**B**), midventricular region (**C**), and apical region (**D**).

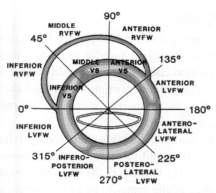

FIGURE 2–6. Short-axis view of the basal region of the heart demonstrating the method of subdividing the myocardial walls into segments using a coordinate system consisting of eight lines that are 45° apart. With this system, the left ventricular free wall (LVFW) is divided into five segments, whereas the ventricular septum (VS) and right ventricular free walls (RVFW) are subdivided into three segments each.

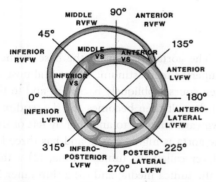

FIGURE 2–7. Short-axis view of the midventricular region of the heart demonstrating the method of subdividing the myocardial walls into segments using a coordinate system consisting of eight lines that are 45° apart. With this system, the left ventricular free wall (LVFW) is divided into five segments, whereas the ventricular septum (VS) and right ventricular free walls (RVFW) are subdivided into three segments each.

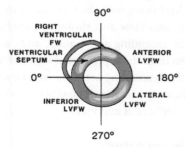

FIGURE 2–8. Short-axis view of the apical region of the heart demonstrating the method of subdividing the myocardial walls into segments using a coordinate system consisting of four lines that are 90° apart. With this system, the left ventricular free wall (LVFW) is subdivided into three segments, whereas the ventricular septum and right ventricular free wall (FW) are subdivided into one segment each.

TABLE 2–5 • TEE Left Ventricle Examination

Views	Structures/Walls
Long-axis (LAX)	• Septum • Posterior wall • Papillary muscles • Trabeculations
Short-axis (SAX)	• Septum (inferior, mid, anterior) • Lateral wall • Posterior wall • Inferior wall
Apical four chamber	• Apex • Lateral wall • Septum • Papillary muscles
Apical two-chamber	• Apex • Posterior wall • Anterior wall
Apical long-axis	• Apex • Septum • Posterior wall
Subcostal four-chamber	• Apex • Septum • Lateral wall
Subcostal short-axis	• Septum • Lateral wall • Posterior wall • Inferior wall

see in other views. The maximum internal dimensions are seen at end systole and should be taken at the peak posterior motion of the interventricular septum (Table 2–5).

Left Atrium

Anatomy. The left atrium is a smooth-walled sac, the walls of which are thicker than those of the right atrium. The chamber receives four pulmonary veins: two (sometimes three) on the right and two (sometimes one) on the left. The interatrial septum divides the left and right atria. It is thinnest in its central portion, the fossa, and varies in thickness elsewhere due to fat deposits. These normally increase with age. The left auricle, or left atrial appendage, arises from the upper anterior part of the left atrium and contains small pectinate muscles. The average dimension of the chamber in the adult is 29–38 mm.

Hemodynamics. The mean pressure in the left atrium ranges from 1 to 10 mm Hg. Oxygenated blood flows from the lungs and enters the atrium through the pulmonary veins.

As left atrial pressure increases over that of the left ventricle, the mitral valve opens, and blood then passes through the mitral valve and enters the left ventricle.

Echocardiographic Views. Maximal dimensions should be measured at end-systole. Measurements may be made from the leading edge of the posterior wall of the aorta to the leading edge of the posterior wall of the left atrium. This chamber is best seen from the parasternal long- and short-axis views; however, it also can be seen from the apical and subcostal views. In the left parasternal long-axis view, the descending aorta can be seen from running posteriorly to the left atrium. Care must be given when measuring the diameter of the left atrium so that the descending aorta is not included in the measurement because this will give an erroneous left atrial diameter. The left atrial appendage can be seen from the transthoracic two-chamber and parasternal short-axis views.

TEE can also be used to evaluate this area and is typically carefully evaluated in patients where the source of embolus is a consideration or when patients may be scheduled for cardioversion.

Right Atrium

Anatomy. The right atrium has two parts: an anterior portion and a posterior portion. The two portions are separated by a ridge of muscle called the crista terminalis. This area is typically not well seen from the transthoracic approach.

The smooth-walled posterior portion of the atrium is derived from the embryonic sinus venosus and receives the inferior and superior vena cavae. Guarding the opening (ostium) of the inferior vena cava is a thin fold of tissue called the eustachian valve, which is sometimes large and complex and forms a network of tissues known as the network of Chiari. The coronary sinus also enters the right atrium anteriorly to the inferior vena cava. The coronary sinus also can be guarded by a thin fold of tissue called the Thebesian valve.

The anterior portion, that represents the embryonic right atrium, is extremely thin and is trabeculated. The right atrial appendage, or right auricle, arises from the superior portion of the right atrium and contains pectinate muscle. The dimensions of the right atrium in adults range from 26 to 34 mm.

Hemodynamics. Deoxygenated blood from the body, head, and heart flows into the right atrium through the inferior vena cava, the superior vena cava, and the coronary sinus, respectively. When pressures in the right atrium increase above the pressures in the right ventricle, the tricuspid valve opens, allowing the blood to flow forward into the right ventricle. Mean pressures in this chamber range from 0 to 8 mm Hg.

Echocardiographic Views. Apical views are best for assessing the right atrium. Others include the subcostal and, to a lesser extent, the parasternal short-axis views.

Right Ventricle

Anatomy. The right ventricle is divided into a posterior inferior inflow portion and an anterior superior outflow portion. The inflow portion contains the tricuspid valve and is heavily trabeculated. The outflow portion, also called the infundibulum, gives rise to the pulmonary trunk. The subpulmonic area is smooth walled.

The right ventricle contains numerous papillary muscles that anchor the tricuspid valve. The ventricle contains numerous bands of muscle. One band, the moderator band, is readily seen in the apex of the ventricle by two-dimensional imaging. Internal diameters range from 7 to 26 mm.

Hemodynamics. Systolic pressures range from 15 to 30 mm Hg, and diastolic pressures range from 0 to 8 mm Hg.

Echocardiographic Views. The right ventricle is seen best from the apical and subcostal views. It also can be seen from the left parasternal long- and short-axis views and right ventricular inflow view.

Aorta

Anatomy. The aorta arises from the base of the heart and enters the superior mediastinum, where it almost reaches the sternum, then courses obliquely backward and to the left over the left bronchus. It then becomes the descending aorta and courses downward anterior to and slightly left of the vertebral column. The aorta is highly elastic and has three layers: (1) a thin inner layer called the tunica intima, (2) a thick middle layer called the tunica media, and (3) a thin outer layer called the tunica adventitia. The diameter of the aortic root measures 2.5–3.3 cm.

Hemodynamics. Maximal velocities of blood flow in adults are 1.0–0.7 m/s.

Echocardiographic Views. The aortic root is seen from the parasternal views. A good portion of the ascending aortic arch can be seen by beginning with the transducer in a standard left parasternal long-axis view and sliding the probe up an intercostal space. The ascending aorta, aortic arch, and descending aorta can be seen from the suprasternal view. As was mentioned earlier, part of the descending aorta also can be seen behind the left atrium in the long-axis view. The subcostal views allow visualization of the aortic root and valve.

Main Pulmonary Artery

Anatomy. The main pulmonary artery is located superior to and originates from the right ventricle. Immediately after leaving the pericardium, it bifurcates into a right pulmonary artery and a left pulmonary artery that enter the right and left lung, respectively.

Hemodynamics. This artery delivers deoxygenated blood from the right ventricle to the lungs. Flow velocities range from 0.6 to 0.9 m/s.

Echocardiographic Views. The artery is best seen from the parasternal short-axis view.

Mitral Valve

Anatomy. The mitral valve is an AV valve. It is located between the left atrium and the left ventricle, and it is a thick yellow-white membrane that originates at the annulus fibrosus, a fibrous ring that surrounds the orifice of the valve. The valve has an anterior leaflet and a posterior leaflet, both of which have sawtooth-like edges. Both leaflets are attached to papillary muscles by chordae tendineae. The surface on the atrial side of the valve is smooth whereas the surface on the ventricular side is irregular the normal mitral valve area is 4–6 cm^2.

Hemodynamics. Flow velocities across the valve range from 9.6 to 1.3 m/s. The valve's function is to prevent backflow of blood from the left ventricle into the left atrium.

Echocardiographic Views. The mitral valve is best seen from the long- and short-axis parasternal views and the apical view. Doppler measurements are best obtained from the apical four- and two-chamber views.

Aortic Valve

Anatomy. The aortic valve consists of three pocket-shaped, thin, smooth cusps named according to their location in relation to the coronary arteries. The cusp near the left coronary artery is the left coronary cusp, the cusp near the right coronary artery is the right coronary cusp, and the cusp that is not near a coronary artery is the noncoronary cusp. Because of its lunar, or half-moon shape, the aortic valve is referred to as semilunar. The normal aortic valve area is 3–4 cm^2.

Hemodynamics. The function of the aortic valve is to prevent backflow of blood from the aorta into the left ventricle. The velocity of flow ranges from 1.0 to 1.7 m/s.

Echocardiographic Views. The valve is best seen from the parasternal views. It also can be seen from the apical four-chamber view with anterior angulation. The best Doppler measurements are obtained from the apical four-chamber view with anterior angulation, from the right parasternal window, and from the suprasternal view.

Tricuspid Valve

Anatomy. The tricuspid valve is an AV valve. It is located between the right atrium and ventricle. The atrial side is smooth, whereas the ventricular side is irregular. As in the mitral valve, it is a thick yellow-white membrane that originates at the annulus fibrosus, a fibrous ring that surrounds the orifice of the valve.

The valve has three leaflets—anterior, posterior, and medial—all of which are sawtooth-like in appearance. Each leaflet is attached to papillary muscles by chordae tendineae.

Hemodynamics. The function of this valve is to prevent backflow of blood from the right ventricle to the right atrium. The velocity of flow ranges from 0.3 to 0.7 m/s.

Echocardiographic Views. The valve is best seen from the parasternal short-axis, parasternal four-chamber, apical four-chamber, and subcostal views. Measurements are best obtained in the parasternal four-chamber view. The best Doppler measurements are taken from the parasternal short-axis and apical four-chamber views.

Pulmonic Valve

Anatomy. The pulmonic valve consists of three thin, smooth pocket S-shaped cusps. Because of its shape, this valve, like the aortic valve, is called semilunar.

Hemodynamics. The function of this valve is to prevent backflow of blood from the main pulmonary artery to the right ventricle. The velocity of flow ranges from 9.6 to 0.9 m/s.

Echocardiographic Views. The pulmonic valve is best seen from the parasternal short-axis view. The best Doppler recordings are taken from the left parasternal short axis.

PHYSIOLOGY

The heart functions as a pump to distribute blood to the body. In order for blood to be adequately distributed, the blood pressure must be maintained. Pressure and flow are controlled by a complex control mechanism that responds to the metabolic requirements of the body.

There are two fluid pumps within the heart, one on the right and one on the left, lying side by side. The right side supplies the pulmonary circulation. From the lungs, blood returns to the left side and ultimately supplies the body via the systemic circulation. The volume pumped by both sides is equal to ensure normal circulation of flow. The blood is pumped from the ventricles during systole and received during diastole, the relaxation phase. The cardiac cycle includes all of the electrical and mechanical events that occur during the cycle of one heartbeat (Fig. 2–9). Each side of the heart has specific characteristics and functions, which are listed as follows.

RIGHT HEART CHARACTERISTICS AND FUNCTIONS

- Blood returns to the right atrium from the superior and inferior vena cava.
- Right heart supplies the pulmonary circulation.

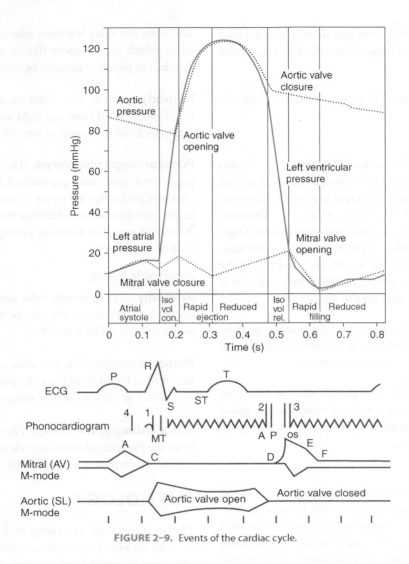

FIGURE 2–9. Events of the cardiac cycle.

- Normal pressure in the right ventricle is approximately 22 mm Hg.
- Blood returning to the right heart has lower oxygen saturation (75%).
- Contains the tricuspid valve that closes during right ventricular systole and contained blood in right ventricle is propelled out of right ventricle outflow tract through the open semilunar pulmonic valve to the pulmonic circulation.

LEFT HEART CHARACTERISTICS AND FUNCTIONS

- LV pressure is approximately 120 mm Hg.
- Blood pumped from the left ventricle has high oxygen saturation (95–100%).
- Left atrium receives blood from the lungs through the pulmonary veins in the back of the left atrium.

- During left atrial systole, the mitral valve opens and allows blood in the left atrium to be propelled into the left ventricle. When ventricular systole occurs, the mitral valve closes and blood is propelled out of the left ventricle through the outflow tract.

The blood supply to the heart is derived from the right and left coronary arteries and their respective tributaries (Fig. 2–10).

CONDUCTION SYSTEM OF THE HEART/INTRINSIC INNERVATION OF THE HEART

The conduction system of the heart is responsible for the initiation, propagation, and coordination of the heartbeat. Fig. 2–11 demonstrates this system.

The sinoatrial (SA) node is also called the pacemaker of the heart. It provides the bursts of electrical impulses that are conducted throughout the walls of the heart. The activation conduction is from the SA node to the AV node, where it is

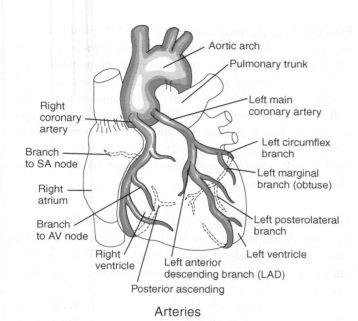

FIGURE 2–10. Anatomic drawing of the heart and vessels.

slows and delays. The impulse is conducted to the ventricles by way of the AV bundle and the right and left bundle branches. It becomes continuous with the fibers of the Purkinje network. The ventricles contract and blood is ejected to the pulmonic and systemic circulation. The heart contains its own intrinsic conduction system; however, its rate is modified by the autonomic nervous system. Fibers from both the sympathetic and the parasympathetic nervous systems are received by the heart. Sympathetic nervous system fibers are received by the atria via the right and left vagus nerves, which contribute to the control of the SA and AV nodes. The parasympathetic nerves are derived from the vagus and come off in the neck as vagal cardiac nerves. They connect to the SA node. Stimulation of the parasympathetic nervous system fibers to the heart causes the following:

- Decrease in the heart rate
- Retardation of transmission between the atria and ventricles
- Decrease in the force of contraction
- Decrease in conduction rate of the nodes and atria

The sympathetic and parasympathetic nervous systems have opposite effects on the heart. The reflex center for both is in the medulla oblongata.

DISEASES AFFECTING THE VALVES

Anomalies or diseases of the valves can be divided into two main categories. Valve anomalies that occur in fetal development are known as congenital anomalies. Valve anomalies that develop after fetal development or in the adult stages are referred to as acquired valve disease. This latter category can be further divided into rheumatic and nonrheumatic heart disease.

Mitral Valve Disease

Stenosis. Mitral valve stenosis results primarily from rheumatic disease. The valves may not become involved for many decades following rheumatic fever. Congenital mitral stenosis can occur but is extremely rare.

M-mode findings include (1) a flattened E–D slope (reduced diastolic filling), (2) anterior motion of the posterior leaflet, (3) thickened leaflets, and (4) an absent A wave in the absence

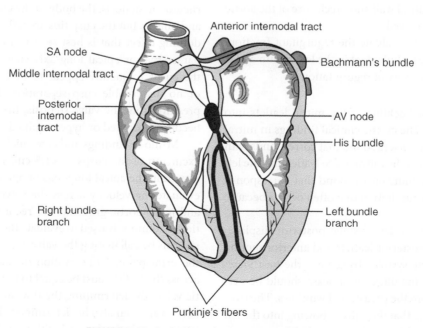

FIGURE 2–11. Intrinsic conduction system of the heart.

of atrial fibrillation. Two-dimensional imaging also indicates thickening and shows doming of the leaflets in diastole.

Doppler measurements reveal a reduced rate of decrease in diastolic flow (reduced diastolic slope), a higher than normal peak velocity of flow, and spectral broadening on Doppler display. Secondary findings and complications include left atrial dilatation, pulmonary hypertension, a left atrial clot, and an exaggerated diastolic dip of the interventricular septum.[3] Color Doppler shows turbulent LV inflow.

Stenosis–Severity of Mitral Stenosis (Valve Area)

Normal	4–6 cm^2
Mild	1.6–2.0 cm^2
Moderate	1.1–1.5 cm^2
Severe	1.0 cm^2 or less

Regurgitation. Mitral regurgitation (shunting back and forth of blood) can occur as a result of mitral annular calcification, rheumatic mitral disease, flail mitral valve leaflet, conditions that may stretch the mitral annulus, such as cardiomyopathies, MI, mitral valve vegetations or other masses on the mitral valve or within the left atrium, papillary dysfunction, and mitral valve prolapse. The hallmark sign of regurgitation is a systolic murmur, most often maximal over the LV apex.

M-mode findings include (1) increased size of the left atrium, (2) exaggerated motion of the interventricular septum, (3) pulsations of the left atrial wall, and (4) preclosure of the aortic valve during systole. The first three findings are the result of volume overload.

Two-dimensional imaging reveals an increase in the size of the left atrium and exaggerated motion of the interventricular septum—all of which are the result of volume overload. In addition, pulsations of the left atrial wall and preclosure of the aortic valve during systole are observed.

Doppler may be used to evaluate the regurgitant fraction. Color Doppler displays the turbulent jet in the left atrium and is useful for estimating the severity of regurgitation.

Prolapse. (Protrusion or buckling of the mitral leaflets into the left atrium in systole.) The classic clinical findings in mitral valve prolapse are a systolic click (a sound that corresponds with the posterior displacement of the mitral valve leaflet into the left atrium) and a late systolic murmur (a sound that corresponds with the resulting mitral regurgitation that often occurs because of the prolapsing leaflets).

M-mode findings include late systolic posterior displacement of the anterior and posterior leaflets and anterior motion of the mitral valve in early systole. To achieve the best views for making the diagnosis, the ultrasound beam should be perpendicular to the valve from the parasternal windows. The two-dimensional findings reveal that the valve is bowing into the left atrium and, in many cases, thickened.

Flail Leaflet. The most common cause of flail leaflet is rupture of the chordae tendineae, which often occurs secondarily to MI. Rupture of the papillary muscle is a less common etiology.

M-mode findings indicate coarse diastolic fluttering and systolic fluttering of the leaflet and visualization of part of the leaflet in the left atrium. Two-dimensional imaging indicates protrusion of the flail leaflet into the left atrium, noncoaptation of the two leaflets, and a systolic and coarse diastolic motion of the flail leaflet. Doppler measurements indicate harsh, turbulent mitral regurgitation.

Annular Calcification. Mitral annular calcification results from the deposition of calcium in the annulus of the mitral valve. This is normally associated with aging. This condition can be caused by mitral regurgitation, conduction abnormalities, aging, or obstruction of the LVOT.

M-mode findings reveal high-density echoes between the valve and the posterior wall of the left ventricle. Two-dimensional imaging reveals high-density bright echoes between the valve and the posterior wall of the left ventricle.

Aortic Valve Disease

Stenosis (Versus Sclerosis). The cause of stenosis of the aortic valve can be congenital, the result of rheumatic heart disease, or degeneration. Degenerative disease is the most common cause of aortic valve stenosis. Clinical symptoms include chest pain, shortness of breath, and syncope. These symptoms do not present until the aortic valve stenosis becomes moderate to severe. Patients with aortic valve stenosis often present with a harsh systolic murmur heard at the right sternal border, which often radiates to the carotids.

The normal aortic valve has three leaflets. In congenital or rheumatic stenosis, the body of the cusps may appear to be thin and pliable, but the cusp tips are tethered, resulting in a systolic doming effect that is best seen in the early systole from a left parasternal or apical long-axis view. In degenerative stenosis, the cusps frequently appear to be bright reflectors with little or no discernable cusp separation. Because of the increased pressure from the valve stenosis, the walls of the left ventricle become thickened or hypertrophied.

M-mode findings indicate thickened cusps and restricted excursion of the cusps to <1.5 cm. Continuous-wave Doppler is used in the apical long-axis or apical "five"-chamber views to evaluate the velocity across the valve. The peak instantaneous and mean aortic gradients are recorded. The continuity equation is commonly used to evaluate the severity of the aortic valve stenosis by calculating the valve area. This equation is based on the principle of "conservation of mass." All blood flow going across the LVOT must be equal to the blood flow across the aortic valve. By determining the flow in the LVOT, the flow in the aortic valve can also be determined. This is measured by calculating the velocity integral of flow in the LVOT and at the aortic

TABLE 2–6 • Criteria Range for Aortic Valve Stenosis

	Mild Aortic Stenosis	Moderate Aortic Stenosis	Severe/Critical Aortic Stenosis
Peak gradient	16–36 mm Hg	37–79 mm Hg	>80 mm Hg
Mean gradient	<20 mm Hg	21–49 mm Hg	>50 mm Hg
Valve area	1.1–1.9 cm^2	0.75–1.0 cm^2	<0.74 cm^2

valve leaflet tips. The diameter of the LVOT is also measured to obtain a cross-sectional area. The continuity equation is as follows: Flow 1 = Flow 2, where Flow 1 = LVOT VTI × LVOT CSA and Flow 2 = AV VTI × AV CSA. The aortic valve area, or AVA, is calculated by dividing LVOT VTI × LVOT CSA by AV VTI. It is important to note that the LVOT VTI is obtained using pulsed-wave Doppler, whereas the AV VTI is obtained using continuous wave Doppler. The LVOT diameter is a two-dimensional measurement. Current equipment normally performs this calculation for the user, but an understanding of these principles is important. The normal aortic valve area is 2.5–4.5 cm^2. The normal diameter of the LVOT ranges from 1.8 to 2.4 cm with an LVOT VTI of 18–22 cm (Table 2–6). Color Doppler can also be used to help identify aortic valve stenosis by demonstrating turbulent flow in the ascending aorta.

Parasternal Long- and Short-Axis Views. These views can be used to help evaluate the aortic valve cusps, making measurements of the LV walls in M-mode or two-dimensional planes. The diameter of the LVOT is usually taken from a left parasternal long-axis view, although the apical long-axis view may also be used.

Apical Views. The apical views are used to obtain Doppler measurements across the valve because the blood flow is parallel to the sound beam and, therefore, well suited to obtain maximal and accurate blood velocities.

Regurgitation. The effects of regurgitation on atria, ventricles, and cardiac vessels result in dilatation of the left ventricle. The condition can be caused by any one of the following: congenital (bicuspid cusp), rheumatic heart disease (the most common cause in adults), or degeneration of the leaflet caused by infection or aortic dilatation (Marfan's syndrome). M-mode findings reveal fluttering of the interventricular septum and diastolic fluttering of the mitral valve. Two-dimensional imaging indicates fine diastolic fluttering of the aortic valve, diastolic fluttering of the mitral valve, and fluttering of the interventricular septum. Spectral Doppler studies reveal diastolic flow, which appears above the baseline when in an apical position.

Tricuspid Valve Diseases

Stenosis. Stenosis of the tricuspid valve is most often caused by rheumatic heart disease. It can be caused by other conditions, which include systemic lupus erythematosus (SLE), carcinoid heart disease, Löffler's endocarditis, metastatic melanoma, and congenital heart disease.[1] In stenotic disease of the tricuspid valve, the effects on atria, ventricles, and vessels cause dilatation of the right atrium.

M-mode findings indicate a reduced diastolic slope and thickening and decreased separation of the leaflets. Two-dimensional imaging reveals the most specific finding, systolic doming, as well as thickening of the leaflets. In Doppler measurements, the sample is placed in the right ventricle, and the results indicate turbulent diastolic flow and slowed reduction in the velocity of flow during diastole.

Doppler is used to qualify and quantitate the severity of stenosis.

Regurgitation. Regurgitation is a common abnormality associated with the tricuspid valve in adults.[1] The primary cause of regurgitation is secondary to pulmonary hypertension. In rare cases, the condition can be caused by rheumatic heart disease, prolapse of the valve, or carcinoid heart disease. A secondary effect is dilatation of the right atrium and ventricle. Continuous-wave Doppler is used to measure the velocity of the regurgitant jet. Pulmonary artery pressure may be calculated by adding the pressure gradient across the tricuspid valve to right atrial pressure (normally 5–10 mm Hg). Generally, a TR (tricuspid valve regurgitation) velocity at 3 m/s or greater indicates pulmonary hypertension.

M-mode findings indicate a dilated right ventricle and anterior motion of the interventricular septum during isovolumetric contraction. Two-dimensional imaging reveals incomplete closure and diastolic fluttering of the leaflets, ruptured chordae, dilatation of the right ventricle, and flattening of the interventricular septum. With Doppler measurements, turbulent flow can be detected in the right atrium during systole.

Pulmonic Valve Disease

Stenosis. The causes of pulmonic valve disease are atherosclerosis, infections, endocarditis, and papillary fibroma. This disease is extremely rare in adults. Continuous-wave Doppler reveals velocities greater than 2 m/s in the main pulmonary artery. Color Doppler reveals turbulent flow distal to the pulmonic valve.

Regurgitation. M-mode findings reveal fluttering of the tricuspid leaflets, and Doppler measurements reveal early diastolic high-velocity, turbulent flow. The cause can be pulmonary hypertension or bacterial endocarditis or secondary to pulmonary valvotomy.

Endocarditis

Endocarditis is an inflammation of the endocardium characterized by vegetations on the surface and in the endocardium.[1]

Types. Endocarditis can be caused by either bacteria or vegetation (fungus-like growth) and, depending on the infecting organism, is classified as acute or subacute. Although the disease can occur in the endocardium of the heart, the infection usually affects the endocardium in specific valves and is more likely to affect the left heart than the right. Infection of the tricuspid and pulmonic valves is usually the result of intravenous (IV) drug abuse.

Bacterial Endocarditis. Predisposing factors for bacterial endocarditis include dental procedures, tonsilloadenoidectomy, cirrhosis, drug addiction, surgery, and burns. Infectious endocarditis is mainly caused by two groups of bacteria: staphylococci and streptococci.[1]

Nonbacterial Endocarditis. Among the nonbacterial forms of the disease are SLE and fungal (mycotic), nonbacterial thrombotic, Löffler's, marantic, and Libman–Sacks endocarditis. The most common manifestation of SLE is vegetation. Although this nonbacterial form of endocarditis primarily involves the mitral valve, it also can affect the mural endocardium. The mycotic form of the disease is usually subacute and can be caused by a variety of fungi—most commonly *Candida*, *Aspergillus*, and *Histoplasma*. In the thrombotic form of nonbacterial endocarditis, the vegetation consists of fibrin and other blood elements.

Löffler's endocarditis is characterized by a marked increase of eosinophils. It primarily affects men in their forties who live in temperate climates. The disease affects both ventricles equally. Thickening of the inflow portions of the ventricles and the apices can be observed, as can formation of mural thrombi. Hemodynamically, diastolic filling is impaired because of increased stiffness of the heart. AV valve regurgitation is a typical finding.

In the marantic form of the disease, the vegetation is nondestructive and sterile. It occurs in patients with malignant tumors and primarily affects the valves on the left side of the heart. Embolus is the most serious complication.

Libman–Sacks endocarditis is characterized by vegetation or verrucae on the echocardium.

Hemodynamic Mechanisms. One common cause of subacute infectious endocarditis occurs when a high-velocity jet consistently hits a surface. Damage results when blood from a high-pressure area flows to a low-pressure area; this is called the Venturi effect. The site where vegetation has formed will usually be in the low-pressure area. When the mitral valve is involved and mitral regurgitation is present, the atrial side of the leaflets is the susceptible area. In this case, the high-pressure area is the ventricle, and because the mitral leaflets fail to coapt, the low-pressure area is the atrial side of the leaflets. The atrial wall that bears the brunt of the regurgitation also may become infected.

When the aortic valve is involved and aortic insufficiency is present, the aorta is the high-pressure area, and the ventricle is the low-pressure area. Vegetations tend to form on the ventricular side of the aortic cusps because the cusps do not close completely in aortic regurgitation. The section of the ventricular wall hit by the regurgitant jet also may be damaged.

In ventricular septal defects (VSDs), the high-pressure area is the left ventricle in left-to-right shunting and the low-pressure area is the right ventricular side of the defect. The right ventricular wall directly across from the defect also can suffer damage and become prone to vegetation.

The presence of a mass on any valve leads to a diagnosis of infection caused by vegetation. However, echocardiography cannot differentiate between a new and an old infection. M-mode patterns indicate shaggy echoes on the infected valve and detect 52% of vegetations. TEE is the imaging modality of choice.

Aortic Valve. Vegetation is seen best in diastole and is attached to the ventricular side of the cusps. This condition can cause reduced cardiac output and acute aortic regurgitation. The best views for two-dimensional imaging are the left parasternal long and short axes.

Mitral Valve. Predisposing factors to vegetational infection of the mitral valve include mitral valve prolapse, rheumatic valvulitis, and dysfunction of the papillary muscles with secondary mitral regurgitation and mitral annular calcification. Infection occurs most commonly on the atrial side of the leaflet.

The best views include the left parasternal short and long axes; the apical two- and four-chamber views also can be used. Vegetations as small as 2 mm in diameter are detectable or can be as large as 40 mm in diameter. Whereas M-mode imaging detects 14–65% of the vegetation, two-dimensional imaging detects 43–100%. Differential diagnoses include myomas, lipomas, and fibromas.

Tricuspid or Pulmonic Valve. Infections of the tricuspid or pulmonic valves are usually caused by IV drug abuse. Such infections are less common than left-sided infections; however, when they occur on the tricuspid valve, the infections can become larger than is typical of left-sided infections. They rarely occur on the pulmonic valve.

Prosthetic Valves

Types. Two types of prosthetic valves are available: mechanical and bioprosthetic. The mechanical types are ball-in-cage, disc-in-cage, and tilting-disc valves. The Starr–Edwards valve is the most common ball-in-cage type. The best view for observing excursion of the ball is the apical view when in the mitral and aortic positions. The disc-in-cage valve has less excursion than the ball-in-cage type. The most common type of tilting-disc valve is the Bjork–Shiley, which consists of one disc that tilts. The less common St. Jude valve contains two tilting discs.

All bioprosthetic valves are made from biological tissue, which include heterografts or xenografts (porcine tissue or bovine pericardial tissue), homografts (human cryopreserved from autopsy), and allografts (patient's own tissue).[1] The most common bioprosthetic valve is the xenograft. A porcine heterograft is the most commonly used tissue; porcine pericardial tissue also can be used. Human homografts and fascia lata tissue are sometimes used as valves.

Malfunctions. The following factors cause both types of prosthetic valves to malfunction: thrombi, regurgitation, stenosis, dehiscence, and vegetation.

Thrombi. Blood clots, the most common cause of valve malfunction, reduce the effective orifice and impair motion of the ball, disc, or leaflet tissue. Their major complication is the potential for an embolus. Two-dimensional imaging is the echocardiographic technique of choice for detecting the presence of a clot. The limitation of the technique is the masking effect produced by the highly reflective nature of the prosthetic valves. In the Bjork–Shiley mitral prosthesis, there is a rounding to the E point on M-mode.

Regurgitation. Regurgitation can occur through the valve or around the sewing ring. Doppler echocardiography is the procedure of choice for detecting the problem. When masking is a problem from apical views, color Doppler is especially useful. Color-flow Doppler not only allows spatial orientation but also demonstrates the direction of blood jets. Secondary echocardiographic findings for aortic prosthetic regurgitation include (1) fluttering of the mitral valve, (2) fluttering of the interventricular septum, and (3) evidence of volume overload in the left ventricle. Doppler echocardiography also is a procedure of choice for detecting paravalvular leaks with a high degree of sensitivity and specificity. In the Bjork–Shiley mitral valve, an early diastolic bump is noted by M-mode and two-dimensional imaging.

Stenosis. All prosthetic valves have some degree of obstruction. Doppler echocardiography can detect a valve with moderate to severe stenosis.

Dehiscence. In dehiscence, the valve becomes detached from its sewing bed. Disruption of suture lines securing the prosthesis to the sewing ring is usually the cause. The result is severe regurgitation, heart failure, or both, which can be detected by a Doppler examination. Two-dimensional imaging demonstrates an unusual rocking motion away from its normal excursion. Cinefluoroscopy can be helpful in assessing abnormal rocking motion.

Vegetation. As was mentioned earlier, vegetation is difficult to assess with echocardiographic techniques because it is often masked by the highly reflective properties of the prosthesis. These infections are usually found on bioprosthetic valves, are extremely mobile, and are more common in the aortic than in the mitral position.

Degeneration. Degeneration is most common in the bioprosthetic valves and usually occurs as a result of calcification of the area where the valve is joined to the surrounding tissue.

DISEASES AFFECTING THE PERICARDIUM

The pericardium is composed of two layers. The inner layer is a serous membrane called the visceral pericardium, which is attached to the surface of the heart. This layer folds back upon itself to form an outer fibrous layer called the parietal pericardium. Between the two layers is the pericardial space, which is filled with a thin layer of fluid throughout. The functions of the pericardium are to (1) fix the heart anatomically,[1] (2) prevent excessive motion during changes in body position, (3) reduce friction between the heart and other organs, (4) provide a barrier against infection, and (5) help maintain hydrostatic forces on the heart. Pericardial disease can be caused by any one of the following: malignant disease that spreads to the pericardium, pericarditis, acute infarction, cardiac perforation during diagnostic procedures, radiation therapy, SLE, or postcardiac surgery.

Effusion

In the normal pericardium, the pressure within the pericardial space is similar to that in the intrapleural pressure and lower than the right and LV diastolic pressures. Increased intrapericardial pressure depends on three factors: the volume of the effusion, the rate at which fluid accumulates, and the characteristics of the pericardium. The normal intrapericardial space contains 15–50 mL of fluid, and it can tolerate the slow addition of as much as 1–2 L of fluid without increasing the intrapericardial pressure. However, if the fluid is added rapidly, the intrapericardial pressure increases dramatically.

Pericardial effusion can be diagnosed using M-mode and two-dimensional techniques. Three diagnostic criteria can be used: (1) posterior echo-free space, (2) obliteration of echo-free space at the left AV groove, and (3) decreased motion of the posterior pericardial motion.

Cardiac tamponade results when intrapericardial pressures increase. This problem is characterized by increased intracardiac pressures, impaired diastolic filling of the ventricles, and reduced stroke volume. The following echocardiographic findings are associated with cardiac tamponade:

- Increased dimensions of the right ventricle during inspiration
- Decreased mitral diastolic slope (E–F)
- Decreased end-diastolic dimension of the right atrium or ventricle
- Posterior motion of the anterior wall of the right ventricle
- Collapse of the right ventricular free wall
- Diastolic collapse of the right atrial wall
- Increased flow velocities across the tricuspid pulmonic valve during inspiration

Several findings can create a false-positive diagnosis of pericardial effusion:

- Epicardial fat located on the anterior wall
- Misinterpretation of normal cardiac structures such as the descending aorta or coronary sinus
- Other abnormal cardiac or noncardiac structures
- Confusion of pleural effusions with pericardial effusions

Pericardial effusion can be differentiated from pleural effusion in several ways. First, in pericardial effusion, a large amount of fluid can collect posterior to the heart without any anterior collection. Second, pericardial effusion tapers as it approaches the left atrium; a pleural effusion does not. Third, if both types of effusion occur simultaneously, a thin echogenic line should be noted between the two collections of fluid. And fourth, the descending aorta lies posterior to a pericardial effusion, whereas it lies anterior to a pleural effusion.

Pericarditis

Pericarditis comes in two forms: acute and constrictive. In acute pericarditis, the pericardium is inflamed. This form of the disease has a variety of etiologies: idiopathic causes, viruses, uremia, bacterial infections, acute MI, tuberculosis, malignancies, and trauma. Echocardiography reveals thickening of the pericardium, with or without pericardial effusion.

In constrictive disease, the pericardium thickens and restricts diastolic filling of the heart chambers. As in the acute form, it has a variety of causes: tuberculosis, hemodialysis used to treat chronic renal failure, connective tissue disorders (eg, SLE, rheumatoid arthritis), metastatic infiltration, radiation therapy to the mediastinum, fungal or parasitic infections, and complications of surgery. Echocardiographic findings may include the following:

- Thickened pericardium
- Flattening of the LV wall in mid and late systole
- A rapid mitral valve E–F slope
- Exaggerated anterior motion of the interventricular septum

- Mid-diastolic premature opening of the pulmonic valve
- Inspiratory dilatation of hepatic veins and the inferior vena cava
- Inspiratory leftward motion of the interatrial and interventricular septa

DISEASES AFFECTING THE MYOCARDIUM

The term cardiomyopathy is used to describe a variety of cardiac diseases that affect the myocardium. Cardiomyopathies have been classified into three categories: (1) hypertrophic, which may or may not obstruct the LVOT, (2) dilated, and (3) restrictive. The classification depends on the anatomical characteristics of the LV cavity as well as systolic ejection and diastolic-filling properties of the left ventricle.

Hypertrophic Cardiomyopathy

Hypertrophic cardiomyopathy is characterized by concentric or asymmetric LV hypertrophy, which results in an increase in LV mass, with normal or reduced dimensions of the LV cavity. Normal systolic function usually is preserved. Although asymmetric hypertrophy can occur anywhere within the left ventricle, the most common site is the proximal portion of the ventricular septum near the outflow tract. Asymmetric septal hypertrophy can be diagnosed when the ratio of septal thickness to posterior wall thickness is 1.3:1.0. When asymmetric hypertrophy is present, obstruction most frequently occurs. Concentric hypertrophy may or may not lead to obstruction. A number of names are used to describe the obstructive forms of cardiomyopathy, including idiopathic hypertrophic subaortic stenosis, muscular subaortic stenosis, asymmetric septal hypertrophy, and hypertrophic obstructive cardiomyopathy.

Several echocardiographic findings, when found in conjunction, are highly specific for the diagnosis of obstructive cardiomyopathy. M-mode and two-dimensional findings include systolic anterior motion of the mitral valve, asymmetric septal hypertrophy, premature midsystolic closure of the aortic valve, septal hypokinesis, and anterior displacement (and its size) of the mitral valve. The left ventricle may be small to normal in size. Doppler examination reveals a decreased E wave to mitral flow with an exaggerated A wave. These findings suggest a decrease in diastolic compliance and an increase in LV end-diastolic pressures. In aortic flow, there is a midsystolic reduction of velocity. Fifty percent of patients demonstrate regurgitation in the mitral valve. Pulsed-wave Doppler is used to determine the obstructed area. At rest, systolic anterior motion of the mitral valve may not be demonstrated. Because this motion is a diagnostic indication for this disease, provocative maneuvers are used to bring it out. Such techniques include the Valsalva maneuver and amyl nitrate and IV isoproterenol administration.

Dilated Cardiomyopathy

Dilated cardiomyopathy is characterized by globally reduced systolic function, with an ejection fraction of less than 40%, increased end-systolic and end-diastolic volumes, and, eventually, congestive heart failure. M-mode findings include increased end-diastolic and end-systolic dimensions of the left ventricle, reduced septal and posterior wall excursion, increased E point-to-septal separation, decreased aortic root movement, and a structurally normal aortic valve that opens slowly and drifts closed during systole because of reduced cardiac output. The principal two-dimensional echocardiographic findings include LV dilatation and dysfunction, abnormal closure of the mitral valve, and dilatation of the left atrium. The abnormal closure of the aortic valve also is noted. Mitral regurgitation is a frequent Doppler finding in dilated cardiomyopathy. Hemodynamically, the left ventricle demonstrates signs of increased diastolic pressure in the left ventricle and decreased compliance. The walls of the left ventricle are normal in size. The right heart also may become enlarged as a result of the increased diastolic pressures in the left heart. The most common complication of dilated cardiomyopathy is the formation of thrombi and a potential cardiac source of emboli.

Dilated cardiomyopathies can be the result of a familiar or X-linked cardiomyopathy, pregnancy, systemic hypertension, ingestion of toxic agents such as alcohol or other drugs, and a variety of viral infections. They also can be of an unknown cause, or idiopathic. This form of cardiomyopathy also can be found in severe CAD.

Restrictive Cardiomyopathy

Restrictive cardiomyopathy falls into two categories: endomyocardial fibrosis and infiltrative myocardial disease, which includes amyloidosis, sarcoidosis, hematochromatosis, Pompe's disease, and Fabry's disease. The characteristic feature of restrictive cardiomyopathy is increased resistance to LV filling. The associated cardiac findings include elevated diastolic pressure in the left ventricle, hypertension and enlargement of the left atrium, and secondary pulmonary hypertension. The echocardiographic features include an increase in the thickness and mass of the LV wall, a small-to-normal-sized LV cavity, normal systolic function, and pericardial effusion. Restrictive cardiomyopathies are most common in East Africa; they account for only 5% of noncoronary cardiomyopathies in the Western world.

Endomyocardial fibrosis involves formation of fibrotic sheets of tissue in the subendocardium. These sheets vary in thickness and result in increased stiffness of the ventricles. The bright reflective characteristic of this tissue is easily seen with two-dimensional echocardiography. Other characteristic echocardiographic findings include a normal-sized left ventricle, increased thickness of the LV wall, thrombus, and left atrial enlargement, which usually occurs because of elevated diastolic pressure of the left ventricle. The right heart is normal in size, with mildly reduced systolic function and increased wall dimensions. Tricuspid regurgitation is present because of the pulmonary hypertension that occurs as a result of elevated pressures in the left heart.

There are two basic varieties of endomyocardial fibrosis. One form, found primarily in temperate regions, results from hypereosinophilia and is, therefore, termed *hypereosinophilic syndrome.* This syndrome, also referred to as Löffler's endocarditis parietalis fibroplastic or Löffler's endocarditis, mainly affects men in their 40s and is characterized by increased eosinophils of more than 1500/mm.[4] The second form, *obliterative endomyocardial fibrosis,*[4] occurs primarily in subtropical climates and is especially common in Uganda and Nigeria. It accounts for 10–20% of all cardiac deaths in those countries. Large pericardial effusions are typical in this cardiomyopathy.

Diastolic Dysfunction

The importance of diastolic function has become apparent over recent years. Many patients with symptoms of congestive heart failure (shortness of breath, edema) have normal systolic function. The inability of the left ventricle to relax properly can result in diastolic heart failure. This is often seen in patients with hypertrophic cardiomyopathies and similar conditions. Doppler echocardiography is the diagnostic tool of choice for evaluating diastolic function.

CARDIAC MASSES

Benign Tumors

Myxomas. Myxomas are neoplasms that arise from the endocardial tissue and typically arise from the left atrium.[1] They are the most common type of benign tumor, accounting for 30–50% of all benign tumors. Three times as many females as males are affected, and 90% of the tumors are found in the atria: 75–86% are found in the left atrium; 9–20% in the right atrium; and 5–11% in the right atrium or left ventricle but rarely in both atria. Ninety percent of myxomas are pedunculated; the most common site of attachment is the interatrial septum near the fossa ovalis. This tumor may be hereditary (autosomal dominant).

M-mode findings reveal echoes behind the anterior leaflet of the mitral valve. Two-dimensional imaging reveals an echogenic mass in the affected chamber. The echo may be brightly echogenic to sonolucent because of hemorrhage or necrosis.

The clinical findings include the following: symptoms similar to those of mitral valve disease, embolic phenomena, no symptoms, symptoms similar to those of tricuspid valve disease, sudden death, pericarditis, MI, symptoms similar to pulmonic valve disease, and a fever of unknown origin.

Rhabdomyomas. Rhabdomyoma is a benign tumor derived from striated muscle most commonly associated with tuberous sclerosis. It is also called myocardial hamartoma and is the most common cardiac tumor found in infants and children. In 90% of the cases, multiple rhabdomyomas are involved. The tumor is yellow gray in appearance, ranges from 1 mm to several centimeters in diameter, and most commonly involves the ventricles. Large tumors may lead to intracavitary obstruction resulting in death.

Lipomas. Lipomas are benign tumors usually containing mature fat cells. They are the second most common benign tumors of the heart. They affect people of all ages and are found equally often in males and females. Most of these tumors are sessile. Fifty percent are located in the subendocardium, and 25% are intramuscular. The most common sites are the left ventricle, right atrium, and interatrial septum.

Fibromas. Fibromas occur in the connective tissue and contain fibrous connective tissue. They are usually well circumscribed and the second most common benign tumors found predominantly in children (most of whom are younger than 10 years). Almost all of these tumors occur in the ventricular myocardium. On the echocardiogram, they typically present as large masses within the interventricular system.

Angiomas. Angiomas are extremely rare. They may occur in any part of the heart.[5]

Teratomas. Teratomas are extremely rare and occur more often in children. They contain all three germ cell layers. They are found most frequently in the right heart but also can occur in the interatrial or interventricular septum.[5]

Malignant Tumors

Primary Cardiac Tumors. Angiosarcomas usually occur in adults and are twice more common in men than in women. They are the fourth most common primary tumors but the most common malignant cardiac tumors. They are soft tissue tumors of the blood vessels and are usually found in the right atrium; the most common site is the interatrial septum. Other primary cardiac tumors are rhabdomyosarcomas, fibrosarcomas, lymphosarcomas, and sarcomas of the pulmonary artery.

Secondary Metastatic Tumors. Metastatic and secondary tumors usually invade the right heart and are far more common than primary tumors. Usually they are clinically silent. However, they can cause superior vena cava syndrome because of obstruction, supraventricular arrhythmias, MI, cardiomegaly, congestive heart failure, or nonbacterial endocarditis, bronchogenic carcinomas, breast carcinomas, malignant melanomas, and leukemias. Spread of these tumors varies. Bronchogenic carcinomas spread via the lymphatic channels, and metastases of malignant melanomas spread through the blood. Usually metastases involve the pericardium or the myocardium.[5]

Cardiac Thrombi

Left Ventricular Thrombi. Thrombi of the left ventricle occur in MIs, LV aneurysms, and cardiomyopathies. They usually form in the apex of the ventricle. Two-dimensional imaging can diagnose clots with 90% sensitivity and specificity. Echocardiography reveals that the clot has distinct margins, is usually located near an akinetic or dyskinetic area, and may protrude within the ventricle or move with the adjacent wall. Protruding thrombi tend to be more echo dense than mural thrombi, whereas mural thrombi have a layered appearance and are often echolucent along the endocardial border.

Thrombi form within the first 4 days after an infarction and occur in 30% of all anterior wall infarctions; they rarely occur in inferior wall infarctions. If they do not dissolve spontaneously, they may disappear with the use of anticoagulants.

Left Atrial Thrombi. Thrombi usually form in the left atrium in the presence of mitral valve disease (stenosis), an enlarged left atrium, and atrial fibrillation—conditions that predispose to blood stasis. The most common site is the atrial appendage. The echocardiographic appearance of these thrombi varies. In many cases, they are attached to the atrial wall and can be round or ovoid in shape. Their borders are often well defined, they demonstrate mobility, and their texture is uniform. Occasionally, a thrombus appears as a flat immobile mass or as a free-floating ball.

Thrombi of the Right Heart. Most thrombi form in the right heart in the presence of right ventricular infarction, cardiomyopathies, or cor pulmonale. They usually are immobile, heterogeneous sessile masses. In addition, secondary thrombi may occur. Their source is embolization from deep vein thrombosis. Echocardiography typically reveals a long, serpentine, apparently free-floating mass with no obvious site of attachment. Patients are at a much higher risk for an embolus when the thrombus in any area of the heart is protruding or free floating.

Other Cardiac Masses. Because a number of foreign objects can mimic a thrombus, one must be aware of their presence and location. For example, right-heart catheters are often seen in both the right atrium and the right ventricle. These appear as highly reflective linear echoes.

Normal cardiac structures also can mimic intracardiac masses. The moderator band seen in the apex of the right ventricle appears as a thick muscular band extending from the free wall of the right ventricle to the interventricular septum. Occasionally, a prominent eustachian valve can be seen in the right atrium at the junction of the inferior vena cava. It appears as a thin, long, mobile structure in the right atrium, which also may contain thin filamentous structures known as the Chiari network that is a remnant of embryonic structures.

The left ventricle also may contain long thin fibers known as false tendons or ectopic chordae tendineae. These filamentous structures traverse the left ventricle and typically are brightly reflective structures of no clinical significance.

DISEASES OF THE AORTA

Aortic Dilatation

The aorta is considered dilated when its diameter is >37 mm. The average diameter of the adult aorta is 33–37 mm. M-mode measurements of the aorta should be taken at the level of the aortic annulus and the sinus of Valsalva. Aortic dilatation is seen most frequently in patients with annuloaortic ectasia or Marfan's syndrome. In these patients, the medial layer of the aorta weakens, and the aorta dilates. The dilatation occurs not only in the wall of the aorta but in the aortic annulus as well. This often leads to aortic insufficiency because the cusps of the aorta are unable to coapt during closure. Two-dimensional echocardiography can easily detect a dilated aorta.

Aortic Aneurysm

An aortic aneurysm can occur anywhere along the thoracic aorta. The most common sites are the arch and descending aorta, with most occurring just beyond the left subclavian artery. Aneurysms of the thoracic aorta often extend into the abdominal aorta. There are several types of aneurysms, that include; saccular (sack-like dilatation), fusiform (spindle-shaped aneurysm), and dissecting (separation of the arterial wall creating a false and true lumen).

A dissecting aortic aneurysm results from intimal tears of the aortic wall. The driving force of the blood destroys the media further and strips the intimal layer from the adventitial layer. Aortic dissections are classified according to the area and extent of the intimal tear. Type I tears extend from the ascending aorta and continue beyond the arch. Type II tears also begin a few centimeters from the aortic valve but are confined to the ascending aorta. Type III tears begin in the descending aorta, usually just distal to the origin of the left subclavian artery. More than 90% of patients with dissecting aneurysms experience severe pain. Dissections occur twice as often in men as in women and usually in the sixth and seventh decade of life. M-mode findings reveal extra linear echoes within the aorta. Two-dimensional imaging is the echocardiographic tool of choice. Two-dimensional imaging allows visualization of the intimal flap, which divides the true lumen of the aorta from the false lumen. Color-flow Doppler can be invaluable in localizing the site of intraluminal communication. Other echocardiographic evidence for dissection includes aortic regurgitation—the most commonly noted complication. Doppler is useful for detecting disturbed flow patterns in the LVOT. The left ventricle may become enlarged because of volume overload from the aortic regurgitation; pericardial effusion can be noted, and left pleural effusion also may

be noted. The diagnosis of dissection should be made when an intima flap is seen in more than one view.

Aneurysms that occur in the sinus of Valsalva are best seen using two-dimensional imaging. They are observed most easily in the short-axis view during diastole. Rupture usually occurs in the right side of the heart, but it also can occur in the left heart and interventricular septum. Sinus of Valsalva aneurysms can be acquired or congenital in nature.

CONGENITAL HEART DISEASE

Aortic Stenosis

Abnormalities of the LVOT are the most common congenital heart disease found in the adult population. Obstruction can occur at the subvalvular, supravalvular, or valvular level. Congenital abnormalities of the aortic valve occur in 1% of the population, with a higher prevalence among males. The most common malformation of the aortic valve is a bicuspid valve. Aortic coarctation, VSD, and isolated pulmonic stenosis are associated with the condition. As the valve ages, it becomes fibrotic and may calcify. By the fourth decade, 50% of all bicuspid aortic valves become stenotic.

Subvalvular stenosis also can occur. There are two types of subvalvular stenosis: discrete and subaortic. In discrete stenosis, a thin membrane obstructs the outflow tract or a more fibromuscular ridge obstructs the flow of blood. Subaortic stenosis, too, is more common in males. Aortic regurgitation is a frequent finding in subaortic stenosis. Discrete subvalvular stenosis is primarily an acquired rather than a congenital problem when it is present in adults.

Supravalvular stenosis also can be classified into two categories. The most frequent supravalvular narrowing is found in the ascending aorta just above the valve. Less frequently, the obstruction involves the ascending aorta, the aortic arch, and the descending aorta. Supravalvular obstruction can be a familial finding, but it also can be sporadic or as a result of rubella infection. When found in association with mental retardation, a diagnosis of Williams' syndrome can be made.

Patients with congenital outflow obstruction usually present with LV systolic hypertension and develop concentric LV hypertrophy. The physical examination reveals a harsh systolic ejection murmur over the right parasternal border. Echocardiography has become the diagnostic tool of choice in making this diagnosis. M-mode echocardiography reveals a thickened valve with an eccentric closure line. Normally, the closure line of the aortic valve is centrally located. In a bicuspid aortic valve, however, the closure line is displaced toward either the anterior or the posterior wall of the aorta. Two-dimensional echocardiography reveals systolic doming of the cusps, which is seen in the left parasternal long-axis view. The left parasternal short-axis view reveals the presence of only two cusps. Pulsed-wave Doppler echocardiography can localize the area of obstruction and determine what type of obstruction is present.

Continuous-wave Doppler examination allows quantification of peak and mean pressure gradients across the obstruction. Color-flow Doppler examination allows assessment of blood flow direction.

Atrial Septal Defects

Atrial septal defects (ASDs) are the second most common congenital abnormality found in adults. There are three classifications of ASDs, depending on their location: ostium secundum defects, ostium primum defects, and sinus venosus defects. Ostium secundum defects make up 70% of all ASDs found in adults. These are located near the fossa ovalis. Women are three times more likely than men to have this defect. Twenty percent of patients with this type of ASD have mitral valve prolapse. Other associated findings include mitral or pulmonic stenosis and atrial septal aneurysm. When an ASD and mitral stenosis exist simultaneously, the condition is called Lutembacher's syndrome. In isolated mitral stenosis, the left atrium is dilated because the valve area is reduced. With ASD, the blood can escape across the atrial defect, thereby preserving the size of the left atrium.

Fifteen percent of all ASDs are of the ostium primum type. These defects occur in the region of the ostium primum or the lower portion of the atrial septum. A commonly associated finding is a clefted anterior mitral valve leaflet.

Sinus venosus ASDs account for the other 15%. The defects occur in the upper portion of the atrial septum near the orifice of the inferior vena cava. The most common finding associated with this defect is partial anomalous pulmonary venous drainage.

Two-dimensional and M-mode echocardiography reveals a volume overload in the right heart. Findings indicative of right-sided volume overload include a dilated right ventricle and a flattening of the septum in diastole. Two-dimensional imaging of the atrial septum allows direct visualization and localization of the defect. The views most commonly used to assess the atrial septum include the parasternal short-axis, the apical four-chamber, and the subcostal views. The latter view is the best one for visualizing the atrial septum. In addition to the secondary findings already described, two-dimensional imaging allows direct visualization of the defect. In septal defects, a dropout of echoes is noted in the area of the defect. On echocardiography, the dropout of echoes is characterized by a bright echo perpendicular to the atrial septum. This finding has been described as the T sign.

Doppler echocardiography also can help detect ASDs. In the absence of elevated pressures in the right heart, blood flows from the higher-pressure left ventricle to the lower-pressure right heart. In the subcostal view, a pulsed Doppler sample gate can be placed in the right heart near the atrial septum. The spectral display will reveal turbulent flow toward the transducer in late systole and throughout diastole. Color-flow Doppler allows visualization of the interatrial shunt by superimposing a color coding on a two-dimensional image.

Contrast echocardiography can be used when imaging and Doppler are unable to identify the atrial defect clearly. When used in conjunction with two-dimensional imaging, 92–100% of ASDs can be detected. Contrast agents injected into a vein enter the right heart, which is often highly opacified. In the presence of an ASD, small amounts of contrast material can be seen crossing the atrial septum into the left atrium and to the left ventricle. When the shunt is left to right, which is normally the case, a negative contrast effect can be noted. Contrast enhancement can be increased by having the patient perform the Valsalva maneuver, or cough.

Patent Foramen Ovale

Patent (open) foramen ovale can be found in 27% of older patients. Left-to-right shunting does not normally occur when pressures are normal. A potential complication of the condition is paradoxical embolus.

Ventricular Septal Defects

VSDs are the most common defects found in infants and children. In the adult, ASDs are much more common. VSDs fall into two major classifications: muscular septal defects and membranous defects. Like ASDs, VSDs are classified according to the region involved.

Muscular Septal Defects. Muscular septal defects are entirely surrounded by muscle. Outlet defects occur in the most superior portion of the septum and make up part of the outflow region of the left ventricle. They are also referred to as outflow defects, subpulmonic or infundibular defects, or bulbar defects. These defects are bordered by the trabecular septomarginalis (right ventricular septal band) and the pulmonary valve annulus. Thus, they are the most difficult VSDs to image and are best seen from the subcostal and high parasternal positions.

A special form of outlet defect occurs above the crista supraventricularis. This defect is known as supracristal ventricular defect; it is also referred to as the doubly committed subarterial defect because of its proximity to both semilunar valves. This defect also is best seen from the subcostal and high parasternal positions. Associated findings in this defect include (1) aortic valve prolapse because of lack of support, usually involving the right coronary cusp, (2) dilatation of the right coronary sinus of Valsalva, and (3) aortic insufficiency. The defect is usually small.

Inlet ventricular defects are bordered superiorly by the tricuspid valve annulus, apically by the tips of the papillary muscles, and anteriorly by the trabecula septomarginalis. They are also referred to as endocardial cushion defects, retrocristal defects, sinus defects, and inflow defects, which can be seen in several planes, including the parasternal, apical, and subcostal views. Because these defects are usually large, they can be confused with a double-inlet ventricle.

Trabecular defects are bordered by the chordal attachments of the papillary muscle to the apex. They extend from the smooth outlet septum to the inlet septum, are heavily trabeculated, and are usually large. They also can be multiple. These defects typically lead to hypertension of the right ventricle and may produce a right-to-left shunt if the pressures in the right heart exceed those in the left. A special type of muscular septal defect that occurs in the muscular septum is characterized by numerous small defects resembling Swiss cheese. This "Swiss cheese" defect occurs primarily in the apex.

Membranous Defects. Membranous septal defects occur in the region bordered by the inlet and outlet septums and the junctions between the right and noncoronary cusps of the aortic valve. This part of the septum is located at the base of the heart. Defects in this area are often referred to as perimembranous because they usually involve part of a surrounding muscular septum. Almost all planes can be used to image these defects, which occur more frequently than the muscular varieties.

Using two-dimensional imaging allows visualization of the septum. When the defect is large, a dropout of echoes is appreciated. In addition, a T artifact is observed. When imaging does not allow localization of the defect, color-flow Doppler can be used. High-velocity turbulent flow usually can be seen as a mosaic color pattern in the area of the jet. Contrast echocardiography also can be used to localize the defect. Agitated solution can be injected into the right heart through a peripheral vein. Even a few bubbles seen entering the left ventricle are indicative of a right-to-left shunt when right-sided pressures are slightly elevated.

Tetralogy of Fallot

In adults, tetralogy of Fallot is the primary congenital disease producing cyanosis. In this condition, four specific findings are noted. The aorta overrides the perimembranous VSD. Infundibular or valvular pulmonic stenosis is present, resulting in right ventricular hypertrophy. M-mode criteria for diagnosing tetralogy of Fallot include a break in the continuity of the anterior wall of the aorta from that of the interventricular septum as well as a narrowing of the right ventricular outflow tract. Two-dimensional imaging, however, allows direct visualization of the cardiac anatomy and is, therefore, the echocardiographic procedure of choice. Imaging often allows visualization of the VSD and gives valuable information about the amount of aortic override. Doppler echocardiography allows quantification of gradients across the obstruction of right ventricular outflow.

Pulmonic Stenosis

Eighty percent of all congenital obstructions of right ventricular outflow occur at the level of the pulmonic valve. The valve is often thickened with fusion of the cusps and can be seen

doming in systole. Right ventricular hypertrophy occurs as a result of the increased resistance to flow. Two-dimensional imaging allows visualization of the valve, which usually appears thickened and with reduced excursion.

Persistent Ductus Arteriosus

Persistent ductus arteriosus (PDA) occurs when the ductus fails to close after birth. In utero, communication exists between the pulmonary circulation and the systemic circulation, the purpose of which in fetal circulation is to direct the flow of desaturated blood away from the coronary and cerebral circulation and toward the placenta. The ductus is located near the isthmus of the aorta near the origin of the left subclavian artery; it extends to the left pulmonary artery just beyond the bifurcation. In the absence of elevated pulmonary pressures, blood flows from the aorta to the pulmonary artery. In adults, the most common symptom of a PDA is dyspnea on exertion. In persistent ductus, the increased blood flow to the lungs results in dilatation of the pulmonary arteries, the left atrium and ventricle, and the aorta. If pulmonary pressure increases, the blood flow may reverse and travel from the pulmonary circulation toward the aorta. This condition is known as Eisenmenger's complex and is characterized by right-to-left shunting.

Coarctation of the Aorta

Coarctation is a stricture or contraction of the aorta. Twice as many men as women are likely to have coarctation of the aorta. Most patients with this condition are asymptomatic. The coarctation is manifested as LV hypertension. On physical examination, a systolic murmur can be heard. The most common site of narrowing occurs in the thoracic aorta just distal to the left subclavian artery. This condition is often found in association with other congenital abnormalities such as VSD, PDA, a bicuspid aortic valve, and mitral valve abnormalities. It is the most common cardiac malformation found in Turner's syndrome.

The suprasternal notch offers the best view of the ascending aorta, the arch, and the descending aorta. Direct visualization of the coarctation is possible using two-dimensional imaging. Doppler echocardiography typically reveals increased velocities across the site of coarctation.

Ebstein's Anomaly

Ebstein's anomaly is characterized by downward displacement of the anterior or septal leaflet of the tricuspid valve into the right ventricle. As a result, the ventricle becomes "atrialized" and loses some of its pumping capacity. Associated findings include secundum-type ASDs, pulmonic stenosis or atresia, VSD, and mitral valve prolapse. Symptoms may not be evident until the patient is between 30 and 40 years of age. The most common complication of this abnormality is failure of the right ventricle.

The M-mode criterion for this anomaly includes visualization of a large tricuspid valve leaflet, simultaneously seen with the anterior leaflet of the mitral leaflet. A delay time in closure of the tricuspid valve of 80 m/s or more to that of closure of the mitral valve is the second M-mode finding. Two-dimensional imaging allows direct visualization of the anatomy. Specific findings in imaging include an apically located tricuspid leaflet and a functionally small right ventricle. Ebstein's anomaly can be diagnosed if the leaflet is displaced 20 mm or more.

HYPERTENSIVE DISEASE

Systemic Hypertension

There are two basic types of systemic hypertension: essential or idiopathic and secondary hypertension. Both affect the diastolic and systolic pressure. The classification of blood pressure is shown in Table 2–7.

The cause of essential hypertension is unknown. Although several mechanisms may come into play, no specific cause has been well described. Secondary hypertension results in high blood pressure associated with any of the following: renal disease, endocrine disease, coarctation of the aorta, pregnancy, neurologic disorders, acute stress, increased intravascular volume, alcohol and other drug abuse, increased cardiac output, and rigidity of the aorta.

The hemodynamic properties of systemic hypertension, whatever the cause, are similar. Initially cardio output increases, as does fluid volume. This increased fluid volume is transferred to the various organs and tissues. Once tissues receive more blood than they need, the blood vessels that deliver the blood constrict. This is known as vasoconstriction, which is an intrinsic property of such systemic vessels as arterioles, and the bicep increases in size when one does curls, so do the arteries. If this state continues, the vessels continue to exert resistance on the incoming blood

TABLE 2–7 • Classification of Blood Pressure*

Normal blood pressure	Less than 120/80
Elevated blood pressure	120-129/less than 80
Stage 1 high blood pressure	130-139 (systolic blood pressure) or 80-89 (diastolic blood pressure)
Stage 2 high blood pressure	140 (systolic blood pressure) or higher or 90 (diastolic blood pressure) or higher

*People who have systolic and diastolic blood pressures in different categories are considered to be in the higher blood pressure category.

Data from Whelton PK, Carey RM, Aronow WS, et al: 2017 ACC/AHA/AAPA/ABC/ACPM/AGS/APhA/ASH/ASPC/NMA/PCNA Guideline for the Prevention, Detection, Evaluation, and Management of High Blood Pressure in Adults: A Report of the American College of Cardiology/American Heart Association Task Force on Clinical Practice Guidelines, Hypertension 2018 Jun;71(6):e13-e115.

(peripheral resistance). As a result, the heartbeats gain greater resistance and the vessel themselves become thicker.

As is the case with any muscle, hypertrophy occurs when stress is exerted. Similar to the bicep increasing in size when one does curls, the heart also increases in size as it is forced to pump blood against increased peripheral resistance. Therefore, the main echocardiographic findings are increased muscle mass of the heart, especially the left ventricle. By M-mode criteria, the walls of the left ventricle are thick. The principal Doppler findings include (1) decreased transmitral E wave, (2) increased A wave, and (3) increased A-to-E-wave ratios.

Pulmonary Hypertension

In normal physiology, the pulmonary blood flow allows passage of blood to the lungs for three basic functions: oxygenation, filtration, and pH balance by excreting carbon dioxide. Blood coming in from the various tissues and organs of the body is directed to the right heart through the superior and inferior vena cavae. Once this deoxygenated blood enters the right atrium, it passes through the tricuspid valve into the right ventricle across the pulmonic valve and into the main pulmonary artery, which bifurcates into a left and right branch and directs blood to the left and right lobes of the lungs. Normally the pulmonary circulation offers little resistance to blood flow. The normal peak systolic pressure ranges from 18 to 25 mm Hg, and the normal diastolic pressure ranges from 6 to 10 mm Hg. Pulmonary artery pressure in excess of 30 mm Hg systolic pressure and 20 mm Hg diastolic pressure represents elevated pulmonary pressures, or pulmonary hypertension.

As with systemic hypertension, pulmonary hypertension has two basic forms: primary and secondary. Primary pulmonary hypertension—also known as idiopathic, essential, or unexplained pulmonary hypertension—has no known discernible cause. Secondary pulmonary hypertension can be the result of any one of the following factors:

- Increased resistance to pulmonary venous drainage
- Elevated LV diastolic pressure
- Left atrial hypertension (mitral stenosis)
- Pulmonary parenchyma disease
- Pulmonary venous obstruction (cor triatriatum or pulmonary veno-occlusive disease

Cor triatriatum is a congenital abnormality in which the common embryonic pulmonary vein is not incorporated into the left atrium. Instead, the pulmonary veins empty into an accessory chamber and communicate with the left atrium through a small opening. The result is obstruction of pulmonary venous flow that simulates mitral stenosis. In pulmonary veno-occlusive disease, the veins and venules of the lung become fibrotic. M-mode findings reveal an absent or decreased A wave in the absence of right ventricular failure: a lack of respiratory variation in the A wave; an extended preejection period; midsystolic closure of the pulmonic valve, also known as midsystolic notch; and reduced ejection time of the right ventricle. Two-dimensional imaging indicates a dilated pulmonary artery and abnormalities in interventricular septal motion.

Doppler measurements reveal the following: a decreased acceleration time, a longer pre-ejection period, a shorter ejection time, and tricuspid regurgitation. The acceleration time is the time interval between the onset of flow and the peak systolic flow. In pulmonary hypertension, the velocity of blood flow increases rapidly and peaks early in systole. This measurement is made by identifying the beginning of the Doppler signal and the peak velocity of the same signal. The time between the two is the acceleration time.

The preejection period is the time interval between the onset of the QRS complex to onset of flow in the pulmonary artery. In pulmonary hypertension, this time period increases.

Ejection time is the time from the onset of flow to the cessation of flow. In pulmonary hypertension, this time period becomes shorter. This measurement is made by taking the time between the beginning and the end of the Doppler signal.

Tricuspid regurgitation occurs in the majority of patients with elevated pressures in the pulmonary artery. Continuous-wave Doppler can be used to localize the regurgitant jet and obtain the peak transtricuspid gradient using the modified Bernoulli equation. The peak gradient is the difference in systolic pressure between the right atrium and right ventricle. Estimation of the pulmonary pressures is accomplished by adding the right atrial pressures, which are determined by visual inspection of the jugular venous pulse. A more common way is to add the constant "10" to the peak systolic transtricuspid gradient. When stenosis of the pulmonic valve is present, however, one cannot determine pulmonary artery pressures using the peak transtricuspid regurgitant gradient.

CORONARY ARTERY DISEASE

The normal right and left coronary arteries supply the heart muscle with oxygenated blood (Table 2–8). The left coronary artery originates from the left coronary sinus of Valsalva, which bifurcates into two branches: the anterior interventricular or descending branch, also known as the left anterior descending branch, and the circumflex branch. The right coronary artery originates from the right coronary sinus of Valsalva.

The coronary anatomy can vary considerably in humans. In 67% of cases, the right coronary artery is the dominant artery. In these cases, this artery supplies the parts of the left ventricle and septum. In 15% of cases, the left coronary artery is the dominant one and supplies blood to all of the left ventricle and septum. In 18% of cases, the two arteries are equal; this situation is called the balanced coronary arterial pattern.

Abnormal Wall Motion

When the blood supply to the heart muscle is interrupted, the muscle is damaged and immediate changes in motion can be observed. The affected area can be identified using the various echocardiographic views. The wall segment should be identified using the ASE's recommendation (see the section on Normal Anatomy).[6]

Complications of Ischemic Heart Disease

Ventricular Aneurysm. One complication of ischemic heart disease is ventricular aneurysm. Although aneurysm can form in any part of the left ventricle, more than 80% form in the apex and are the result of an anterior infarction. Of the 5–10% that form in the posterior wall, nearly half are false aneurysms.

The echocardiographic appearance of aneurysms includes thin walls that do not thicken in systole, a bulging wall, and dyskinetic motion to the affected area.

TABLE 2–8 • Normal Branches of the Coronary Arteries

Coronary Artery	Major Branches	Area Supplied
Left coronary	Left anterior descending	Anterior left ventricular wall Anterior two-thirds of apical septum Anteroapical portions of left ventricle Anterior-lateral papillary muscle Midseptum Bundle of His Anterior right ventricular papillary muscle
	Circumflex*	Lateral left ventricular wall Left atrium
Right coronary	Numerous branches	Anterior right ventricular wall Posterior third (or more) of the interventricular septum Diaphragmatic wall of right ventricle Atrioventricular node

*If the circumflex terminates at the crux of the heart, it supplies the entire left ventricle and interventricular septum.

There are three types of ventricular aneurysms: anatomically true, functionally true, and anatomically false aneurysms. An anatomically true aneurysm is composed of fibrous tissue, may or may not contain a clot, and protrudes during both diastole and systole. Its mouth is wider or as wide as its maximum diameter, and its wall is the former LV wall. An anatomically true aneurysm almost never ruptures once healed. A functionally true aneurysm also consists of fibrous tissue but protrudes only during ventricular systole.

An anatomically false aneurysm always contains a clot. Its mouth is considerably smaller than its maximum diameter, and it protrudes during both systole and diastole and may even expand. Its wall is composed of parietal pericardium. Because a false aneurysm often ruptures, immediate surgery is usually required.

Ventricular Septal Defect. A VSD occurs when a rupture occurs in the septum. Several echocardiographic techniques can be used to make the diagnosis. Two-dimensional imaging allows direct visualization of the defect. With contrast echocardiography with imaging, contrasting material can be seen filling the right ventricle and entering the left ventricle as blood moves back and forth through the defect. Negative contrast effect also can be noted. Doppler measurements can detect turbulent high-velocity signals on the right side of the ventricular septum. The best views include the left parasternal long- and short-axis views and the apical four-chamber view. Color Doppler can demonstrate communication between the left and right ventricles. The color jet appears as a mosaic pattern of high-velocity flow.

Thrombus. Thrombus, the most common complication of infarction, usually occurs in the apex in areas of dyskinesia.

It can be laminar, lay close to the wall of the ventricle, or protrude into the cavity and be highly mobile. The diagnosis should be made when the thrombus is seen in several views.

Valve Dysfunction. An infarction is most likely to affect the mitral valve. Mitral regurgitation results if the papillary muscle is ruptured, if it becomes fibrosed, or if the mitral annulus is affected, resulting in incomplete closure of the leaflets.

Right Ventricular Involvement. Involvement of the right ventricle occurs primarily when the infarction is in the inferior wall or when the proximal right coronary artery is obstructed. Echocardiography reveals that the ventricle is dilated and its free wall moves abnormally.

References

1. Allen MN. *Echocardiography*. 2nd ed. New York: Lippincott; 1999.
2. Williams PL, Warwick R, Dyson M, eds. *Gray's Anatomy*. 37th ed. New York: Churchill Livingstone; 1989.
3. Driscoll DJ, Fuster V, McGoon DC. Congenital heart disease in adolescents and adults: atrioventricular canal defect. In: Brandenburg RO, Fuster V, Giulani ER, et al, eds. *Cardiology: Fundamentals and Practice*. Chicago: Year Book Medical Publishers; 1987.
4. *Report of the American Society of Echocardiography Committee on Nomenclature and Standards Identification of Myocardial Wall Segments*. 1982.
5. Braunwald E. *Heart Disease: A Textbook of Cardiac Medicine*. 3rd ed. Philadelphia: WB Saunders; 1988.
6. Feigenbaum H. *Endocardiopathy*. 4th ed. Philadelphia: Lea & Febiger; 1986.

Questions

GENERAL INSTRUCTIONS: For each question, select the best answer. Select only one answer for each question unless otherwise specified.

1. Which heart groove or sulci separates the atria from the ventricles?

    (A) interventricular

    (B) interatrial

    (C) anterior interventricular

    (D) coronary or atrioventricular

Identify the coronary arteries in Fig. 2–12.

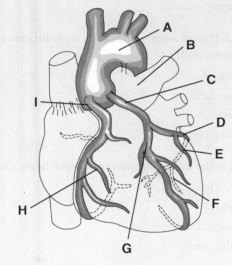

FIGURE 2–12. Anatomic drawing of the heart and vessels.

2. _____ left posterolateral branch

3. _____ left circumflex branch

4. _____ pulmonary trunk

5. _____ left marginal branch

6. _____ AV node branch

7. _____ left main coronary artery

8. _____ right coronary artery

9. _____ aortic arch

10. _____ left anterior descending branch

11. Which of the following is *not* an indication for stress echocardiography?

    (A) screening of new patients for CAD

    (B) assessing states before and after intervention

    (C) determining prognosis after MI

    (D) unstable angina

12. Which of the following cardiology examination requires a physician to perform?

    (A) echocardiography

    (B) stress echocardiography

    (C) TEE

    (D) color-flow Doppler

13. What is the purpose of the pericardium?

    (A) allowing the heart to move freely with each beat

    (B) facilitating ejection and volume changes

    (C) containing the heart within the mediastinum

    (D) serving as a barrier to infection

    (E) all of the above

14. What is the largest cardiac chamber?

    (A) right atrium

    (B) right ventricle

    (C) left atrium

    (D) left ventricle

15. The left atrium receives how many pulmonary veins?

    (A) one

    (B) two

    (C) three

    (D) four

16. What is crista terminalis?

    (A) anterior portion of the right atrium

    (B) posterior portion of the right atrium

    (C) a ridge of muscle separating the right atrium

    (D) a heart groove or sulci

17. **Which valve is located between the left atrium and the left ventricle?**

    (A) tricuspid

    (B) mitral

    (C) aortic

    (D) foramen ovale

18. **Which of the following is *not* a right heart characteristic and/or function?**

    (A) supplies blood to the pulmonary circulation

    (B) normal pressure in the ventricle is approximately 140 mm Hg

    (C) blood returning to the right heart has a lower oxygen saturation

    (D) contains the tricuspid valve

19. **Mitral valve stenosis results primarily from which of the following?**

    (A) atherosclerosis

    (B) endocarditis

    (C) hypertension

    (D) rheumatic disease

20. **Vegetations are more commonly associated with which of the following?**

    (A) pulmonary hypertension

    (B) aneurysms

    (C) endocarditis

    (D) mitral valve disease

21. **Which of the following is not a type of bioprosthetic heart valve?**

    (A) xenograft

    (B) heterograft

    (C) homograft

    (D) Bjork–Shiley valve

22. **Which of the following would indicate pericardial effusion?**

    (A) 5–10 mL of fluid

    (B) 10–15 mL of fluid

    (C) 15–50 mL of fluid

    (D) 75–100 mL of fluid

23. **The term *cardiomyopathy* is used to describe which of the following?**

    (A) pericardial effusion

    (B) variety of cardiac diseases that affect the pericardium

    (C) variety of cardiac diseases that affect the myocardium

    (D) variety of cardiac diseases that affect the endocardium

24. **What is the most common type of benign tumor of the heart?**

    (A) myxoma

    (B) rhabdomyoma

    (C) lipoma

    (D) fibroma

25. **What is the most common malignant cardiac tumor?**

    (A) teratoma

    (B) rhabdomyoma

    (C) carcinoma

    (D) angiosarcoma

26. **Which type of aneurysm results from intimal tears of the aortic wall?**

    (A) saccular

    (B) fusiform

    (C) pseudo

    (D) dissecting

27. **What is the most common congenital heart disease?**

    (A) ASDs

    (B) VSDs

    (C) muscular septal defects

    (D) abnormalities of the LVOT

28. **What is the primary congenital disease in adults that produces cyanosis?**

    (A) pulmonic stenosis

    (B) coarctation of the aorta

    (C) PDA

    (D) tetralogy of Fallot

29. **Which of the following is *not* a characteristic of cardiomyopathy?**

    (A) dilatation

    (B) pericarditis

    (C) restrictive

    (D) hypertrophic

30–36. Identify the structures in Fig. 2–13.

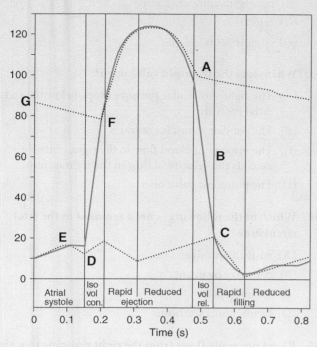

FIGURE 2–13. Events of the cardiac cycle.

30. _____ aortic valve closure

31. _____ aortic valve opening

32. _____ aortic pressure

33. _____ LV pressure

34. _____ mitral valve closure

35. _____ left atrial pressure

36. _____ mitral valve opening

37. In stenotic diseases of the tricuspid, which of the following is dilated?

   (A) left atrium

   (B) left ventricle

   (C) right atrium

   (D) right ventricle

38. In tricuspid valve disease, what is the primary cause of regurgitation?

   (A) carcinoid heart disease

   (B) prolapse of the valve

   (C) rheumatic heart disease

   (D) secondary to pulmonary hypertension

39. Which of the following is not a type of endocarditis?

   (A) Ebstein's anomaly

   (B) bacterial

   (C) mycotic

   (D) Löffler's

40. Which of the following is *not* a clinical symptom associated with aortic valve stenosis?

   (A) chest pain

   (B) dyspnea on exertion

   (C) shortness of breath

   (D) syncope

41. Which of the following is the bicuspid valve with two major leaflets?

   (A) tricuspid valve

   (B) aortic valve

   (C) pulmonic valve

   (D) mitral valve

42. What is a classic finding in mitral valve prolapse?

   (A) systolic doming

   (B) fluttering of the mitral valve

   (C) pulmonary edema

   (D) systolic click

43. What is the most common cause of a flail leaflet?

   (A) rupture of the chordal tendineae

   (B) rupture of the papillary muscle

   (C) annular calcification

   (D) congenital defect

44. Which cardiac examination provides the highest resolution?

   (A) TTE

   (B) contrast TTE

   (C) stress echocardiography

   (D) TEE

45. In which cardiac sinus is a thin fold of tissue guard called the thebesian valve?

   (A) sinus of Morgagni

   (B) aortic sinus

   (C) coronary sinus

   (D) sinus of Valsalva

46. **What is the average length of an adult heart?**

    (A) 12 cm

    (B) 8–9 cm

    (C) 6 cm

    (D) 16 cm

47. **The AV node is located in which triangular region of the right atrium?**

    (A) posterior region

    (B) anterior region

    (C) triangular region

    (D) triangle of Koch

48. **Which vessel drains the head and parts of the upper extremities?**

    (A) aorta

    (B) superior vena cava

    (C) inferior vena cava

    (D) portal venous system

49. **Which of the following views would *best* demonstrate all four cardiac chambers simultaneously?**

    (A) left parasternal

    (B) right parasternal

    (C) subcostal

    (D) suprasternal

50. **Which of the following is used to denote the three orthogonal planes for two-dimensional echocardiographic imaging?**

    (A) long axis, short axis, and four chamber

    (B) apical, subcostal, and parasternal

    (C) suprasternal, right sternal border, and left sternal border

    (D) anterior, posterior, and coronal

51. **Which of the following abnormalities are usually *best* demonstrated with the subcostal four-chamber view?**

    (A) ASDs and VSDs

    (B) mitral regurgitation and tricuspid regurgitation

    (C) mitral stenosis and tricuspid stenosis

    (D) aortic insufficiency and pulmonic insufficiency

52. **Which of the following terms is used to describe the control that suppresses near-field echoes and enhances the intensity of the far-field echoes?**

    (A) attenuation

    (B) time-gain compensation

    (C) reject

    (D) compression

53. **When does the tricuspid valve open?**

    (A) The right ventricular pressure drops below the right atrial pressure.

    (B) The papillary muscle contracts.

    (C) The velocity of blood flow in the right ventricle exceeds the velocity of flow in the right atrium.

    (D) The pulmonic valve opens.

54. **Which of the following is *not* a remnant of the fetal circulation?**

    (A) eustachian valve

    (B) coronary ligament

    (C) foramen ovale

    (D) ligamentum arteriosus

55. **Blood normally flows from the right ventricle to which of the following?**

    (A) pulmonary artery

    (B) aorta

    (C) right atrium

    (D) pulmonary vein

56. **A pulmonary vein is normally attached to which of the following?**

    (A) right ventricle

    (B) left ventricle

    (C) left atrium

    (D) right atrium

57. **Which of the following statements regarding cardiac anatomy is false?**

    (A) The heart tends to assume a more vertical position in tall thin people and a more horizontal position in short, heavy people.

    (B) The ligamentum arteriosum runs from the left pulmonary artery to the descending aorta.

    (C) The coronary arteries arise from the sinuses within the pockets of the left and right coronary cusps of the aortic valve.

    (D) The left ventricle constitutes most of the ventral surface of the heart.

58. LV ejection time can be assessed from an M-mode echocardiogram by measuring the distance between which of the following?

    (A) aortic valve opening and closing points

    (B) mitral D and C points

    (C) R wave and T wave

    (D) mitral valve closure and aortic valve opening

59. Often, what is the best two-dimensional view for examining patients with chronic obstructive pulmonary disease?

    (A) parasternal

    (B) apical

    (C) suprasternal

    (D) subcostal

60. What are the two best transducer positions for Doppler investigation of systolic blood flow across the aortic valve?

    (A) parasternal and suprasternal

    (B) apical and right sternal border

    (C) suprasternal and subcostal

    (D) subcostal and apical

61. When should the size of the left atrium be measured on the M-mode?

    (A) at end systole

    (B) at the peak of the R wave

    (C) with the onset of aortic valve opening

    (D) at the beginning of the P wave

62. Doming of any cardiac valve on two-dimensional echocardiography is consistent with which of the following?

    (A) regurgitation

    (B) decreased cardiac output

    (C) stenosis

    (D) congenital malformation

63. Two-dimensional images are best obtained when the ultrasound beam is directed _____ to the structure of interest. Doppler signals are best obtained when the ultrasound beam is directed _____ to the flow of blood.

    (A) oblique; perpendicular

    (B) parallel; perpendicular

    (C) perpendicular; parallel

    (D) perpendicular; oblique

64. Right ventricular systolic pressure overload can be caused by which of the following?

    (A) pulmonary insufficiency

    (B) an ASD

    (C) aortic stenosis

    (D) pulmonary hypertension

65. LV measurements should be obtained from the parasternal long-axis view at the level of which of the following?

    (A) mitral valve annulus

    (B) tips of the mitral leaflets

    (C) chordae tendineae

    (D) papillary muscle

66. Which of the following cannot cause paradoxical interventricular septal motion?

    (A) left bundle branch block

    (B) postpericardiotomy

    (C) LV volume overload

    (D) severe tricuspid regurgitation

67. In a patient with volume overload of the right ventricle, the onset of ventricular systole is likely to show the interventricular septum moving

    (A) toward the right ventricular free wall

    (B) toward the LV wall

    (C) laterally

    (D) not at all

68. A murmur that is associated with a thrill is likely to be which of the following?

    (A) organic in origin

    (B) insignificant

    (C) functional

    (D) the result of an ASD

69. The Valsalva maneuver and the inhalation of amyl nitrite are techniques that are sometimes used during an echocardiographic examination when checking for which of the following?

    (A) mitral valve prolapse or systolic anterior motion of the mitral valve

    (B) aortic stenosis or mitral stenosis

    (C) aortic stenosis or aortic regurgitation

    (D) VSD or pulmonic stenosis

70. **Clubbing of the fingers and nail beds is a sign of which of the following?**

    (A) cyanotic heart disease

    (B) Marfan's syndrome

    (C) Barlow's syndrome

    (D) increased cardiac output

71. **Even though two-dimensional echocardiography has largely replaced M-mode echocardiography for cardiac diagnosis, M-mode still has the advantage of which of the following?**

    (A) defining spatial relationships of cardiac structures

    (B) providing enhanced temporal resolution

    (C) providing dynamic assessment of the velocity of blood flow

    (D) providing superior lateral resolution

72. **When attempting a parasternal short-axis view, if the left ventricle appears oval rather than circular, where should the echocardiographer move the transducer?**

    (A) medially

    (B) laterally

    (C) to a higher intercostal space

    (D) to a lower intercostal space

73. **A Doppler tracing of the mitral valve in which the A point is higher than the E point indicates which of the following?**

    (A) high cardiac output

    (B) low cardiac output

    (C) decreased LV compliance

    (D) high LV end-diastolic pressures

74. **Which of the following is usually not a secondary finding in patients with mitral stenosis?**

    (A) a dilated left atrium

    (B) a dilated right atrium

    (C) an LV thrombus

    (D) a left atrial thrombus

75. **Which of the following is most likely to *not* be demonstrated on the Doppler signal obtained from the apex in a patient with mitral stenosis?**

    (A) an increased diastolic peak velocity

    (B) spectral broadening

    (C) a decreased E–F slope

    (D) a peak gradient occurring in late diastole

76. **Torn chordae tendineae will cause which of the following?**

    (A) aortic insufficiency

    (B) MI

    (C) mitral insufficiency

    (D) mitral stenosis

77. **Which of the following cannot produce false-positive signs of mitral valve prolapse on an M-mode?**

    (A) pericardial effusion

    (B) premature ventricular contractions

    (C) improper placement of the transducer

    (D) hypertrophic obstructive cardiomyopathy

78. **Which of the following is a secondary echocardiographic finding in mitral regurgitation?**

    (A) a dilated left atrium

    (B) LV hypertrophy

    (C) a hypokinetic left ventricle

    (D) a dilated aortic root

79. **The degree of mitral regurgitation is best estimated by measuring which of the following?**

    (A) width and length of the systolic jet by color Doppler

    (B) peak velocity of the continuous-wave Doppler systolic mitral signal

    (C) pressure half-time of the continuous-wave Doppler diastolic signal

    (D) integral of the continuous-wave systolic curve

80. **Which of the following is least likely to occur as a sequela of rheumatic fever?**

    (A) mitral stenosis

    (B) mitral insufficiency

    (C) aortic stenosis

    (D) pulmonic stenosis

81. **The two-dimensional echocardiogram of a patient with combined mitral and aortic stenosis is most likely to demonstrate which of the following?**

    (A) a dilated left atrium and LV hypertrophy

    (B) a dilated left atrium and a dilated left ventricle

    (C) a small left atrium and a small left ventricle

    (D) systolic anterior motion of the mitral valve and LV hypertrophy

82. **Why is the M-mode of the mitral valve in mitral stenosis often missing an A wave?**

    (A) high initial diastolic pressures in the left ventricle

    (B) concurrent atrial fibrillation

    (C) decreased compliance of the left ventricle

    (D) a dilated left atrium

83. **A Doppler tracing that demonstrates a late diastolic mitral inflow velocity (A point) that is higher than the initial diastolic velocity (E point) can be seen with which of the following pathologies?**

    (A) aortic insufficiency

    (B) hypertrophic cardiomyopathy

    (C) mitral regurgitation

    (D) a VSD

84. **If the two-dimensional examination demonstrates a markedly dilated and hyperkinetic left ventricle and a left atrium of normal size, one should suspect the presence of which of the following?**

    (A) mitral regurgitation

    (B) aortic regurgitation

    (C) a VSD

    (D) aortic stenosis

85. **Which group of echocardiographic findings would give a definitive diagnosis of mitral stenosis?**

    (A) a decreased E–F slope, a dilated left atrium, and a small left ventricle

    (B) a thickened mitral valve, a dilated left atrium, and a small left ventricle

    (C) a decreased E–F slope, a thickened mitral valve, and diastolic doming of the mitral valve

    (D) a thickened mitral valve and a mitral diastolic velocity >1.5 m/s

86. **A patient with mitral stenosis will usually not have which of the following?**

    (A) a diastolic rumble on auscultation

    (B) an increased E–F slope on M-mode

    (C) a history of rheumatic fever

    (D) a dilated left atrium

87. **To obtain the true circumference of the mitral valve, one should obtain a short-axis view at the level of which of the following?**

    (A) papillary muscle

    (B) chordae tendineae

    (C) tips of the mitral leaflets

    (D) mitral annulus

88. **Which of the following is not a secondary echocardiographic finding of mitral stenosis?**

    (A) a dilated left atrium

    (B) a dilated right atrium

    (C) a dilated left ventricle

    (D) a left atrial thrombus

89. **Which of the following is a successful mitral valve commissurotomy *least* likely to demonstrate?**

    (A) doming of the mitral valve

    (B) mitral valve thickening

    (C) an increase in pressure half-time

    (D) a dilated left atrium

90. **Which of the following can be suggested by LV dilatation in a patient with mitral stenosis?**

    (A) severe mitral stenosis

    (B) concomitant mitral regurgitation

    (C) aortic stenosis

    (D) hypertrophic cardiomyopathy

91. **Early diastolic closure of the mitral valve is usually a sign of which of the following?**

    (A) severe acute aortic regurgitation

    (B) a left bundle branch block

    (C) poor function of the left ventricle

    (D) first-degree A–V block

92. **Which one of the following conditions cannot accelerate degenerative calcification of the mitral annulus?**

    (A) systemic hypertension

    (B) aortic stenosis

    (C) hypertrophic obstructive cardiomyopathy

    (D) a VSD

93. **A mitral valve pressure half-time of 220 ms is consistent with which of the following mitral valve areas?**

    (A) 0.6 cm^2

    (B) 1 cm^2

    (C) 2.2 cm^2

    (D) 5 cm^2

154. **Which of the following statements regarding left atrial myxomas is *not* true?**

    (A) They usually attach to the interatrial septum.

    (B) They may be pedunculated.

    (C) They do not recur once they are surgically removed.

    (D) Clinically, they can mimic mitral stenosis.

155. **The QP/QS ratio is used to evaluate the severity of which of the following?**

    (A) pulmonic stenosis

    (B) VSDs

    (C) aortic stenosis

    (D) systemic hypertension

156. **Which of the following would best describe the pulsed Doppler pattern of a patent ductus arteriosus if the sample volume were placed in the pulmonary artery from a short-axis view of the base of the heart?**

    (A) systolic flow below baseline

    (B) continuous flow (systolic and diastolic) above baseline

    (C) diastolic flow above baseline

    (D) a biphasic systolic flow pattern below baseline

157. **Which of the following is the best way to detect a small ASD?**

    (A) two-dimensional echocardiography

    (B) contrast injection echocardiography

    (C) M-mode echocardiography

    (D) pulsed-wave Doppler echocardiography

158. **What is the most common type of ASD?**

    (A) primum

    (B) secundum

    (C) fenestrated

    (D) sinus venosus

159. **Which of the following is consistent with a VSD with right-to-left shunting?**

    (A) Ebstein's anomaly

    (B) tetralogy of Fallot

    (C) Eisenmenger's syndrome

    (D) a double-outlet right ventricle

160. **Which of the following is not associated with Ebstein's anomaly?**

    (A) an abnormally large tricuspid valve

    (B) infundibular pulmonic stenosis

    (C) "atrialization" of the right ventricle

    (D) an ASD

161. **The echocardiogram of a patient with an endocardial cushion defect might exhibit which of the following?**

    (A) a muscular VSD and tricuspid valve vegetation

    (B) a hypokinetic left ventricle and mitral valve vegetation

    (C) overriding of the aorta and subpulmonic stenosis

    (D) ostium primum ASD and an inlet VSD

162. **An echocardiographic diagnosis of coarctation of the aorta can be made by detecting a high-velocity Doppler jet in which of the following?**

    (A) left branch of the pulmonary artery

    (B) aortic arch, proximal to the subclavian artery

    (C) descending thoracic aorta

    (D) abdominal aorta

163. **Which of the following is *not* one of the four principal components of tetralogy of Fallot?**

    (A) a VSD

    (B) an override of the aorta

    (C) an obstruction of pulmonary blood flow

    (D) an ASD

164. **Which of the following describes cor triatriatum?**

    (A) It is a fairly common congenital abnormality.

    (B) It is a congenital malformation in which the right atrium is divided by a fibrous membrane, resulting in three atrial chambers.

    (C) It results in mitral stenosis.

    (D) It is a condition in which the pulmonary veins drain into the right atrium.

165. **Which of the following echocardiographic findings is most commonly associated with left bundle branch block?**

    (A) LV hypertrophy

    (B) a hypercontractile interventricular septum

    (C) paradoxical septal motion

    (D) a dilated left ventricle

166. The echocardiographic pattern of the mitral valve in Fig. 2–14 is consistent with which of the following?

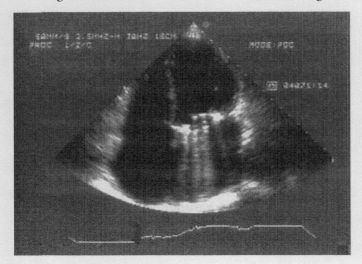

FIGURE 2–14. Apical four-chamber view.

(A) mitral stenosis

(B) mitral valve vegetation

(C) a mechanical prosthetic valve

(D) a calcified mitral valve annulus

167. The M-mode pattern in Fig. 2–15 suggests which of the following about the ejection fraction of the left ventricle?

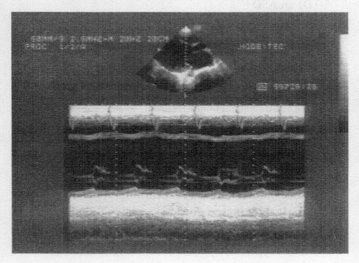

FIGURE 2–15. M-mode echocardiogram at the level of the mitral valve.

(A) normal

(B) mildly increased

(C) significantly increased

(D) significantly decreased

168. What other hemodynamic information could be derived from the M-mode (see Fig. 2–15)?

(A) cardiac output is increased

(B) LV end-diastolic pressure is increased

(C) the systolic ejection period is prolonged

(D) atrial flutter is present

169. The Doppler tracing in Fig. 2–16 demonstrates which of the following?

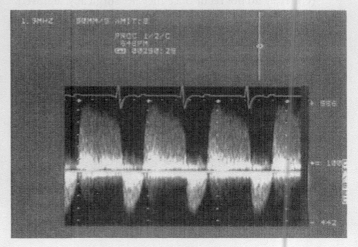

FIGURE 2–16. Continuous-wave Doppler tracing obtained from the apical position.

(A) aortic stenosis and aortic insufficiency

(B) mitral stenosis and mitral regurgitation

(C) tricuspid stenosis and tricuspid regurgitation

(D) mitral stenosis and aortic stenosis

170. The echocardiographic findings in Fig. 2–17 indicate that the patient probably has a history of which of the following?

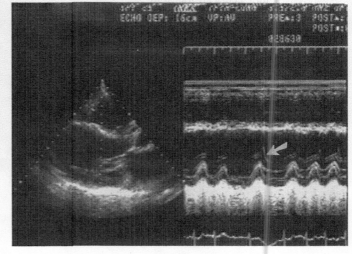

FIGURE 2–17. Split-screen display of a two-dimensional long-axis (left) and a correlating M-mode pattern (right). Note M-mode scan plane indicated by cursor (arrow).

(A) hypertension

(B) diabetes mellitus

(C) rheumatic fever

(D) CAD

171. What is the arrow in Fig. 2–17 pointing to?

   (A) a side-lobe artifact
   (B) papillary muscle
   (C) chordae tendineae
   (D) the anterior mitral leaflet

172. Fig. 2–18 demonstrates echoes within the LV cavity. These echoes are which of the following?

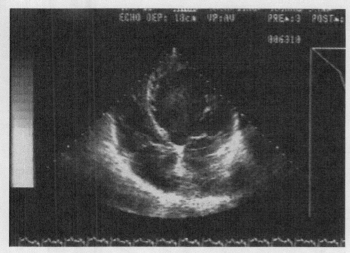

FIGURE 2–18. Apical four-chamber view showing a dilated left ventricle.

   (A) artifactual
   (B) caused by a mural thrombus
   (C) caused by stagnant blood
   (D) caused by a high near-gain setting

Questions 173–179: Match the numbered structures in Fig. 2–19 with the correct term given in Column B.

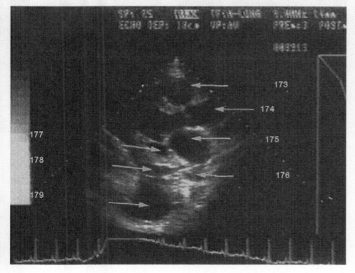

FIGURE 2–19. Parasternal long-axis view with an increased depth setting.

COLUMN A	COLUMN B
173. _____	left ventricle
174. _____	coronary sinus
175. _____	left atrium
176. _____	right ventricle
177. _____	pericardial effusion
178. _____	descending aorta
179. _____	pleural effusion aortic root right atrium

180. What is demonstrated in Fig. 2–20?

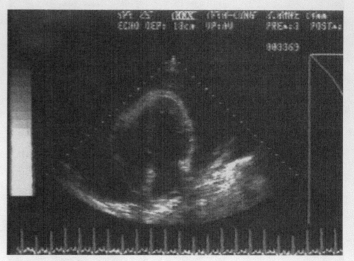

FIGURE 2–20. Apical four-chamber view.

   (A) a large pleural effusion
   (B) pneumomediastinum
   (C) ascites
   (D) a large pericardial effusion

181. The echocardiographic examination of this patient should include analysis of the motion of which of the following?

   (A) interventricular septum
   (B) right ventricular wall
   (C) LV wall
   (D) tricuspid valve

182. Color Doppler interrogation of the aortic valve shown in Fig. 2–21 is most likely to demonstrate which of the following?

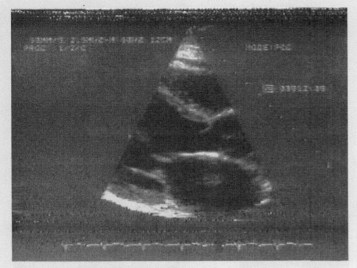

FIGURE 2–21. Narrow sector parasternal long-axis view.

(A) a narrow diastolic jet directed at the anterior mitral leaflet

(B) a diastolic jet filling the LVOT and extending deep into the left ventricle

(C) a normal pattern of blood flow

(D) a narrow systolic jet directed at the anterior mitral leaflet

183. The arrow in Fig. 2–22 is pointing to which of the following?

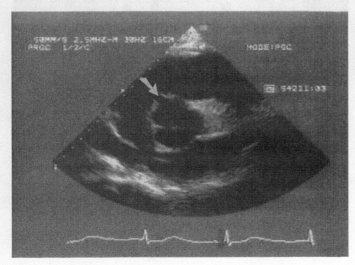

FIGURE 2–22. Short-axis view of the base of the heart.

(A) a fistula between the aorta and right ventricle

(B) the coronary sinus

(C) the left main coronary artery

(D) the origin of the right coronary artery

184. The right ventricular outflow tract is located medial to the arrow in Fig. 2–22.

(A) true

(B) false

185. The contrast study in Fig. 2–23 shows which of the following?

(A) left-to-right shunting at the atrial level

(B) no shunting of blood

(C) right-to-left shunting at the atrial level

(D) right-to-left shunting at the ventricular level

186. A secondary finding noted on Fig. 2–23 is a moderate-sized pericardial effusion.

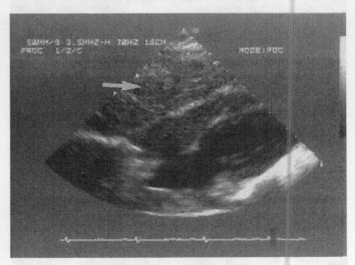

FIGURE 2–23. Subcostal four-chamber view with contrast injection.

(A) true

(B) false

187. The arrow in Fig. 2–23 is pointing to which of the following?

(A) lung tissue

(B) liver parenchyma

(C) a mediastinal tumor

(D) the spleen

188. The absence of an A wave and midsystolic notching of the pulmonic valve on the M-mode in Fig. 2–24 is consistent with which of the following?

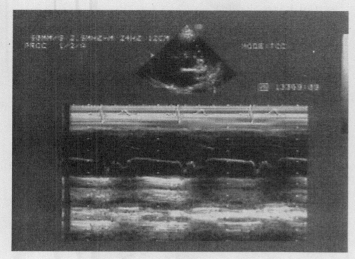

FIGURE 2–24. M-mode of the pulmonic valve.

(A) pulmonic stenosis
(B) tricuspid stenosis
(C) mitral stenosis
(D) pulmonary hypertension

189. What other abnormality should be ruled out in the presence of the abnormality noted on the M-mode of the tricuspid valve in Fig. 2–25?

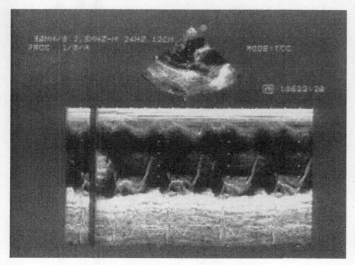

FIGURE 2–25. M-mode of the tricuspid valve.

(A) tricuspid stenosis
(B) pulmonary hypertension
(C) mitral valve prolapse
(D) ASD

190. An 85-year-old woman with a long history of chest pain is sent for an echocardiogram. The M-mode of the mitral valve is shown in Fig. 2–26. The M-mode of the aortic valve would be likely to demonstrate which of the following?

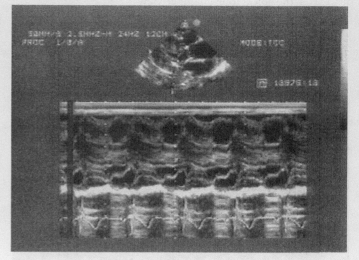

FIGURE 2–26. M-mode echocardiogram at the level of the mitral valve.

(A) diastolic fluttering
(B) delayed opening
(C) midsystolic notching
(D) systolic fluttering

191. An extremely tall, slender young man was referred for an echocardiogram because he has a murmur. Echocardiographic findings in Fig. 2–27 include which of the following?

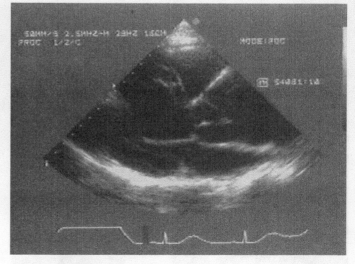

FIGURE 2–27. Parasternal long-axis view.

(A) a bicuspid aortic valve
(B) a cleft mitral valve
(C) a dilated aortic root
(D) LV hypertrophy

192. **Which echocardiographic view would be best for further evaluation of this abnormality?**

    (A) the long-axis suprasternal view

    (B) the short-axis view of the base of the heart

    (C) the apical four-chamber view

    (D) the subcostal four-chamber view

193. **The left ventricle in Fig. 2–28 demonstrates which of the following?**

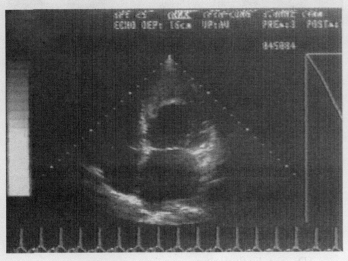

FIGURE 2–28. Apical four-chamber view.

    (A) hypertrophic cardiomyopathy

    (B) an infiltrative tumor

    (C) a large apical thrombus

    (D) a myxoma

194. **Which of the following is true about the mitral valve shown in Fig. 2–29?**

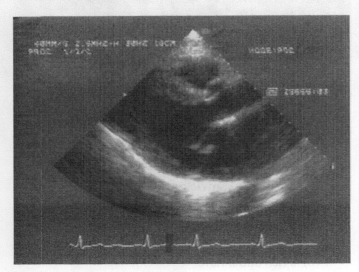

FIGURE 2–29. Parasternal long-axis view.

    (A) It is normal.

    (B) It is flail.

    (C) It is stenotic.

    (D) It is prolapsing.

195. **What is the arrow in Fig. 2–30 pointing to?**

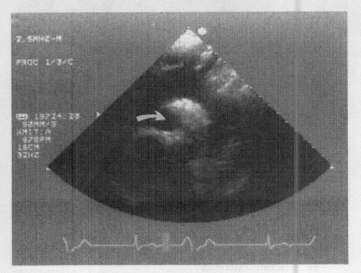

FIGURE 2–30. Suprasternal notch long-axis view of the aorta and transverse arch.

    (A) left subclavian artery

    (B) right pulmonary artery

    (C) superior vena cava

    (D) left pulmonary vein

196. **Posterior to this structure is an echo-free space, which represents which of the following?**

    (A) the left atrium

    (B) a pleural effusion

    (C) pericardial effusion

    (D) the superior vena cava

197. The curved arrow in Fig. 2–31 is directed at which of the following?

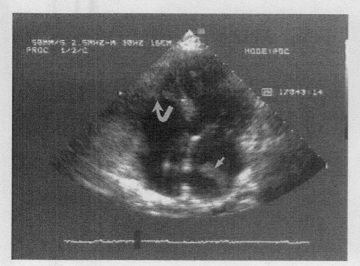

FIGURE 2–31. Apical four-chamber view.

(A) a pacemaker wire
(B) the Chiari network
(C) false chordae tendineae
(D) the moderator band

198. The straight arrow in Fig. 2–31 is pointing to a structure that most likely represents which of the following?

(A) a right atrial myxoma
(B) a left atrial thrombus
(C) the left pulmonary vein
(D) the eustachian valve

199. The echocardiographic findings in the long-axis view presented in Fig. 2–32 include which of the following?

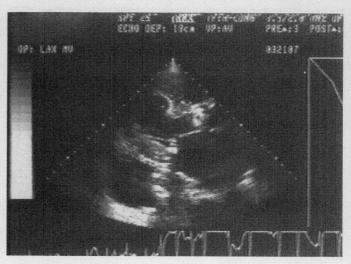

FIGURE 2–32. Parasternal long-axis view with slightly increased depth setting.

(A) a dilated left atrium, mitral stenosis, and a pericardial effusion
(B) aortic stenosis, a calcified mitral annulus, and basal septal hypertrophy
(C) a dilated coronary sinus, LV hypertrophy, and mitral valve vegetation
(D) a dilated aortic root, a dilated left ventricle, and a thickened mitral valve

200. What are these findings most consistent with?

(A) rheumatic heart disease
(B) congenital heart disease
(C) subacute bacterial endocarditis
(D) an aged heart

201. The mitral valve diastolic waveforms in Fig. 2–33C are not uniform. Which of the following causes this?

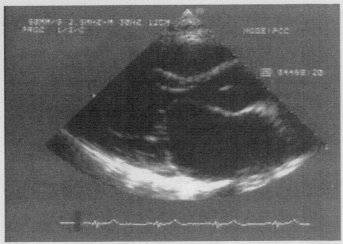

A

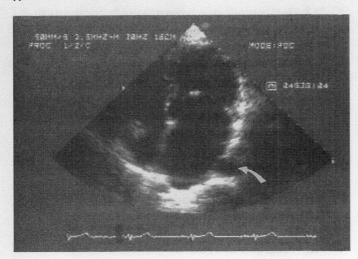

B

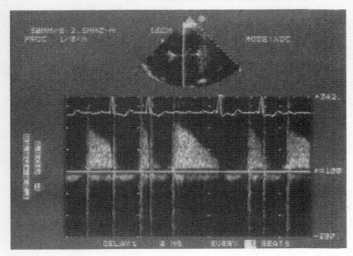

C

FIGURE 2–33. **(A)** Parasternal long-axis view; **(B)** apical four-chamber view; **(C)** continuous-wave Doppler tracing of mitral inflow from the apical position.

(A) high end-diastolic pressure of the left ventricle
(B) faulty technique
(C) inspiration
(D) atrial fibrillation

The following study is of a 58-year-old woman who vaguely remembers a childhood illness that included pain in her joints. She presented with a transient ischemic attack and atrial fibrillation. For questions 202–204, refer to Figs. 2–33A, B, and C.

202. What does the mitral valve demonstrate?

(A) systolic prolapse
(B) diastolic doming
(C) myxomatous degeneration
(D) hyperkinesis

203. Which chamber is significantly dilated?

(A) the left atrium
(B) the left ventricle
(C) the right atrium
(D) the right ventricle

204. What is most likely to be revealed by auscultation of this patient?

(A) a midsystolic click
(B) a systolic ejection murmur
(C) a systolic rumble
(D) an opening snap

205. What is the arrow in Fig. 2–33B pointing to?

(A) coronary sinus
(B) inferior vena cava
(C) descending aorta
(D) left pulmonary vein

206. The pressure half-time derived from the Doppler tracing of the mitral valve in Fig. 2–33C can be used to estimate which of the following?

(A) the mitral valve area
(B) the mitral valve gradient
(C) the severity of aortic insufficiency
(D) the ejection fraction

118. **(B)** Mitral valve vegetation. IV drug abusers have an increased incidence of endocarditis because of microorganisms that enter the bloodstream via unsterile needles. Vegetations usually form on the valves of the right side of the heart, but they may settle on left-sided valves as well. One complication of valvular vegetation is an embolic event.

119. **(B)** Presence of paravalvular regurgitation. The spatial orientation of color Doppler allows for a quick assessment of blood flow in the region surrounding the prosthetic valve.

120. **(A)** May exhibit high Doppler velocities. The normal Doppler velocities across any prosthetic valve will be slightly higher than those of a native valve. A Starr–Edwards, or ball-in-cage, valve tends to exhibit the highest velocities.

121. **(A)** An example of a mechanical heart valve. The Bjork–Shiley is a tilting-disc mechanical heart valve.

122. **(C)** TEE. This is a major application in the evaluation of prosthetic heart valves, particularly in the mitral position.

123. **(D)** Hancock. This valve is an example of a heterograft (bioprosthetic) valve.

124. **(C)** Abnormal rocking motion of the valve. Valve dehiscence refers to a condition in which the prosthetic valve loosens or separates from the sewing ring and causes an abnormal rocking motion and a paravalvular leak.

125. **(C)** It often makes anticoagulation unnecessary. Mechanical valves require constant anticoagulation. Women during childbearing years would, therefore, be more likely to receive a bioprosthetic valve, which would not require anticoagulation.

126. **(A)** These patients are at a higher risk for endocarditis. Because bacteremias occur during dental or surgical procedures, prophylactic antibiotics are often administered to susceptible patients (such as mitral valve prolapse patients) in an attempt to prevent bacterial endocarditis.

127. **(C)** A "swinging heart" on the two-dimensional examination. Excessive motion of the heart can sometimes be noted with massive pericardial effusion.

128. **(A)** It impairs diastolic filling. The rigid and fibrotic pericardial sac impairs diastolic filling of the cardiac chambers.

129. **(A)** Pressure in the pericardial cavity rises to equal or exceed the diastolic pressure in the heart. Tamponade occurs when intrapericardial pressures rise and impair cardiac filling. Although cardiac tamponade is usually seen in association with a large pericardial effusion, a small effusion may cause tamponade if the rate of accumulation of pericardial fluid exceeds the ability of the pericardium to accommodate the increased volume.

130. **(D)** In Dressler's syndrome, a pericardial effusion develops as a result of renal disease. Dressler's syndrome, also known as postmyocardial infarction syndrome, is the development of pericardial effusion 2–10 weeks after infarction.

131. **(D)** A pericardial effusion. Neoplasms from the thoracic region often lead to pericardial effusion.

132. **(D)** Mitral valve prolapse. The descending aorta, a calcified mitral annulus, and ascites can cause echo-free spaces that may be misleading on an echocardiogram. Although a large effusion in which the heart exhibits excessive motion may lead to false mitral valve prolapse, which will not lead to a false-positive diagnosis of pericardial effusion.

133. **(A)** Pulmonic stenosis. Diastolic collapse of the right ventricular walls is a good indicator of tamponade. Pulmonic stenosis, or any other form of right ventricular pressure overload, leads to thickening of the right ventricular walls. A thickened wall is unlikely to collapse in diastole.

134. **(C)** There is a large acoustic mismatch between lung tissue and pericardial tissue. A greater mismatch between two structures results in brighter reflected echoes from the interface between them. Because there is an extremely large acoustic mismatch between lung (air) and pericardium (tissue), the interface created by the two will cause a bright echo to appear on the echocardiogram.

135. **(C)** Decreasing overall gain and increasing depth setting. Decreasing the gain allows for differentiation between the pericardium and epicardium, and increasing the depth setting helps define the borders of the effusion.

136. **(D)** Descending aorta. Because the descending aorta lies posterior to the pericardial effusion and anterior to the pleural effusion, it often aids in differentiating between the two.

137. **(A)** Constrictive pericarditis. The pericardium limits cardiac motion. When the pericardium is surgically removed (eg, in constrictive pericarditis), the heart expands and exhibits excessive motion.

138. **(A)** Excessive cardiac motion. Again, because the pericardium limits cardiac motion, the heart exhibits excessive motion when the pericardium is surgically removed.

139. **(C)** Reduced compliance of the left ventricle. Systemic hypertension causes pressure overload of the left ventricle. As in all pressure-overload situations (eg, aortic stenosis), the LV hypertrophies and may become noncompliant, leading to diastolic dysfunction.

140. **(B)** LV hypertrophy. This condition can be present in the absence of an obstruction.

141. **(D)** Endomyocardial biopsy. Several echocardiographic signs are suggestive of amyloid heart disease, but a definitive diagnosis can be made only with an endomyocardial biopsy performed in the catheterization laboratory.

142. **(B)** Sarcoidosis. This is an infiltrative process that can lead to restrictive cardiomyopathy.

143. **(A)** Increased systolic velocity in the LVOT. Velocities are low because of decreased cardiac output.

144. **(A)** It is more likely to affect the right ventricle than the left ventricle. Cardiac contusion may be seen following a blunt trauma to the chest (such as a steering-wheel injury). Because the right ventricle is the most anterior structure of the heart, it is the one most susceptible to injury.

145. **(A)** An apical aneurysm with a mural thrombus. Apical aneurysms sometimes develop following an anterior wall MI. Because aneurysms are a likely site for thrombus, choice A is the most likely answer.

146. **(C)** Two-dimensional demonstration of an ejection fraction lower than 50%. The ejection fraction is a measure of systolic LV function.

147. **(C)** LAD. This artery supplies the anterior wall of the left ventricle and the anterior portion of the interventricular septum.

148. **(D)** They have a narrow neck. The best way to differentiate a true aneurysm from a pseudoaneurysm is to look at the width of its neck. Pseudoaneurysms tend to have a narrow neck because they result from a tear in the myocardium.

149. **(B)** A reduced ejection fraction. An E point-to-septal separation of more than 10 mm correlates with a reduced ejection fraction.

150. **(B)** Akinetic. Lack of systolic thickening and motion is referred to as akinesis.

151. **(D)** Occlusion of the left anterior descending coronary artery. Blood to the inferior wall of the left ventricle is usually supplied by the right coronary artery.

152. **(B)** Severe mitral regurgitation. Doppler interrogation of a patient with ruptured papillary muscle will usually demonstrate this condition.

153. **(D)** It is used in diagnosing ischemic heart disease. Stress echocardiography is used as an adjunct to standard stress testing in diagnosing patients with suspected CAD. Resting wall motion is compared to wall motion during and after stress.

154. **(C)** They do not recur once they are surgically removed. Although characterized as a benign tumor, a myxoma may recur if some cells remain after excision of the tumor.

155. **(B)** VSDs. The QP/QS ratio refers to the ratio of pulmonary-to-systemic blood flow. It can be calculated echocardiographically to determine the magnitude of left-to-right shunting of blood.

156. **(B)** Continuous flow (systolic and diastolic) above baseline. Shunting of blood from the aorta to the pulmonary artery occurs in both systole and diastole.

157. **(B)** Contrast injection echocardiography. Even a small ASD can be detected by noting the presence or absence of microbubbles.

158. **(B)** Secundum. ASDs occur most commonly in the area of the foramen ovale, where they are termed *ostium secundum defects.*

159. **(C)** Eisenmenger's syndrome. In this syndrome, the pulmonary vascular resistance is equal to or greater than the systemic vascular resistance, leading to right-to-left shunting.

160. **(B)** Infundibular pulmonic stenosis. In Ebstein's anomaly, the tricuspid valve is large and partially adherent to the walls of the right ventricle so that the valve orifice is displaced apically. Therefore, most of the right ventricle functions as part of the right atrium. It is frequently associated with an ASD. Infundibular pulmonic stenosis is not part of the spectrum of this disorder.

161. **(D)** Ostium primum ASD and an inlet VSD. Endocardial cushion defects occur when the atrial and ventricular components of the cardiac septum fail to develop properly.

162. **(C)** Descending thoracic aorta. Coarctation of the aorta is a constrictive malformation of the aortic arch, usually located just distal to the origin of the left subclavian artery. The obstruction increases the velocity of blood flow beyond the point of constriction.

163. **(D)** An ASD. The fourth component is right ventricular hypertrophy.

164. **(B)** It is a congenital malformation in which a fibrous membrane divides the left atrium into an upper and lower chamber. Cor triatriatum is a rare abnormality in which an embryonic membrane in the left atrium fails to regress. It can be detected echocardiographically by noting a linear echo traversing the left atrium. Doppler echocardiography will detect high-velocity flow across a hole in the membrane.

165. **(C)** Paradoxical septal motion. Left bundle branch block often causes this motion.

166. **(C)** A mechanical prosthetic valve. This high echogenicity of the mitral valve is characteristic of a mechanical prosthetic valve.

167. **(D)** It is significantly decreased. The M-mode demonstrates a dilated and hypokinetic left ventricle. The markedly increased E point-to-septal separation is consistent with a decreased LV ejection fraction.

168. **(B)** LV end-diastolic pressure is increased. There is a mitral valve B notch, which is consistent with high end-diastolic pressure in the left ventricle.

169. **(A)** Aortic stenosis and aortic insufficiency. The systolic waveform below baseline is consistent with moderate aortic stenosis. A mitral regurgitation waveform would

be wider and is usually of higher velocity. The diastolic waveform above baseline is too high a velocity to be caused by mitral or tricuspid stenosis and is consistent with aortic insufficiency.

170. **(D)** CAD. The interventricular septum is hypokinetic and more echogenic than the posterior LV wall. These findings are consistent with an old MI.

171. **(C)** Chordae tendineae. The M-mode cursor in this long-axis view is directed beyond the tips of the mitral leaflets at the level of the chordae tendineae—the level at which LV measurements are obtained.

172. **(C)** Caused by stagnant blood. The cloud of fuzzy smoke-like echoes in the left ventricle is the result of blood stasis. It is usually seen when there is a severe decrease in LV contractibility.

173–179. If you are having a difficult time orienting yourself to an echocardiographic image, find a structure that is easy for you to recognize and work your way from there. For example, if you can identify the aortic root, you can then follow the anterior wall of the root as it continues into the interventricular septum. The posterior wall of the root will follow into the anterior mitral leaflet, and so on. **173.** Right ventricle. **174.** Aortic root. **175.** Left atrium. **176.** Descending aorta. **177.** Left ventricle. **178.** Pericardial effusion. **179.** Pleural effusion.

180. **(D)** A large pericardial effusion. A massive circumferential pericardial effusion is demonstrated in this four-chamber view.

181. **(B)** Right ventricular wall. The presence of tamponade should be ruled out in patients with pericardial effusion, especially a massive one. A fairly specific echocardiographic sign of tamponade is diastolic collapse of the right ventricle, the right atrium, or both.

182. **(B)** A diastolic jet filling the LVOT and extending deep into the left ventricle. This long-axis view demonstrates a flail right coronary cusp of the aortic valve. The cusp is seen extending into the LVOT in diastole. Color Doppler would be likely to demonstrate severe aortic insufficiency, which choice B describes.

183. **(D)** The origin of the right coronary artery. With slight superior angulation from a standard short-axis view of the aortic valve, the ostia and proximal segments of the right coronary artery can be visualized.

184. **(B)** False. The right ventricular outflow tract is located lateral to the origin of the right coronary artery.

185. **(A)** Left-to-right shunting at the atrial level. There is a washout effect in the right atrium as blood from the left side of the heart enters the contrast-filled right atrium.

186. **(B)** False. A pericardial effusion would appear on a subcostal four-chamber view as an echo-free space anterior to the right ventricle.

187. **(B)** Liver parenchyma. To obtain a subcostal four-chamber view, the transducer is placed on the abdomen and angled in a cephalic direction. Therefore, liver parenchyma will occupy the near field of the image.

188. **(D)** Pulmonary hypertension. An absent A wave and midsystolic notching (flying W sign) are consistent with this condition.

189. **(C)** Mitral valve prolapse. The M-mode in Fig. 2–25 demonstrates late-systolic tricuspid valve prolapse. Tricuspid valve prolapse almost always occurs in patients with concomitant mitral valve prolapse.

190. **(C)** Midsystolic notching. Fig. 2–26 is an example of systolic anterior motion of the mitral valve. This is one classic echocardiographic sign of hypertrophic obstructive cardiomyopathy. The midsystolic obstruction of the LVOT will often be demonstrated on the M-mode of the aortic valve as well as by midsystolic notching.

191. **(C)** A dilated aortic root. This patient exhibits characteristic findings of Marfan's syndrome, a connective tissue disorder. There is a linear echo near the aortic valve suggesting aortic root dissection, another complication of Marfan's syndrome. This syndrome often causes ascending aortic dilatation as well as myxomatous degeneration of the aortic and mitral valves.

192. **(A)** The long-axis suprasternal view. Because the aortic root is dilated, echocardiographic evaluation should follow the length of the aorta to determine the extent of the aneurysm. The suprasternal long-axis view allows for visualization of the aortic arch and the proximal portion of the descending aorta. Further investigation should include a modified apical two-chamber view for evaluating the thoracic aorta and a subcostal approach for interrogating the abdominal aorta.

193. **(C)** A large apical thrombus. This thrombus is seen filling the apex, with a piece of the medial segment protruding into the left ventricle. Most thrombi are associated with anterior infarctions and are located in the apex in the majority of cases.

194. **(B)** It is flail. The tip of the posterior leaflet can be seen protruding into the left atrium, which is consistent with a flail mitral valve.

195. **(B)** Right pulmonary artery. The artery is seen in its short axis.

196. **(A)** The left atrium. This atrium can sometimes be visualized posterior to the right pulmonary artery on the suprasternal long-axis view.

197. **(D)** The moderator band. This is a muscular strip located in the apical third of the right ventricle. It is sometimes misdiagnosed as a right ventricular apical thrombus.

198. **(B)** A left atrial thrombus. This is seen protruding into the left atrium. (The bright linear echo in the right atrium originates from a pacemaker wire.)

199. **(B)** Aortic stenosis, a calcified mitral annulus, and basal septal hypertrophy. The aortic valve is markedly calcified; there is a bright echo posterior to the mitral valve, representing a calcified mitral annulus; and the base of the interventricular septum is hypertrophied. The posterior echo-free space represents pleural effusion, as opposed to a pericardial effusion, because it does not taper at the descending aorta.

200. **(D)** An aged heart. When seen together, these findings usually indicate signs of aging.

201. **(D)** Atrial fibrillation. The ECG at the top of the Doppler tracing indicates this fibrillation. The variations from beat to beat reflect the altering lengths in diastolic filling periods that occur with atrial fibrillation.

202. **(B)** Diastolic doming. The mitral valve is bulging into the left ventricle in diastole because the valve is stenotic and cannot accommodate all the blood available for delivery into the left ventricle.

203. **(A)** The left atrium. Even without using the centimeter markers as a gauge, one can determine that the left atrium is dilated. In the long-axis view, the aortic root and left aorta should be approximately the same size. The apical four-chamber view is extremely useful for assessing relative chamber size. The right and left atria should be roughly the same size (although the left atrium is usually slightly larger), and they should be smaller than the ventricles.

204. **(D)** An opening snap. The opening snap often affords the first clue to the diagnosis of mitral stenosis.

205. **(C)** Descending aorta. A portion of the aorta can be seen lying behind the left atrium on the apical four-chamber view.

206. **(A)** The mitral valve area. The pressure half-time, or the time it takes for the initial pressure drop of the mitral valve to be halved, can be used to measure the mitral valve area. A pressure half-time of 220 ms has been shown to correlate with a valve area of 1 cm^2.

207. **(C)** LV hypertrophy. The LV walls are thickened and exhibit increased echogenicity.

208. **(B)** A thickened mitral valve, a prominent interatrial septum, a small left ventricle, and pericardial effusion. The mitral valve and interatrial septum are slightly thickened, there is a small-to-moderate-sized pericardial effusion, and the left ventricle is small.

209. **(D)** Amyloid cardiomyopathy. This patient exhibits classic features of this disease. The infiltrative process of the disease causes thickening of the ventricles, interatrial septum and valves. Pericardial effusion is another finding sometimes associated with this disease.

210. **(B)** An endomyocardial biopsy. This has been shown to be helpful in identifying amyloid cardiomyopathy.

211. **(B)** VSD. The short-axis and modified four-chamber views demonstrate a gap in the posterior aspect of the midsection of the interventricular septum. Given the patient's history and the irregular borders on the echocardiogram, one can assume that this defect is acquired rather than congenital.

212. **(A)** Color-flow Doppler imaging. This is particularly useful for quickly determining the location and quantifying the extent of abnormal blood flow in patients with VSDs.

213. **(A)** Coronary sinus. When imaged from the apical two-chamber view, the coronary sinus appears as a circular structure in the AV groove. By rotating to a four-chamber view and angling posteriorly, one can follow the coronary sinus as it courses along the length of the posterior AV groove.

214. **(B)** Deoxygenated blood. The coronary sinus carries venous blood to the right atrium.

215. **(A)** Anteriorly. By tilting the scan plane anteriorly from this posteriorly directed apical four-chamber view, the aorta and LVOT can be imaged.

216. **(C)** Prolapse of the posterior leaflet. The posterior mitral leaflet bulges beyond the plane of the mitral annulus, which is consistent with prolapse.

217. **(A)** A systolic curve below baseline >3 m/s. Mitral valve prolapse, especially to the degree shown in this study, is most likely to be accompanied by some degree of mitral regurgitation, which is detected from the apical window with Doppler echocardiography by noting a systolic curve below baseline usually >3 m/s.

218. **(B)** False. The arrow is pointing to the lateral wall of the left ventricle.

219. **(C)** Artifactual. A dropout of echoes in the interatrial septum is not an uncommon finding when visualized from the apical four-chamber view. If this were a true ASD, a T sign would likely be noted.

220. **(A)** Slight thickening of the valve with a normal opening. This thickening is noted best in diastole. The leaflets appear to open widely in systole. (They open in close proximity to the walls of the aortic root.)

221. **(C)** 36 mm Hg. Using the simplified Bernoulli equation, the peak aortic gradient can be obtained by squaring the peak velocity (in this case 3 m/s) and then multiplying by 4.

222. **(B)** Congenital aortic stenosis. In this disorder, the valve may be thin or minimally thickened, and M-mode may demonstrate a normal opening if the cursor was directed at the body of the leaflets rather than at the restricted tips. The best way to determine if congenital aortic stenosis is present is by noting Doppler evidence of increased velocities across the valve.

223. **(A)** Systolic doming. This occurs in congenital aortic stenosis because the body of the leaflets expands to

accommodate systolic flow while the tips of the leaflets restrict blood flow. (Normally, the tips of the aortic valve open wide and lie parallel to the aortic root in systole.)

224. (C) It is exhibiting shaggy irregular echoes. The mitral valve has a mass of shaggy echoes with irregular borders attached to it.

225. (B) Subacute bacterial endocarditis. Because of the patient's history and the echocardiographic demonstration of an irregular mass attached to the mitral valve, this is the most likely diagnosis.

226. (B) Increased. Unlike calcium, which tends to inhibit valve opening, vegetations are likely to increase valve excursion. Because calcium and vegetations can look similar, echocardiographically this difference can aid in the diagnosis.

227. (A) Systolic waveform below baseline. A mitral valve vegetation will usually cause the mitral valve to be regurgitant. Mitral regurgitation can be detected by continuous-wave Doppler from the apical four-chamber view by noting systolic flow below baseline.

228. (D) It prolapses into the left atrium and left ventricle. In Fig. 2–38A, the mass is in the left atrium. In Figs. 2–38B and C, the mass appears in the left ventricle. Therefore, one could deduce that the mass is prolapsing into the left atrium in systole and into the left ventricle in diastole.

229. (B) The posteromedial papillary muscle. On the opposite wall of the left ventricle, one can see the anterolateral papillary muscle. Between the two papillary muscles, the tip of the mitral valve vegetation can be seen protruding into the left ventricle.

Associated Disease[6,59]

- Bicuspid aortic valve (found in as many as 50% of patients with coarctation of the aorta)
- Additional levels of left heart obstruction
- Ventricular septal defects
- Transposition of the great arteries
- Double-outlet right ventricle

Natural History. If unrelieved, as many as 80% of patients die before reaching the age of 50 years.[6]

Neonatal coarctation (ductal-dependent systemic blood flow lesion) will present in shock after closure of the ductus

Treatment.[6,13] Early repair seems to decrease probability of residual systemic hypertension.

- Surgical resection of constricted area and primary anastomosis (end to end) or subclavian artery flap to widen aortic lumen. Surgery is the dominant treatment for native coarctation in the neonate.
- Balloon angioplasty and stent placement are commonly used for treatment of native coarctation in older children and adults, and to treat recurrent coarctation.[61,62]

Postoperative Echocardiographic Evaluation

- Assessment of the lumen size and pressure gradient in the area of the re-anastomosis
- PW Doppler spectral tracing of the descending aortic flow may continue to appear somewhat blunted

Hypoplastic Left Heart Syndrome

A spectrum of left-sided hypoplasia in which the left atrium, mitral valve, left ventricle, aortic valve, and aorta may be hypoplastic, stenotic, or atretic. Frequently associated with an atrial septal defect through which pulmonary venous return flows into the right atrium and a patent ductus arteriosus, which in turn supplies the descending aorta.[26]

This is a ductal-dependent systemic blood flow lesion.

Treatment[63]

- Prostaglandins started in the immediate neonatal period to ensure patency of the ductus arteriosus and maintain systemic blood flow
- Norwood procedure
- Cardiac transplantation

Pulmonary Stenosis

Anatomy. Obstruction may occur at various levels along the RV outflow tract and the pulmonary arterial system. Types are listed as follows[6,24]:

- Valvular stenosis: fusion or dysplasia of cusps
- Infundibular stenosis: hypertrophy of muscle bands in the RV outflow tract; usually associated with a ventricular septal defect or valvular pulmonary stenosis[26]
- Double-chamber right ventricle: hypertrophied anomalous muscle bundles in the right ventricle, effectively dividing the right ventricle into two chambers with a communication between them; associated with valvular pulmonary stenosis, perimembranous ventricular septal defects, and subaortic stenosis[44,64]
- Peripheral pulmonary stenosis: may occur as a distinct shelf in the PA, discrete narrowing of the PA branches, or as diffuse tapered narrowing of the PA branches[65]

Hemodynamics. Increased resistance to RV outflow results in a pressure overload to this chamber. The RV walls thicken. Blood flow into the pulmonary arterial system is at high velocity and turbulent. Eddy currents produced distal to the obstruction may cause poststenotic dilatation of the PA.[26]

Clinical Presentation.[6] Patients are usually asymptomatic.

- Auscultation: systolic ejection murmur
- ECG: RV hypertrophy
- Chest x-ray: prominent PA trunk; large right atrium

Key Echocardiographic Concepts

- 2D visualization and measurement of pulmonary valve annulus in candidate for balloon angioplasty of valvular stenosis[66]
- 2D visualization of anomalous muscle bundle and orifice from parasternal and subcostal views[66]
- Measure the diameter of main and branch PAs
- Doppler estimation of pressure gradient from all available positions[67]
- Assess RV function, free wall hypertrophy, systolic pressure (based on TR jet estimation)
- Assess tricuspid valve morphology and annulus size
- Determine the presence of a ductus arteriosus
- Accentuation of the "a wave" on M-mode[6]

Natural History[6]

- Increased risk of endocarditis
- Mild valvular and peripheral stenosis (RV pressure <50 mm Hg and a pressure gradient of <40 mm Hg) is considered benign and may or may not progress.
- Severe stenosis (RV pressure >100 mm Hg and a pressure gradient >60 mm Hg) requires relief.[68]
- Infundibular stenosis and anomalous muscle bundles tend to become progressively more obstructive.

Treatment. When the patient becomes symptomatic or pressure gradient exceeds 60 mm Hg[13]

- Balloon valvuloplasty: to relieve valvular and peripheral stenosis[55]
- Surgical valvotomy[6]
- Surgical resection of infundibular muscle or anomalous muscle bundles

Postoperative Echocardiographic Evaluation

- Assess patency of area of former obstruction
- Assess presence and severity of pulmonary insufficiency

Pulmonary Atresia With Intact Ventricular Septum

Anatomy. There is an imperforate membrane or thick fibrous band in place of a pulmonary valve or complete absence of the main PA in the absence of a ventricular septal defect.[65,69]

Hemodynamics. Life is dependent on a persistent patent ductus arteriosus. Main and branch PAs are usually normal in size.

Clinical Presentation.[6] Severe cyanosis and hypoxemia are seen in the neonate.

- Auscultation: possibly the murmur of a persistent ductus arteriosus
- ECG: RV hypertrophy; right-axis deviation
- Chest x-ray: decreased pulmonary vascular markings

Key Echocardiographic Concepts[6,66]
- 2D delineation of anatomy
  - RV outflow tract, location, and size of main PA and branches (subcostal coronal and parasternal short axis)
  - Assessment of tricuspid valve anatomy and annulus diameter (annulus predicts outcome—z score of <3 associated with lower likelihood of tolerating RV decompression)[70,71]
  - Associated malformations
- Contrast echocardiography to delineate anatomy
- Doppler and color-flow delineation of flow patterns

Associated Disease[66]
- Persistent ductus arteriosus
- Atrial septal defect or patent foramen ovale
- Malformations of the tricuspid valve
- Coronary arterial sinusoids (interrogate myocardium by color and Doppler at low Nyquist limit)

Natural History
- Death when the persistent ductus arteriosus closes or becomes insufficient to sustain minimal blood oxygenation requirements[6]

Treatment[6,13]
- Prostaglandin: to keep the ductus arteriosus patent
- Palliation with a surgically created systemic-to-pulmonary shunt
- Surgical reconstruction and/or placement of prosthetic valve
- May need to follow single ventricle palliative route (Glenn–Fontan)

Postoperative Echocardiographic Evaluation
- Evaluate patency of systemic-to-pulmonary shunt
- Evaluate patency of reconstructed area

Left Ventricular Inflow Obstruction

Anatomy. Left ventricular inflow is obstructed by a membrane in the left atrium or a decrease in the mitral orifice size. Various forms exist, listed as follows.[26,44]:

- Cor triatriatum: rare; LA membrane immediately superior to the fossa ovalis and LA appendage
- Supravalvular ring: more common than cor triatriatum; LA membrane immediately superior to the mitral valve annulus; usually associated with other mitral valve anomalies[36,72]
- Valvular mitral stenosis: rare; dysplastic valve leaflets, chordae and papillary muscles
- Parachute mitral valve: all chordae insert onto a single papillary muscle
- Arcade mitral valve: chordae insert onto multiple papillary muscles; may be regurgitant
- Double orifice mitral valve: rare; tissue bridge divides mitral valve into two halves and chordae from each half inserting onto a particular papillary muscle; may be regurgitant; associated with atrioventricular malformation[73]
- Mitral valve hypoplasia: small mitral valve annulus and leaflets
- Mitral Atresia: imperforate mitral valve may be associated with a large ventricular septal defect, straddling tricuspid valve, or double-outlet right ventricle

Hemodynamics. Obstruction to left ventricular inflow results in a buildup of pressure in the left atrium causing it to dilate. Pulmonary veins become congested because they cannot empty easily into the left atrium.

Clinical Presentation[6]
- Physical exam: history of recurrent respiratory infections
- Auscultation: diastolic murmur heard best at the apex
- ECG: LA enlargement
- Chest x-ray: LA enlargement; increased pulmonary vascular markings; right heart enlargement

Key Echocardiographic Concepts

- Delineation of anatomy by 2D:
  Supravalvar area (cor triatriatum/supravalvar mitral ring)
  Annulus size
  Anatomy of papillary muscles
- Doppler estimation of pressure gradient
- Estimation of orifice size by application of the continuity equation

Associated Disease[6]

- Other levels of left heart obstruction
- Secundum and primum atrial septal defects
- Transposition of the great arteries
- Double-outlet right ventricle

Natural History.

The degree of obstruction depends on the valve area, the cardiac output, and the heart rate.[74] Left ventricle inflow obstruction eventually develops into pulmonary vascular obstructive disease.[7]

Treatment[6,74]

- Valvular: balloon valvuloplasty (in attempt to delay surgery); commissurotomy or valve replacement
- Cor triatriatum and supramitral ring: surgical excision of membrane[66]

Postoperative Echocardiographic Evaluation

- Evaluate residual stenosis and regurgitation

Tricuspid Atresia

Anatomy. A dense band of tissue replaces the tricuspid valve preventing direct communication between the right atrium and ventricle. A large atrial septal defect or patent foramen ovale must coexist to provide an outlet to the right atrium (obligatory shunt).[44] The right ventricle is usually small.[13]

Type I: Normally related great arteries; ventricular septal defect or patent ductus arteriosus is path of pulmonary blood flow.

Type II: Transposed great arteries; ventricular septal defect is the path for systemic blood; any restriction causes subaortic stenosis.[75]

Hemodynamics. Deoxygenated systemic venous blood returns to the right atrium and is shunted into the left atrium, where it mixes with oxygenated pulmonary venous return. This mixing of deoxygenated blood with the pulmonary venous return results in a desaturation of the oxygenated blood and, therefore, cyanosis. The right atrium and left heart are generally dilated because of increased flow volume. Because the right ventricle receives blood only indirectly through a ventricular septal defect, it is generally small.[24]

Clinical Presentation.[6,24] Patients are cyanotic with a history of hypoxic spells.

- Physical exam: clubbing of the fingers; delayed growth; hyperactive cardiac impulse at the apex
- Auscultation: single first heart sound; no murmur
- ECG: left ventricular hypertrophy; left axis deviation
- Chest x-ray: decreased vascular markings

Key Echocardiographic Concepts

- 2D visualization of dense fibrous band across tricuspid annulus and absence of tricuspid valve leaflets
- Dilated right atrium[44]
- Atrial septal defect (determine size and effective shunting) or single atrium
- Small right ventricle or RV outflow tract
- Relationship of great arteries (normally related versus dextrotransposition of the great arteries)

Associated Disease[6,24]

- Atrial septal defect or patent foramen ovale
- Ventricular septal defect and pulmonary stenosis
- Pulmonary atresia
- Transposition of the great vessels (coarctation is common in this group—30%)[75]

Natural History

- Early death without intervention[6]

Treatment[1]

- PA band (surgical palliation to restrict flow to the pulmonary bed)
- Systemic-to-pulmonary shunt (surgical palliation to increase flow to the pulmonary bed)
- Balloon atrial septostomy (interventional catheterization to increase interatrial shunting)
- Park blade septostomy (interventional catheterization to increase interatrial shunting)
- Fontan procedure: definitive physiologic correction; the right atrium is connected to the PA by placement of a patch or conduit in the hope of increasing pulmonary flow[35]

Postoperative Echocardiographic Evaluation

- Assess right atrial contractility and adequacy of flow through the PA

Tricuspid Hypoplasia/Stenosis

Anatomy. There is a small tricuspid valve annulus, usually associated with critical pulmonary stenosis, pulmonary atresia with intact interventricular septum, or Ebstein's anomaly.[44]

Imperforate Tricuspid Valve

Anatomy. Membrane exists in place of a tricuspid valve, which may be surgically opened.[44]

MALFORMATION OF THE TRICUSPID VALVE

Ebstein's Anomaly of the Tricuspid Valve

Anatomy. The septal leaflet is tethered to the interventricular septum and attaches at least 8 mm distal to the tricuspid valve annulus.[32] Other tricuspid leaflets may also adhere to the ventricular wall and be dysplastic.[76] This malformation results in a large "functional" right atrium and small "functional" right ventricle. In Ebstein's anomaly, the tricuspid valve is "off-set" relative to the anterior leaflet of the mitral valve >0.8 mm/m^2.[77] The dysplastic nature of the leaflets and chordae prevents effective coaptation resulting in varying degrees of tricuspid insufficiency and stenosis.[44] Contractility of the right ventricle is affected by its size.

Hemodynamics. The right atrium is dilated because of the volume overload that results from the tricuspid regurgitation. The size of the right ventricle varies with the severity of tricuspid valve leaflet displacement.

Clinical Presentation.[6,24,76] Cyanosis, dyspnea, or exertion, and profound weakness or fatigue may be present.

- Physical exam: prominent left chest
- Auscultation: systolic and diastolic murmurs; loud, widely split first heart sound—"sail sound"; triple or quadruple rhythm
- ECG: right atrial hypertrophy; right bundle branch block; Wolff–Parkinson–White syndrome; paroxysmal supraventricular tachycardia
- Chest x-ray: enlarged heart; decreased pulmonary vascular markings; right atrial enlargement

Key Echocardiographic Concepts

- 2D delineation of the anatomy of the tricuspid valve and degree of displacement and tethering of each leaflet from parasternal short axis, apical four-chamber and subcostal long- and short-axis views[78]
- Determination of the size of the functional right ventricle—if less than 35% of the size of the anatomic right ventricle, prognosis is poor[32]
- Severity of tricuspid regurgitation
- Tricuspid valve closure delayed greater than 90 m/s after mitral valve closure on M-mode[32]

Associated Disease[6,76,78]

- Persistent patent ductus arteriosus
- Atrial septal defect or patent foramen ovale with right-to-left shunting

- Mitral valve prolapse
- Pulmonary stenosis
- Pulmonary atresia with intact ventricular septum
- Congenitally corrected transposition of the great vessels
- Ventricular septal defect

Natural History[6,76,78]

- Increased risk of endocarditis
- Prognosis is better with a larger functional right ventricle
- Prognosis is good if the child survives infancy but generally is poor if there are associated lesions

Treatment[6,76,78]

- Annuloplasty: repair of the valve annulus to make it smaller
- Valve replacement
- Valve repair
- Plication of some of the atrialized portion of the right ventricle

Postoperative Echocardiographic Evaluation

- Assess RV function and residual tricuspid insufficiency and/or stenosis

COMPLEX CONGENITAL HEART DISEASE

Tetralogy of Fallot

Anatomy. In this malformation, a large anterior malaligned ventricular septal defect is associated with malalignment of the aorta, so that the aortic root overrides the septal defect. The malalignment of the aortic root contributes to the infundibular pulmonary stenosis that occurs as part of this malformation.[66]

Hemodynamics. The large size of the ventricular septal defect allows equalization of left and RV pressures, so that the shunting through the defect is bidirectional. The overriding aorta receives blood from both ventricles, thereby mixing deoxygenated with oxygenated blood.

Clinical Presentation.[6,24] Cyanosis and a history of "tet spells" (transient cerebral ischemia resulting in limpness, paleness, and unconsciousness); history of squatting may present.

- Physical exam: prominent left chest, "clubbing" of fingers in older patients, RV heave
- Auscultation: single second heart sound; systolic ejection murmur
- ECG: RV hypertrophy; right axis deviation
- Chest x-ray: boot-shaped heart with decreased vascular markings

Key Echocardiographic Concepts[66]

- Assessment of cardiac position
- Assessment of atrial level communication and pulmonary venous return
- 2D visualization of large perimembranous ventricular septal defect and assessment of degree of aortic override
- 2D assessment of degree and levels of RV outflow obstruction
- Size of pulmonary valve annulus and morphology
- Size of PA and branches from high parasternal short axis and suprasternal notch views (aneurysmally dilated in cases of absent pulmonic valve)[79]
- Thickened RV free wall
- 2D delineation of coronary artery (rule out anomalous origin of left anterior descending artery [LAD] from the right coronary artery or other prominent branches crossing the RV outflow tract) and aortic arch anatomy to determine surgical approach[80]

Associated Disease[6,32,66,79]

- Valvular pulmonary stenosis or pulmonary atresia
- Congenitally absent pulmonic valve
- Right-sided aortic arch
- Atrioventricular malformation (Ebstein's malformation, mitral stenosis, common atrioventricular valve)
- Coronary artery anomalies
- Persistent left superior vena cava

Natural History.[6] Severe infundibular stenosis may result in a fatal "tet spell," in which the infundibulum becomes totally occluded. Recognition and surgical treatment have had a tremendous impact on the natural history of this disease, leaving now a population of adults with repaired tetralogy of Fallot that needs adequate imaging for follow-up.

Treatment[6]

- Palliation by surgical creation of a systemic-to-pulmonary shunt
- Patch closure of ventricular septal defect and possible myomectomy of the RV outflow tract, pulmonary valvotomy (valve sparing technique) or transannular patch repair

Postoperative Echocardiographic Evaluation

- Evaluation of patency of surgically created systemic-to-pulmonary shunt
- Evaluation of residual RV outflow obstruction and residual shunting around ventricular septal defect patch
- Evaluation of ventricular function
- Evaluation of degree of pulmonary regurgitation

Transposition of the Great Arteries

Anatomy. The aorta arises from the embryologic right ventricle, and the PA arises from the embryologic left ventricle. Terminology is listed as follows:

- D-transposition of the great arteries (D-TGA, frequently referred to simply as transposition of the great arteries or complete transposition): the ventricles are concordant with the atria; however, the aorta originates from the right ventricle and the PA originates from the embryologic left ventricle.
- Congenitally corrected transposition of the great arteries (L-transposition): ventricular inversion with the great vessels originating from the incorrect ventricle; blood flow sequence is normal; however, there is a high incidence of associated congenital heart disease.

Hemodynamics

- D-TGA: Blood flows in two parallel circuits. It flows from the systemic veins into the right atrium, through the tricuspid valve, into the right ventricle and out the aorta, to return again through the systemic veins. Pulmonary venous return flows into the left atrium, through the mitral valve into the left ventricle, and out the PA, to return again through the pulmonary veins. In short, deoxygenated blood flows in a continuous loop, and oxygenated blood flows in a separate continuous loop. Unless a communication exists between the systemic and pulmonary circulations (ie, an obligatory shunt), this situation is incompatible with life. In the newborn period, a left-to-right shunt occurs at the level of the foramen ovale and through a persistent ductus arteriosus, allowing mixing of oxygenated with deoxygenated blood.
- Congenitally corrected TGA: Blood flows in the normal sequence—from the systemic veins into the right atrium, through the mitral valve into the left ventricle, and out the PA, returns to the left atrium via the pulmonary veins, courses through the tricuspid valve, into the right ventricle and out the aorta.

Clinical Presentation for D-TGA.[6,24] Newborns become cyanotic, as the ductus arteriosus closes.

- Physical exam: normal weight, healthy-looking infant
- Auscultation: no murmurs; single second heart sound
- ECG: RV hypertrophy
- Chest x-ray: cardiomegaly; narrow mediastinum (egg on a string); increased vascular markings

Key Echocardiographic Concepts[81]

- Identify situs by delineating anatomic atrial landmarks on 2D

- Identify ventricular morphology (embryologic origins) by delineating anatomic landmarks on 2D
- Identify great vessel morphology and relationship (will course in parallel fashion)
- Identify and evaluate magnitude of shunt through the obligatory shunt defect(s)
- Delineate coronary artery anatomy for consideration of surgical approach[80]
- Identify and evaluate associated congenital heart disease

Associated Disease for D-TGA[32,81]

- Patent ductus arteriosus: obligatory shunt; most commonly associated with heart disease
- Aortic arch anomalies: coarctation, hypoplastic segment, interrupted aortic arch
- Atrial septal defect or patent foramen ovale: obligatory shunt
- Ventricular septal defect: obligatory shunt; with or without juxtaposed atrial appendages
- Outflow tract obstruction: fixed or dynamic; morphology of aortic and pulmonary valves; degree of aortic or pulmonary regurgitation
- Straddling atrioventricular valve: chordae from one atrioventricular valve attach into both ventricles
- Atrioventricular malformation: rare
- Pulmonary origin of coronary artery

Natural History. Patients with D-TGA must be palliated or repaired on an emergent basis because occlusion of the obligatory shunt would result in immediate death. The mortality rate in the absence of intervention is 95% at the end of 2 years of life.[16]

Patients with congenitally corrected transposition may never know they have congenital heart disease unless there is associated congenital heart disease, in which case, the natural history is determined by the associated disease.

Treatment[6,32,34]

Prostaglandin E₁ Treatment. Palliation; to keep ductus arteriosus patent until arterial switch can be performed.

Balloon Atrial Septostomy (Rashkind Procedure). Palliative interventional catheterization technique in which a distended balloon catheter is torn across a patent foramen ovale or small atrial septal defect creating a large atrial septal defect. Atrial level shunt is the most important site for adequate mixing.

Arterial Switch (Jatene Procedure). Surgical procedure in which the great arteries are taken off their trunks and moved so that each is re-anastomosed to the trunk that will restore a normal blood flow sequence; coronary arteries also are removed and re-implanted into the neoaorta.

Rastelli Procedure (Intraventricular Repair and Extracardiac Conduit). Surgical procedure in which a tunnel is constructed through a large ventricular septal defect so that the left ventricular outflow is directed to the aortic valve and a valved conduit is placed between the right ventricle and PA.

Mustard Procedure (Atrial Switch). The atrial switch (Mustard and Senning, see later) is no longer performed as a first line of choice for surgical repair; however, many adult patients with this type of repair survive. Surgical excision of the interatrial septum and placement of a baffle made of pericardium or synthetic material to redirect right atrial flow through the mitral valve into the left ventricle and allow pulmonary venous return to flow around the baffle into the tricuspid valve.

Senning Procedure (Atrial Switch). Surgical reconstruction of the atrial wall and interatrial septum to create an intra-atrial baffle redirecting venous flow through the atria.

Postoperative Echocardiographic Evaluation. Evaluation of left ventricular function.

- Balloon atrial septostomy: 2D visualization of definitive tear in the interatrial septum and calculation of atrial septal defect size to interatrial septal length ratio[16]
- Arterial switch operation: evaluate anastomotic sites of great arteries for possible constriction, assess intracardiac shunting and regional wall motion and coronary artery flow[6]
- Mustard and Senning procedures: rule out superior vena cava or pulmonary venous obstruction and baffle leaks[6,12] by PW Doppler, color-flow Doppler, or contrast echocardiography[40]

Truncus Arteriosus

Anatomy.[6,24] A rare malformation in which a single large great artery (common trunk) arises from the heart through a single semilunar valve and receives outflow from both ventricles. In most cases, the common trunk overrides the large ventricular septal defect, which must be present. The valve of the common trunk frequently has more than three cusps. Pulmonary circulation occurs in one of the following ways:

- Type I: main pulmonary trunk arises from the common trunk (usually from the posterior aspect) and bifurcates into right and left branches
- Type II: right and left PAs arise separately from the left posterolateral aspect of the common trunk
- Type III: right and left PAs arise separately from lateral aspects of the common trunk
- Type IV: no PAs exist; pulmonary circulation is through bronchiole arteries arising from the descending aorta

Hemodynamics.[6] The large ventricular septal defect causes equalization of pressures between the ventricles. Flow into the pulmonary circulation is at systemic pressures because the PAs arise from the aorta, and there is no pulmonary valve. There may be decreased flow to the pulmonary circulation if there is stenosis of the pulmonary branches or in type IV.

Clinical Presentation.[6,24] Patients are cyanotic.

- Physical exam: early congestive heart failure or hypoxic spells
- Auscultation: single second heart sound; systolic ejection click and murmur
- ECG: biventricular hypertrophy
- Chest x-ray: cardiomegaly; biventricular enlargement; wide mediastinum

Key Echocardiographic Concepts

- 2D delineation of anatomy:
  - Presence of atrial communication
  - Location and size of ventricular septal defect
  - Atrioventricular valve anatomy
  - Morphology of truncal valve
  - Evaluation of size of PAs
  - Additional sources of pulmonary blood flow
  - Aortic arch anatomy and branching
  - Coronary artery anatomy (relation to PA and truncal valve leaflets)
  - Associated lesions
- Color-flow and PW Doppler:
  - Truncal valve (rule out stenosis or insufficiency)
  - PAs (suprasternal notch views may be most helpful)
- Assessment of function and size of ventricles

Associated Disease.[6] Usually, truncus arteriosus is an isolated lesion.

- Right aortic arch
- Truncal valve stenosis and/or insufficiency
- Aortic arch anomalies
- Persistent patent ductus arteriosus
- Coronary ostial anomalies
- Absence of a branch PA on the side of the arch
- Persistent LSVC
- Anomalous pulmonary venous connections

Natural History.[6] If left untreated, death in infancy from heart failure or later from pulmonary vascular obstructive disease will result. Without intervention, survival beyond 1 year is unusual.

Treatment[6]

- Complete surgical repair involves closure of the ventricular septal defect and removal of the PAs from the aorta and placement of a valved conduit between the right ventricle and PAs. If coarctation or interrupted aortic arch is present, these are corrected at the same time.

Postoperative Echocardiographic Evaluation

- Evaluate truncal valve (now aortic valve) function
- Evaluate competency of the conduit valve and evaluate PA branches for stenosis
- Look for residual lesions (ventricular septal defects)
- Ventricular size and function
- Evaluate aortic arch

ANOMALIES OF THE CORONARY ARTERIES

Kawasaki's Syndrome (Mucocutaneous Lymph Node Syndrome)

Definition. Kawasaki's disease is an acute systemic vasculitis of unknown cause. It is a common form of acquired heart disease in the pediatric population. The acute phase of the illness features microvascular angiitis, endarteritis, and perivascular inflammation of coronary arteries. The subacute phase may have persistent panvasculitis of the coronary arteries. The convalescent phase shows resolution of the microvascular angiitis replaced by intimal thickening of the coronary arteries. In addition, the inflammatory process may involve pericarditis, myocarditis, and endocarditis.[82]

The proximal branches seem to be most frequently involved. Distal aneurysms may occur in addition, although rarely without proximal involvement.[83]

Clinical Presentation.[84] There is no diagnostic test for Kawasaki's disease, so the diagnosis is made clinically. It begins as a febrile illness of more than 5 days in children between 1 and 5 years. In addition to the fever, at least four of the following five findings are noted:

- Physical exam: (1) nonexudative bilateral conjunctivitis; (2) dry, fissured lips, strawberry tongue; (3) polymorphous truncal rash; erythema of palms and soles; (4) desquamation of fingertips and toes; (5) anterior cervical lymphadenopathy of 1.5 cm or greater.

Diagnosis can be made with fewer than four of five criteria in the presence of echocardiographic evidence of coronary involvement.

- Lab tests: elevated white count, platelet count, erythrocyte sedimentation rate, α_2-globulin, immunoglobulin E, transaminase, and lactic acid dehydrogenase
- ECG: infrequent, minimal changes

TABLE 3–1 • Echocardiographic Views Used to Evaluate Coronary Artery Anatomy	
Coronary Artery	**Echocardiographic View**
Proximal right, left main, proximal left anterior descending, proximal left circumflex	Parasternal short axis High parasternal short axis (caudal angle) Subcostal four coronal
Distal right coronary	Subcostal coronal (acute margin of heart) Subcostal short axis (sagittal) Posterior apical four chamber (posterior atrioventricular groove)
Posterior descending	Parasternal short axis Subcostal coronal Apical four chamber
Left circumflex	Parasternal short Parasternal long Subcostal sagittal
Distal left anterior descending	Parasternal long Parasternal short Subcostal coronal

(Data from references 5 and 46.)

Key Echocardiographic Concepts

Acute Phase[80,85]
- Left ventricular dysfunction
- Valvular regurgitation
- Pericardial effusion

Convalescent Phase
- 2D demonstration of saccular or fusiform coronary aneurysms (Table 3–1)
- Segmental wall motion abnormalities

Natural History. The majority of aneurysms resolve; however, those with diameters larger than 8 mm are at increased risk for thrombosis, which may result in myocardial infarction.[85] Other factors related to aneurysm regression are age younger than 1 year at diagnosis, saccular aneurysm, and distal aneurysm location. Giant aneurysms are more frequently associated with late sudden death from infarction.

Follow-up. Serial echocardiographic exams are performed at 2 weeks and again at 6–8 weeks after diagnosis. This is the time at which transient changes in coronary ectasia or dilatation will resolve or that aneurysms obtain their maximal size. Imaging of coronary arteries should be performed with the highest transducer frequency possible.

Treatment. Patients are treated with intravenous immunoglobulin and high-dose aspirin per day until defervescence, and then the aspirin is changed to a low dose for 6–8 weeks to decrease risk of thrombosis.

With persistent aneurysms, coronary angiography is indicated at intervals to determine whether coronary artery bypass surgery is indicated.[6]

Anomalous Origin of the Left Coronary Artery

Anatomy. A rare malformation in which the left coronary artery originates from the main PA rather than from the aortic root.[80]

Hemodynamics. In the newborn period, the myocardium of the left ventricle is inadequately perfused with oxygen because the blood flowing into the left coronary artery is deoxygenated blood from the PA when pulmonary vascular resistance is high; however, this does not cause ischemia. During the transitional period, when pulmonary vascular resistance and pressure decrease, flow in the left coronary becomes retrograde (from right coronary to left coronary via collaterals) and left coronary artery perfusion pressure decreases. This is the usual stage at presentation. Some may pass this stage and present as adults once myocardial ischemia is produced from "steal" phenomenon (left coronary artery drains right coronary blood into the PA).

Clinical Presentation.[80] It is symptomatic in infancy.

- Physical exam: irritable, dyspneic, tachypneic
- Auscultation: mitral insufficiency murmur
- ECG: left ventricular hypertrophy with anterolateral myocardial infarction and deep Q wave in lead I and aVL
- Chest x-ray: enlarged heart

Key Echocardiographic Concepts[80]

- 2D visualization of left coronary artery originating from the PA
- 2D visualization of a dilated right coronary artery originating from the right sinus of Valsalva
- PW Doppler or color-flow demonstration of diastolic flow entering the main PA just distal to the pulmonary valve
- Decreased left ventricular contractility
- Mitral insufficiency

Natural History. In the absence of intervention, permanent myocardial damage occurs.

Treatment. Surgery to reimplant the left coronary artery into the aortic root is recommended.[80]

Coronary Arteriovenous Fistula

Anatomy. A variably tortuous coronary artery courses along the surface of the heart or within the myocardium to empty into a cardiac chamber or great vessel. Generally, it is the right coronary artery (60%) that is involved, and the site of drainage is usually a right heart structure.[80]

Hemodynamics. Rather than perfusing the myocardium, blood from the coronary artery flows into the cardiac chamber or vessel into which it empties. The amount of blood that is "stolen" from the myocardium is small, evidenced by the rare presentation of myocardial ischemia. The physiology is more of a shunt and if fistula is large may cause symptoms of volume overload even in infancy.

Clinical Presentation. Generally, patients remain asymptomatic and are diagnosed after investigation of a murmur or incidentally during echocardiographic exam.[84,86]

- Auscultation: atypical continuous murmur

Key Echocardiographic Concepts[87]
- 2D demonstration of a dilated coronary artery
- 2D demonstration of origin, course, and site of drainage of the fistula
- Color-flow Doppler visualization and PW Doppler confirmation of a continuous, turbulent jet entering a cardiac chamber or great vessel in a location in which shunt lesions do not enter
- PW Doppler demonstration of turbulent late systolic, early diastolic flow in a dilated coronary artery supplying the fistula

Natural History[87]
- Spontaneous closure may occur
- Bacterial endocarditis
- Congestive heart failure due to volume overload and myocardial ischemia

Treatment. Elective surgical ligation of the fistula.[87]

Postoperative Echocardiographic Evaluation. Check for residual flow through the fistula.

VENOUS MALFORMATIONS

Persistent Left Superior Vena Cava

Anatomy. In this relatively common malformation (0.5% of the general population and 3–5% of patients with congenital heart disease), a superior vena cava persists in the left chest and travels in front of the LPA and between the LA appendage and left pulmonary veins. The left superior vena cava may empty into coronary sinus (62%), pulmonary venous atrium (21%), common atrium (17%), or rarely into a left-sided pulmonary vein. In most cases, there is also a right superior vena cava, and in 45–60% of cases, a communication exists between the two superior venae cavae.[88]

Hemodynamics. Systemic venous blood returns to the cardiac chamber to which the left superior vena cava connects. Deoxygenated blood mixes with oxygenated blood (right-to-left shunt) if the left superior vena cava drains into a left heart structure.

Key Echocardiographic Concepts[35]
- 2D and color-flow visualization of the left superior vena cava (from a high left parasagittal view)
- Dilated coronary sinus
- Contrast echocardiography to assess for unroofed coronary sinus or drainage into the left atrium[89]
- Absent or small innominate vein

Associated Disease[88]
- Atrial septal defect
- Complex congenital heart disease

Total Anomalous Pulmonary Venous Return

Anatomy. All of the pulmonary veins drain into systemic venous channels. The types of anomalous drainage are listed as follows[35,90]:

- Supracardiac: pulmonary veins drain in a confluence behind the left atrium and through a vertical vein empty into the innominate vein, superior vena cava, or occasionally the azygous vein. The vertical vein travels usually in front of the PA.
- Cardiac: pulmonary veins drain into the right atrium or coronary sinus
- Infracardiac: pulmonary veins form a collection behind the heart and by a common vein descend below the diaphragm and empties into the portal vein, ductus venosus or hepatic vein, reentering the heart through the inferior vena cava. On echocardiogram there is the appearance of an inverted Christmas tree.
- Mixed: a combination of any of the above

Hemodynamics. There is increased flow into a systemic vein, right atrium, or coronary sinus,[90] and ultimately, the right heart. There is an obligatory right-to-left shunt at the atrial level with complete mixing (all chambers will have the same saturation)[24,91]

Clinical Presentation Without Obstruction.[24] There is mild cyanosis; usually asymptomatic.

- Physical exam: poor growth; prominent left chest; RV heave and hepatomegaly
- Auscultation: fixed, widely split second sound
- ECG: RV hypertrophy
- Chest x-ray: enlarged right heart; increased pulmonary vascular markings; snowman- or figure 8–shaped mediastinum

Clinical Presentation in the Presence of Obstruction.[24] Patients are acutely ill; there is cyanosis; symptomatic with respiratory distress during the newborn period.

- Physical exam: tachypnea; dyspnea; RV failure
- Auscultation: no murmurs
- ECG: RV hypertrophy
- Chest x-ray: normal size heart; increased pulmonary vascular markings

Key Echocardiographic Concepts[36,90]
- Determine the number of pulmonary veins, their connections, and drainage by 2D and color Doppler
- Visualization of all systemic venous return to the heart including left innominate vein, superior vena cava, inferior vena cava, and coronary sinus
- Assessment of position and patency of the atrial septum
- Color-flow Doppler interrogation of anomalous venous structures to rule out obstruction, direction of flow direction, as well as restriction of the atrial septum by color-flow and spectral Doppler
- Assessment of RV dysfunction and RV or pulmonary hypertension

Associated Disease
- Atrial septal defect

Natural History.[24] Obstruction of the common vein or entry into a systemic venous structure will result in pulmonary edema and right heart failure, complete obstruction will cause death. Eventually, pulmonary vascular obstructive disease will develop.

Treatment. Surgical anastomosis of the common vein with the left atrium and closure of the atrial communication are the indicated treatment.

Postoperative Echocardiographic Evaluation
- Assessment of RV size and function
- Evaluate area of anastomosis and individual pulmonary veins to rule out obstruction. Usually apical views are the best for assessment of the pulmonary venous confluence;

individual veins are best seen in subcostal, high parasternal, and suprasternal views.

- Evaluation of right heart and PA pressure

TRANSESOPHAGEAL ECHOCARDIOGRAPHY

Transesophageal echocardiography (TEE) is a more invasive echo technique that requires sedation of the patient. A biplane or multiplane echo probe, similar to an endoscope, allows visualization of the heart from the esophagus and stomach. Most of the ultrasound's limiting factors are removed in this technique like lung and bone, allowing for much better imaging and resolution.

Indications: TEE is becoming a standard of care in the operating room during pediatric cardiovascular procedures. It enables the surgeon to delineate anatomy before surgery and evaluate repair effectiveness after surgery and is known to demonstrate anatomic details missed by transthoracic imaging and alter the surgical plan.[92] TEE allows the probe to be left in the patient for the entire procedure with continuous monitoring, although images and hemodynamics are better assessed once reduced or the patient is off cardiopulmonary bypass. Comparison of the preoperative and postoperative left ventricular systolic function has proved helpful in perioperative medical management. Intraoperative TEE is most commonly performed by the echocardiographer or an anesthesiologist.

Routine TEE is performed in cases where acceptable images are not obtained by transthoracic echocardiography (TTE) due to poor acoustic windows (large patients, open chest after surgery, etc.). TEE is superior to TTE in most of these cases, allowing better visualization of valve apparatus, interatrial septum, and most other cardiac structures. Anterior structures such as the RV outflow tract, pulmonary valve, or anterior muscular ventricular septal defects or structures close to an adjacent airway (like the LPA and transverse aortic arch) can be difficult to visualize.

TEE is invaluable in situations where assessment of intracardiac vegetations or thrombus is required in patients with poor echocardiographic windows, as well as in the guidance of catheterization procedures such as device closure of atrial and ventricular septal defects or stenting and ballooning complex venous baffles or outflow tract obstruction.[93]

The review of the guidelines for TEE in children is beyond the scope of this chapter but may be accessed by the interested reader from the American Society of Echocardiography.[94]

HYPERTENSION

Long recognized as a contributor to heart disease in adults, hypertension is being diagnosed much more frequently in pediatric patients than in the recent past. Echocardiography is required to assess the effect on the heart.

Clinical Presentation

- Normally asymptomatic and usually noted during routine examinations

Hemodynamics

- In adults, systolic and diastolic pressures may be elevated.

Key Echocardiographic Findings

- Long-standing hypertension can result in left ventricular hypertrophy and increased left ventricular mass, resulting in impaired left ventricular filling.
- Careful evaluation of the patency of the aortic arch is required to exclude clinically unrecognized coarctation of the aorta

Natural History

- Untreated hypertension will result in myriad cardiac abnormalities, including left ventricular outflow obstruction, coronary artery disease, stroke, and kidney failure.

CHEST PAIN AND FATIGUE

Chest pain and fatigue are fairly common complaints among older children and adolescents. The cause is seldom cardiac and usually not serious. However, if cardiac causes are present, they are generally serious.

Causes of Cardiac Chest Pain in Children

1. Congenital coronary abnormalities (rare, associated with exercise, explained by ischemia)
   a. Anomalous coronary origin (left main coronary artery from right coronary artery—left main coronary artery is compressed between great vessels)
   b. Coronary fistula (rare—may cause ischemia from steal phenomenon)
2. Acquired coronary disease
   a. Kawasaki's disease (residual critical narrowing of coronary arteries)
   b. Emboli
3. Aortic stenosis
4. Cardiomyopathy
   a. Hypertrophic cardiomyopathy
   b. Dilated cardiomyopathy
5. Pericarditis
6. Rhythm abnormalities

As previously stated, these are rare, but their seriousness requires that the echo exam for chest pain in children must be accurate and comprehensive. Particular attention should be paid to the coronary arteries.

Fatigue in children is also rarely cardiac related, but some cardiac findings may include the following:

- Dilated cardiomyopathy
- Hypertrophic cardiomyopathy
- Shunts
- Aortic stenosis
- Pulmonic stenosis

As in cases of chest pain, a complete echo exam is required to rule out any cardiac source.

References

1. Anderson R, Ho SY. Echocardiographic diagnosis and description of congenital heart disease: anatomic principles and philosophy. In: St. John Sutton M, Oldershaw PJ, eds. *Textbook of Adult and Pediatric Echocardiography and Doppler.* Boston: Blackwell Scientific; 1989:573-606.
2. Silverman NS, Araujo LML. An echocardiographic method for the diagnosis of cardiac situs and malpositions. *Echocardiography.* 1987;4:35-57.
3. Foale R, Stefanini L, Rickards A, et al. Left and right ventricular morphology in complex congenital heart disease defined by two-dimensional echocardiography. *Am J Cardiol.* 1982;49:93.
4. Sutherland GR, Smallhorn JF, Anderson RH, et al. Atrioventricular discordance: cross-sectional echocardiographic morphological correlative study. *Br Heart J.* 1983;50:8.
5. Tani L, Ludomirsky A, Murphy DJ, et al. Ventricular morphology: echocardiographic evaluation of isolated ventricular inversion. *Echocardiography.* 1988;5:39-42.
6. Adams FH, Emmanouilides GC, Riemenschneider TA, eds. *Moss' Heart Disease in Infants, Children, & Adolescents.* 4th ed. Baltimore: Williams & Wilkins; 1989.
7. Hatle L, Angelsen B. *Doppler Ultrasound in Cardiology: Physical Principles and Clinical Applications.* 2nd ed. Philadelphia: Lea & Febiger; 1985.
8. Sahn DJ, Valdes-Cruz LM. Ultrasound Doppler methods for calculating cardiac volume flows, cardiac output and cardiac shunts. In: Kotler MN, Steiner RM, eds. *Cardiac Imaging: New Technologies and Clinical Applications.* Philadelphia: FA Davis; 1986:19-31.
9. Cloez JL, Schmidt KG, Birk E, Silverman NS. Determination of pulmonary to systemic blood flow ratio in children by a simplified Doppler echocardiographic method. *J Am Coll Cardiol.* 1987;11:825-830.
10. Stevenson JG. Doppler evaluation of atrial septal defect, ventricular septal defect, and complex malformations. *Acta Paediatr Scand.* 1986;329 (suppl):21-43.
11. Stevenson JG. The use of Doppler echocardiography for detection and estimation of severity of patent ductus arteriosus, ventricular septal defect and atrial septal defect. *Echocardiography.* 1987;4:321-346.
12. Silverman NH, Schmidt KG. The current role of Doppler echocardiography in the diagnosis of heart disease in children. *Cardiol Clin.* 1989;7:265-297.
13. Fuster V, Driscoll DJ, McGoon DC. Congenital heart disease in adolescents and adults. In: Brandenburg RO, Fuster V, Giulani ER, McGoon DC, eds. *Cardiology: Fundamentals and Practice.* Chicago: Year Book Medical; 1987:1386-1458.
14. Bustamante-Labarta M, Perrone S, Leon de la Fuente R, et al. Right atrial size and tricuspid regurgitation severity predict mortality or

transplantation in primary pulmonary hypertension. *J Am Soc Echocardiogr.* 2002;15:1160-1164.

15. Kosturakis D, Goldberg SJ, Allen HD, et al. Doppler echocardiographic prediction of pulmonary arterial hypertension in congenital heart disease. *Am J Cardiol.* 1984;53:1110-1114.

16. Marantz P, Capelli H, Ludomirsky A, et al. Echocardiographic assessment of balloon atrial septostomy in patients with transposition of the great arteries: prediction of the need for early surgery. *Echocardiography.* 1988;5:99-104.

17. Weyman AE, Dillon JC, Feigenbaum H, et al. Echocardiographic patterns of pulmonic valve motion with pulmonary hypertension. *Circulation.* 1974;50:905-910.

18. Stevenson JG. Comparison of several noninvasive methods for estimation of pulmonary artery pressure. *J Am Soc Echo.* 1989;2:157-171.

19. Yock PG, Popp RL. Noninvasive estimation of right ventricular systolic pressure by Doppler ultrasound in patients with tricuspid regurgitation. *Circulation.* 1984;70:657-662.

20. Beard JT, Byrd BF. Saline contrast enhancement of trivial Doppler tricuspid regurgitation signals for estimating pulmonary artery pressure. *Am J Cardiol.* 1988;62:486-488.

21. Masuyama T, Kodama D, Kitabatake A, et al. Continuous wave Doppler echocardiographic detection of pulmonary regurgitation and its application to noninvasive estimation of pulmonary artery pressure. *Circulation.* 1986;74:484-492.

22. Friedberg MK, Feinstein JA, Rosenthal DN. A novel echocardiographic Doppler method for estimation of pulmonary arterial pressures. *J Am Soc Echocardiogr.* 2006;19:559-562.

23. Kitabatake A, Inoue M, Asao M, et al. Noninvasive evaluation of pulmonary hypertension by a pulse Doppler technique. *Circulation.* 1983;68:302-309.

24. Fink, BW. *Congenital Heart Disease: A Deductive Approach to Its Diagnosis.* 2nd ed. Chicago: Year Book Medical; 1985.

25. Sahn DJ, Allen HD. Real-time cross-sectional echocardiographic imaging and measurement of the patent ductus arteriosus in infants and children. *Circulation.* 1978;58:343-354.

26. Seward JB, Tajik AJ, Edwards WD, Hagler DJ. *Two-Dimensional Echocardiographic Atlas.* vol I: *Congenital Heart Disease.* New York: Springer; 1987.

27. Smallhorn JF. Patent ductus arteriosus—evaluation by echocardiography. *Echocardiography.* 1987;4:101-118.

28. Smallhorn JF, Huhta JC, Anderson RH, et al. Suprasternal cross-sectional echocardiography in assessment of patent ductus arteriosus. *Br Heart J.* 1982;48:321-330.

29. Kyo S. Congenital heart disease. In: Omoto R, ed. *Color Atlas of Real-Time Two-Dimensional Doppler Echocardiography.* 2nd ed. Philadelphia: Lea & Febiger; 1987:149-209.

30. Ritter SB. Application of Doppler color flow mapping in the assessment and the evaluation of congenital heart disease. *Echocardiography.* 1987;4:543-556.

31. Snider AR. Doppler echocardiography in congenital heart disease. In: Berger M, ed. *Doppler Echocardiography in Heart Disease.* New York: Marcel Dekker; 1987.

32. Armstrong, WF. Congenital heart disease. In: Feigenbaum H, ed. *Echocardiography.* 4th ed. Philadelphia: Lea & Febiger; 1986:365-461.

33. Perry SB, Keane JF, Lock JE. Interventional catheterization in pediatric congenital and acquired heart disease. *Am J Cardiol.* 1988;61:109G-117G.

34. NeSmith J, Philips J. The sonographer's beginning guide to surgery for congenital heart disease. *J Am Soc Echo.* 1988;1:384-387.

35. Sanders SP. Echocardiography and related techniques in the diagnosis of congenital heart defects. Part I: Veins, atria and interatrial septum. *Echocardiography.* 1984;1:185-217.

36. Schmidt KG, Silverman NH. Cross-sectional and contrast echocardiography in the diagnosis of interatrial communications through the coronary sinus. *Int J Cardiol.* 1987;16:193-199.

37. Lin F, Fu M, Yeh, S, et al. Doppler atrial shunt flow patterns in patients with secundum atrial septal defect: determinants, limitations and pitfalls. *J Am Soc Echo.* 1988;1:141-149.

38. Fraker TD, Harris PJ, Behar VS, et al. Detection and exclusion of interatrial shunts by two-dimensional echocardiography and peripheral venous injection. *Circulation.* 1979;59:379-384.

39. Valdez-Cruz LM, Sahn DJ. Ultrasonic contrast studies for the detection of cardiac shunts. *J Am Coll Cardiol.* 1984;3:978-985.

40. Van Hare GF, Silverman NH. Contrast two-dimensional echocardiography in congenital heart disease: techniques, indications and clinical utility. *J Am Coll Cardiol.* 1989;13:673-686.

41. Hsiao JF, Hsu LA, Chang CJ, et al. Late migration of septal occluder device for closure of atrial septal defect into the left atrium and mitral valve obstruction. *Am J Cardiol.* 2007;99:1479-1480.

42. Meier B. Iatrogenic atrial septal defect, erosion of the septum primum after device closure of a patent foramen ovale as a new medical entity. *Catheter Cardiovasc Interv.* 2006;68:165-168.

43. Baykut D, Doerge SE, Grapow M, et al. Late perforation of the aortic root by an atrial septal defect occlusion device. *Ann Thorac Surg.* 2005;79:e28.

44. Sanders SP. Echocardiography and related techniques in the diagnosis of congenital heart defects. Part II: Atrioventricular valves and ventricles. *Echocardiography.* 1984;1:333-391.

45. Goldfarb BL, Wanderman KL, Rovner M, et al. Ventricular septal defect with left ventricular to right atrial shunt: documentation by color flow Doppler and avoidance of the pitfall of the diagnosis of tricuspid regurgitation and pulmonary hypertension. *Echocardiography.* 1989;6:521-525.

46. Ritter S, Rothe W, Kawai D, et al. Identification of ventricular septal defects by Doppler color flow mapping. *Clin Res.* 1988; 36:311A.

47. Stevenson JG, Kawabori I, Dooley T, et al. Diagnosis of ventricular septal defects by pulsed Doppler echocardiography. *Circulation.* 1978;58:322-326.

48. Murphy DJ, Ludomirsky A, Huhta JC. Continuous-wave Doppler in children with ventricular septal defect: noninvasive estimation of interventricular pressure gradient. *Am J Cardiol.* 1986;57:428-432.

49. Schmidt KG, Cassidy SC, Silverman, NH. Doubly committed subarterial ventricular septal defects: echocardiographic features and surgical implications. *Am Coll Cardiol.* 1988;12:1538-1546.

50. Silverman NH, Zuberbuhler JR, Anderson RH. Atrioventricular septal defects: Cross-sectional echocardiographic and morphologic comparisons. *Int J Cardiol.* 1986;13:309-331.

51. Lai W, Mertens L, Cohen M, et al. *Echocardiography in pediatric and congenital heart disease from fetus to adult.* Wiley-Blackwell; 2009.230-248.

52. Chambers J. Low "gradient," low flow aortic stenosis. *Heart.* 2006;92:554-558.

53. Brenner JI, Baker KR, Berman MA. Prediction of left ventricular pressure in infants with aortic stenosis. *Br Heart J.* 1980;44:406-410.

54. Rakowski H, Sasson Z, Wigle ED. Echocardiographic and Doppler assessment of hypertrophic cardiomyopathy. *J Am Soc Echo.* 1988;1:31-47.

55. McKay RG. Balloon valvuloplasty for treating pulmonic, mitral, and aortic valve stenosis. *Am J Cardiol.* 1988;61:102G-108G.

56. Sweeney MS, Walker WE, Cooley DA, et al. Apicoaortic conduits for complex left ventricular outflow obstruction: 10-year experience. *Ann Thorac Surg.* 1986;42:609-611.

57. Marek J, Fenton M, Khambadkone S. Aortic arch anomalies: Coarctation of the aorta and interrupted aortic arch. In: Lai W, Mertens L, et al, eds. *Echocardiography in Pediatric and Congenital Heart Disease—From Fetus to Adult.* Wiley-Blackwell; 2009: 339-361.

58. Huhta JC, Gutgesell HP, Latson LA, et al. Two-dimensional echocardiographic assessment of the aorta in infants and children with congenital heart disease. *Circulation.* 1984;70:417-424.

59. Nihoyannopoulos P, Karas S, Sapsford RN, et al. Accuracy of two-dimensional echocardiography in the diagnosis of aortic arch obstruction. *J Am Coll Cardiol.* 1987;10:1072-1077.

60. George B, DiSessa TG, Williams R, et al. Coarctation repair without cardiac catheterization in infants. *Am Heart J.* 1987;114: 1421-1425.

61. Pfammatter JP, Ziemer G, Kaulitz R, et al. Isolated aortic coarctation in neonates and infants: results of resection and end to end anastomosis. *Ann Thorac Surg.* 1996;62:778-782.

62. Redington AN, Booth P, Shore DF, Rigby ML. Primary balloon dilatation of coarctation of the aorta in neonates. *Br Heart J.* 1990;64:277-281.

63. Bash SE, Huhta JC, Vick GW, et al. Hypoplastic left heart syndrome: is echocardiography accurate enough to guide surgical palliation? *J Am Coll Cardiol.* 1986;7:610-616.

64. Cassidy SC, Van Hare GF, Silverman NH. The probability of detecting a subaortic ridge in children with ventricular septal defect or coarctation of the aorta. *Am J Cardiol.* 1990;66:505-508.

65. Burrows PE, Freedom RM, Rabinovitch M, et al. The investigation of abnormal pulmonary arteries in congenital heart disease. *Radiol Clin North Am.* 1985;23:689-717.

66. Smallhorn J. Right ventricular outflow tract obstruction. In: St. John Sutton M, Oldershaw P, eds. *Textbook of Adult and Pediatric Echocardiography and Doppler.* Boston: Blackwell Scientific; 1989:761-790.

67. Frantz EG, Silverman NH. Doppler ultrasound evaluation of valvar pulmonary stenosis from multiple transducer positions in children requiring pulmonary valvuloplasty. *Am J Cardiol.* 1988;61:844-849.

68. Tynan M, Anderson RH. Pulmonary stenosis. In: Anderson RH, Baker EJ, MacCarthy FJ, et al, eds. *Pediatric Cardiology.* 2nd ed. London: Harcourt; 2002:1461-1479.

69. Levine J. Pulmonary atresia with intact ventricular septum. In: Lai W, Mertens L, et al, eds. *Echocardiography in Pediatric and Congenital Heart Disease—from Fetus to Adult.* Wiley-Blackwell; 2009:264-279.

70. Minich LL, Tani LY, Ritter S, et al. Usefulness of the preoperative tricuspid/mitral valve ratio for predicting outcome in pulmonary atresia with intact ventricular septum. *Am J Cardiol.* 2000;85:1319-1324.

71. Hanley FL, Sade RM, Blackstone EH, et al. Outcomes in neonatal pulmonary atresia with intact ventricular septum. A multi-institutional study. *J Thorac Cardiovascular Surg.* 1993;105:406-423.

72. Sullivan ID, Robinson PJ, DeLeval M, et al. Membranous supravalvular mitral stenosis: a treatable form of congenital heart disease. *J Am Coll Cardiol.* 1986;8:159-164.

73. Lipshultz SE, Sanders SP, Mayer JE, et al. Are routine preoperative cardiac catheterization and angiography necessary before repair of ostium primum atrial septal defect? *J Am Coll Cardiol.* 1988;11:373-378.

74. Geggel RL, Fyler DC. Mitral valve and left atrial lesions. In: Keane J, Lock J, Fyler D, eds. *Nadas' Pediatric Cardiology.* 2nd ed. St. Louis, MO: Saunders Elsevier 2006:697-714.

75. Keane JF, Fyler DC. Tricuspid atresia. In: Keane J, Lock J, Fyler D, eds. *Nadas' Pediatric Cardiology.* 2nd ed. St. Louis, MO: Saunders Elsevier 2006:753-758.

76. Zuberbuhler JR, Anderson RH. Ebstein's malformation of the tricuspid valve: morphology and natural history. In: Anderson RH, Neches WH, Park SC, Zuberbuhler JR, eds. *Perspectives in Pediatric Cardiology.* Mt. Kisco, NY: Futura Publishing; 1988:99-112.

77. Shiina A, Seward JB, Edwards WD, et al. Two-dimensional echocardiographic spectrum of Ebstein anomaly: detailed anatomic assessment. *J Am Coll Cardiol.* 1984;3:356-370.

78. Silverman NS, Birk E. Ebstein's malformation of the tricuspid valve: cross-sectional echocardiography and Doppler. In: Anderson RH, Neches WH, Park SC, Zuberbuhler JR, eds. *Perspectives in Pediatric Cardiology.* Mt. Kisco, NY: Futura Publishing; 1988:113-125.

79. McIrvin DM, Murphy DJ, Ludomirsky A. Tetralogy of Fallot with absent pulmonary valve. *Echocardiography.* 1989;6:363-367.

80. Caldwell RL, Ensing GJ. Coronary artery abnormalities in children. *J Am Soc Echo.* 1989;2:259-268.

81. Smallhorn J. Complete transposition. In: St. John Sutton M, Oldershaw P, eds. *Textbook of Adult and Pediatric Echocardiography and Doppler.* Boston: Blackwell Scientific; 1989:791-808.

82. Yutani C, Go S, Kamiya T, et al. Cardiac biopsy of Kawasaki disease. *Arch Pathol Lab Med.* 1981;105:470-473.

83. Neches WH. Kawasaki syndrome. In: Anderson RH, Neches WH, Park SC, Zuberbuhler JR, eds. *Perspectives in Pediatric Cardiology.* Mt. Kisco, NY: Futura Publishing; 1988:411-424.

84. Lloyd TR, Mahoney LT, Marvin WJ, et al. Identification of coronary artery to right ventricular fistulae by color flow mapping. *Echocardiography.* 1988;5:115-120.

85. Meyer RA. Echocardiography in Kawasaki disease. *J Am Soc Echo.* 1989;2:269-275.

86. Keane JF, Fyler DC. Vascular fistulae. In: Keane J, Lock J, Fyler D, eds. *Nadas' Pediatric Cardiology.* 2nd ed. St. Louis, MO: Saunders Elsevier; 2006:799-804.

87. Velvis H, Schmidt KG, Silverman NH, et al. Diagnosis of coronary artery fistula by two-dimensional echocardiography pulsed Doppler ultrasound and color flow imaging. *J Am Coll Cardiol.* 1989;14:968-976.

88. Zellers TM, Hagler DJ, Julsrud PR. Accuracy of two-dimensional echocardiography in diagnosing left superior vena cava. *J Am Soc Echo.* 1989;2:132-138.

89. Huhta, JC, Smallhorn JF, Macartney FJ, et al. Cross-sectional echocardiographic diagnosis of systemic venous return. *Br Heart J.* 1980;44:718-723.

188 CHAPTER 3 Pediatric Echocardiography

90. Van Hare GF, Schmidt KG, Cassidy SC, et al. Color Doppler flow mapping in the ultrasound diagnosis of total anomalous pulmonary venous connection. *J Am Soc Echo*. 1988;1:341-347.

91. Keane JF, Fyler DC. Total anomalous pulmonary venous return. In: Keane J, Lock J, Fyler D, eds. *Nadas' Pediatric Cardiology*. 2nd ed. St. Louis, MO: Saunders Elsevier; 2006:773-781.

92. Randolph GR, Hagler DJ, Connoly HM, et al. Intraoperative transesophageal echocardiography during surgery for congenital heart defects. *J Thorac Cardiovasc Surg*. 2002;124:1176.

93. van der Velde EA. Echocardiography in the catheterization laboratory. In: Lock JE, Keane JF, Perry SB, eds. *Diagnostic and Interventional Catheterization in Congenital Heart Disease*. Norwell, MA: Kluwer Academic Publishers; 2000:355.

94. Fyfe DA, Ritter SB, Snider AR, et al. Guidelines for transesophageal echocardiography in children. *J Am Soc Echocardiogr*. 1992;5:640.

Questions

GENERAL INSTRUCTIONS: For each question, select the best answer. Select only one answer for each question unless otherwise specified.

1. What is the most common type of atrial septal defect?

   (A) primum

   (B) secundum

   (C) sinus venosus

   (D) single atrium

2. Which transducer position is most helpful in the 2D visualization of atrial septal defects?

   (A) left parasternal

   (B) apical

   (C) subxiphoid

   (D) right parasternal

3. Partial anomalous pulmonary venous return is most commonly associated with which type of atrial septal defect?

   (A) secundum

   (B) primum

   (C) sinus venosus

   (D) coronary sinus

4. What is the most common congenital heart lesion in the pediatric population?

   (A) mitral stenosis

   (B) atrial septal defect

   (C) ventricular septal defect

   (D) pulmonary stenosis

5. A "T-sign" artifact demonstrated by _____ is useful in the detection of ventricular septal defects.

   (A) M-mode

   (B) 2D

   (C) PW Doppler

   (D) CW Doppler

   (E) color-flow Doppler

6. A small muscular ventricular septal defect may be most easily localized by which of the following?

   (A) M-mode

   (B) 2D

   (C) PW Doppler

   (D) CW Doppler

   (E) color-flow Doppler

7. Which of the following will *not* cause a reversal of flow in the descending aorta during diastole?

   (A) large patent ductus arteriosus with severe pulmonary hypertension (suprasystemic pulmonary pressures)

   (B) severe aortic insufficiency

   (C) surgically created systemic-to-pulmonary shunt with normal PA pressures

   (D) large patent ductus arteriosus with normal PA pressures

8. Which of the following may be associated with valvar aortic stenosis?

   (A) patent ductus arteriosus

   (B) coarctation of the aorta

   (C) ventricular septal defect

   (D) pulmonary stenosis

   (E) all of the above

9. Which of the following is the most commonly associated findings in patients with coarctation of the aorta?

   (A) ventricular septal defect

   (B) bicuspid aortic valve

   (C) patent ductus arteriosus

   (D) aortic stenosis

   (E) mitral stenosis

10. In the normally related heart, where does the aortic valve lie?

    (A) anterior and to the left of the pulmonary valve

    (B) anterior and to the right of the pulmonary valve

    (C) posterior and to the right of the pulmonary valve

    (D) posterior and to the left of the pulmonary valve

11. Which of the following surgical procedures is *not* frequently used to treat transposition of the great arteries?

    (A) Senning procedure

    (B) Mustard procedure

    (C) arterial switch procedure

    (D) Fontan procedure

12. Which of the following is also known as the arterial switch procedure?

    (A) Rashkind procedure

    (B) Mustard procedure

    (C) Jatene procedure

    (D) Senning procedure

13. When the aorta and PA are transposed, they course _____ as they exit the heart.

    (A) parallel to each other

    (B) perpendicular to each other

    (C) wound around each other

    (D) in no particular relationship to each other

14. Balloon atrial septostomy is most commonly performed in infants who have which of the following?

    (A) Ebstein's anomaly of the tricuspid valve

    (B) transposition of the great arteries

    (C) truncus arteriosus

    (D) tetralogy of Fallot

15. Of all children who suffer from Kawasaki's disease, what percentage will develop coronary artery aneurysms?

    (A) 2%

    (B) 15%

    (C) 50%

    (D) 75%

16. Which of the following groups is most likely to develop coronary artery aneurysms as a complication of Kawasaki's disease?

    (A) toddlers

    (B) infants

    (C) adolescents

    (D) adults

17. Which of the following is useful in the assessment of PA pressure?

    (A) peak Doppler gradient through a patent ductus arteriosus

    (B) peak Doppler gradient of tricuspid regurgitation

    (C) end-diastolic Doppler gradient of pulmonary insufficiency

    (D) AcT-to-ET ratio calculated from an RV outflow tract velocity curve

    (E) all of the above are useful in estimating PA pressure

18. A child with tetralogy of Fallot is upset and crying during the echocardiogram. The Doppler gradient through the RV outflow tract will be _____ than if the child were sleeping peacefully.

    (A) greater

    (B) less

    (C) not affected by the patient's activity

    (D) none of the above

19. A 3-year old child with Kawasaki's disease undergoes an echocardiogram. Which of the following views is *not* really necessary in the 2D evaluation of the coronary arterial system?

    (A) subcostal transverse

    (B) parasternal short axis

    (C) apical five chamber

    (D) all views are helpful

20. Which of the following Doppler findings is *not* characteristic of coarctation of the aorta?

    (A) forward flow through the descending aorta extending throughout diastole

    (B) normal or slightly increased velocity of flow in the aorta proximal to the left subclavian artery

    (C) rapid acceleration and deceleration of the Doppler signal taken from the descending aorta

    (D) Doppler signal from the descending aorta does not return to baseline during diastole

21. Careful echocardiographic evaluation of a child with complex congenital heart disease reveals absence of the inferior vena cava above the level of the renal arteries. The aorta is to the left of the spine. What is this child's situs mostly likely to be?

   (A) solitus
   (B) inversus
   (C) LA isomerism
   (D) right atrial isomerism

22. Which of the following characteristics will be demonstrated on the aortic valve M-mode tracing from a patient with discrete membranous subaortic stenosis?

   (A) asymmetric closure line
   (B) early closure and partial reopening
   (C) gradual closure (drifting closed)
   (D) prolonged ET

23. Which of the following should *not* be included in the differential diagnosis when a Doppler tracing such as that in Fig. 3–1 is obtained from the descending aorta?

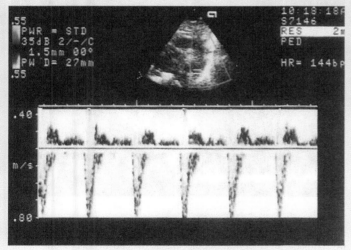

FIGURE 3–1. Pulsed Doppler spectral tracing of flow in the descending aorta as obtained from the suprasternal notch view.

   (A) patent ductus arteriosus
   (B) severe aortic regurgitation
   (C) arteriovenous malformation
   (D) aortic to pulmonary window
   (E) coarctation of the aorta

24. An echocardiogram was requested for a premature infant in the neonatal intensive care unit who appeared clinically to be in congestive failure and in whom a murmur was heard. The color-flow Doppler image in Fig. 3–2 was taken from the ductus view, which is a parasternal sagittal view. The closed aortic valve may be appreciated in the center of the image. What does this image demonstrate?

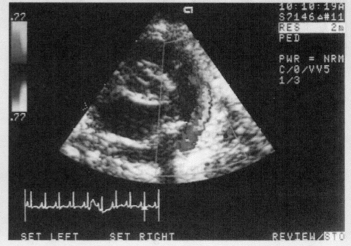

FIGURE 3–2. Color-flow Doppler image of a modified short-axis parasternal view, known as the "ductus view." The patient is a premature infant in congestive heart failure in whom a murmur is heard.

   (A) a small patent ductus arteriosus
   (B) a moderate patent ductus arteriosus
   (C) a large patent ductus arteriosus
   (D) no ductus arteriosus

25. **The image in Fig. 3–3 was taken from an 8-month-old female child with trisomy 21. The color-flow Doppler image was taken from the subcostal four-chamber view. What does the image demonstrate?**

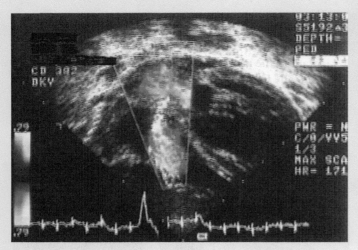

FIGURE 3–3. Color-flow Doppler image of a subcostal four-chamber view presented with the apex down (anatomically correct) presentation. The patient is an 8-month-old female with trisomy 21.

(A) a left-to-right shunt through a primum atrial septal defect

(B) a right-to-left shunt through a primum atrial septal defect

(C) a left-to-right shunt through a secundum atrial septal defect

(D) a right-to-left shunt through a secundum atrial septal defect

26. **The images presented in Fig. 3–4 were taken from the cardiac apex of a cyanotic infant. What do these images demonstrate?**

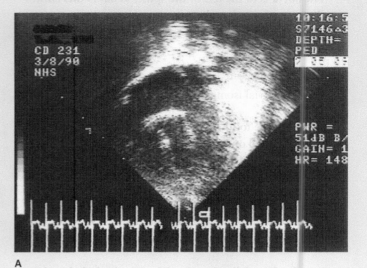

A

B

FIGURE 3–4. Apical four-chamber view presented with the apex down. (A) 2D image. (B) Color-flow Doppler image. The patient is a cyanotic infant.

(A) a normal heart

(B) an isolated inflow ventricular septal defect

(C) single atrium

(D) tricuspid atresia with ventricular septal defect

27. The color-flow Doppler image presented in Fig. 3–5 was taken from an 8-year-old boy with a systolic murmur. The image is of the parasternal short-axis view during early systole and demonstrates a left-to-right shunt through which of the following?

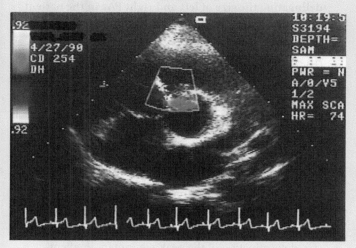

FIGURE 3–5. Color-flow Doppler image of the parasternal short-axis view at the level of the semilunar valves taken in early systole. The patient is an 8-year-old boy in whom a systolic murmur may be heard.

(A) inflow ventricular septal defect

(B) membranous ventricular septal defect

(C) muscular ventricular septal defect

(D) doubly committed subarterial ventricular septal defect

28. The 2D image in Fig. 3–6 was taken from the cardiac apex. What does the image demonstrate?

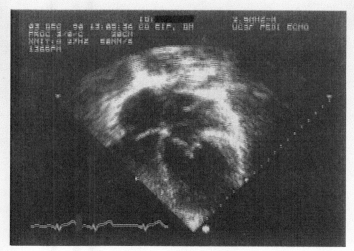

FIGURE 3–6. 2D image of the apical four-chamber view presented with the apex down.

(A) a normal apical four-chamber view

(B) tricuspid atresia

(C) Ebstein's anomaly of the tricuspid valve

(D) ventricular inversion

29. The 2D image of the parasternal long-axis view presented in Fig. 3–7 was taken during diastole. What does the image demonstrate?

(A) a normal heart

(B) valvular aortic stenosis

(C) discrete membranous subaortic stenosis

(D) idiopathic hypertrophic subaortic stenosis

30. If the left ventricular outflow tract of the patient presented in Fig. 3–7 was interrogated by PW Doppler, what is the most proximal location at which an increase in velocity would be detected?

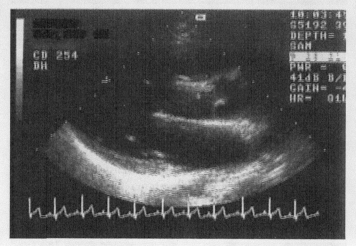

FIGURE 3–7. 2D image of a parasternal long-axis view taken in diastole.

(A) just proximal to the aortic valve

(B) at the aortic valve

(C) just distal to the aortic valve

(D) in the aortic root

TABLE 4–1 • Intersegmental Fissures

Fissures	Location	Landmark
Right intersegmental	Divides the right lobe into anterior and posterior segments	Right hepatic vein
Left intersegmental	Divides the left lobe into medial and lateral segments	Left hepatic vein Ligament of Teres Left portal vein Middle hepatic vein
Middle intersegmental (Main lobar fissure)	Divides the liver into right and left lobes	Oblique plane connecting gallbladder fossa and IVC

TABLE 4–2 • Couinaud's Anatomy

Segments	Location	Supplied by Branches of
1	Caudate lobe	Right and left portal veins
2	Lateral segment of left lobe–superior	Ascending segment of LPV
3	Lateral segment of left lobe–inferior	Descending segment of the LPV
4	Medial segment of the left lobe–quadrate	Horizontal segment of the LPV
5	Anterior segment of the right lobe	Anterior branch of the RPV
6	Posterior segment of the right lobe–inferior	Posterior branch of the RPV
7	Posterior segment of the right lobe–superior	Posterior branch of the RPV
8	Anterior segment of the right lobe–superior	Anterior branch of the RPV

***Falciform Ligament.* (see Fig. 4–3B).** The falciform ligament is a fold of peritoneum, which contains the ligamentum of teres. It extends from the umbilicus to the diaphragm and attaches the liver to the anterior abdominal wall and diaphragm. It divides the right and left lobe of the liver on the diaphragmatic surface. Sonographically it is seen as a round, hyperechoic area in the left lobe of the liver.

Coronary Ligament. The coronary ligament is contiguous with the falciform ligament. It connects the posterior surface of the liver to the diaphragm.

Main Lobar Fissure (Middle Intersegmental Fissure). The main lobar fissure separates the right and left lobes of the liver. It is visualized sonographically as an echogenic linear line extending from the portal vein to the neck of the gallbladder. Table 4–1 is a guide to the anatomic structures useful in defining segmental anatomy.

Liver Vessels—Hepatic Veins, Portal Vein, Hepatic Artery

The liver has a dual blood supply system. It receives blood from both the hepatic artery and the portal vein. The main portal vein blood carries nutrients from the gastrointestinal (GI) tract, gallbladder, pancreas, and spleen. The majority of the total blood supplied to the liver is from the main portal vein.

Hepatic Veins. There are three hepatic veins: right, middle, and left. They follow a superior posterior course and drain deoxygenated blood into the IVC. Hepatic veins are nonpulsatile, increase in size as they course superiorly toward the IVC, and the walls are less echogenic than the portal veins (Tables 4–2 and 4–3).

Portal Vein. The portal vein is formed posterior to the pancreatic neck by the confluence of the splenic vein and superior

mesenteric vein (SMV). It follows a cephalic right oblique course and enters into the liver at the porta hepatis also known as the portal triad. The portal triad contains (1) portal vein, (2) hepatic artery, and (3) bile duct. The main portal vein lies anterior to the IVC, cephalic to the head of the pancreas, and caudal to the caudate lobe. The main portal vein bifurcates in the liver into the right and left portal veins.

Right Portal Vein. The right portal vein is larger than the left portal vein. It follows a posterior caudad course and further divides into anterior and posterior branches.

TABLE 4–3 • Differentiation between the Portal Vein and Hepatic Veins

Portal Veins	Hepatic Veins
Walls are more echogenic because of collagen within the wall	Caliper changes in size with respiration
Branches horizontally and orientates toward the portal hepatic	Branches vertically and orientates toward the IVC
Decreases in caliper as it courses away from the portal hepatis	Increases in caliper as it courses toward the IVC

Left Portal Vein. The left portal vein follows a cephalic anterior course to supply blood to the left lobe of the liver. It is the umbilical portion of the portal vein.

Hepatic Artery. The hepatic artery originates from the celiac axis and courses transversely. The hepatic artery and the common bile duct are anterior to the portal vein as they enter the liver at the portal hepatis, with the common bile duct slightly more lateral. The hepatic artery is at the same level as the hepatoduodenal ligament and is superior to the head of the pancreas.

Common Bile Duct. The common bile duct is formed by the confluence of the common hepatic duct and the cystic duct. The superior portion of the biliary duct, which is anterior to the right portal vein is the common hepatic duct. The common bile duct follows an oblique posterocaudal course and travels along the dorsal aspect of the pancreatic head before it joins with the main pancreatic duct, and together they enter into the second portion of the duodenum.

Liver Function Tests

1. Aspartate aminotransferase (AST), formerly known as serum glutamic-oxaloacetic transaminase (SGOT): This is increased with hepatocellular disease and is useful in detecting acute hepatitis before jaundice occurs and following in the course of hepatitis. It is not increased in cases of such chronic liver disease as cirrhosis or obstructive jaundice. It is increased in liver cell necrosis due to viral hepatitis, toxic hepatitis, and other forms of acute hepatitis.

2. Alanine aminotransferase (ALT), formerly known as serum glutamic pyruvic transaminase (SGPT): This enzyme is increased with hepatocellular disease and is used to assess jaundice. It rises higher than AST in cases of hepatitis and takes 2–3 months to return a normal level.

3. Alkaline phosphatase (ALP): Normally found in serum. Its level rises in liver and biliary tract disorders when bile excretion is impaired. Obstruction of bile can be caused by either a biliary or liver disorder such as; obstructive jaundice, biliary cirrhosis, acute hepatitis, and granulomatous liver disease.

4. Ammonia: Normally metabolizes in the liver and is excreted as urea; increased in hepatocellular disease.

5. Alpha-fetal protein (α-AFP): A protein normally produced by the fetal liver and yolk sac, GI tract, scrotal and hepatocellular (hepatomas) germ cell neoplasms, and other cancers in adults. AFP level is used to monitor chemotherapy treatment and prenatal diagnosis neural tube defects in the fetus, rarely in other cases.

6. Bilirubin: Derived from the breakdown of red blood cells into hemoglobin. Excreted by the liver in bile (main pigment). When destruction of red blood cells increases greatly or when the liver is unable to excrete normal amounts, the bilirubin concentration in the serum increases. If it is increased too high, jaundice may occur. Levels of indirect and direct bilirubin may determine intrahepatic and extrahepatic obstruction.

   Direct bilirubin (conjugated bilirubin): It is elevated when there is an obstruction of the biliary system. obstructive jaundice.

   Indirect bilirubin (unconjugated bilirubin): Excessive destruction of red blood cells/hemolysis associated with anemias and liver disease; elevation of the total bilirubin occurs with hepatitis, hepatic metastasis.

7. Hematocrit: Volume percentage of erythrocytes in the whole body; a drop-in hematocrit can indicate a hematoma due to liver trauma or bleeding elsewhere in the body.

8. Leukocytosis: A substantial increase in white blood cells above the normal range indicates an inflammatory process or abscess.

9. Prothrombin time (PT): Prothrombin is converted to thrombin in the clotting process by action of vitamin K that is absorbed in the intestines and stored in the liver. When liver function is compromised by liver disease, prothrombin is decreased and can cause uncontrolled hemorrhage.

10. Urinary bile and bilirubin: Bile and bilirubin are not normally found in the urine. There may be spillover into the blood when there is obstructive liver disease and excessive red cell destruction. Bile pigments are found in the blood when there is a biliary obstruction. Bilirubin is found alone when there is an excessive amount of red blood cell destruction.

11. Urinary urobilinogen: This test is used to differentiate between a complete obstruction of the biliary tract versus an incomplete obstruction of the biliary tract.

    Urobilinogen is a product of hemoglobin breakdown and can be elevated in cases of liver disease, hemolytic disease, or severe infections. Urobilinogen does not increase or there is no excess amount found in urine in cases of complete biliary obstruction.

12. Fecal urobilinogen: Traces of urobilinogen are normally found in fecal matter, but an increase or decrease in normal amounts may indicate hepatic digestive abnormalities. An increase may suggest an increase in hemolysis. A decrease is seen with complete obstruction of the biliary system.

Diffuse Hepatocellular Disease. There is a decrease in liver function with an increase in the liver enzymes; the increase in the liver enzymes is directly related to the amount of hepatocytic necrosis. Total bilirubin levels may be elevated with increase PT (blood clotting factor). Diffuse liver disease has a varied sonographic appearance depending on whether it is acute or chronic (Tables 4–4 and 4–5).

TABLE 4–4 • Diffuse Liver Disease

Diffuse Liver Disease	Clinical Findings/Etiology	Laboratory Data	Sonographic Appearance
Fatty liver—accumulation of fat within the hepatocytes	ETOH abuse, steroids, malignancy, diabetes mellitus, protein malnutrition, hepatitis	Increased LFTs because of hepatocellular disease	Progressive disease—enlarged left and caudate lobe, increase liver echogenicity with decrease through transmission as the disease progresses, decreases visualization of vessel walls
Acute viral hepatitis—diffuse inflammatory process of the liver, most common types HAV, HBV, and HCV	Malaise, nausea, fever, pain, may be jaundiced, enlarged tender liver	Increased bilirubin, ALT higher levels than AST, alkaline phosphatase	Hepatosplenomegaly, hypoechoic liver parenchyma, renal cortex more echogenic than the liver, increased echogenicity of portal vein walls, thickening gallbladder wall
Chronic viral hepatitis most common types HBV and HCV	Malaise, nausea, fever, pain, may be jaundiced, enlarged tender liver in the early stages	Increase—bilirubin, ALT, AST, alkaline phosphatase	Liver parenchyma is coarse and echogenic, the walls of the portal system blend with the liver echogenicity
Cirrhosis—diffuse fibrotic process that involves the entire liver, most commonly caused ETOH abuse, HBV or HBC	Fatigue, weight loss, diarrhea, dull RUQ pain, increased abdominal girth if ascites is present	LFTs depend upon the stage and function of the liver, the following values are increased: ALT, AST, alkaline phosphatase, serum and urine conjugated bilirubin values	Late features—small nodular echogenic liver with decrease through transmission, caudate lobe may be spared in severe cases—ascites, portal hypertension, collateral vessels, patent umbilical vein
Chronic (passive) hepatic congestion	History of heart failure, acute phase causes RUQ pain	Normal or slightly abnormal LFTs	Acute disorder—hepatomegaly, dilatation of IVC, hepatic veins—reverse flow during systole, slightly pulsatile portal vein
Glycogen storage disease—autosomal recessive disorder of carbohydrate metabolism, Von Gierke's disease is the most common type	Usually occurs in infancy or young childhood, hypoglycemia	Decreased glucose-6-phosphatase	Hepatomegaly, fatty liver infiltration with diffuse increased liver echogenicity

Causes of Jaundice

Medical jaundice (nonobstructive)

Hepatocellular diseases—Disturbances within the liver cells that interfere with excretion of bilirubin:

Hepatitis

Drug-induced cholestasis

Fatty liver (most common cause ETOH abuse)

Cirrhosis

Hemolytic disease—An increase in red blood cell destruction that results in the increase of indirect bilirubin (nonobstructive jaundice):

Sickle-cell anemia

Cooley's anemia

Surgical jaundice (obstructive)—Interference with the flow of bile caused by obstruction of the biliary tract. There are many causes of obstruction, some of the causes are

Choledocholithiasis

Pancreatic pseudocyst

Mass in the head of the pancreas

Hepatoma

Metastatic carcinoma

Cholangiocarcinoma

Mass in the porta hepatis

Enlarged lymph nodes at the level of the porta hepatis

Vascular Abnormalities Within the Liver

Portal Hypertension

Etiology:

Intrahepatic—Most common cause is cirrhosis, Budd–Chiari syndrome

Extrahepatic—thrombosis, occlusion and compression of portal or splenic veins, CHF

TABLE 4–5 • Focal Disease of the Liver

Tumors	Clinical Findings	Laboratory Values	Sonographic Appearance
Cysts, congenital	Usually asymptomatic—if cysts become large hepatomegaly and jaundice may occur	Normal LFTs	Round, smooth thin walls, anechoic, increased through transmission
Polycystic disease	More than 50% associated with renal cystic disease	Normal LFTs	Multiple cysts of various sizes in the liver parenchyma
Acquired cysts Echinococcal cyst (hydatid)—caused by a parasite	Usually asymptomatic—may cause pain if cysts become large	Jaundice and increased alkaline phosphatase if cysts cause biliary obstruction	Depends on the level of maturity—solitary cysts which may have thick or calcified walls, mother-daughter cysts, honeycomb appearance or solid in appearance
Infection Abscess (pyogenic)	Fever, pain, nausea, vomiting, diarrhea, pleuritic pain	Leukocytosis, elevated LFTs, anemia	Usually found in the right lobe, solitary, variable size, anechoic to echogenic or complex may have calcifications or shadowing from gas
Fungal infection—Candidiasis	Immunocompromised; ie, AIDS, organ transplant, malignancy; RUQ pain, fever	Varied—depending on the cause	Hepatomegaly, fatty infiltrations, focal lesions. "Wheel within a wheel,"* becomes more hypoechoic
Hematoma	RUQ pain, hypotension	Decreased hematocrit, leukocytosis	Varied depending on age—mostly cystic (fresh blood), echogenic, mixed appearance, irregular shape
Benign solid tumors Cavernous hemangioma (most common)	Usually asymptomatic, more prevalent in women	Normal LFTs	Varied—usually small, round in the right lobe, subcapsular, usually homogeneous with increased through transmission
Focal nodular hyperplasia (FNH)	Usually asymptomatic, increased incidence in women on oral contraceptives	Normal LFTs	Varied—usually echogenic, usually found in the right lobe, similar in appearance as adenomas, hepatomas
Liver cell adenoma	Usually asymptomatic, or as a palpable mass, increased incidence in women on oral contraceptives or men on steroids	Normal LFTs	Varied—most often found in the right lobe, subcapsular, hyperechoic may have areas of hemorrhage
Infantile hemangioendothelioma	Usually occurs before 6 months of age, abdominal mass, congestive heart failure secondary to arteriovenous shunting	Normal AFP excludes the mass being malignant	Varied—hyperechoic, hypoechoic or mixed echogenicity
Malignant tumors Hepatocellular carcinoma (HCC) hepatoma-associated with longstanding cirrhosis Hepatic angiosarcoma (rarely seen in people 60–80 years of age) Hepatoblastoma—usually found during infancy or childhood	Acute—palpable mass, rapid liver enlargement, jaundice, weight loss Chronic—portal hypertension, ascites, splenomegaly, Budd–Chiari syndrome Abdominal enlargement, hepatomegaly, weight loss, nausea, vomiting, precocious puberty	Increased AST, ALT, alkaline phosphatase, 70% of the time AFP will be present Abnormal LFTs, elevated AFP	Varied—hypoechoic in early stage and becomes hyperechoic, may be singular or multiple Varied—heterogeneous, hyperechoic or cystic with internal septations
Metastatic lesions—more common than primary malignancies	Primary sites—gastrointestinal tract, breast, lungs Causes symptoms 50% of the time	LFTs usually abnormal, increase in total bilirubin, alkaline phosphatase	Varied—hyperechoic, hypoechoic, complex, target lesions, anechoic

*Reproduced with permission from Brooke JR, Ralls PW, Chernesky M: Sonography of the Abdomen, Ultrasound Quarterly April 1995;13(1):60

Clinical findings:

    Formation of collateral venous channels

    Splenomegaly

    GI tract bleeding caused by opening of low-pressure vascular channels

    Ascites

Sonographic findings:

    Dilatation of the portal vein (>13 mm)

    Dilatation of SMV and splenic vein (>10 mm)

    Formation of collaterals (portal vein, splenic vein, SMV can be normal size)

    Varices—esophageal, splenorenal, gastrorenal, intestinal

    Portafugal (reversal) blood flow

    Splenomegaly

    Recanalization of the umbilical vein >3 mm

Portal Vein Obstruction

Etiology:

    Thrombosis, invasion of the portal vein by tumor

Clinical findings:

    Hepatocellular carcinoma (HCC), pancreatic or GI cancer or lymphoma

Sonographic findings:

    Nonvisualization of the portal vein

    Echoes within the portal vein

    Dilatation of the splenic and SMV (proximal to the level of obstruction)

Budd–Chiari Syndrome

Etiology:

    Obstruction of the hepatic veins caused by thrombosis or compression from a liver mass

Clinical findings:

    Abdominal pain

    Jaundice

    Abnormal liver function tests

    Hepatomegaly

    Ascites

Sonographic findings:

    Reduced or nonvisualization of the hepatic veins

    Hepatic veins proximal to the obstruction may be dilated

    Large and hypoechoic caudate lobe

    Ascites

    Abnormal Doppler blood flow

Shear Wave Elastography of the Liver

This technique utilizes a central pulse into the first 5–8 cm of the right lobe of the liver followed by calculations of the speed of propagation of the beam perpendicular to the pulse. Shear wave elastography (SWE) is quantitated in m/s. It has its major application in assessment of liver fibrosis prior to consideration of antiviral treatment of hepatitis C.

SWE of the liver needs to be performed after the patient is NPO for 6–8 hours. Each measurement needs to be done while the patient suspends respiration. Ten samples are usually obtained with the median value used. This value is compared to data obtained from large European centers. The exact value used to determine suitability for treatment may vary slightly and may depend on the scanner used. Metavir scores range from F0 (no fibrosis) to F5 (severe fibrosis).

Sonography of Transjugular Intrahepatic Portosystemic Shunt

Transjugular intrahepatic portosystemic shunt (TIPS) is a procedure performed on patients with portal hypertension or cirrhosis. The procedure consists of placement of a metallic shunt with fluoroscopic guidance using the internal jugular vein as an access site. Once the catheter with the preloaded shunt is directed into a major hepatic vein, usually the right, the catheter is directed toward the main portal vein and pushed through the liver. Once the shunt is deployed, there is flow from the portal vein directly into a hepatic vein.

Duplex color Doppler sonography is used to confirm patency of the TIPS and determines the relative velocity in the proximal, mid, and distal portion of the TIPS. In general, velocities within the TIPS can range from 90 to 190 cm/s. Intimal hyperplasia or thrombus can obstruct the shunt.

Sonography of Liver Transplant

Sonography has an important role in assessing the flow within liver transplants. It is also used for guided biopsy/aspiration of intrahepatic lesions or perihepatic collections. Sonography is also used for preoperative assessment of candidates for liver transplants to ensure patency of the main portal vein and to determine whether there are any intrahepatic masses.

Duplex color Doppler sonography of a patient with a liver transplant includes assessment of flow (spectral and color Doppler) of the main portal vein, right and left portal veins, main hepatic artery, right and left hepatic artery, right, middle, and left hepatic veins, IVC, and splenic artery and vein. Spectral waveforms obtained from these vessels determine direction and relative velocity of flow. Waveforms obtained from the hepatic veins correlate with "liver compliance," which is diminished in cirrhosis and passive liver congestion or rejection. Normal values for velocities of the blood flow in these vessels have been reported.

In addition, the shape of the waveforms suggests "downstream" resistance. For example, the waveform from the main hepatic artery can demonstrate a "spikey" appearance early after transplantation only to become less resistant as the anastomosis matures. The interested reader should consult the reference suggested in this study guide for further information regarding this topic. Prior to considering whether the patient is a candidate for liver transplantation, vascular Doppler assessment of the patency of the main portal vein is needed. After the liver transplant, it is imperative to confirm adequate flow in the hepatic arteries. This topic is extensively covered in Chapter 11.

GALLBLADDER

Gross Anatomy

The gallbladder is mostly intraperitoneal and is located in the gallbladder fossa, which is on the visceral surface of the liver. It lies between the right and left lobes of the liver and posterior and caudal to the main lobar fissure. The gallbladder is a pear-shaped structure with a thin wall that is <3 mm. It is approximately 8 cm in length, with a transverse diameter <5 cm. The gallbladder is divided into three main segments: fundus, body, and neck. The fundus is the most anterior segment, while the neck has a fixed anatomic relationship to the right portal vein and main lobar fissure. The neck tapers to form the cystic duct. The spiral valves of Heister are located in the cystic duct, and stones may collect here.

The right and left hepatic ducts join to form the common hepatic duct whose function is to transport bile to the gallbladder. Bile enters and exits the gallbladder via the cystic duct. The cystic duct unites with the common bile duct to transport concentrated bile to the second portion of the duodenum.

Function

The three main functions of the gallbladder are to concentrate bile, store the concentrated bile, and transport the bile to the duodenum. The release of the hormone cholecystokinin is stimulated when food enters into the stomach, especially fatty foods and dairy products. Cholecystokinin stimulates the gallbladder to contract and the sphincter of Oddi to relax and open. The intraductal pressure decreases with the contraction of the gallbladder and the opening of the sphincter of Oddi. The bile flows to the small intestine, which aids in the digestion of food by breaking down fatty foods and dairy products.

Gallbladder Variants and Anomalies

Junctional Fold. Is the most common variant, which is a fold or kinking located on the posterior gallbladder wall between the body and neck.

Phrygian Cap. A fold located in the fundal portion of the gallbladder (Fig. 4–5).

Hartmann's Pouch. A small sac located between the junctional fold and the neck of the gallbladder. It is an area where stones may collect (see Fig. 4–5)

Septation. A thin wall or partition into the lumen of the gallbladder. This is seen as a thin linear hyperechoic structure within the gallbladder.

Congenital anomalies are rare; the gallbladder can have an ectopic location and be found intrahepatic.

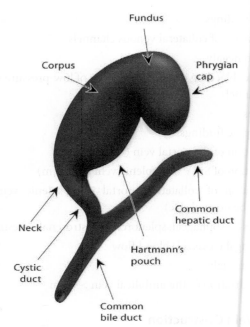

FIGURE 4–5. Gallbladder with variants.

Laboratory Values of Biliary Tract Disease

White Blood Count (WBC). Increases in cases of infection, acute cholecystitis, chronic cholecystitis, cholangitis

Serum Bilirubin. Increases in cases where the biliary system becomes obstructed, gallbladder carcinoma

Abnormal Liver Function Tests

Serum ALP. Increases in cases of post hepatic jaundice

PT. The clotting time is longer in patients with acute cholecystitis, carcinoma of the gallbladder, and prolonged common bile duct obstruction.

AST and ALT are abnormal in cases of cholecystitis, choledocholithiasis, and any injury to the bile ducts.

Sonographic Nonvisualization of the Gallbladder. The most common reason for not visualizing the gallbladder on a sonogram is normal physiological contraction of the gallbladder caused by the patient not being NPO. The gallbladder may not be identified in patients who have had a cholecystectomy, ectopic gallbladder, chronic cholecystitis with the gallbladder lumen filled with gallstones, solid mass obliterating the gallbladder, intrahepatic obstruction, or a porcelain gallbladder. Agenesis of the gallbladder is very rare. When the gallbladder in not identified on ultrasound, the gallbladder fossa should be documented. This can be accomplished by locating the right portal vein and following the main lobar fissure from the right portal vein to the gallbladder fossa region.

Causes of a Large Gallbladder (Hydrops). A large gallbladder can be caused by prolonged fasting, intravenous hyperalimentation, a cystic obstruction, or obstruction of the common bile duct. A Courvoisier gallbladder is a large gallbladder caused by an obstruction at the distal portion of the common bile duct. The patient has "painless" jaundice, elevated serum bilirubin, and abnormal liver function tests. The obstruction is usually caused by a malignancy in the area of the distal CBD (pancreatic head carcinoma, common duct carcinoma, duodenal carcinoma, ampulla of Vater carcinoma) or diabetes and post vagotomy.

Causes of a Small Gallbladder. A common cause of a small gallbladder is that the patient has eaten. Other causes include: intrahepatic biliary obstruction (bile is unable to enter into the gallbladder) chronic cholecystitis; liver disease that destroys the liver parenchyma and, therefore, decreases the production of bile; and in extremely rare cases, congenital hypoplasia of the gallbladder.

Causes of Low-Level Echoes in the Gallbladder Lumen/With Mobility

Biliary Sludge. The most common cause of sludge is stasis of bile attributable to cholecystitis, extrahepatic obstruction, hyperalimentation, or in patients who have been NPO for a long period of time. Sludge is a common precursor to gallstones. Sludge appears as low-level nonshadowing echoes in the dependent portion of the gallbladder that moves with a change in the patient position. Other causes of mobile low-level echoes within the gallbladder lumen include; blood, pus and viscous bile. Intraluminal echoes that do not shadow or are nonmobile include: polyps, cholesterosis, artifacts, septi (junctional fold), and gallbladder carcinoma.

Pathology of the Gallbladder
Reasons for Gallbladder Wall Thickening >3 mm (Table 4–6)

Cholelithiasis (Gallstones). Patients may present asymptomatic or with right upper quadrant (RUQ) pain and a history of

TABLE 4–6 • Reasons for Gallbladder Wall Thickening >3 mm

Diffuse Thickening	Focal Thickening	Pseudo Thickening
Physiologic due to postprandial	Adenomyomatosis	Gain setting too high
		Time-gain compensation set inappropriate
Ascites	Polyps—cholesterol, papillary	Beam averaging artifact
Acute hepatitis	Gallbladder carcinoma—primary and secondary	Sludge
Congestive heart failure	Metastatic wall masses	
Cholecystitis		
Hypoalbuminemia		
AIDS		
Sepsis		

nausea and vomiting after eating. Cholecystitis is sometimes present. The following sonographic characteristics need to be present in order to diagnose gallstones:

1. Echogenic foci—Echogenic due to the acoustic mismatch between the stones and bile
2. Posterior acoustic shadowing—Most of the sound is absorbed (attenuated), producing a shadow.
3. Gravity dependent—Stones are gravity dependent and move to the most dependent portion of the GB when the patient position is changed.

Structures That Can Mimic Gallstones
- Gas in the duodenum
- Surgical clips from post-cholecystectomy
- Valves of Heister and folds in gallbladder

Shadowing from the spiral valves of Heister—refraction artifact from the cystic duct

Bowel—usually not a clean shadow

Air in the biliary tree—from previous surgery or GB fistula

Low-level echoes in the gallbladder lumen—no shadowing

Polyps. Polyps are not gravity dependent and do not move with changing patient position.

Adenomyomatosis. Hyperplastic change in the gallbladder wall (see Table 4–6).

Causes of gallstones in children include hemolysis; for example, sickle cell disease, cystic fibrosis, malabsorption syndrome (Crohn's disease), hepatitis, and congenital biliary anomalies (choledochal cyst, biliary atresia).

Mirizzi Syndrome. Refers to a common hepatic duct obstruction caused by a stone in the cystic duct with a normal common bile duct. Most patients present with clinical findings of RUQ pain, jaundice and fever.

Acute Cholecystitis. Acute cholecystitis is inflammation of the gallbladder wall with decreased gallbladder function. Acute cholecystitis is usually caused by an obstruction at the level of the cystic duct, bacterial infection in the biliary system, or pancreatic enzyme reflux. Clinically, the patient may present with acute RUQ pain that may radiate to the right scapular area. Patient may have a sonographic Murphy's sign which is a focal pain over the gallbladder when compressed by the transducer, this should not be confused with clinical Murphy's sign in which tenderness occur with a sudden stop in inspiratory effort when pressure is applied to the RUQ. Sonographic findings may include diffuse gallbladder wall thickening >3 mm; gallstones; "halo" sign suggestive of subserosal edema; cystic artery along the anterior gallbladder wall; transverse diameter >5 cm; sludge; and pericholecystic fluid. The laboratory findings in acute cholecystitis may include elevated serum bilirubin and abnormal liver function test results.

Complications of Acute Cholecystitis

Empyema—Pus in the Gallbladder. Clinically, the patient presents sicker than with acute cholecystitis, and sonographically, there will be low-level echoes in the gallbladder lumen with thickening gallbladder wall.

Emphysematous Cholecystitis—Rare occurrence caused by gas forming bacteria in the wall of the gallbladder

Gangrene of the Gallbladder—Caused by absence of blood supply to the gallbladder

Perforation of the Gallbladder—Caused by infection and gallstones

Pericholecystic Abscess—Usually caused by perforation of the gallbladder

Ascending Cholangitis—Caused by spreading of the inflammation of the gallbladder

Acalculous Cholecystitis—Less than 5% of patients with cholecystitis will not have gallstones. The cause of acalculous cholecystitis is a combination of bile stasis and direct vascular changes. The etiology of this combination: trauma, patients who are NPO for long period of time

Chronic Cholecystitis—Caused by recurrent or chronic inflammatory changes of the gallbladder. It is the most common cause of symptomatic gallbladder disease and is associated with gallstones in 90% of the cases. Clinically, the patient presents with intermittent RUQ pain and intolerance to fatty and fried foods. Laboratory findings can include elevated AST, ALT, ALP, and increase in direct serum bilirubin. The sonographic appearance includes small or normal size gallbladder, gallstones, sludge, and thicken echogenic gallbladder wall. A positive WES sign may be imaged: the double arc and shadowing are caused by W-echo from the gallbladder wall, E-echo from the gallstone, S-shadowing from gallstones.

Complications:

Bouveret's syndrome

Mirizzi's syndrome

Fistula between the gallbladder and duodenum

Causes of pericholecystic fluid include acute cholecystitis, pericholecystic abscess, ascites, pancreatitis, peritonitis, and acquired immunodeficiency syndrome (AIDS).

Porcelain Gallbladder—Porcelain gallbladder is defined as an intramural calcification of the gallbladder wall, which occurs in association with chronic cholecystitis in most cases. The etiology is unknown and has an increased incidence of gallbladder carcinoma. The sonographic appearance of porcelain gallbladder includes the following:

- Curvilinear echogenic structure in the gallbladder fossa with posterior acoustic shadowing. The gallbladder wall of porcelain gallbladder can be so calcific that the distal acoustic shadow obscures the visualization of the posterior wall.

- Hyperechoic anterior and posterior gallbladder wall with distal acoustical shadowing

- Convex or Irregular gallbladder wall with areas of echo densities and shadowing

Benign Tumors of the Gallbladder—Benign tumors of the gallbladder are rare. They represent overgrowth of the epithelial lining. Patients are usually asymptomatic.

Adenoma—The most common of the benign gallbladder tumors. They are frequently located in the fundus portion of the gallbladder and <1 cm in size. Sonographically they appear as low-level echo masses that do not shadow or move to the dependent portion of the gallbladder.

Adenomyomatosis (a form of hyperplastic cholecystosis)—Characterized by:

- Hyperplasia of the epithelial and muscular surfaces of the gallbladder wall

- Epithelial and intramural diverticula (Rokitansky–Aschoff sinuses [RAS])

There are various types and the most common type is usually located at the fundus. They may also be annular or they can be either diffuse or segmental

Sonographic appearance:

Diffuse or segmental wall thickening

Intraluminal diverticula (RS sinuses) may be filled with bile, sludge or stones and appear either as anechoic or echogenic with distal shadowing or comet tail artifact. The reverberations are the sonographic appearance that differentiates this disease from an adenoma.

Cholesterolosis (strawberry gallbladder)—A form of hyperplastic cholecystosis. The gallbladder usually appears normal on ultrasound.

Polyps—Small echo-densities attached to the gallbladder wall by a stalk; they do not shadow or move to the dependent portion of the gallbladder.

Carcinoma of the Gallbladder—The most common biliary malignancy. Pancreatic cancer is the most common malignant cause to obstruct the biliary tree. Most carcinomas of the gallbladder are adenomas. They usually do not occur until the sixth or seventh decade and are more common in women than men. Previous gallbladder disease; for example, inflammatory disease or gallstones are often precursors. Gallstones are usually present. Most patients have direct extension into the liver and surrounding structures (lymphatic). Signs and symptoms are similar to chronic cholecystitis (may be asymptomatic, loss of appetite, nausea, vomiting, intolerance to fatty foods and dairy products.) Sonographic appearance usually includes gallstones in addition to:

Solid mass filling the gallbladder lumen (most common type)

Localized thickened gallbladder wall with a small gallbladder lumen

Fungating mass projecting from the gallbladder wall into the lumen

Secondary findings:

Liver metastasis

Regional lymphadenopathy

BILE DUCTS

Gross Anatomy

The intrahepatic radicles converge to form the main right and left hepatic ducts at the porta hepatis. The right and left hepatic ducts unite to form the common hepatic duct.

The common hepatic duct joins the cystic duct to form the common bile duct. The common bile duct courses along the hepatoduodenal ligament (ligament that attaches the liver to the duodenum), behind the duodenal bulb and posterior aspect of the pancreatic head to enter the second portion of the duodenum. The common bile duct joins with the main pancreatic duct at the ampulla of Vater (Fig. 4–6).

The common hepatic duct is always anterior the right portal vein, except in cases normal variant or congenital anomalies. The normal common bile duct lumen measures ≤6 mm; the walls are not included in the measurement. The normal diameter of the common bile duct may increase 1 mm per decade starting at the sixth decade. This is due to the common bile duct becoming ecstatic with age. An enlarged common bile duct after a cholecystectomy is normal; if a patient is symptomatic (jaundiced or RUQ pain), a retained stone or a postoperative stricture must be ruled out.

Bile Duct Measurements in a Fasting Patient

Common Hepatic Duct ≤ 4 or 5 mm

Common Bile Duct ≤ 6 mm

Sonographic Appearance of the Biliary System.
The cystic duct and intrahepatic ducts (right and left hepatic ducts)

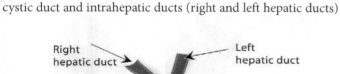
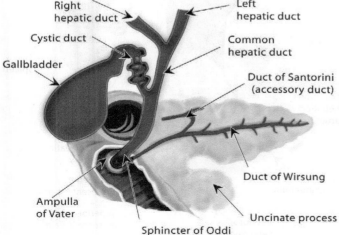

FIGURE 4–6. Gallbladder and biliary ducts anatomy.

TABLE 4–7 • Types of Biliary Obstruction	
Biliary Obstruction without Dilatation	**Dilatation without Biliary Obstruction**
Obstruction occurred within 12–24 hours before exam—ducts may not be dilated yet	Postop cholecystectomy
	Stone in biliary tree has passed

are not usually visualized on ultrasound unless they are dilated. The extrahepatic ducts (common hepatic duct and common bile duct, which are also known as the common ducts) are routinely visualized on ultrasound.

Sonographic Criteria for Intrahepatic Dilatation

The bile duct courses anterior to the portal veins. When dilated, a "parallel channel sign" or "double-barrel shotgun sign" is imaged.

Increased numbers of tubular structures are imaged in the periphery of the liver.

Stellate formation of the tubes near the porta hepatis.

Posterior acoustic enhancement distal to the ducts.

The sonographic appearance of the biliary system varies depending on the level of obstruction. Ducts dilate proximal to the level of obstruction. Intrahepatic dilatation may be the only sonographic indication of an obstruction (Table 4–7). There may be intrahepatic dilatation with common bile duct dilatation with a normal gallbladder or intrahepatic and common bile duct dilatation with a small gallbladder (Table 4–8). The cause of the latter is chronic cholecystitis.

Biliary Atresia—The most common fatal liver disorder in children in the United States. There are two forms. In atresia of the intrahepatic radicles, there is nonvisualization of the biliary radicles and gallbladder. In atresia of the extrahepatic radicles, there is an anastomosis of the biliary tree to the jejunum (second part of the small intestine), there will be dilatation of the intrahepatic radicles, and occasionally, the

TABLE 4–8 • Level of Obstruction Causing Intrahepatic Dilatation	
Common Bile Duct and Gallbladder Normal Size	**Common Bile Duct—Dilated With Enlarged Gallbladder**
Bile duct tumor (cholangiocarcinoma, Klatskin tumor)	Stones in the common bile duct
Sclerosing cholangitis	Chronic pancreatitis
Biliary atresia	Mass of the head of the pancreas (carcinoma)
Choledochal cyst	

TABLE 4–15 • Renal Cystic Masses

Cystic Masses	Clinical Findings	Sonographic Findings
Simple cyst	1. Seen in 50% of patients over the age of 55 2. Usually originates in the renal cortex 3. Asymptomatic unless they are large and obstruct the collecting system 4. Unilocular	1. Anechoic 2. Thin walls 3. Round 4. Increased through acoustical transmission
Atypical cyst	1. Septated or multilocular 2. Septations have no pathological significance	Fulfills all of the criteria for a simple cyst but, will have internal echogenic lines, ie, septations
Parapelvic cyst	1. Originates from renal parenchyma and is seen in the renal hilum 2. May present with hypertension and pain	1. Fulfills the criteria for a simple cyst but located within the renal pelvis 2. Solitary and large 3. Does not communicate with the collecting system
Peripelvic cysts	1. Originates in the renal pelvis 2. May develop from the lymphatic system or obstruction	1. Small, multiple, and irregular shape 2. May appear as dilated renal pelvis 3. Does not communicate with the collecting system
Inflammatory cysts	1. Simple cysts that have become infected 2. An increase in leukocytosis 3. Pain	1. Complex pattern of internal echoes from inflammatory debris 2. Slightly thickens walls, not as thick as chronic abscess
Hemorrhagic cysts	1. 6% of all renal cysts will hemorrhage 2. Increases incidence in polycystic disease	Complex echo pattern dependent upon state of hemorrhage
Calcified cysts	2% of all cysts will calcify	1. Anechoic 2. Smooth round borders that are echogenic or have echogenic foci 3. Calcified walls attenuate sound making it difficult to visualize the complete cyst
Renal abscess (carbuncle)	1. Fever, chills, flank pain 2. Elevated white blood count	1. May appear solid early in the course 2. Complex echo pattern due to debris 3. Walls are thick and irregular 4. Gas may produce a dirty shadow
Hydronephrosis	Obstruction 1. Intrinsic—within the collecting system by a stone or stricture 2. Extrinsic—a mass compresses the ureter or bladder outlet	The calices, infundibula and renal pelvis dilate due to the obstruction of urine flow. Minor dilatation (grade 1)—slight splaying of the collecting system Moderate dilatation (grade 2)—increased dilatation of the collecting system with thinning of the parenchyma Severe dilatation (grade 3)—huge anechoic collecting system with lose of shape and very little parenchyma
Pyonephritis	Pus in the dilated collecting system complication of hydronephrosis that occurs secondary to urinary stasis and infection	Dilated pelvicaliceal system filled with internal echoes, shifting urine-debris level, may have shadowing caused by gas-forming organisms
Renal sinus disease Renal sinus lipomatosis	More common in older patients; may be secondary to chronic calculus disease and inflammation. The renal sinus is replaced by fatty tissue	In replacement lipomatosis, the kidney is enlarged, the renal sinus appears hypoechoic because of fat (one of the few times that fat appears hypoechoic instead of echogenic)

TABLE 4–16 • Solid Renal Masses

Tumors	Clinical Findings	Sonographic Findings
Benign Solid Tumors		
Angiomyolipoma, also called renal hamartoma (tumor composed of fat, muscle, and blood vessels)	More common in women than men (2:1). Symptoms are flank pain, hematuria, and hypertension	Discrete highly echogenic mass found in the cortex
Adenomas (benign counter part of renal cell carcinoma)	Asymptomatic or painless hematuria, usually found on autopsy	Small well-defined isoechoic or hypoechoic mass found in the cortex
Connective tissue tumors 1. Hemangiomas 2. Fibromas 3. Myomas 4. Lipomas	Gross hematuria	These tumors present as homogenous echogenic lesions relating to their vascularity and fat content
Malignant Solid Tumors		
Hypernephroma (also known as adenocarcinoma, renal cell carcinoma [RCC], and Grawitz's tumor)	1. Affect males more than females (2:1) commonly after the age of 50 2. Hematuria 3. An arteriogram of the kidney demonstrates a mass with increased vascular supply with irregular branching 4. Metastases to bone, heart, and brain	1. Unilateral, solitary and encapsulated 2. Varied echogenicity from hypoechoic to echogenic 3. Look for metastases via the bloodstream infiltrating the renal vein and inferior vena cava 4. Look for metastases to the contralateral kidney, ureter, peritoneum, liver, and spleen
Transitional cell carcinoma (affects the urothelium and may be located anywhere within the urinary system)	1. Occurs in the renal pelvis 2. Usually asymptomatic, may have pain or palpable mass 3. Painless hematuria 4. Known to be invasive	1. Invasive tumor not well-defined or encapsulated within the renal pelvis 2. Occasionally appears as a bulky discrete mass 3. Hypoechoic or isoechoic
Renal lymphoma	1. Relatively common in patients with widely disseminated lymphomatous malignancy	1. Solid mass with low-level internal echoes 2. May appear similar to renal cysts but will not demonstrate increase through acoustic transmission
Wilms' tumor (nephroblastoma)	1. Most common malignancy of renal origin in children 2. Abdominal mass, hypertension, nausea 3. Hematuria	1. Early on encapsulated later on it may extend into the perirenal area 2. Varied sonographic appearance depending upon the amount of necrosis and/or hemorrhage

Nephrolithiasis may be composed of uric acid, cystine, or calcium. Sonographically, renal calculi appear as highly reflective echogenic foci. A high-frequency transducer with proper settings of the focal zones is necessary to document posterior shadowing. Using tissue harmonics can also assist in seeing posterior acoustic shadowing. The "twinkle sign" is a color artifact that has been seen with urinary stones. The "twinkle sign" is described as rapidly changing colors that are seen posterior to an echogenic reflector, ie, stones. A Staghorn calculus is large stones located in the central portion of the kidney, the collecting system, and takes the shape of the calyces. Renal obstruction may be secondary to stones located in the collecting system.

Laboratory Values. In cases of chronic obstruction, there is an increase in serum creatinine and BUN levels. In acute obstruction, there are no specific lab values. Urine may show hematuria and/or bacteria.

Signs and Symptoms. Renal colic, flank pain, nausea, and vomiting.

Renal Failure

Renal failure is the kidneys' inability to filter metabolites from the blood resulting in decreased renal function, which may be either acute or chronic. Laboratory findings are increased serum BUN and serum creatinine levels.

Etiology

Prerenal Causes. Renal hypoperfusion secondary to a systemic cause can occur as a result of vascular disorders leading to renal failure and includes the following conditions.

Nephrosclerosis. Arteriosclerosis of the renal arteries, resulting in ischemia of the kidney. Nephrosclerosis develops rapidly in patients with severe hypertension.

Infarction. This may result from occlusion or stenosis of the renal artery.

Renal Artery Stenosis. Any narrowing of the renal artery will affect the blood flow to the kidney, resulting in atrophy of the kidney and decreased renal function.

CHF. This may cause renal hypoperfusion secondary to heart failure.

Thrombosis. Thrombosis of the renal vein will increase the intravascular pressure and, thus, decrease blood flow to the kidney.

Sonography. Doppler of the renal artery is employed to detect arterial blood flow patterns either directly from the renal artery or indirectly from parenchyma flow patterns.

Renal Parenchymal Disease—Infection and Inflammatory Disease

Acute Tubular Necrosis. Of the acute renal medical diseases, this is the most common cause of acute renal failure. The destruction of the tubular epithelial cells of the proximal and distal convoluted tubules may occur as a result of ingestion or inhalation of toxic agents, ischemia caused by trauma, hemorrhage, acute interstitial nephritis, cortical necrosis, and diseases of the glomeruli.

Pyelonephritis. Infection is the most common disease of the urinary tract, and the combination of parenchymal, caliceal, and pelvic inflammation constitutes pyelonephritis. Bacteria ascending from the urinary bladder or adjacent lymph nodes to the kidney usually cause infection of the kidney.

Glomerulonephritis. Etiology is unknown, but it frequently follows other infections.

Metabolic Disorders. Diabetes mellitus, amyloidosis, gout, and nephrocalcinosis (deposit of calcium in the renal parenchyma) are metabolic disorders associated with renal failure.

Chronic Nephrotoxicity. This is caused by exposure to radiation, heavy metals, industrial solvents, and drugs.

Sonography. In acute renal failure, the kidney may be normal sized or enlarged. There may be decreased definition between the medullary/cortical junctions. As the case progresses from acute to chronic, the echogenicity will increase. There is no definite correlation between the echogenicity of the kidney, the kidney size, and degree of decreased renal function. Patients in end-stage renal failure will have small echogenic kidneys that are difficult to image sonographically.

Postrenal Causes. These include urinary tract obstruction, which cause hydronephrosis, and may be congenital or acquired intrinsically and extrinsically.

Sonography. There are varying degrees of the dilation of the renal sinus, calyces, infundibulum, and pelvis.

Renal Medical Diseases (Table 4–17)

Type I. There is increased cortical echogenicity with a decrease in corticomedullary differentiation. Type I diseases are those caused by glomerular infiltrate, such as acute and chronic glomerulonephritis, acute lupus nephritis, nephrosclerosis, any type of nephritis, and renal transplant rejection. All these disorders can cause the echogenicity of the renal cortex to be greater than the liver and spleen. As the disease progresses to the chronic state, the kidney becomes smaller, the cortex becomes more echogenic, and eventually the medulla will become equally echogenic.

Type II. There is distortion of normal anatomy involving cortex and medullary pyramids; sonographically, there is a decrease in the corticomedullary differentiation in either a focal or diffuse manner. The type II pattern is seen with such focal lesions as cysts, abscesses, hematomas, bacterial nephritis (lobar nephroma), infantile polycystic disease, adult polycystic disease, chronic pyelonephritis, and chronic glomerulonephritis.

Renal Transplants

The renal transplant is typically supplied by one or two main renal arteries that are surgically anastomosed to the internal iliac artery. The veins ae similarly anastomosed to the iliac veins. Common disorders following renal transplants include acute/chronic rejections, drug toxicity, and acute tubular nervous (ATN). Duplex Doppler (spectral) assessment can provide vital information regarding the flow within these major vessels and their branches. The complications of renal transportation that are readily amenable to sonography are extensively covered in Chapter 11.

The transplanted kidney is placed within the iliac fossa. A baseline sonogram is performed within 48 hours postoperatively to document the exact location, size, and sonographic appearance of the transplanted kidney. The most serious sign of transplant rejection is renal failure. Clinical signs of renal rejection include, fever, pain, and decreased urine output. The laboratory results are the same as renal failure, elevated BUN, and serum creatinine.

Acute rejection of the transplanted kidney may be caused by acute tubular necrosis or arterial obstruction. Differentiating between the different causes of renal failure is important to ensure proper treatment is administered.

In cases of acute rejection, the kidney appears sonographically as an enlarged kidney with increased cortical echogenicity, decreased renal sinus echogenicity, irregular sonolucent areas in the cortex, enlarged and decreased echogenicity of the pyramids, distortion of the renal outline, and indistinct corticomedullary junction.

Rejection caused by acute tubular necrosis usually results in a normal sonogram. In rejection caused by acute renal arterial occlusion, the sonographic appearance seems grossly normal. However, duplex Doppler studies may reveal an absence of or decreased diastolic flow.

TABLE 4–17 • Renal Medical Diseases

Disease	Clinical Findings	Sonographic Appearance
Acute pyelonephritis	Ninety percent are female, dysuria, urinary frequency, fever, leukocytosis, bacteriuria	Normal or enlarged kidneys, may have mild hydronephrosis; enlarged corticomedullary area with decreased echogenicity and loss of definition between the cortex and medulla; low level echoes may be produced by multiple small abscesses and areas of necrosis in the cortex and medulla
Chronic pyelonephritis	Affects male and females; usually caused by recurrent urinary tract infection or inadequately treated pyelonephritis; proteinuria	Normal or small kidneys; parenchymal thinning; increased echogenicity due to fibrosis
Acute lobar nephronia (acute focal bacterial nephritis)	Inflammatory mass without drainable pus results from gram-negative bacteria that ascends from ureteral reflux; fever, chills, flank pain	Poorly defined cystic mass containing echoes that may disrupt the corticomedullary junction; unable to differentiate from an abscess
Xanthogranulomatous pyelonephritis	Rare form of inflammatory disease found in patients with long-standing renal calculi	Enlarged kidneys with multiple anechoic or hypoechoic areas
Glomerulonephritis	Glomerular disease results from an immunological reaction in which antigen-antibody complexes in the circulation are trapped in the glomeruli. It is the most common cause of renal failure. In the acute stage—oliguria, edema, increased BUN, increased creatinine and increased serum K. In the chronic state—polyuria, proteinuria to such a high extent that 50% of patients develop nephritic syndrome.	Increased echogenicity of the renal cortex with a decrease of the renal size as the disease progresses
Acute tubular necrosis	Most common cause of acute renal failure may result from ischemia, decreased blood flow to and from the kidney, renal transplant. It may be toxin induced or result from trauma/surgery.	Enlarged kidney, especially in the anteroposterior diameter; normal renal parenchyma; renal medullary pyramids will appear more prominent and anechoic

Perinephric fluid collections, commonly associated with the transplanted kidneys, are lymphocele, urinoma, abscess, and hematoma (Table 4–18).

URETERS

The ureters are located in the retroperitoneal cavity and course along the anterior surface of the psoas muscle along the medial side. The ureters are approximately 6 mm in diameter. The three most common places for obstruction to occur are at the UPJ, as they cross over the pelvic brim, and at the junction into the bladder. In the pelvis, the ureters are anterior to the iliac vessels.

Urine can be imaged entering into the urinary bladder with the use of color Doppler. Color Doppler is used because the ureteral jet will cause a Doppler shift because of the continued changes in the turbulent flow in the urine. If the bladder has recently been overly distended, ureteral jets may not be imaged because of the specific gravity of the urine in the ureters and in the bladder being similar, thus causing no Doppler shift. Ureteral jets occur at regular intervals, approximately every 2–3 seconds. They appear as bursts of color entering from the base of the bladder flowing toward the center of the bladder and lasting for a fraction of a second. The absence or decrease of a ureteral jet indicates the presence of an obstruction.

TABLE 4–18 • Perinephric Fluid Collections

Type	Clinical Findings	Sonographic Appearance
Abscess (renal carbuncle is a confluence of several small abscesses.)	Flank pain, high white blood count, fever	Usually echogenic with irregular thickened walls, may have shadowing within caused by gas
Hematoma	Drop in hematocrit	Same sonographic appearance as an abscess depending upon the age and amount of clot/liquification
Urinoma	An encapsulated collection of extravasated urine	Usually anechoic, may have low-level echoes if superimposed with infection
Lymphocele	Collection of lymphatic fluid	Usually anechoic, may have low-level echoes if superimposed with hemorrhage

Abscess, hematoma, urinoma, and lymphocele are commonly associated with renal transplant, although it is not exclusive.

Congenital Anomalies of the Ureters

These include double or bifid ureter, narrowing, strictures, diverticuli, and hydroureter caused by a congenital defect, as in a polycystic kidney, or acquired, as in a low ureteral obstruction.

Megaureter in Childhood (Primary-Nonobstructive, Nonrefluxing Megaureter)

This includes prune belly syndrome (Eagle–Barrett syndrome), deficiency of the abdominal musculature, and urinary tract abnormalities (large hypotonic bladder, undescended testes, hydroureter), and retroperitoneal fibrosis, which fixes the ureter and prevents peristalsis, leading to functional obstruction.

Secondary Megaureter

This is caused by reflux of urine or obstruction. Ureteral abnormalities are viewed in Table 4–19.

URINARY BLADDER

Gross Anatomy

The urinary bladder is a thin-walled triangular structure that is located directly posterior to the pubic bone. The apex of the bladder points anteriorly and is connected to the umbilicus by the median umbilical ligament, the remains of the fetal urachus. The ureters enter at a posteroinferior angle, and the urethra extends from the bladder neck to the exterior of the body. The trigone is the area of the bladder between the neck and apex. It contains three orifices: two for the ureters and one for the urethra.

A normal distended urinary bladder on ultrasound is imaged as a midline symmetrical anechoic structure. The bladder wall is imaged as a thin, smooth, echogenic line that measures between 3 and 6 mm in thickness. The normal bladder volume varies and can usually reach 500 mL without any major discomfort.

Bladder stones can develop in the bladder or form in the kidney. Patients passing a urinary tract stone present with renal colic, flank pain, and hematuria. Sonographically, the bladder stone appears as an echogenic focus with posterior acoustic shadowing. Calculi are gravity dependent (calculi moves to the dependent portion of the bladder when the patient is placed in a decubitus position). Ureteral jets are usually normal; rarely do the calculi obstruct the ureter.

During a pelvic ultrasound examination, the bladder wall thickness, irregularities of the wall, bladder shape, and lumen should be evaluated. There may be an extrinsic mass; for example, a fibroid or enlarged prostate, compressing the bladder and causing bladder distortion. Table 4–20 reviews abnormalities that will distort the wall and shape of the bladder.

ADRENAL GLANDS

Gross Anatomy

The adrenal glands are part of the endocrine system and consist of two distinct regions: the medulla, which is surrounded by the cortex. The adrenal glands are triangle-shaped structures located superior and anteromedial to the upper pole of the kidney. They measure $5 \times 5 \times 1$ cm but at birth are proportionately much larger. Gerota's fascia encloses the kidneys, adrenals, and perinephric fat.

The right adrenal gland lies posterior and lateral to the IVC, lateral to the right crus of the diaphragm, and medial to the right lobe of the liver. To image the right adrenal gland the patient is typically placed in a left lateral decubitus position (right side up). The right adrenal gland is located between the right lobe of liver, IVC, and right kidney.

The left adrenal gland lies medial to the spleen, lateral to the aorta, and posterior to the tail of the pancreas. Sonographically, the normal adrenal glands in adults are difficult to visualize because of their small size and the echo texture being similar to the surrounding retroperitoneal fat. To image the left adrenal gland, the patient lies in a right lateral decubitus position (left side up) the transducer is placed in a coronal position. The left adrenal glands lie—between the spleen, aorta, and left kidney,

TABLE 4–19 • Ureteral Abnormalities

Abnormality	Clinical Finding	Sonographic Appearance
Posterior urethral valves syndrome (PUV): A flap of mucosal tissue covers the opening in the area of the prostatic urethra, causing a urinary outlet obstruction.	Most common cause of urinary obstruction in the male infant and are the second most common cause of hydronephrosis in the neonate. Decreased urine output, failure to thrive and severe cases renal failure in infants. Older patients will experience decreased urine output, dysuria, and urinary tract infections (UTIs).	Distended bladder with a thickened wall bilateral hydroureters seen medial and posterior to the bladder and in severe cases hydronephrosis. The bladder may have a "keyhole" appearance with dilation of the proximal portion of the urethra.
Ureterocele: A cystic dilation of the distal portion of the ureter with narrowing of the ureteric orifice; can be either congenital or acquired.	Patients are usually asymptomatic and the cysts are usually small. Ureteroceles may cause obstruction and infection of the upper urinary tract. If large they may cause bladder outlet obstruction.	An anechoic thin-walled structure of variable size and shape projecting into the bladder.

TABLE 4–20 • Urinary Bladder Abnormalities

Abnormality	Clinical Findings	Ultrasound Findings
Urachal cysts: The urachus connects the apex of the bladder with the allantois (an embryological structure with no function after birth) through the umbilical cord. Normally, it fibroses at birth, but it may, in part or in whole, remain patent. The urachus lies in the Retzius space (anterior to the urinary bladder)	A urachal cyst remains clinically asymptomatic until an infection develops, and then there is vague abdominal pain or urinary complaints.	An anechoic tubular structure in the lower mid-abdominal anterior wall. It may extend from the umbilicus to the bladder.
Diverticula of the bladder: Pouchlike envaginations of the bladder wall. They can be either congenital or acquired.	The diverticula constitute a site of urinary stasis that tends to become infected	Diverticula vary greatly in size and may appear separate from the bladder. They are round, well-defined, thin-walled cystic masses. To help delineate it from an adnexal mass, have the patient void; it should disappear.
Reduplication: Complete reduplication of the bladder is rare	Unilateral reflex, obstruction or infection	Two bladders will be visualized separated by a peritoneal fold with two urethras and two external openings.
Reflux: Vesicoureteral reflux is a common urinary tract abnormality in children secondary to anomalies such as ectopic, posterior urethral valves, prune belly syndrome, neurogenic bladder, and primary congenital abnormalities of the bladder	Reflux may be a cause of chronic renal failure with scarring and atrophic changes in the kidney	Cysto-Conray (20%) is injected into the bladder. Each kidney is scanned while the contrast is injected. With each increasing grade of reflux, there is increasing renal collecting system dilation.
Bladder neck obstruction: The lower portion continuous with the urethra is called the neck.	In the male bladder, neck obstruction commonly is secondary to benign prostatic hypertrophy (BPH) or carcinoma. With prolonged obstruction the bladder wall will become thickened and trabeculated.	A thickened and irregular-walled bladder
Cystitis: Infection or inflammation of the bladder. More common in females because of the shorter urethra.	Secondary to diverticula, urethral obstruction, fistulas, cystocele, bladder neoplasm, pyelonephritis, neurogenic dysfunction, bladder calculi, trauma, pregnancy, rectal/vaginal fistula	In cases of long-standing infection or inflammation (chronic), the bladder walls may show inflammatory changes and thickening. In cases of a neurogenic bladder, low-level echoes may be seen in the bladder producing a pus–urine fluid level.
Primary benign tumor (uncommon): papilloma, epithelial, leiomyoma, neurofibroma, adenoma (associated with cystitis)	Patients present with painless hematuria, dysuria, frequent urination	Ultrasound cannot distinguish between a benign and malignant tumor. Small to massive solid tumors are seen projecting from the bladder wall, some may evaginate the bladder wall and may be smooth or irregular in contour. May mimic benign prostatic hypertrophy or cystitis. Outflow obstruction and hydronephrosis also need to be evaluated.
Primary malignant tumor: 95% are transitional cell carcinoma (TCC); 5% are squamous cell carcinoma	Invasive growths, with 40% having metastases to lymph nodes and invasion of the prostate and seminal vesicles. They are usually not detected until they have metastasized. Patients present with hematuria, urinary frequency, dysuria	Ultrasound cannot distinguish between a benign and malignant tumor. Small to massive solid tumors are seen projecting from the bladder wall, some may evaginate the bladder wall, and may be smooth or irregular in contour. May mimic benign prostatic hypertrophy or cystitis. Outflow obstruction and hydronephrosis also need to be evaluated.

TABLE 4–21 • Adrenal Gland Malfunctions

Malformations	Clinical Findings	Sonographic Findings
Adrenal Cortex		
Adrenocortical hyperfunction Cushing's syndrome	Increased corticosteroid production produces diabetes mellitus, protuberant abdomen from muscle weakening and loss of elastic tissue, rounded faces, mild hypertension, cardiac enlargement, and edema.	Varied—the adrenal glands may appear normal, diffusely enlarged, solid, cystic, or complex, with focal areas of necrosis or hemorrhage.
Conn's syndrome—benign	Hyperaldosteronism caused by an increase of aldosterone producing sodium retention, which leads to essential hypertension, increased thirst, and urination.	Varied—the adrenal glands may appear normal, diffusely enlarged, solid, cystic, or complex with focal areas of necrosis or hemorrhage.
Adenomas—may be functional or nonfunctional	Benign tumors associated with Cushing's and Conn's syndrome. May present with hypertension, diabetes, hyperthyroidism, and renal cell carcinoma.	Round or oval in shape usually larger than 1 cm, hypoechoic.
Adrenocortical hypofunction Addison's disease—rare condition	Decreased hormonal production causing hypotension, malaise, weight loss, changes in skin pigmentation, loss of body hair, and menstrual irregularity. 80% are attributable to idiopathic destruction, probably autoimmune in nature, and 20% are caused by tuberculosis.	Varied normal or hyperechoic may be small because of the destruction of cortical tissue.
Adrenal Medulla		
Pheochromocytoma—rare vascular tumors	Paroxysmal or sustained hypertension, angina, cardiac arrhythmias, anxiety, nausea, vomiting, and headaches. These features are caused by the concentration of catecholamines released into circulation. Large tumors may lead to heart failure and death.	Well-defined large, highly vascular masses that can be cystic, solid, or heterogeneous with calcifications.
Neuroblastoma	A highly malignant tumor that arises from the sympathetic nervous tissue or adrenal medulla. Children can be asymptomatic or have weight loss, fever episodes of tachycardia, sweats, and headaches with a palpable abdominal mass.	Varied presentation—large echogenic, heterogeneous mass with areas of cystic degeneration and focal calcifications. The kidney will be displaced posteriorly and inferiorly.
Adrenal Masses		
Adrenal metastases	Most commonly from bronchogenic CA, lung adenocarcinoma, breast or stomach carcinoma.	Metastases to the adrenals vary in size and echogenicity.
Adrenal cysts—rare	None—patients are usually asymptomatic	Round or oval in shape, anechoic with increased through acoustical transmission. Adrenal cysts tend to become calcified, which appear as an echo-free structure, with an echogenic back wall with posterior shadowing (no through acoustic transmission).
Adrenal hematomas	Most often seen in infants caused by trauma from birth, prematurity or hypoxia. In adults, it is caused by trauma or anticoagulant therapy.	Varies depending upon the age of the bleed initially the hematoma is echogenic, and then it becomes sonolucent to complex and then calcified.

and these structures are used as sonographic landmarks. Computed tomography (CT) is the imaging modality of choice. Adrenal tumors may be identified on a sonogram usually by their displacement and/or compression of adjacent structures. See Table 4–21 for adrenal gland malfunctions.

Right Adrenal Pathology Will Displace

Anteriorly	*Posteriorly*
The retroperitoneal fat line	The right kidney
The IVC	
The right renal vein	

Left Adrenal Pathology Will Displace

Anteriorly	*Posteriorly*
The splenic vein	The left kidney

Adrenal Cortex The adrenal cortex, which produces steroid hormones, is subdivided into three zones listed from outer to inner: (1) the zona glomerulosa, which produces mineralocorticoids (for the regulation of aldosterone to regulate electrolyte metabolism); (2) the zona fasciculata, which produces glucocorticoids (for the regulation of cortisol, which is an anti-stress and anti-inflammatory hormone); and (3) the zona reticularis, which produces gonadocorticoids (for regulation of the secretion of androgens and estrogens, which are the sex hormones of an individual).

The adrenal cortical hormones are regulated by the adrenocorticotropic hormones (ACTH) of the anterior pituitary gland. A *decrease* in adrenal cortical function leads to an increased ACTH, which then stimulates the adrenal cortex. An *increase* in concentration of adrenal hormones leads to a drop in ACTH secretion, which leads to a drop in the activity of adrenal cortex.

The adrenal cortex may be affected either by lesions that produce an excess of steroid hormones or by lesions that produce a deficiency. The adrenocortical hormone levels may be abnormal (increased or decreased production) as a result of a pituitary tumor, which can cause the overproduction or underproduction of ACTH.

Adrenal Medulla

The adrenal medulla produces epinephrine (adrenalin) and norepinephrine. These hormones have a wide range of effects.

Epinephrine dilates the coronary vessels and constricts the skin and kidney vessels. It increases coronary output, raises oxygen consumption, and causes hyperglycemia.

Norepinephrine constricts all arterial vessels except the coronary arteries (which dilate). It is the essential regulator of blood pressure.

Epinephrine, in particular, is responsible for the fight orflight reaction. It stimulates the metabolic rate, allowing energy that is more available.

GASTROINTESTINAL TRACT

Sonography is not routinely used to image the GI tract because of the air within the bowel lumen. Normal bowel patterns can be imaged and recognize bowel peristalsis on abdominal sonographic examination. Knowledge of the GI tract is essential for identifying the location of the pathology. The appendicitis can be detected when there is a noncompressible tubular structure in the right lower quadrant that measures over 6 mm in thickness. Complicated appendicitis can be diagnosed when there are periappendiciteal fluid collections.

Sometimes an echogenic fecalith also present. Rarely, the appendix is involved in neoplastic growth. Another cause of an appendicular mass is a mucocele of the appendix where there are multiple layers of inflammatory tissue that surround the appendix, giving an "onion skin" appearance.

Gross Anatomy

The GI tract is composed of the esophagus, the stomach, the small intestine, and the colon.

The esophagus is a tubular structure that extends from the pharynx to the stomach. Its main function is to bring food and water to the stomach. The gastroesophageal junction (GEJ) can be identified slightly to the left of midline on a sagittal scan. Sonographically, it appears round with an echogenic center with a hypoechoic rim also referred to as a "target sign" or "bull's eye" located posterior to the left lobe of the liver and anterior to the aorta.

The stomach lies between the esophagus and the duodenum. The opening between the stomach and the duodenum is called the pyloric orifice. The main function of the stomach is to break down food to chyme, which then passes through to the duodenum. Sonographically, the fluid-filled stomach is imaged as an anechoic structure with echogenic foci and thin walls. The small intestine lies between the stomach and the colon and is divided into three parts: duodenum, jejunum, and the ileum. The main function of the small intestine is to absorb food.

The ileocecal valve connects the distal portion of the ileum to the first section of the colon, the cecum. The appendix is located in the right lower quadrant as a tubular structure that extends from the cecum. The ascending colon ascends from the cecum along the right side of the body to the posterior inferior surface of the liver. The ascending colon bends to the left and forms the hepatic flexure. The transverse colon extends across the body from the hepatic flexure to the splenic flexure. The splenic flexure is located posterior and inferior to the spleen and bends inferiorly forming the descending colon, which courses along the left side to the body and terminates at the sigmoid colon.

The sigmoid is the narrowest portion of the colon, and the distal end forms the rectum. The anal canal is the distal end of the rectum, which expels solid waste products (feces) from the body.

DIAPHRAGM

Gross Anatomy

The diaphragm is a dome-shaped muscle separating the thorax from the abdominal cavity. The diaphragm covers the superior and lateral border of the liver on the right side and the spleen on the left side. Sonographically, the diaphragm is identified as a thin, echogenic, curvilinear interface between the lungs and liver (spleen).

The *subphrenic space* is between the liver (or spleen) and the diaphragm and is a common site for abscess.

CRURA OF THE DIAPHRAGM

The diaphragmatic crura are right and left fibromuscular bundles that attach to the lumbar vertebra at the level of L3 on the right and L1 on the left. They act as anchors to the diaphragm.

The left crus can be visualized anterior to the aorta above the level of the celiac artery. Below the celiac artery, the crura extend along the lateral aspects of the vertebral columns. The right crus is visualized posterior to the caudate lobe and the IVC.

FLUID COLLECTIONS

Ascites

Ascites is an abnormal accumulation of serous fluid in the peritoneum. The most common cause for ascites in the United States is cirrhosis and accounts for about 80 percent of causes.[3] Ascites are categorized into:

- Transudative—anechoic/freely mobile usually benign, free-floating bowel in the abdomen
- Exudative—internal echoes/loculated—associated with infection and malignancy

- Bowel matted or fixed to posterior abdominal wall—associated with malignancy
- Nonmobile fluid associated with coagulated hematoma (trauma)

Pathology Associated With Ascites

- CHF
- Infection (inflammatory process)
- Kidney failure
- Liver failure/disease—end-stage fatty liver, cirrhosis
- Malignancy
- Ruptured aneurysm
- Pyogenic peritonitis
- Tuberculosis
- Portal venous system obstruction
- Obstruction of lymph nodes
- Obstruction of vessels—Budd–Chiari syndrome
- Acute cholecystitis
- Postoperative

Clinical Presentation

The clinical presentation of ascites is a distended abdomen. In cases of massive ascites, respiratory distress will also be present.

Sonographic Findings

Accumulations occur (supine position) in the following order:

1. Inferior tip—right lobe liver
2. Superior portion—right flank
3. Pelvic cul de sac
4. Right and Left paracolic gutter
5. Morison's pouch
   - Ascites is found inferior to the diaphragm
   - Gross (massive) ascites—extrahepatic portion falciform ligament seen attaching the liver to anterior abdominal wall
   - Ascites may cause a downward displacement of the liver
   - May cause gallbladder wall to appear to thicken
   - Liver may appear more echogenic
   - May see patent umbilical vein
   - Changing patient's position to observe fluid movement may be useful
   - Disproportional accumulation in lesser sac suggestive of adjacent organ pathology (ie, acute pancreatitis, pancreatic CA)

Abscess

An abscess is an encased collection of pus (acute/chronic). A cavity formed by liquefactive necrosis within solid tissue.

Pathology Associated With Abscesses

- Penetrating trauma (wounds)
- Postsurgical procedures
- Retained products of conception
- Pelvic inflammatory disease
- Chronic bladder disease
- Sepsis—blood-borne bacterial infection
- Long-standing hematomas
- Postcholecystectomy—site of the gallbladder fossa
- GI tract—peptic ulcer perforation; bowel spill during surgery (peritonitis)
- Urinary tract infection
- Infected ascites with septa/debris
- Amebic abscess—may be densely echogenic

Clinical Presentation. Pain, spiking fever, chills, elevated white blood cell count, solitary or multiple sites, tenderness

Hepatic Abscess Intrahepatic

Abscesses are most often associated in the Western hemisphere with cholangitis; also seen with sepsis and penetrating trauma to the liver.

- Location: within liver parenchyma
- Differential diagnosis: solid tumor, usually round lesion with scattered internal echoes, variable through transmission

Subhepatic

Abscess associated with cholecystectomy

- Location: inferior to liver; fluid collection anterior to right kidney (Morison's pouch); gallbladder fossa (post cholecystectomy)

Subphrenic

Abscess associated with bacterial spill into peritoneum during surgical procedure; bowel rupture; peptic ulcer perforation; trauma

- Location: fluid collection superior to the liver, inferior to diaphragm; transmission variable; gas (dirty shadowing)

General Sonographic Findings. A variable, complex, solid, cystic lesion with septa, debris, and scattered echoes; through transmission may be good; mass/cyst with shaggy/thick irregular walls; mass displacing surrounding structures; complex mass with dirty shadowing from within. *Presence of gas within a mass suggests an abscess (may also be attributable to fistulous communication with bowel or airway or outside air).*

General Differential Diagnosis. Necrosing tumor with fluid center (these usually have thicker walls and *no gas*).

Ascites Versus Abscess

A localized area of ascites may be mistaken for an abscess. Place the patient in the erect or Trendelenburg position; ascites will shift to the dependent portion, but an abscess will not, unless it contains air; the air/fluid level will shift.

Pleural Effusion

Pleural effusions are nonspecific reactions to an underlying pulmonary or systemic disease such as cirrhosis. Obtaining fluid for analysis may allow a more specific diagnosis.

Sonographic appearance shows a pleural effusion usually as an echo-free (anechoic), wedge-shaped area that lies posteromedial to the liver and posterior to the diaphragm. Occasionally, pleural effusions contain internal echoes, sometimes indicating the presence of a neoplasm. These echoes may be caused by blood or pus (empyema), especially when the collection is loculated. Loculated effusions do not always lie adjacent to the diaphragm and may be loculated anywhere on the chest wall. Sometimes effusions lie between the lung and the diaphragm and are known as subpulmonic. Right-sided pleural effusions can be assessed easily on a view demonstrating the diaphragm and the liver. Effusions on the left side are more difficult to see in the supine position but can be seen more readily with the patient in an oblique position and imaging through the spleen.

RETROPERITONEUM

The retroperitoneum is the area between the posterior portion of the parietal peritoneum and the posterior abdominal wall, extending from the diaphragm to the pelvis.

Divisions

The retroperitoneum is divided into three areas by the renal fossa (Gerota's fascia). Fig. 4–8 demonstrates the division of the retroperitoneum into anterior perirenal and posterior perirenal spaces.

1. The anterior perirenal space contains the retroperitoneal portion of the intestines and the pancreas.
2. The perirenal space contains the kidneys, ureters, adrenal glands, aorta, IVC, and retroperitoneal nodes.
3. The posterior perirenal space contains the posterior abdominal wall, iliopsoas muscle, and quadratus muscle.

Pathology

The retroperitoneal area is subject to infection, bleeding, inflammation, and tumors.

Anterior Perirenal Space. Pancreatic pathology, carcinoma of the duodenum, ascending and descending colon causing bowel thickening or infiltration resulting in a "bull's eye."

Perirenal Space. Kidney diseases, adrenal diseases, invasion or displacement of the IVC, aortic aneurysms, ureteral abnormalities, sarcoma, liposarcoma, aortic, and retroperitoneal adenopathy.

Posterior Perirenal Space. Renal transplant is usually performed in this extraperitoneal space within the iliac fossa, using the iliac vessels for anastomosis.

Primary Retroperitoneal Tumors

Primary retroperitoneal tumors are mostly malignant; rapidly growing; and larger tumors are more likely to show evidence of necrosis and hemorrhage. Concurrence of mass with ascites indicates invasion of peritoneal surfaces.

Liposarcoma. Originates from fat. Liposarcoma has a complex echogenic pattern with thick walls.

Fibrosarcoma. Originates from connective tissue. Fibrosarcoma has a complex mostly sonolucent pattern, invading surrounding tissues.

Rhabdomyosarcoma. Originates from muscle. It occurs as a solid, complex, or homogeneous echogenic mass, invading surrounding tissue.

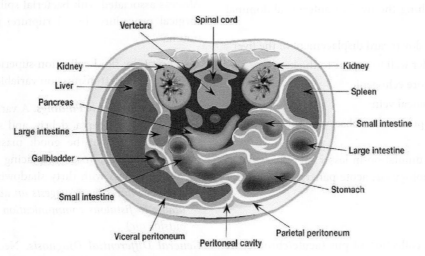

FIGURE 4–8. Cross-sectional anatomy of the retroperitoneal compartments.

Leiomyosarcoma. Originates from smooth muscle. It occurs as a complex echo-dense mass that may have areas of necrosis and cystic degeneration.

Teratoma. Originates from all three germ cell layers. Most teratomas occur in the area of the upper pole of the left kidney. Ninety percent are benign. They are complex with echogenic and cystic areas. Fifty percent occur in children.

Neurogenic Tumors. Originate from nerve tissue and occur mostly in the paravertebral region. They are heterogeneous and echogenic.

Secondary Retroperitoneal Tumors

Secondary retroperitoneal tumors are primary recurrences from previously resected tumors or recurrent masses from previous renal carcinoma.

Ascitic fluid along with a retroperitoneal tumor usually indicates seeding or invasion of the peritoneal surface. Evaluation of the para-aortic region should be made for extension to the lymph nodes. The liver should also be evaluated for metastatic involvement.

Retroperitoneal Fibrosis

Retroperitoneal fibrosis is the formation of thick sheets of connective tissue extending from the perirenal space to the dome of the bladder. It encases, rather than displaces, the great vessels, ureters, and lymph channels, causing obstruction. Severe uropathy may ensue. The etiology of retroperitoneal fibrosis is usually idiopathic, but it may sometimes be associated with aortic aneurysm.

Clinical Findings. The clinical findings in retroperitoneal fibrosis include hydronephrosis, hypertension, anuria, fever, leukocytosis, anemia, nausea and vomiting, weight loss, malaise, palpable abdominal or rectal mass, and abdominal, back, or flank pain. It is more frequent in males than females, and most common at age 50 through the 60s.

Sonographic Findings. Retroperitoneal fibrosis appears as thick masses anterior and lateral to the aorta and IVC, extending from renal vessels to the sacral promontory. The anterior to hypoechoic sheets have smooth, well-defined anterior margins and irregular, poorly defined posterior margins. The differential diagnosis includes lymphoma, nodal metastases, and retroperitoneal sarcoma or hematoma.

Retroperitoneal Fluid Collections. Collections of fluids in the retroperitoneum include abscesses, hematomas, urinomas, lymphoceles, and cysts.

LYMPHATIC SYSTEM

Gross Anatomy

The lymphatic system arises from veins in the developing embryo and is closely associated with veins throughout most parts of the body. Lymphatic vessels assist veins in their function by draining many of the body tissues and, thus, increasing the amount of fluid returning to the heart. The lymph vascular network does not form a closed-looped system such as the blood vascular system. Lymph vessels begin as tiny, colorless, unconnected capillaries in the connective tissues. These merge to form progressively larger vessels that are interrupted at various sites by small filtering stations called lymph nodes. The lymph fluid from the entire body ultimately drains into the IVC.

This lymphatic network has tremendous clinical significance. Interruption of lymph drainage in an area generally creates considerable swelling (edema) owing to the accumulation of fluids. In addition, the lymph vessels offer a variety of routes for cancer cells to move from one site to another (metastasis).

Lymph Nodes

Lymph nodes contain lymphocytes and reticulum cells, their function being one of filtration and production of lymphocytes and antibodies. All the lymph passes through nodes, which act as filters not only for bacteria but also for cancer cells. Enlargement of lymph nodes is a usual sign of an ongoing bacterial or carcinogenic process. Normal lymph nodes measure <1 cm in size. The parietal nodes follow the same course as the prevertebral vessels, while the visceral nodes are more superficial and generally follow the same course that the organ-specific vessels follow. Sonographically, we can evaluate lymph nodes in the pelvis, retroperitoneum, porta hepatis, perirenal, and prevertebral vasculature.

Function. The functions of the lymph nodes are (1) the formation of lymphocytes, (2) the production of antibodies, and (3) the filtration of lymph.

Sonographic Appearance. To visualize lymph nodes, they must be at least 2 cm in size. They are very homogeneous. Lymph nodes are typically hypoechoic, but there is no through transmission. Lymphomas have a nonspecific appearance but in general the following are true:

- Adenopathy secondary to lymphoma is usually sonolucent.
- Adenopathy secondary to metastatic disease is usually complex.
- Posttherapy enlarged nodes are usually very echogenic but may develop cystic areas secondary to necrosis.

Periaortic nodes have specific characteristics: They may drape the great vessels anteriorly (obscuring sharp anterior vascular border); may have a lobular, smooth, or scalloped appearance; and with mesenteric involvement, they may fill most of the abdomen in an irregular complex necrosis.

Para-aortic nodes may displace the celiac axis and SMA anteriorly. Enlarged nodes posterior to the aorta will displace the great vessels away from the spine; this is referred to as the floating aorta sign. The "sandwich" sign occurs when nodes surround the mesenteric vessels.

Sonographic Technique. Concentrates on the preverte-bral vessels, aorta, IVC; porta hepatic (can produce *biliary obstruction*); spleen size; iliopsoas muscles; urinary bladder contour; perirenal; retroperitoneum; and pelvis.

Para-aortic lymph nodes are involved with lymphoma in 25% of cases and 40% with Hodgkin's disease. The sono-graphic appearance of these lymphomatous nodes varies from hypoechoic to anechoic with no increased through transmis-sion. Occasionally, anechoic nodal masses may resemble cystic structures. Nodal enlargement secondary to other neoplasms or inflammatory processes, such as retroperitoneal fibrosis, may be indistinguishable from lymphomatous lymphadenopathy. Para-aortic or paracaval nodes frequently obscure the sharp anterior vascular border or compress the aorta or IVC. Placing a patient in a decubitus position demonstrating the aorta and IVC facilitates sonographic imaging of the retroperitoneal area down to the aortic bifurcation.

Tumors of Lymphoid Tissue

Lymphomas (Tumors of Lymphoid Tissue). *Hodgkin's disease* (40%) is a malignant condition characterized by generalized lymphoid tissue enlargement (eg, enlarged lymph nodes and spleen). Twice as many males as females are affected. It usually occurs between the ages of 15 and 34, or after 50. Histopatho-logic classification: Reed–Sternberg (RS) cells and multinucle-ated cells are present.

Non-Hodgkin's disease (60%) is further subdivided into nod-ular and diffuse histopathologies. It is a heterogeneous group of diseases that consists of neoplastic proliferation of lymphoid cells that usually disseminate throughout the body. It occurs in all age groups with the incidence increasing with age.

Mesenteric nodal involvement in <4% in patients with Hodgkin's disease but >50% in non-Hodgkin's patients. Lym-phomatous cellular infiltration of the greater omentum may be seen as a uniformly thick, hypoechoic band-shaped structure. The appearance of mesenteric nodes can resemble that of retro-peritoneal nodes.

Mesenteric masses may also appear as multiple cystic or sep-arated masses that may resemble fluid-filled bowel loops. Peri-hepatic nodes, celiac axis nodes, splenic-hilar, and renal-hilar nodes may also be demonstrated sonographically. Although most are hypoechoic to anechoic, inhomogeneous areas of increased echogenicity can be found in areas of focal necrosis within large nodes. Nodes can encase or invade adjacent organs and produce significant organ displacement, whereas portal nodes produce biliary obstruction.

Extranodal Lymphoma. The liver, kidneys, GI tract, pancreas, and thyroid may show lymphomatous involvement.

Hepatic Lymphoma. Hepatic lymphomatous involvement pres-ents as multiple hypoechoic or anechoic focal parenchy-mal defects. Although these anechoic lesions may resemble cystic structures, they rarely demonstrate enhanced posterior acoustic transmission or peripheral refractory shadowing. Hepatic abscesses, metastases from sarcomas or melanomas, focal areas of cholangitis, radiation fibrosis, and extensive hemosiderosis have presented with findings sonographically indistinguishable from hepatic lymphoma.

Renal Lymphomas. Less than 3% of all non-Hodgkin's lympho-mas present with renal involvement, mainly Burkitt's lym-phoma or diffuse histiocystic lymphomas.

GI Lymphoma. Fifteen percent of non-Hodgkin's lymphomas may present with GI involvement. Sonographic features include a relatively hypoechoic mass with central echogenic foci. The sonographic appearance is nonspecific for lym-phomatous involvement; gastric carcinoma or gastric wall edema may have the same sonographic appearance.

Pancreatic Lymphoma. Ten percent of non-Hodgkin's patients present with pancreatic involvement—portions of tissue rep-resented by focal hypoechoic or anechoic masses.

Thyroid Lymphoma. Lymphomatous thyroid masses also pres-ent in the same manner.

Inflammatory Conditions

There are three inflammatory conditions of the lymphatic system: acute and chronic lymphadenitis and infectious mononucleosis.

Common primary tumors with metastases to lymph are those of the breast, lung, melanoma, prostate, cervix, and uterus.

Sonographic Pitfalls

1. Enlarged nodes can mimic aortic aneurysm at lower gain settings on longitudinal scans; transverse scans are needed to differentiate.

2. Aneurysms enlarge fairly symmetrically, whereas enlarged nodes tend to drape over prevertebral vessels.

3. Bowel can mimic enlarged nodes so check for peristalsis; nodes are reproducible, whereas bowel is not.

RETROPERITONEAL VERSUS INTRAPERITONEAL MASSES

The retroperitoneal location of a mass is confirmed when there is any of the following:

- Anterior renal displacement
- Anterior displacement of dilated ureters
- Anterior displacement of the retroperitoneal fat ventrally and often cranially, whereas hepatic and subhepatic lesions produce inferior and posterior displacement. The direc-tion of displacement may permit diagnosis of the anatomi-cal origin of RUQ masses.
- Anterior vascular displacement—aorta, IVC, splenic vein, SMV

Contrast-Enhanced Sonography

The recent availability and Food and Drug Administration (FDA) approval of microbubble contrast for sonography has extended the diagnostic accuracy of sonography in several areas including evaluation of focal liver lesions (FLL), traumatic abdominal organ laceration, assessment of renal lesions (particularly in patients with impaired renal function) vesicoureteral reflex in children with recurrent urinary tract infection. The oscillations of microbubbles are optimally seen using harmonic imaging. Perfusion characteristics (wash-in/wash-out/vascularity) can be determined and are relatively specific for FLLs. Hepatic neoplasms tend to wash-out quickly; hemangiomas continued to fill-in form the periphery, focal nodular hyperplasia (FNH) demonstrate a central scar. For trauma patients. Contrast-enhanced ultrasonography (CEUS) can detect liver/renal/splenic laceration. In children with recurrent urinary tract infections, intravascular placement of microbubble contrast can identify reflux into the renal collecting systems.

Sonographically Guided Procedures

Sonography provides real-time guidance for a variety of biopsy procedures and drainages. The echogenic nature of metallic needles provides an excellent source of high-level echoes to observe the location of the needle shaft and tip relative to the area of interest. Thus, sonographic guidance is used for paracentesis, thoracentesis, thyroid, liver, and renal biopsies. Placement of drainage catheters with sonography has become standard as well as guided placement of central lines in patients in intensive care units (ICUs).

References

1. Crossin JD, Mauradali D, Wilson SR. US of liver transplants: normal and abnormal 1. *RadioGraphics*. 2003:1093-1114.

2. Kanterman RY, Darcy MD, Middleton WD, et al. Doppler sonography findings associated with transjugular intrahepatic portosystemic shunt malfunction. *AJR*. 1997;168:467-472.

3. Runyon BA. Care of patients with ascites. *N. Engl J Med*. 1994;330:337.

4. Rumack CM, Wilson SR, Charboneau JW. *Diagnostic Ultrasound*. 3rd ed. St. Louis: Elsevier Mosby; 2005.

5. Tortora GJ. Derrickson B. *Principles of Anatomy and Physiology*. 11th ed. Hoboken: John Wiley & Sons; 2006.

6. Barr F. *Elastography: A Practical Approach*. New York: Thieme; 2017.

Questions

234

GENERAL INSTRUCTIONS: For each question, select the best answer. Select only one answer for each question unless otherwise instructed.

1. What three structures comprise the portal triad?

   (A) portal vein, portal artery, and common bile duct

   (B) hepatic artery, portal vein, and bile duct

   (C) hepatic vein, portal artery, and cystic duct

   (D) hepatic artery, portal artery, and bile duct

2. A 4-year-old boy presents with high blood pressure, hematuria, and a palpable left flank mass. An ultrasound examination is performed, and a solid renal mass is identified. This finding is most characteristic of which of the following?

   (A) hypernephroma

   (B) IPKD

   (C) neuroblastoma

   (D) nephroblastoma

3. A patient presents with ampulla of Vater obstruction, distention of the gallbladder, and painless jaundice. Which of the following is this presentation associated with?

   (A) hydropic gallbladder

   (B) choledochal cyst

   (C) Courvoisier's sign

   (D) Mirizzi's syndrome

4. Which of the following will long-standing cystic duct obstruction give rise to?

   (A) porcelain gallbladder

   (B) hydropic gallbladder

   (C) septated gallbladder

   (D) gallbladder septations

5. While performing an ultrasound examination, the sonographer finds that both kidneys measure 5 cm in length. They are very echogenic. One should consider the possibility of all of the following *except*

   (A) chronic glomerulonephritis

   (B) chronic pyelonephritis

   (C) renal vascular disease

   (D) renal vein thrombosis

6. Staghorn calculus refers to a large stone within which of the following?

   (A) pancreas

   (B) urinary bladder

   (C) renal pelvis of the kidney

   (D) neck of the gallbladder

7. What GI peptide hormone stimulates gallbladder contraction?

   (A) gastrin

   (B) cholecalciferol

   (C) cholestyramine

   (D) cholecystokinin

8. What is the name of the portion of the liver that is *not* covered by the peritoneum?

   (A) quadrate lobe

   (B) intraperitoneal

   (C) Riedel's lobe

   (D) bare area

9. What is the normal thickness of the gallbladder wall?

   (A) 15 mm

   (B) 10 mm

   (C) 3 cm

   (D) 3 mm

10. Where does the pancreatic head lie?

    (A) caudad to the portal vein and medial to the SMV

    (B) cephalad to the portal vein and medial to the SMV

    (C) caudad to the portal vein and anterior to the IVC

    (D) cephalad to the portal vein and anterior to the IVC

11. Identify the sonographic pattern that best describes hydronephrosis.

    (A) distortion of the reniform shape

    (B) multiple cystic space masses throughout the kidneys

    (C) fluid-filled pelvocalyceal collecting system

    (D) fluid-filled pararenal space

12. A patient presents with a dilated intrahepatic duct, dilated gallbladder, and a dilated common bile duct. This is most characteristic of which one of the following levels of obstruction?

    (A) proximal common bile duct

    (B) distal common bile duct

    (C) distal common hepatic duct

    (D) cystic duct

13. What is the most common location of pancreatic pseudocyst?

    (A) lesser sac

    (B) porta hepatis area

    (C) groin

    (D) splenic hilum

14. Which of the following is true about the extrahepatic portion of the falciform ligament?

    (A) courses between the IVC and the gallbladder

    (B) is visualized when massive ascites is present

    (C) connects the liver to the lesser sac

    (D) is visualized when peritonitis is present

15. The SMA arises 1 cm below the celiac trunk and courses

    (A) 1 cm before it bifurcates

    (B) inferiorly and lateral to the head of the pancreas

    (C) anterior and parallel to the aorta

    (D) transversely and caudad

16. The division by using Couinaud's sections into right and left lobes of the liver is

    (A) main lobar fissure

    (B) ligamentum venosum

    (C) falciform ligament

    (D) hepatoduodenal ligament

    (E) hepatic arteries

17. Which of the following is the portion of the pancreas that lies posterior to the superior mesenteric artery and vein?

    (A) head

    (B) neck

    (C) uncinate process

    (D) body

18. Which vessel courses along the posterior surface of the body and tail of the pancreas?

    (A) SMA

    (B) left renal vein

    (C) splenic vein

    (D) splenic artery

19. Sonographically, where can the GEJ be visualized?

    (A) anterior to the IVC and posterior to the right lobe of the liver

    (B) anterior to the aorta and posterior to the left lobe of the liver

    (C) lateral to the head of the pancreas

    (D) anterior to the stomach and medial to the spleen

20. Which of the following describes adenomyomatosis of the gallbladder?

    (A) a congenital anomaly that presents itself in the fourth or fifth decade

    (B) an inflammation of the gallbladder and biliary ducts

    (C) associated with chronic hepatitis

    (D) proliferation of the mucosal layer, which extends into the muscle layer

    (E) a malignant process that involves the gallbladder wall and lumen

21. What is the most common cause of acute pyelonephritis?

    (A) hypertension

    (B) *Escherichia coli*

    (C) *Klebsiella*

    (D) hydronephrosis

22. A renal sonogram is performed, and an echogenic well-defined mass is identified in the renal cortex. This is characteristic of which of the following?

    (A) angiomyolipoma

    (B) column of Bertin

    (C) adenocarcinoma

    (D) pyonephrosis

23. The gastroduodenal artery is a branch of which of the following?

    (A) aorta

    (B) celiac axis

    (C) common hepatic artery

    (D) left gastric artery

24. Identify the vessel that is seen anterior to the aorta and posterior to the SMA.

    (A) splenic vein
    (B) common hepatic artery
    (C) left renal vein
    (D) left renal artery

25. The liver is covered by a thick membrane of collagenous fibers intermixed with elastic elements. What is this membrane called?

    (A) Glisson's capsule
    (B) Gerota's fascia
    (C) Bowman's capsule
    (D) adipose capsule

26. Which of the following can cause anterior displacement of the splenic vein?

    (A) pancreatitis
    (B) pseudocysts
    (C) left adrenal hyperplasia
    (D) aneurysm

27. Which one of the following vessels originates from the celiac axis and is very tortuous?

    (A) splenic artery
    (B) hepatic artery
    (C) right gastric artery
    (D) gastroduodenal artery

28. When accessory spleens are present, where are they usually located?

    (A) at the superior margin of the spleen
    (B) on the posterior aspect of the spleen
    (C) near the kidney
    (D) near the splenic hilum

29. What is a fold at the fundal portion of the gallbladder usually called?

    (A) Hartmann's pouch
    (B) junctional fold
    (C) valves of Heister
    (D) Phrygian cap

30. The IVC forms at the confluence of which of the following vessels?

    (A) right and left carotid veins
    (B) right and left common iliac veins
    (C) right and left lumbar veins
    (D) right and left renal veins

31. Diffuse thickening of the gallbladder wall can be seen sonographically in all of the following except

    (A) acute cholecystitis
    (B) hepatitis
    (C) CHF
    (D) portal hypertension

32. A gallbladder sonographic examination is performed, and a small gallbladder with intrahepatic dilatation is seen. This may indicate that the level of obstruction is at the level of which of the following?

    (A) neck of the gallbladder
    (B) common bile duct
    (C) cystic duct
    (D) common hepatic duct

33. What is the maximum inner diameter of the main pancreatic duct in young adults?

    (A) 10 mm
    (B) 5 mm
    (C) 2 mm
    (D) 3 cm

34. Which of the following is produced by the endocrine function of the pancreas?

    (A) insulin
    (B) lipase
    (C) amylase
    (D) trypsin

35. Which laboratory test is used to assess renal function?

    (A) serum creatinine
    (B) serum bilirubin
    (C) AST
    (D) ALP

36. Adult polycystic disease may be characterized by all of the following except

    (A) it is autosomal dominant disease
    (B) it may be associated with cysts in the liver, pancreas, and spleen
    (C) bilateral small and echogenic kidneys
    (D) usually does not produce any symptoms until the third or fourth decade of life

37. What is the best sonographic window to image the left hemidiaphragm?

    (A) liver
    (B) spleen
    (C) stomach
    (D) left kidney

38. A patient in the late stages of sickle cell anemia will have a spleen that is which of the following?

    (A) enlarged and lobulated
    (B) enlarged and echogenic
    (C) small and hypoechoic
    (D) small and echogenic

39. Bilateral hydronephrosis frequently occurs in all of the following *except*

    (A) urinoma
    (B) PUV
    (C) late pregnancy
    (D) fibroid uterus

40. In a patient with acute hepatitis, what is the appearance of the liver parenchyma sonographically?

    (A) hypoechoic
    (B) echogenic
    (C) complex
    (D) normal

41. What is a hypertrophied column of Bertin?

    (A) benign tumor of the kidney
    (B) malignant tumor of the lower urinary tract
    (C) renal variant
    (D) a common cause of hydronephrosis

42. What is a ureterovesical junction?

    (A) junction between the renal pelvis joins the proximal ureter
    (B) junction between the distal ureter and the base of the bladder
    (C) junction between the renal pyramids and the distal calyces
    (D) junction between the ejaculatory ducts and urethra

43. What is the landmark for the posterolateral border of the thyroid?

    (A) trachea
    (B) esophagus

    (C) strap muscle
    (D) common carotid artery

44. Which of the following is *not* a clinical sign of renal disease?

    (A) oliguria
    (B) palpable flank mass
    (C) jaundice
    (D) hypertension

45. Acute hydroceles may be caused by all of the following *except*

    (A) infarction
    (B) tumor
    (C) testicular torsion
    (D) trauma

46. What is the most common malignancy of the adrenal gland in children?

    (A) adrenal adenoma
    (B) neuroblastoma
    (C) nephroblastoma
    (D) pheochromocytoma

47. If a mass in the area of the pancreatic head is found, what other structure should be examined sonographically?

    (A) liver
    (B) IVC
    (C) spleen
    (D) kidney

48. What is the most common primary carcinoma of the pancreas?

    (A) insulinoma
    (B) cystadenocarcinoma
    (C) adenocarcinoma
    (D) pancreatic pseudocyst

49. The ligament of venosum separates which two lobes of the liver?

    (A) right and left lobes
    (B) medial portion of the left lobe and the lateral portion of the left lobe
    (C) caudate lobe and left lobe of the liver
    (D) anterior portion of the right lobe and the posterior portion of the right lobe

50. **What is the most common benign neoplasm of the liver?**

    (A) hemangioma

    (B) angiomyolipoma

    (C) FNH

    (D) abscess

51. **Which of the following may develop in patients with right-sided heart failure and elevated systemic venous pressure?**

    (A) fatty liver

    (B) portal-systemic anastomoses

    (C) FLLs

    (D) dilatation of the intrahepatic veins

52. **Which of the following separates the right and left lobes of the liver?**

    (A) coronary ligament

    (B) main lobar fissure

    (C) falciform ligament

    (D) ligament of venosum

53. **Which of the following is *not* a retroperitoneal structure?**

    (A) kidney

    (B) pancreas

    (C) aorta

    (D) spleen

54. **Which of the following statements is *true* about the portal vein?**

    (A) It is formed by the union of the common hepatic duct and the cystic duct.

    (B) It is only imaged sonographically when there is liver pathology.

    (C) It is formed by the union of the splenic vein and SMV.

    (D) It is very pulsatile.

55. **The common bile duct is joined by the pancreatic duct as they enter the**

    (A) first portion of the duodenum

    (B) second portion of the duodenum

    (C) third portion of the duodenum

    (D) fourth portion of the duodenum

56. **A patient presents with empyema of the gallbladder. What should the sonographer expect to find?**

    (A) pus within the gallbladder

    (B) common bile duct obstruction

    (C) stones within the gallbladder

    (D) abscess surrounding the gallbladder

57. **Identify the laboratory value that is specific for a hepatoma of the liver.**

    (A) ALP

    (B) α-AFP

    (C) serum amylase

    (D) bilirubin

58. **If the prostate is found to be enlarged, which of the following should the sonographer also check?**

    (A) spleen for enlargement

    (B) scrotum for hydroceles

    (C) kidneys for hydronephrosis

    (D) liver for metastases

59. **The body of the pancreas is bound on its anterior surface by which of the following?**

    (A) atrium of stomach

    (B) greater sac

    (C) splenic vein

    (D) common bile duct

60. **On a transverse scan, the portal vein is seen as a circular anechoic structure**

    (A) anterior to the IVC

    (B) posterior to the aorta

    (C) medial to the head of the pancreas

    (D) inferior to the head of the pancreas

61. **Hyperthyroidism associated with a diffuse goiter is associated with which of the following?**

    (A) papillary carcinoma

    (B) Graves' disease

    (C) Hashimoto's thyroiditis

62. **Identify the part of the pancreas that lies anterior to the IVC and posterior to the SMV.**

    (A) head

    (B) neck

    (C) body

    (D) uncinate process

63. In a dissecting aneurysm, the dissection is through which of the following?

    (A) adventitia

    (B) media

    (C) intima

    (D) all three layers

64. The adrenal gland can be divided into which of the following parts?

    (A) pelvis and sinus

    (B) cortex and medulla

    (C) major and minor calices

    (D) head and tail

65. Where can a patent umbilical vein be found?

    (A) ligamentum venosum

    (B) main lobar fissure

    (C) ligamentum teres

    (D) intersegmental ligament

66. All of the following are characteristic for dilated intrahepatic bile ducts *except*

    (A) the parallel channel sign

    (B) irregular borders to dilated bile ducts

    (C) echo enhancement behind dilated ducts

    (D) decreasing size as they course toward the porta hepatis

67. A retroperitoneal abscess may be found within in all of the following *except*

    (A) the rectus abdominis muscle

    (B) the psoas muscle

    (C) the iliacus muscle

    (D) the quadratus lumborum muscle

68. Dilatation of the intrahepatic biliary ducts without dilatation of the extrahepatic ducts may be caused by all of the following *except*

    (A) a Klatskin tumor

    (B) enlarged portal lymph nodes

    (C) a cholangiocarcinoma

    (D) a pancreatic carcinoma

69. A 42-year-old woman presents post cholecystectomy with RUQ pain, elevated serum bilirubin (mainly conjugated), and bilirubin in her urine. Which of the following is this best characteristic of?

    (A) hepatitis

    (B) stone, tumor, or stricture causing obstruction of the bile duct

    (C) small common duct stone <5 mm in diameter

    (D) ALP will be normal

70. What is a cause of a small gallbladder?

    (A) prolonged fasting

    (B) insulin-dependent diabetes

    (C) chronic cholecystitis

    (D) hydrops

71. Identify the vessel that is located superior to the pancreas.

    (A) IVC

    (B) SMA

    (C) splenic vein

    (D) celiac axis

72. A tumor in the retroperitoneal space will displace surrounding organs in what position?

    (A) anterior

    (B) posterior

    (C) medial

    (D) lateral

73. Which of the following can cause anterior displacement of the abdominal aorta?

    (A) enlarged adrenal gland

    (B) kidney mass

    (C) aortic aneurysm

    (D) enlarged lymph nodes

74. Sonographically, how do enlarged lymph nodes most commonly appear?

    (A) as solid masses

    (B) as complex masses

    (C) as cystic masses with increased through transmission

    (D) as hypoechoic masses with no increased through transmission

75. Which of the following best describes hepatofugal blood flow?

    (A) blood flows away from the liver

    (B) turbulent blood flow

    (C) intermittent blood flow

    (D) blood flows toward the liver

76. **What anatomic landmarks can be used to sonographically locate the left adrenal gland?**

    (A) aorta, stomach, and spleen

    (B) aorta, spleen, and left kidney

    (C) IVC, spleen, and left kidney

    (D) IVC, stomach, and left kidney

77. **Which of the following most likely appears as nonshadowing, nonmobile, echogenic foci imaged within the gallbladder lumen?**

    (A) polyps

    (B) calculi

    (C) biliary gravel

    (D) thin bile

78. **What is hydrops of the gallbladder?**

    (A) a small contracted gallbladder

    (B) a gallbladder with a thickened wall

    (C) a thick-walled gallbladder filled with stones

    (D) an enlarged gallbladder

79. **Which of the following most likely causes jaundice in a pediatric patient?**

    (A) hepatitis

    (B) fatty infiltration

    (C) biliary atresia

    (D) cirrhosis

80. **The majority of primary retroperitoneal tumors are malignant. Which of the following is an example of a primary retroperitoneal tumor?**

    (A) hepatoma

    (B) hypernephroma

    (C) leiomyosarcoma

    (D) adenocarcinoma

81. **Compare the echogenicities of the following structures and place them in increasing echogenic order.**

    (A) renal sinus < pancreas < liver < spleen < renal parenchyma

    (B) renal sinus < liver < spleen < pancreas < renal parenchyma

    (C) pancreas < liver < spleen < renal sinus < renal parenchyma

    (D) renal parenchyma < liver < spleen < pancreas < renal sinus

82. **In comparison to the normal echotexture in adults, the pancreas in children will be relatively**

    (A) more echogenic

    (B) less echogenic

    (C) the same echogenicity

    (D) larger and less echogenic

83. **The kidneys, the perinephric fat, and the adrenal glands are all covered by which of the following?**

    (A) a true capsule

    (B) Gerota's fascia

    (C) peritoneum

    (D) Glisson's capsule

84. **What is the largest major visceral branch of the IVC?**

    (A) portal vein

    (B) hepatic veins

    (C) renal veins

    (D) inferior mesenteric vein

85. **The spleen is variable in size, but it is considered to be which of the following?**

    (A) concave superiorly and inferiorly

    (B) convex superiorly and concave inferiorly

    (C) concave superiorly and convex inferiorly

    (D) convex superiorly and inferiorly

86. **A malignant solid renal mass can be all of the following except**

    (A) renal cell carcinoma

    (B) adenocarcinoma of the kidney

    (C) oncocytoma

    (D) transitional cell carcinoma

87. **Which one of the following statements correctly describes the anatomic location of structures adjacent to the spleen?**

    (A) The diaphragm is superior, lateral, and inferior to the spleen.

    (B) The fundus of the stomach and lesser sac are medial and posterior to the splenic helium.

    (C) The left kidney lies inferior and medial to the spleen.

    (D) The pancreas lies anterior and medial to the spleen.

88. Which of the following sonographic findings are associated with hematoceles?

    (A) a cyst along the course of the vas deferens

    (B) a blood-filled sac that surrounds the testicle, secondary to trauma or surgery

    (C) dilated veins caused by obstruction of the venous return

    (D) a condition in which the testicles have not descended

89. When scanning a 22-year-old patient to rule out cholelithiasis, a single echogenic lesion is seen within the liver. What is this most characteristic of?

    (A) a cavernous hemangioma

    (B) a hematoma

    (C) a hepatic cyst

    (D) an abscess

90. What are normal measurements of the thyroid gland?

    (A) 3–4 cm in anteroposterior and length dimensions

    (B) 2–3 cm in anteroposterior dimensions and 4–6 cm in length

    (C) 1–2 cm in anteroposterior dimensions and 4–6 cm in length

    (D) 3–5 cm in anteroposterior dimensions and 6–8 cm in length

91. Ascites can be caused by all of the following *except*

    (A) malignancy

    (B) nephritic syndrome

    (C) CHF

    (D) adenomyomatosis

92. What is the best way to delineate a dissecting aneurysm on sonography?

    (A) Begin scanning in the transverse section and document serial scans.

    (B) Show an intimal flap pulsating with the flow of blood.

    (C) Scan the patient in a decubitus position to document the aorta and inferior vena cava simultaneously.

    (D) Document the renal arteries.

93. Obstructive jaundice may be diagnosed sonographically by demonstrating which of the following?

    (A) a mass in the head of the pancreas with a dilated common bile duct

    (B) an enlarged liver

    (C) a fibrotic and atrophic liver

    (D) cholangitis

94. Where would a subhepatic abscess be located?

    (A) superior to the liver

    (B) inferior to the liver, anterior to the right kidney

    (C) inferior to the liver, posterior to the right kidney

    (D) adjacent to the porta hepatis

95. Which of the following is *not* a remnant of the fetal circulation?

    (A) ligamentum teres

    (B) ligamentum venosum

    (C) falciform ligament

    (D) coronary ligament

96. Which of the following is a major branch of the common hepatic artery?

    (A) gastroduodenal artery

    (B) coronary artery

    (C) esophageal artery

    (D) left gastric artery

97. A 44-year-old patient presents with painless jaundice and a palpable RUQ mass, which is most characteristic of which of the following?

    (A) acute hepatitis

    (B) cirrhosis

    (C) porcelain gallbladder

    (D) Courvoisier's gallbladder

98. A common anatomical variant is a bulge of the lateral border of the left kidney. What is this called?

    (A) duplex kidney

    (B) dromedary hump

    (C) column of Bertin

    (D) Bowman's capsule

99. Which of the following *cannot* be imaged in a case of end-stage liver disease?

    (A) ascites

    (B) small atrophied liver

    (C) biliary dilatation

    (D) portal hypertension

100. The head of the pancreas is located anterior to which of the following vessels?

    (A) IVC
    (B) aorta
    (C) SMA
    (D) splenic vein

101. What is the lesser sac located between?

    (A) pancreas and the IVC
    (B) stomach and pancreas
    (C) abdominal wall and stomach
    (D) liver and right kidney

102. Where are the renal pyramids found?

    (A) cortex
    (B) medulla
    (C) renal pelvis
    (D) renal sinus

103. Which of the following is chronic renal disease associated with?

    (A) an enlarged kidney with a small contralateral kidney
    (B) unilateral hydronephrosis
    (C) small echogenic kidneys
    (D) renal carbuncle

104. A 50-year-old woman with a long history of alcoholism presents with increased abdominal girth. Which of the following is the most probable finding on a sonogram of the abdomen?

    (A) liver metastases
    (B) massive ascites with a small echogenic liver
    (C) hepatoma
    (D) gallstones with a mass in the lumen of the gallbladder

105. Chronic active hepatitis is a progressive destructive liver disease that eventually leads to which of the following?

    (A) liver cysts
    (B) hepatoma
    (C) cirrhosis
    (D) pancreatitis

106. A 6-year-old child presents with recurrent fever, right-upper-quadrant pain, and jaundice. An abdominal sonogram is performed. The liver and gallbladder appear normal, but a 2-cm cyst is seen communicating with the common bile duct. What does this cystic structure most likely represent?

    (A) a choledochal cyst
    (B) a pseudocyst
    (C) an aortic aneurysm
    (D) a mucocele

107. A 35-year-old woman presents with a tender neck, and on physical exam, an enlarged thyroid is found. An enlarged inhomogeneous thyroid with irregular borders is seen on the sonogram. What is this most characteristic of?

    (A) a malignant lesion
    (B) Graves' disease
    (C) cyst
    (D) Hashimoto's thyroiditis

108. What is calcification of the gallbladder wall called?

    (A) Cholesterolosis
    (B) Courvoisier's gallbladder
    (C) hydropic gallbladder
    (D) porcelain gallbladder

109. A 60-year-old man presents with an abdominal pulsatile mass and high blood pressure. What is this most characteristic of?

    (A) an aneurysm
    (B) a mesenteric cyst
    (C) gallstones
    (D) Budd–Chiari syndrome

110. Identify the vessel that may be imaged posterior to the IVC.

    (A) right renal vein
    (B) right renal artery
    (C) left renal vein
    (D) left renal artery

175. **Which of the following is usually the cause of an aneurysm?**

    (A) degenerative joint disease

    (B) atherosclerosis

    (C) hypertension

    (D) diabetes

176. **What is the arrow in Fig. 4–31 pointing to?**

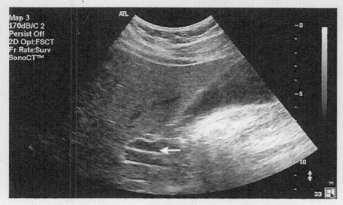

FIGURE 4–31. Magnified sagittal sonogram of the porta hepatis area.

    (A) common hepatic duct

    (B) hepatic artery

    (C) common bile duct

    (D) portal vein

177. **What are the sonographic findings shown in Fig. 4–32 consistent with?**

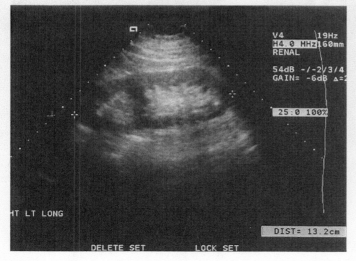

FIGURE 4–32. Long-axis view of the left kidney. *(Used with permission from Shpetim Telegrafi, MD, New York University.)*

    (A) column of Bertin

    (B) prominent renal pyramid

    (C) junctional parenchymal defect

    (D) duplex collecting system

178. **What is the arrowhead in Fig. 4–33 pointing to?**

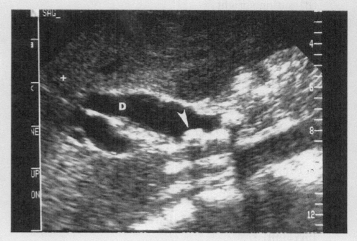

FIGURE 4–33. Magnified oblique sonogram of the porta hepatis area.

    (A) calculi in the common bile duct

    (B) calculi in the neck of the gallbladder

    (C) air in the bile system

    (D) a Klatskin tumor

179. **A renal ultrasound is performed on a 30-year-old patient with right flank pain, elevated BUN, and creatinine. The findings in Fig. 4–34 are consistent with all of the following *except***

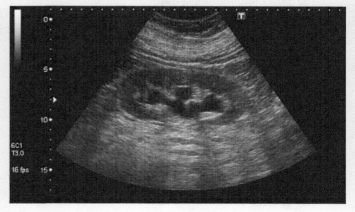

FIGURE 4–34. Long-axis scan through the left kidney. *(Used with permission from Shpetim Telegrafi, MD, New York University.)*

    (A) a stone in the ureter

    (B) an enlarged prostate

    (C) gallstones

    (D) the posterior urethra valve (PUV)

180. Sonographers are sometimes asked to assist in sonographic-guided needle thoracentesis. What is the recommended position for the patient?

    (A) Trendelenburg position
    (B) sitting upright
    (C) Sims position
    (D) recumbent position

181. Patients with hyperthyroidism caused by Graves' disease is most likely to have which of the following biochemical markers?

    (A) increased triiodothyronine (T_3) and thyroxine (T_4)
    (B) decreased T_3 and T_4
    (C) high thyroid-stimulating hormone (TSH)
    (D) no changes in T_3 and T_4

182. What is the sonographic characteristic of Hashimoto's thyroiditis?

    (A) atrophic thyroid tissue with homogeneous echo-texture
    (B) multiple hypoechoic micronodules
    (C) bilateral enlargements of the thyroid with multiple small cyst
    (D) hypertrophy of the thyroid gland with homogeneous echo-texture

183. Which of the following is associated with an increase with the biochemical marker CEA?

    (A) post radioimmunotherapy
    (B) bowel decompression surgery
    (C) follicular cyst of the ovaries
    (D) relapse of colorectal cancer

184. A 35-year-old man was found to have an abdominal mass, and a sonographically guided fine needle aspiration biopsy is required. What kind of anesthesia is normally used for this type of procedure?

    (A) topical
    (B) regional
    (C) general
    (D) local

185. Pneumobilia is most likely seen after which of the following procedures?

    (A) cholecystectomy
    (B) barium enema
    (C) gallstone lithotripsy
    (D) endoscopic retrograde cholangiopancreatography (ERCP)

186. Which of the following anatomical structures is *not* seen anterior to the IVC in the abdomen?

    (A) main lobar fissure
    (B) main portal vein
    (C) left hepatic vein
    (D) right renal artery

187. Hashimoto's disease is a chronic disease of which of the following glands?

    (A) pancreas
    (B) thyroid
    (C) adrenal
    (D) prostate

188. What is the most common cause for acute pancreatitis in the United States?

    (A) smoking and alcohol abuse
    (B) cocaine and marijuana
    (C) cholelithiasis and pancreatic tumor
    (D) cholelithiasis and alcoholism

189. Fig. 4–35 suggests that the patient has which of the following?

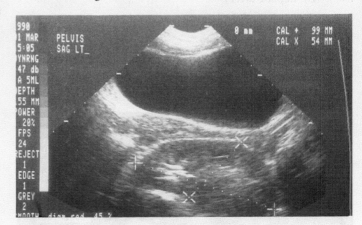

FIGURE 4–35. Sagittal sonogram through the pelvis.

    (A) horseshoe kidney
    (B) unilateral renal agenesis
    (C) three kidneys
    (D) pelvic kidney

190. A patient presents with a history of epigastric pain and elevated lipase. What does the arrows in Fig. 4–36 point to?

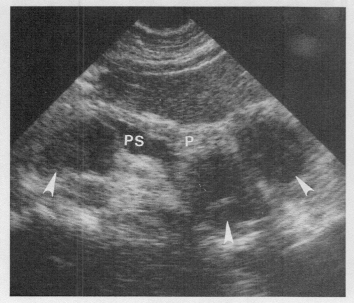

FIGURE 4–36. Transverse sonogram through the pancreatic region.

(A) lymph nodes
(B) mesenteric cysts
(C) pseudocyst
(D) abscesses

191. What is the arrow in Fig. 4–37 pointing to?

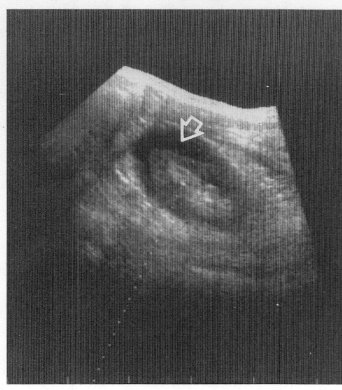

FIGURE 4–37. Longitudinal sonogram through the kidney.

(A) a pseudocyst
(B) perirenal fluid
(C) a dromedary hump
(D) pleural effusion

192. What are the findings in Fig. 4–38 most consistent with?

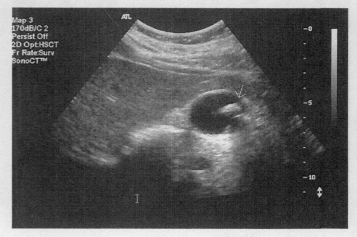

FIGURE 4–38. Left decubitus scan through the upper abdomen.

(A) acute cholecystitis with gallstones
(B) porcelain gallbladder with gallstones
(C) biliary sludge
(D) adenomyomatosis

193. Identify the artifact shown in Fig. 4–39 (arrow).

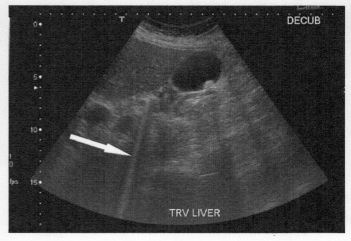

FIGURE 4–39. Left decubitus scan through the upper abdomen.

(A) comet tail
(B) noise
(C) distal acoustic shadow
(D) refraction

194. What is the arrowhead in Fig. 4–40 pointing to?

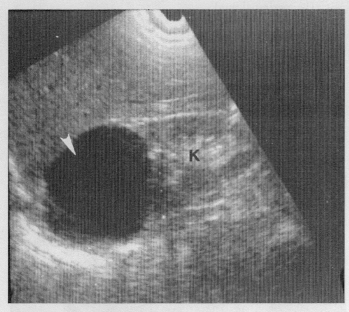

FIGURE 4–40. Long-axis view through a kidney.

(A) the gallbladder

(B) an upper pole hydronephrosis

(C) a renal cyst

(D) an aneurysm

195. The patient in Fig. 4–40 will most likely present with which of the following?

(A) flank pain

(B) fever

(C) nausea and vomiting

(D) no symptoms

196. What are the calipers in Fig. 4–41 measuring?

(A) antrum of stomach

(B) lymph node

(C) pancreatic pseudocyst

(D) body of pancreas

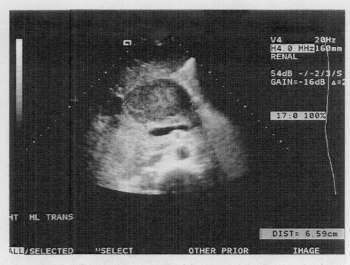

FIGURE 4–41. Transverse sonogram of the upper abdomen. *(Used with permission from Shpetim Telegrafi, MD, New York University.)*

197. A 35-year-old man presents with RUQ pain and recurrent attacks of pancreatitis. His laboratory results would be expected to indicate which of the following?

(A) increased BUN

(B) decreased serum amylase

(C) increased lipase

(D) increased indirect bilirubin

198. Sonographically, one can recognize fatty infiltration of the liver by all of the following *except*

(A) hepatomegaly

(B) parenchymal echoes are echogenic

(C) a focal mass

(D) decreased through transmission

199. Obstruction of the common bile duct by a mass in the head of the pancreas will lead to which of the following?

(A) a dilated gallbladder with dilated biliary radicles

(B) a contracted gallbladder with dilated biliary radicles

(C) dilated biliary radicles with normal or shrunken gallbladder

(D) portal hypertension

200. A 41-year-old man presents with epigastric pain and a history of alcoholism. The findings in Fig. 4–42 include which of the following?

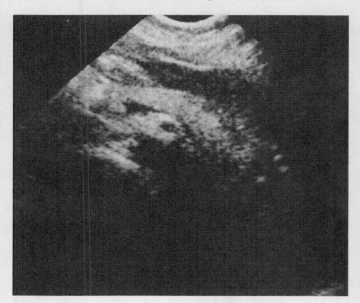

FIGURE 4–42. Transverse sonogram of the upper abdomen.

(A) fatty pancreas

(B) adenocarcinoma

(C) metastatic disease to the pancreas

(D) chronic pancreatitis

201. A 50-year-old woman presents with painless hematuria. A longitudinal view of the left kidney is imaged in Fig. 4–43. What are the findings most consistent with?

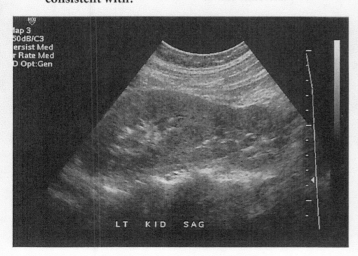

FIGURE 4–43. A longitudinal sonogram of the left kidney.

(A) transitional cell carcinoma

(B) renal cell carcinoma

(C) adenoma

(D) angiolipoma

202. What is the most common medical disease that causes acute renal failure?

(A) acute tubular necrosis

(B) renal infarction

(C) diabetes

(D) hypertension

203. What is Fig. 4–44 consistent with?

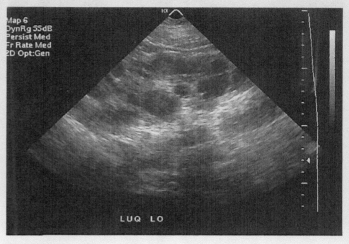

FIGURE 4–44. Longitudinal sonogram of the kidney.

(A) adult polycystic kidneys

(B) hydronephrosis

(C) medullary sponge kidney

(D) medullary cystic disease

204. A pelvic sonogram is performed. What is Fig. 4–45 consistent with?

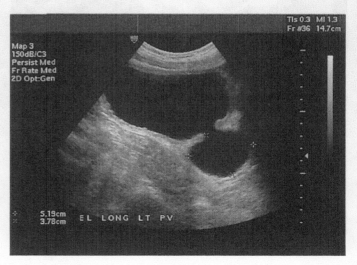

FIGURE 4–45. Left sagittal sonogram of the pelvis.

(A) diverticula

(B) a Foley catheter balloon

(C) a ureterocele

(D) a bladder cyst

205. What are the arrows in Fig. 4–46 pointing to?

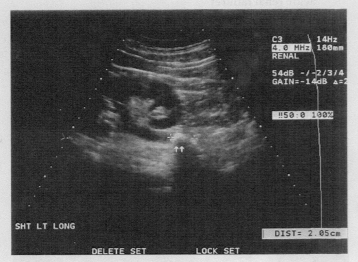

FIGURE 4–46. Longitudinal scan of the left kidney. *(Used with permission from Shpetim Telegrafi, MD, New York University.)*

(A) thrombus

(B) polyp

(C) bowel

(D) calculi

206. Fig. 4–47 is a midline longitudinal scan of the abdomen. What is the abnormality?

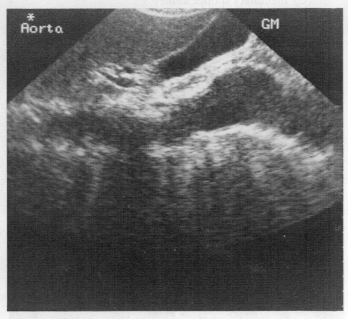

FIGURE 4–47. Midline longitudinal scan of the abdomen.

(A) an ectopic gallbladder

(B) aneurysmal dilatation of the distal abdominal aorta

(C) occlusion of abdominal aorta by thrombus

(D) a dissecting aneurysm

207. What term is used to describe onset of pain while scanning over the gallbladder?

(A) Kehr's sign

(B) candle sign

(C) Murphy's sign

(D) Chandelier's sign

208. What is the most likely diagnosis that can be made by the findings shown in Fig. 4–48?

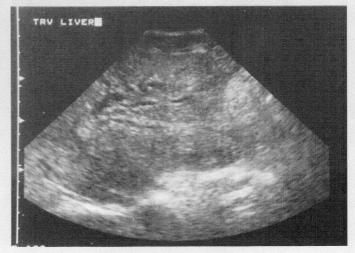

FIGURE 4–48. Transverse sonogram of the liver.

(A) biliary obstruction caused by cholelithiasis

(B) biliary obstruction caused by pancreatitis

(C) distended portal vein caused by portal hypertension

(D) obstruction of the distal common duct caused by a pancreatic tumor

209. Which one of the following statements concerning the sonographic patterns of periaortic lymph nodes is *not* correct?

(A) They may drape or mantle the great vessels anteriorly.

(B) They may displace the SMA posteriorly.

(C) They may displace the great vessels anteriorly.

(D) They may have lobar, smooth, or scalloped appearance.

210. Which of the following findings is *not* represented in Fig. 4–49?

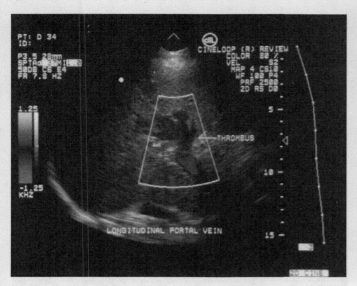

FIGURE 4–49. Longitudinal sonogram of the portal vein.

(A) diabetes

(B) hepatitis

(C) malignancy

(D) chronic pancreatitis

211. What is the blood flow in Fig. 4–50 consistent with?

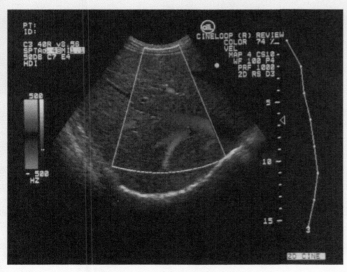

FIGURE 4–50. Transverse sonogram of the upper liver.

(A) right-sided heart failure

(B) cirrhosis

(C) normal blood flow in the hepatic and portal veins

(D) cavernous transformation of the portal vein

212. What is the arrow in Fig. 4–51 pointing to?

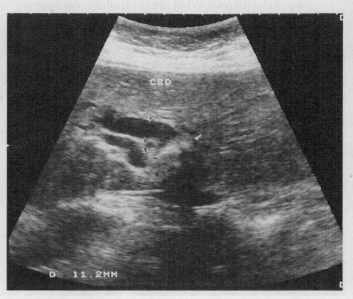

FIGURE 4–51. Oblique sonogram of the liver.

(A) a mass in the head of the pancreas

(B) C-loop of duodenum

(C) bowel mass

(D) calculi

213. What are the calipers in Fig. 4–51 measuring?

(A) common hepatic duct

(B) common bile duct

(C) main portal vein

(D) hepatic vein

214. What are the findings in Fig. 4–51 most consistent with?

(A) mass in the head of the pancreas

(B) intrahepatic obstruction

(C) choledocholithiasis

(D) liver trauma

271. The findings in Fig. 4–81 are associated with all of the following *except*

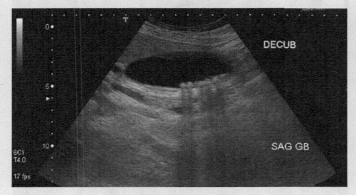

FIGURE 4–81. Longitudinal scan of the gallbladder.

(A) an increase in ALP
(B) an increase in SGOT
(C) sickle cell disease
(D) an increase α-AFP

272. The findings in Fig. 4–82 are consistent with which of the following diagnoses?

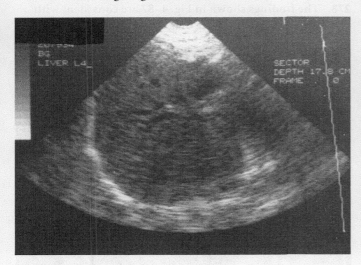

FIGURE 4–82. Longitudinal scan of the liver.

(A) Budd–Chiari syndrome
(B) hepatitis
(C) dilated biliary radicles
(D) gallstones

273. The findings in Fig. 4–83 are consistent with which of the following diagnoses?

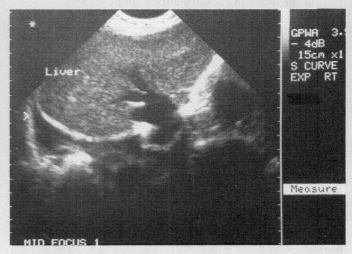

FIGURE 4–83. Transverse scan of the liver.

(A) portal hypertension
(B) CHF
(C) fatty liver disease
(D) cirrhosis

274. Which of the following ligaments are visualized in Fig. 4–84?

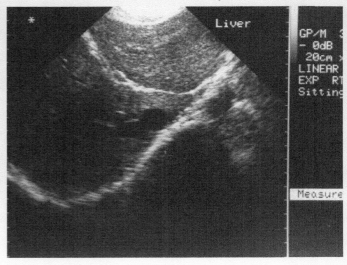

FIGURE 4–84. Transverse scan of the liver.

(A) middle lobar ligament
(B) ligament venosum
(C) coronary ligament
(D) round ligament

275. Fig. 4–85 is an upright coronal image of the lower left hemithorax of a 12-year-old child with a fever. Which of the following abnormalities can be seen?

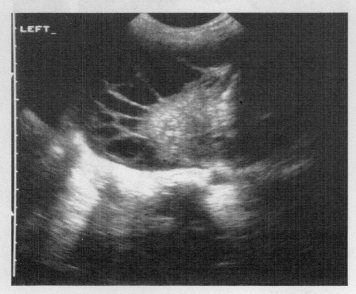

FIGURE 4–85.   An upright coronal image of the lower left hemithorax of a 12-year-old child with a cough and fever.

(A) loculated pleural effusion

(B) nonloculated pleural effusion

(C) hydronephrotic kidney

(D) herniated bowel

276. Which of the following is the most likely diagnosis of the patient in Fig. 4–85?

(A) simple effusion

(B) cystic lung mass

(C) obstructed bowel

(D) empyema

277. A patient presents with RUQ pain, fever, nausea, and leukocytosis. The findings in Fig. 4–86 are most consistent with which of the following diagnoses?

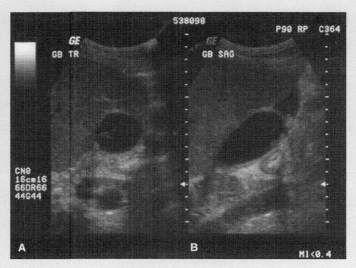

FIGURE 4–86.   (A) Transverse image of the gallbladder. (B) Long-axis image of the gallbladder.

(A) gallbladder carcinoma

(B) chronic cholecystitis

(C) adenomyomatosis

(D) acute cholecystitis

278. The findings shown in Fig. 4–87 are consistent with which of the following diagnoses?

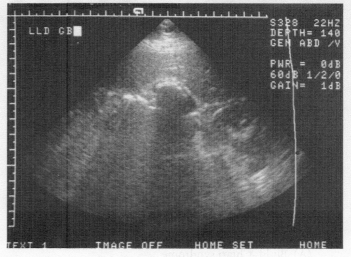

FIGURE 4–87.   Longitudinal scan of the right upper quadrant.

(A) chronic cholecystitis with cholelithiasis

(B) adenomatosis

(C) postprandial gallbladder contraction

(D) duodenal bulb

279. A patient presents with an increase in direct bilirubin, ALT, and ALP. What are the findings in Fig. 4–88 suggestive of?

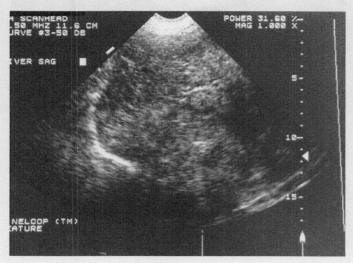

FIGURE 4–88. Longitudinal scan of the liver.

(A) liver metastases

(B) hepatoma

(C) cirrhosis

(D) fatty infiltrations

280. A patient presents with vague RUQ pain and normal liver function laboratory test results. The echogenic mass in Fig. 4–89 is suggestive of a liver

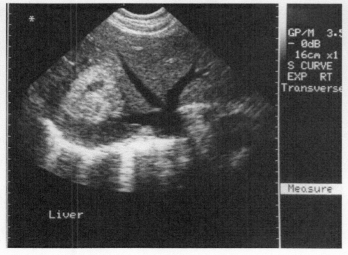

FIGURE 4–89. Transverse scan of the liver.

(A) abscess

(B) hematoma

(C) hepatoma

(D) hemangioma

281. Where is the echogenic mass shown in Fig. 4–89 located?

(A) posterior segment of the right lobe

(B) anterior segment of the right lobe

(C) anterior segment of the left lobe

(D) medial segment of the right lobe

282. Which of the following terms describes the malformation variant in the gallbladder that involves an acutely angulated pouch of the fundus?

(A) Phrygian cap

(B) duplication of the gallbladder

(C) Hartmann's pouch

(D) junctional fold

283. Identify the vessels being imaged in Fig. 4–90 in the order in which they appear (anterior to posterior).

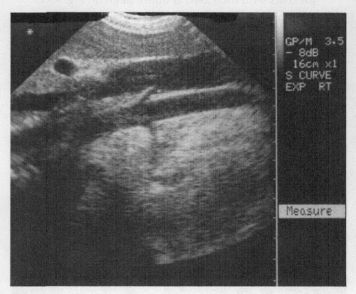

FIGURE 4–90. Coronal scan of the midabdomen.

(A) IVC, portal vein, left renal vein, right renal vein

(B) IVC, aorta, right hepatic artery, splenic artery

(C) IVC, aorta, left renal vein, right renal vein

(D) IVC, aorta, right renal artery, left renal artery

284. Which of the following statements does *not* differentiate the portal veins from the hepatic veins?

(A) portal veins become larger as they approach the diaphragm.

(B) portal veins have echogenic borders.

(C) portal veins bifurcate into the right and left branches.

(D) the main portal vein is part of the portal triad.

285. Horseshoe kidney may be confused sonographically with which of the following?

(A) carcinoma of the head of the pancreas

(B) lymphadenopathy

(C) hypernephroma

(D) gastric mass

286. A 53-year-old man with a history of liver cirrhosis presents with increased abdominal girth. Fig. 4–91 demonstrates a thickened gallbladder wall, which is most often associated with which of the following?

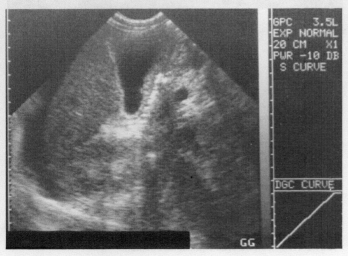

FIGURE 4–91. Longitudinal scan of the liver and gallbladder.

(A) calculous cholecystitis

(B) pancreatitis

(C) portal hypertension

(D) adjacent ascites

287. What is the arrow in Fig. 4–92 pointing to?

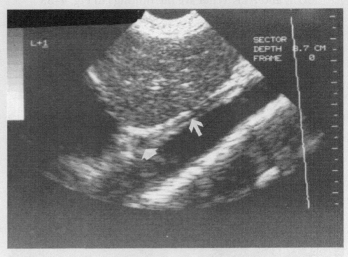

FIGURE 4–92. Longitudinal scan of the aorta.

(A) IVC

(B) SMA

(C) celiac

(D) right crus of the diaphragm

288. The left crus of the diaphragm may be confused with which of the following?

(A) left adrenal gland

(B) aorta

(C) splenic vein

(D) SMA

289. What is the long arrow in Fig. 4–93 pointing to?

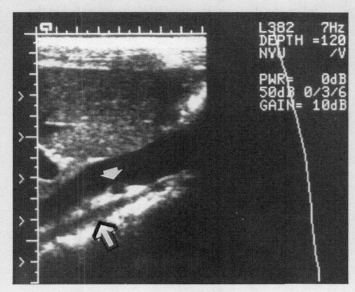

FIGURE 4–93. Longitudinal scan of the inferior vena cava.

(A) IVC
(B) psoas muscle
(C) lumbar artery
(D) right crus of diaphragm

290. What is the short arrow in Fig. 4–93 pointing to?

(A) right renal vein
(B) right renal artery
(C) left renal vein
(D) left renal artery

291. What is the arrow in Fig. 4–94 pointing to?

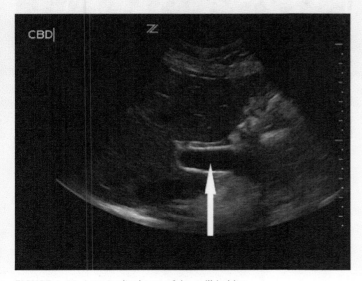

FIGURE 4–94. Longitudinal scan of the gallbladder.

(A) hepatic artery
(B) common duct
(C) hepatic vein
(D) portal vein

292. What is the lumen seen anterior and parallel to the arrow in Fig. 4–94?

(A) common duct
(B) cystic duct
(C) left renal vein
(D) hepatic vein

293. There appear to be two echogenic masses in Fig. 4–95. One is anterior to the diaphragm (indicated by the calipers), and the other one is posterior to the diaphragm (indicated by the arrow). Which of the following usually causes this phenomenon?

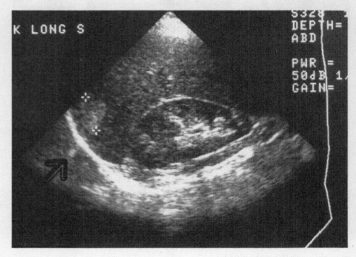

FIGURE 4–95. Longitudinal scan of the right upper quadrant.

(A) slice-thickness artifact
(B) reflection
(C) mirror-image artifact
(D) refraction

294. A 38-year-old man, who is an intravenous drug abuser, with a known mediastinal mass is seen in Fig. 4–96A and B. What does Fig. 4–96A show?

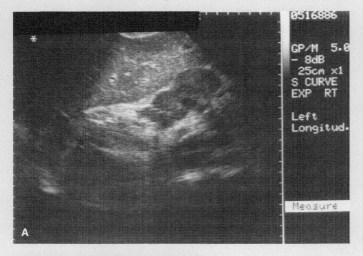

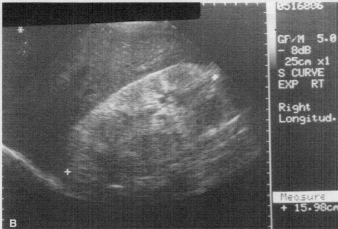

FIGURE 4–96. **(A)** Sagittal scan of the right upper quadrant. **(B)** Sagittal scan through the right kidney.

   (A) a mass near the head of the pancreas
   (B) periportal lymphadenopathy
   (C) chronic cholecystitis
   (D) Klatskin tumor

295. Which of the following is demonstrated in Fig. 4–96B?

   (A) a normal kidney
   (B) a kidney consistent with acute renal insufficiency
   (C) a kidney consistent with chronic renal insufficiency
   (D) renal cell carcinoma

296. A sonogram is performed on a 32-year-old woman with a history of pancreatic carcinoma. Which of the following diagnoses is most likely represented in the scan in Fig. 4–97?

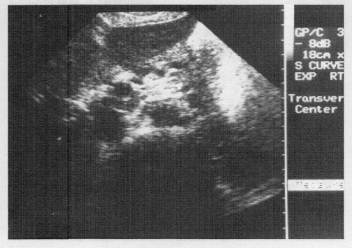

FIGURE 4–97. Transverse scan of the abdomen.

   (A) celiac nodes
   (B) an aortic aneurysm
   (C) horseshoe kidney
   (D) gastric lesion

297. What type of aneurysm is demonstrated in Fig. 4–98?

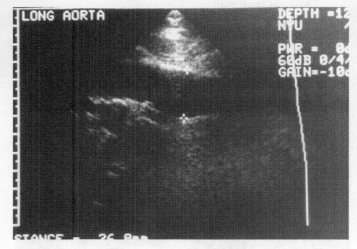

FIGURE 4–98. Longitudinal scan through the abdominal aorta.

   (A) fusiform
   (B) saccular
   (C) cylindrical
   (D) berry

298. What is the arrow in Fig. 4–99 pointing to?

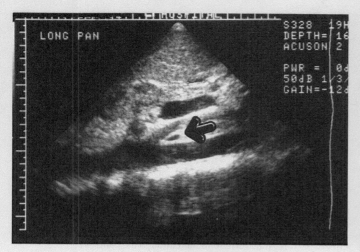

FIGURE 4–99. Longitudinal scan through the abdominal aorta.

(A) right renal artery

(B) right renal vein

(C) left renal artery

(D) left renal vein

299. What is the arrow in Fig. 4–100 pointing to?

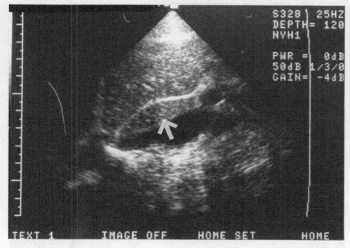

FIGURE 4–100. Sagittal scan through the right upper quadrant.

(A) head of the pancreas

(B) body of the pancreas

(C) caudate lobe of the liver

(D) medial aspect of the left lobe

300. What is the thin black arrow in Fig. 4–101 pointing to?

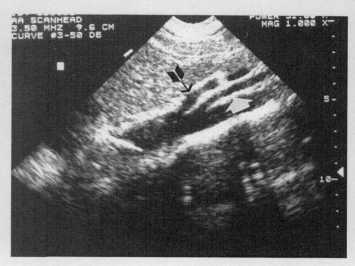

FIGURE 4–101. Sagittal scan through the right upper quadrant.

(A) celiac artery

(B) SMA

(C) portal vein

(D) left gastric artery

301. What is the white arrowhead in Fig. 4–101 pointing to?

(A) celiac artery

(B) SMA

(C) portal vein

(D) left gastric artery

302. What is the name of the vessel that lies posterior to the pancreas in Fig. 4–101?

(A) splenic vein

(B) aorta

(C) portal vein

(D) left renal vein

303. What is the arrow in Fig. 4–102 pointing to?

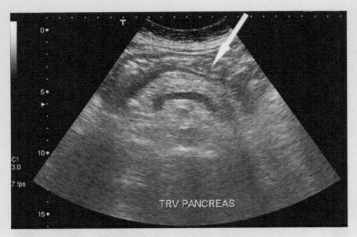

FIGURE 4–102. Transverse scan through the pancreas.

(A) stomach

(B) pancreas

(C) C-loop of the duodenum

(D) gastroduodenal artery

304. What is the arrow in Fig. 4–103 pointing to?

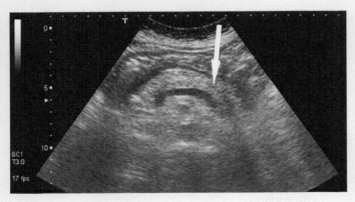

FIGURE 4–103. Transverse sonogram through the pancreas.

(A) normal head of pancreas

(B) normal stomach

(C) pancreatic duct

(D) normal tail of the pancreas

305. What is the arrow in Fig. 4–104 pointing to?

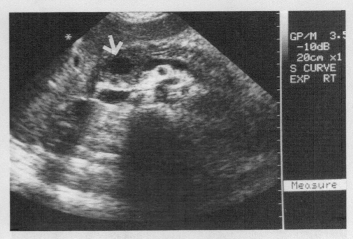

FIGURE 4–104. Transverse sonogram through the pancreas.

(A) gastroduodenal artery

(B) common bile duct

(C) portal vein

(D) SMV

306. Which of the following structures defines the anterolateral aspect of the head of the pancreas?

(A) gastroduodenal artery

(B) IVC

(C) splenic vein

(D) common bile duct

307. What are the arrows in Fig. 4–105 pointing to?

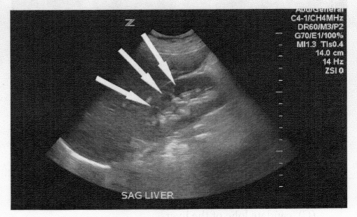

FIGURE 4–105. Long-axis image of the right kidney.

(A) peripelvic cysts

(B) extrapelvic cysts

(C) parapelvic cysts

(D) renal pyramids

308. What is demonstrated in this color Doppler image of the bladder in Fig. 4–106?

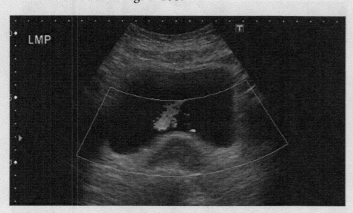

FIGURE 4–106. Short-axis sonogram through the urinary bladder.

(A) acute obstructive uropathy

(B) ureteral dilatation

(C) diverticular jet effect

(D) color Doppler flow

309. What is the finding seen within the urinary bladder of the patient imaged in Fig. 4–106?

(A) ureteral jet

(B) thickened Foley catheter

(C) bladder aneurysm

(D) ureteral venous flow

310. Ureteral jets will not be seen in which of the following?

(A) extrapelvic cyst

(B) obstructive hydronephrosis

(C) renal artery aneurysm

(D) parapelvic cyst

311. A 30-year-old patient with a history of biliary disease presents with fever, pain, and leukocytosis. An abdominal sonogram is performed. The areas labeled "A" in Fig. 4–107 are consistent with which of the following diagnoses?

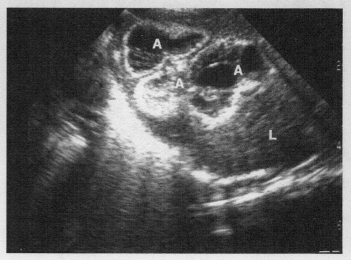

FIGURE 4–107. Sonogram of the urinary bladder.

(A) hematomas

(B) complicated cysts

(C) abscesses

(D) echinococcal disease

312. A patient presents with polycystic liver disease. What other organ should also be evaluated by sonogram?

(A) kidneys

(B) pancreas

(C) gallbladder

(D) adrenal glands

313. Identify the vessel with a postprandial low-resistive blood flow.

(A) celiac artery

(B) hepatic artery

(C) splenic artery

(D) SMA

ligament. The falciform ligament divides the left lobe of the liver into medial and lateral segments. The main lobar fissure divides the liver into right and left lobes.

50. (A) The most common benign neoplasm of the liver is a hemangioma, which is also called a cavernous hemangioma. It can be either single or multiple and is more commonly found in women and in the right lobe of the liver.

51. (D) Blood from the hepatic veins drain into the IVC, which delivers deoxygenated blood to the right atrium of the heart. Right-side heart failure will produce venous congestion of the liver, which will lead to marked dilation of the intrahepatic veins.

52. (B) The main lobar fissure separates the right and left lobes of the liver. The ligamentum of venosum separates the anterior portion of the caudate lobe from the left lobe of the liver, and the ligament of teres (round ligament) is a cord-like ligament that is located in the free margin of the falciform ligament. The falciform ligament divides the left lobe of the liver into medial and lateral segment.

53. (D) The spleen is an intraperitoneal structure. Retroperitoneal structures include the kidney, pancreas, great vessels, adrenal glands, psoas muscles, and duodenum.

54. (C) The splenic vein and SMV join together to form the portal vein. The junction of the splenic vein and SMV occurs posterior to the neck of the pancreas.

55. (B) The common bile duct unites with the main pancreatic duct just before entering the second portion of the duodenum.

56. (A) Empyema of the gallbladder is a complication of acute cholecystitis. The patient presents with high spiking fever, chills, and leukocytosis. The walls of the gallbladder are thickened, and the lumen is filled with pus and debris. There may be a "dirty" shadow caused by the gas, which is formed by the bacteria.

57. (B) A cause of an increase in α-AFP in a nonpregnant patient is a hepatoma of the liver.

58. (C) If the prostate is found enlarged, one should check the kidneys for hydronephrosis. An enlarged prostate gland is a common cause of bladder neck obstruction in older men.

59. (A) The anterior wall of the body of the pancreas is the posterior wall of the antrum of the stomach.

60. (A) On a transverse scan, the portal vein is seen as a circular structure anterior to the IVC and superior to the head of the pancreas.

61. (B) The most common cause of hyperthyroidism is Graves' disease that is an autoimmune disease where by the immune system attacks the thyroid and causes diffuse enlargement of the thyroid gland.

62. (D) A prominent uncinate process is anterior to the IVC and posterior to the SMV.

63. (C) A dissecting aortic aneurysm is when there is a tear through the intima layer and a blood-filled channel forms within the aortic wall. Patients are usually hypertensive males and have a known aneurysm.

64. (B) The adrenal glands can be divided into the cortex and medulla. The cortex has three zones, and each zone secretes a different type of steroid hormone, while the medulla secretes epinephrine and norepinephrine.

65. (C) The ligament of teres is formed embryologically from the portal sinus branch of the umbilical vein. This canal closes after birth. Recanalization of the umbilical vein is associated with end-stage cirrhosis and portal hypertension.

66. (D) The parallel channel sign, irregular borders, and echo enhancement posterior to the dilated ducts are all characteristic of dilated intrahepatic bile ducts. It is common bile duct near the porta hepatis that is the first to dilate and is greatest in size.

67. (A) The rectus abdominis muscle arises from the pelvis lines, but it lines the anterior abdominal wall; therefore, it is not located in the retroperitoneal cavity.

68. (D) A Klatskin tumor originates at the junction of the right and left hepatic ducts. Cholangiocarcinoma is a primary adenocarcinoma located in the intrahepatic ducts. A Klatskin tumor, cholangiocarcinoma, and enlarged portal lymph nodes will only cause intrahepatic obstruction. Pancreatic carcinoma will initially obstruct the common bile duct before intrahepatic dilatation occurs.

69. (B) Direct or conjugated bilirubin elevated levels are seen in cases of obstructive jaundice. The laboratory results suggest obstructive jaundice, and one must check for the causes of the obstruction.

70. (C) Prolonged fasting and diabetes, especially in one who is insulin dependent, are causes of enlarged gallbladder. Ascites is a nonbiliary cause of diffuse thickening of the gallbladder wall. Chronic cholecystitis is a cause of a small gallbladder.

71. (D) The celiac axis originates within the first 2 cm of the abdominal aorta; therefore, it is located superior to the pancreas. All of the vessels listed are used as landmarks for locating and imaging the pancreas.

72. (A) Retroperitoneal masses tend to cause anterior and cranial displacement of surrounding organs. The direction of the displacement is one way to distinguish between a retroperitoneal versus a peritoneal mass.

73. (D) Enlarged paraspinal lymph nodes may displace the aorta anteriorly, causing the aorta to appear to be "floating."

74. (D) Sonographically, enlarged nodes appear as hypoechoic masses with no demonstration of through transmission, because of its composition.

75. **(A)** Hepatofugal (portafugal) blood flow is the reversal of blood flow, that is, blood flow away from the liver. This may be caused by portal hypertension or liver disease.

76. **(B)** Anatomical landmarks helpful in locating the left adrenal gland are the aorta, spleen, left kidney, and left crus of the diaphragm.

77. **(A)** Gallbladder polyps can be distinguished from calculi by the absence of shadowing and mobility.

78. **(D)** Hydrops is dilatation of the gallbladder, which may be caused by an obstruction in the cystic duct. The gallbladder is palpable, and the patient may be asymptomatic or may present with pain, nausea, and vomiting. The intrahepatic and extrahepatic ducts are not dilated.

79. **(C)** The most common cause of jaundice in the pediatric patient is biliary atresia, a narrowing and obstruction of the intrahepatic bile duct.

80. **(C)** Examples of primary retroperitoneal tumors imaged sonographically are leiomyosarcomas, neurogenic tumors, fibrosarcomas, rhabdomyosarcomas, and teratomatous tumors.

81. **(D)** A series of relative echogenicity has been established. Going from least echogenic to most: renal parenchyma < liver < spleen < pancreas < renal sinus.

82. **(D)** The pancreas in children will be relatively less echogenic and larger in size relative to the body size. The echogenicity of the pancreas increases with age because there is an increase in body fat deposition, which increases the amount of body fat within the parenchyma of the pancreas.

83. **(B)** The kidneys are covered by three layers: the true capsule is the most internal layer that covers only the kidney; the perinephric fat is the middle layer, which is between the kidney and adrenal gland; and Gerota's fascia surrounds the kidneys, perinephric fat, and the adrenal glands.

84. **(B)** The middle, right, and left hepatic veins originate in the liver and drain directly into the IVC at the level of the diaphragm. They are the largest major visceral branches of the IVC.

85. **(B)** The spleen is variable in size, but it is considered to be convex superiorly and concave inferiorly.

86. **(C)** Hypernephroma is a malignant solid renal tumor, which is also called renal cell carcinoma or adenocarcinoma of the kidney. Transitional cell carcinoma is the most common tumor to the collecting system. Oncocytoma is a rare benign renal tumor.

87. **(C)** The left kidney lies inferior and medial to the spleen. The diaphragm is superolateral, and posterior to the spleen, and the stomach, tail of the pancreas; splenic flexure is medial to the spleen.

88. **(B)** A hematocele is a condition in which blood fills the scrotal sac. Sonographically, an acute hematocele appears with thickened scrotal walls and fluid within the scrotal sac without increased through transmission. It is usually a result of trauma or surgery.

89. **(A)** A cavernous hemangioma is the most common benign hepatic neoplasm, and the most common sonographic appearance is an echogenic round or oval with well-defined borders.

90. **(C)** The normal thyroid gland measures 1–2 cm in anteroposterior dimension and 4–6 cm in length.

91. **(D)** Ascites in most cases is secondary to a primary disease process. Some of the causes of ascites include CHF, nephritic syndromes, and infections, for example tuberculosis, trauma, and malignancy. Adenomyomatosis is a benign gallbladder condition, where their proliferation of the mucosal lining of the gallbladder into the muscle layer. Diverticulum of the muscle layer occurs, and bile may collect there and cause ring-down artifacts.

92. **(B)** Sonographically, the best way to diagnose a dissecting aneurysm is by documenting the intimal flap moving with the pulsations of blood through the aorta.

93. **(A)** A mass in the head of the pancreas with a dilated common bile duct is suggestive of obstructive jaundice.

94. **(B)** A subhepatic abscess would be located inferior to the liver and anterior to the right kidney. This space is also referred to as Morrison's pouch. Other common sites for abscesses are the subphrenic, perinephric, intrarenal, intrahepatic, pelvic, and around lesions at the site of surgery.

95. **(D)** The ligamentum venosum is a remnant of the fetal ductus venosus; the ligament of teres and the falciform ligament are remnants of the fetal umbilical vein. The coronary ligaments define the bare area of the liver.

96. **(A)** The gastroduodenal artery is a major branch of the common hepatic artery.

97. **(D)** Patients with Courvoisier gallbladder present with painless jaundice and a palpable right-upper-quadrant mass. The obstruction of the common bile duct is usually caused by enlargement of the head of the pancreas. Patients with acute hepatitis and cirrhosis do have painless jaundice. The jaundice is not caused by obstruction of the biliary system. It is caused by destruction of the liver parenchyma. Porcelain gallbladder is calcification of the gallbladder wall.

98. **(B)** A dromedary hump is a cortical bulge of the lateral border of the left kidney. A junctional parenchymal defect is a distinct division between the upper and lower pole of the kidney. A column of Bertin is prominent indentations of the renal sinus. All of these variants have a mass effect on ultrasound. A Phrygian cap is a fold between the fundus and body of the gallbladder.

99. **(C)** Ascites, small liver, portal hypertension, and nodular liver borders may all be present with end-stage liver disease. The bile ducts will not be dilated because of the fibrotic liver parenchyma.

100. (A) The head of the pancreas is located anterior to the IVC.

101. (B) The lesser sacs are located between the stomach and pancreas.

102. (B) The renal pyramids are located in the medulla of the kidney.

103. (C) In chronic renal disease, both kidneys are small and echogenic.

104. (B) A long history of alcoholism is a major cause of cirrhosis and ascites often is seen secondarily to cirrhosis.

105. (C) Chronic active hepatitis may progress to cirrhosis. The etiology of chronic active hepatitis is usually idiopathic but may be viral or immunologic.

106. (A) Choledochal cyst is a rare focal cystic dilatation of the common bile duct caused by an anomalous junction of the common bile duct with the main pancreatic duct. The reflux of the pancreatic enzymes causes a weakness of the common bile duct wall and an outpouching of the wall. Choledochal cysts may be associated with gallstones, cirrhosis, and pancreatitis. Clinically, the patient presents with pain, fever, abdominal mass, or jaundice.

107. (D) Hashimoto's thyroiditis is chronic inflammation of the thyroid. It is a common cause of hypothyroidism in regions where there is a lack of iodine. The entire thyroid gland is involved, and sonographically, the thyroid is enlarged with irregular borders with decreased heterogeneous echoes. People with Graves' disease present with hyperthyroidism, bulging eyes, and skin thickening. The thyroid is enlarged with increased vascularity. Malignant tumors of the thyroid are rare and have varied appearance on ultrasound, from a single small solid nodule to hypoechoic to being isoechoic with the thyroid tissue. In 50% of cases, there will be calcification.

108. (D) Calcification of part or the entire wall of the gallbladder is called a porcelain gallbladder. It is associated with chronic cholecystitis and gallstones. These patients have a higher risk of carcinoma of the gallbladder.

109. (A) Patients typically are diagnosed with an aortic aneurysm by a pulsatile mass noted on physical examination. They usually have a history of smoking and vascular disease, such as hypertension. On ultrasound, it is important to measure the diameter of the lumen and the location of the aneurysm in reference to the renal arteries.

110. (B) The right renal artery courses posterior to the IVC and may be imaged as a round anechoic structure posterior to the IVC on a longitudinal scan.

111. (A) The retroperitoneal space is the area between the posterior portion of the parietal peritoneum and the posterior abdominal wall muscle.

112. (A) When there is extrinsic pressure and obstruction of the common bile duct (ie, a mass in the head of the pancreas), the gallbladder and biliary tree will be enlarged.

113. (C) The serum amylase and lipase both elevate upon the onset of pancreatitis, but amylase reaches its maximum value within 24 hours. Lipase remains elevated for a longer period of time.

114. (B) HPS is more commonly seen in males between the ages of 1 week and 6 months. The pylorus is the channel between the stomach and duodenum. When the muscle of the pylorus is thickened, it prevents food from entering the stomach. The child typically presents with projectile vomiting, dehydration, and a palpable olive-size mass in the epigastric region. The diagnosis of HPS is made if the length of the pylorus is greater than 18 mm, the anterior to posterior diameter is greater than 15 mm, or the muscle thickness is greater than 4 mm.

115. (B) Neuroblastoma is a malignant tumor of the adrenal medulla that is found in children.

116. (B) Chronic pancreatitis. Enlarged lymph nodes are hypoechoic with no increase in through transmission. Aortic aneurysm, crus of the diaphragm, and bowel may all appear sonographically as hypoechoic. Chronic pancreatitis is imaged as echogenic.

117. (D) Budd–Chiari syndrome is caused by thrombus in the hepatic veins or in the IVC causing obstruction of blood flow to the heart. The obstruction may be congenital or acquired. Budd–Chiari is associated with renal cell carcinoma, primary carcinoma of the liver, or prolonged usage of oral contraceptives. It is characterized by abdominal pain, massive ascites, and hepatomegaly. Sonographically, the right lobe of the liver may be small with normal or enlarged caudate lobe. There will either be absence of blood flow in the hepatic veins and IVC or abnormal blood flow pattern on Doppler.

118. (D) In response to the increased pressure in the portal vein, which is associated with portal hypertension, there may be recanalization of the umbilical vein, which is located within the ligamentum of teres.

119. (B) A pelvic kidney is a kidney that has failed to ascend to the renal fossa. It is located in the pelvis but has the same sonographic appearance as a kidney located in the renal fossa.

120. (A) The UPJ is where the renal pelvis narrows and joins the proximal portion of the ureter.

121. (B) According to Platt et al, an RI of the renal artery greater than 0.70 is 90% accurate in diagnosing renal obstruction.

122. (C) Cushing's syndrome is an adrenal disease where there is oversecretion of glucocorticoids.

123. (D) Body and tail. Islet cell tumors of the pancreas are well-circumscribed solid masses with low-level echoes and are frequently found in the body and tail of the pancreas and rarely in the head of the pancreas.

124. **(C)** The celiac artery has three branches: the common hepatic artery, left gastric artery, and splenic artery.

125. **(A)** The most common benign mass of the spleen is a cavernous hemangioma. The most common malignant tumor of the spleen is an angiosarcoma. Congenital cysts of the spleen are rare, and lymphomas are not benign masses.

126. **(B)** The parietal peritoneum lines the abdominal cavity. Organs are intraperitoneal if they are surrounded by peritoneum or retroperitoneal if only their anterior surface is covered.

127. **(C)** A normally functioning transplanted kidney will have the same sonographic appearance as a normal kidney located in the renal fossa.

128. **(D)** When food containing fat enters the small intestines, cholecystokinin is released into the bloodstream, which activates the contraction of the gallbladder and the relaxing of the sphincter of Oddi.

129. **(B)** A transplanted kidney is usually placed in the pelvis along the iliopsoas margin and anterior to the psoas muscle. The ureter of the donor kidney is anastomosed to the bladder. The donor renal artery is anastomosed to the external iliac artery, while the renal vein is connected to the internal iliac vein.

130. **(A)** Klatskin tumors arise at the junction of the right and left hepatic ducts and causes dilation of the intrahepatic ducts with no dilatation of the extrahepatic ducts.

131. **(D)** Pancreas. The liver, spleen, hepatic veins, and gallbladder are located in the peritoneal cavity. The great vessels, pancreas, adrenal glands, and kidneys are not surrounded by peritoneum; therefore, they are located in the retroperitoneal cavity.

132. **(C)** The splenic artery originates from the celiac axis and courses along the superior aspect of the pancreas body and tail.

133. **(C)** Artifacts result from a variety of sources including thickness and side-lobe artifacts, reverberation artifacts, electronic noise, and range in ambiguity effects. Edge effects cause acoustic shadowing owing to reflection and refraction of sound.

134. **(B)** When ascites is present, it acts as an acoustic window. Therefore, the liver will appear more echogenic. There is always posterior acoustic enhancement when the sound travels through fluid.

135. **(A)** All ultrasound equipment is calibrated at 1540 m/s, the speed of sound in soft tissue. When the ultrasound beam goes through a fatty tumor with a lower propagation speed, the tumor will appear *farther* away than its actual distance.

136. **(D)** A fluid collection located between the diaphragm and the spleen may represent a subphrenic abscess.

137. **(B)** If a mass is solid, displacement of adjacent organs will aid in helping to evaluate the origin of the mass. In a retroperitoneal sarcoma, the kidney, spleen, and pancreas would be displaced anteriorly.

138. **(C)** Splenomegaly may be caused by congestion, that is, portal thrombosis, trauma, infection, Hodgkin's disease, lymphoma, neoplasms, storage diseases, and polycythemia vera.

139. **(A)** Adenomyomatosis is a benign infiltrative disease that causes a diffuse thickening of the gallbladder wall. It does not cause enlargement of the gallbladder.

140. **(D)** Posterior to the kidneys are the quadratus lumborum muscles, diaphragm, psoas muscle, and twelfth rib.

141. **(D)** Patients with chronic cirrhosis will have a small nodular fibrotic liver, which impedes blood flow through the liver causing collateral vessel development and portal hypertension. Ascites, peripheral edema, and splenomegaly are usually secondary to the increase in pressure in the portal vein. Liver failure causes jaundice and an increase in the clotting time. Sonographically, the liver is small and echogenic.

142. **(C)** Ureteral jets are not present if there is an obstructive hydronephrosis. A bladder tumor or PUVs may obstruct urine from exiting the body. In cases of severe obstruction, the increased pressure in the urinary bladder may cause the ureters and renal collecting system to dilate. A parapelvic cyst usually does not cause hydronephrosis.

143. **(B)** An extrarenal pelvis extends from the renal pelvis to outside the renal capsule. One way to differentiate an extrarenal pelvis from hydronephrosis is to place the patient prone. The pressure will collapse the extrarenal pelvis.

144. **(C)** The long narrow arrow points to the heart. The aorta and the IVC enter the thoracic cavity to the heart.

145. **(A)** The short wide arrow is pointing to the aorta, which enters the thoracic cavity to the heart. The aorta lies posterior to the left lobe of the liver.

146. **(A)** The arrow is pointing to a round anechoic structure anterior and slightly to the left of the spine, which is the aorta.

147. **(B)** Simple cysts are present in 50% of all adults older than 50 years. They are usually of no clinical significance and may be located anywhere in the kidney. Fig. 4–11 of the left kidney documents a small upper pole cyst with a larger cyst of the lower pole.

148. **(A)** The most common causes of a fatty liver are alcohol abuse and obesity. Diabetes, chemotherapy, cystic fibrosis, and tuberculosis are other causes of fatty liver infiltration. The liver varies in appearance depending on the severity of the fatty changes. The liver parenchyma will have an increase in echogenicity with a decrease in acoustic penetration. In cases of severe fatty infiltration, there will be a decrease in the echogenicity of the portal

vessel walls caused by the increase in the echogenicity of the liver parenchyma. There may be difficulty in visualization of the diaphragm because of the increase of the liver parenchyma.

149. **(B)** SMA arises from the abdominal aorta. It is seen posterior to the pancreas.

150. **(A)** Acute cholecystitis is usually associated with gallstones. Sometimes there may be cholecystitis without gallstones, which is referred to as acalculous cholecystitis. The sonographic appearance will be the same except for the presence of echogenic foci with posterior shadowing within the gallbladder lumen.

151. **(C)** Cystic artery. The sonographic characteristics of acute cholecystitis include an enlarged gallbladder with a transverse diameter >5 cm, gallbladder wall >5 mm, pericholecystic fluid, a positive Murphy's sign, and an enlarged cystic artery. Not all of the sonographic criteria will be present in every case of cholecystitis.

152. **(A)** The pleural sac surrounds the lungs. The internal pleura (visceral pleura) line the lungs, while the external pleura (parietal pleura) line the inner surface of the chest wall. A pleural effusion is fluid superior to the diaphragm in the pleural sac. The diaphragm must be identified to differentiate fluid in the pleural space verses fluid in the abdominal cavity (ascites).

153. **(C)** The liver is a common site for metastatic involvement. The most common primary sites include the colon, breast, and lungs. Metastatic lesions to the liver have varied sonographic appearances. They may be hypoechoic, echogenic, and well-defined or cause a diffuse echogenic hepatic pattern.

154. **(B)** The arrow is pointing to a normal hepatic vein, which drains into the IVC.

155. **(B)** The arrow is pointing to the right renal artery, which lies posterior to the IVC.

156. **(B)** The quadratus lumborum muscle is posterior to the kidney and courses lateral to the psoas muscle. It protects the posterior and lateral abdominal wall.

157. **(C)** The falciform ligament extends from the umbilicus to the diaphragm and can only be imaged sonographically when massive ascites is present.

158. **(C)** A multicystic (dysplastic) kidney is a common cause of a palpable neonatal mass. It is usually unilateral. Bilateral multicystic pathology is not compatible with life.

159. **(D)** The main lobar fissure is a landmark used to document the gallbladder fossa when there is nonvisualization of the gallbladder. It appears sonographically as an echogenic linear structure that extends from the portal vein to the neck of the gallbladder.

160. **(A)** The most common primary neoplasm of the pancreas is an adenocarcinoma.

161. **(D)** The arrowhead is pointing to an enlarged pancreatic duct. The normal measurement of the pancreatic duct is <2 mm.

162. **(A)** Sonographically, acute pancreatitis may appear normal or diffusely enlarged with a decrease in echogenicity. The pancreatic duct may be enlarged. Hemorrhagic pancreatitis appearance depends on the age of the hemorrhage. Usually there will be a well-defined mass in the head of the pancreas. Phlegmonous pancreatitis typically has an ill-defined hypoechoic mass on ultrasound. Chronic pancreatitis on a sonogram is usually atrophied and is very echogenic. There may be dilatation of the main pancreatic duct secondary to a stone in the duct.

163. **(C)** Aortic aneurysm with a small thrombus in the proximal aorta and partial occlusion documented by color Doppler on both a transverse and a longitudinal view.

164. **(B)** The SMA is a ventral branch of the aorta. It courses parallel and anterior to the abdominal aorta.

165. **(A)** The sonographic appearance of acute pancreatitis varies depending on the severity of the inflammation. The echogenicity is hypoechoic and usually less than the liver. The pancreas may be enlarged with a dilated pancreatic duct.

166. **(A)** The arrow is pointing to a medullary pyramid.

167. **(C)** Gallstones (calculi) sonographically appear as mobile echogenic foci with posterior shadowing.

168. **(D)** Acoustic shadowing.

169. **(D)** The common bile duct is a sonolucent tubular structure that is imaged anterior to the portal vein.

170. **(C)** The upper limits of the normal common bile duct (CBD) is 8 mm. The CBD diameter increases in size after the age of 50 years by approximately 1 mm per decade.

171. **(B)** Pneumobilia is air in the biliary tract. Air in the biliary tract may be caused from chronic cholecystitis, biliary-enteric fistula, or a surgical complication. Sonographically, pneumobilia appears as echogenic foci usually found in the region of the porta hepatis. There may be motion and weak posterior acoustic shadowing of the foci.

172. **(A)** Liver metastatic disease has various sonographic appearances. It may present as multiple echogenic masses of varying sizes. Malignant masses tend to have irregular borders and invade the surrounding tissue. Metastasis of the liver may present as a well-defined mass, hypoechoic mass, or a cystic lesion. Primary sites include the colon and breast.

173. **(D)** The spleen appears normal.

174. **(C)** The common bile duct is formed from the confluence of the common hepatic duct and the cystic duct.

175. **(B)** Atherosclerosis is the most common cause of an aneurysm.

CASE 3

History: 51-year-old man with elevated liver function tests. Sagittal and transverse gray scale (A, B, C) sonograms of the liver.

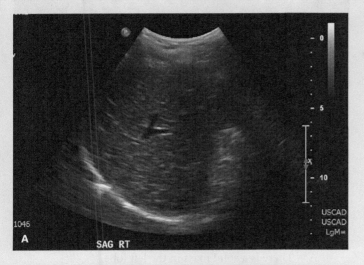

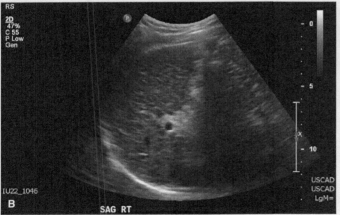

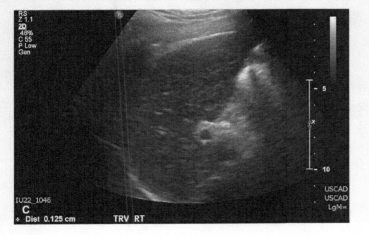

3-1. **Which of the following are true statements concerning this patient's sonogram?**

A. The liver texture is normal.

B. The liver texture is diffusely irregular.

C. The liver is fatty replaced.

D. There are innumerable metastatic lesions.

3-2. **What do the calipers measure?**

A. hepatic artery

B. portal vein

C. common bile duct

D. pancreatic duct

3-3. **Which of the following can be included in the diagnostic possibilities?**

A. normal liver

B. fatty change

C. hepatitis

D. metastatic disease

CASE 4

History: 51-year-old man with elevated liver function tests. Transverse gray scale (A) and (B), Color Doppler (C) and arterial CT scan (D)

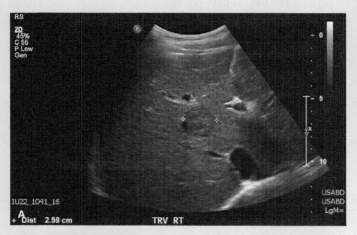

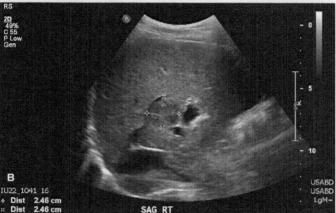

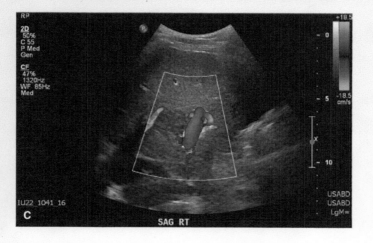

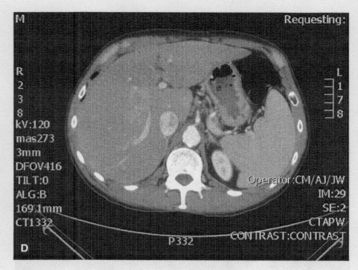

4-1. Which of the following statements are true concerning this patient's imaging studies?

A. There is a solid mass in the left lobe.

B. There is a solid mass in the anterior segment of the right lobe.

C. There is a solid mass in the posterior segment of the right lobe.

D. There are no masses within the liver.

4-2. Based on the imaging findings, what is the most likely diagnosis?

A. HCC

B. hemangioma

C. metastatic lesion

D. all of the above are possible

4-3. Which of the following are shown in the arterial-phase CT scan?

A. peripheral "cloud-like" enhancement

B. central vascularity

C. nothing

D. diffuse metastatic disease

CASE 5

History: 62-year-old man S/P liver transplant with elevated liver function tests. Transverse gray scale (A) and color Doppler (B, C) images of main and right portal veins.

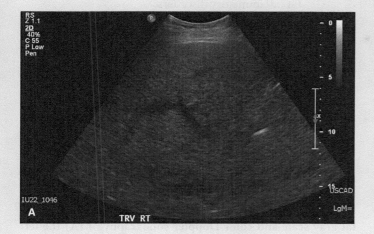

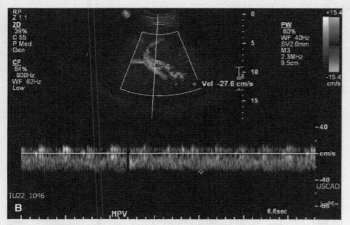

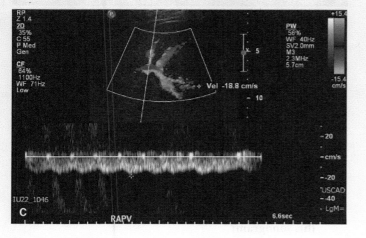

5-1. Which of the following abnormal findings are shown in the images?

  A. reversed flow in the main portal vein

  B. abnormal liver texture

  C. both A and B

  D. none of the above

5-2. Which of the following are possible causes of this finding?

  A. rejection

  B. arterial thrombosis

  C. diffuse infiltration by tumor

  D. faulty anastomosis of portal vein

5-3. What is the most likely diagnosis?

  A. portal hypertension

  B. liver steatosis

  C. both A and B

  D. none of the above

CASE 6

History: 53-year-old with history of inflammatory bowel disease. Sagittal gray scale (A, B) and color Doppler (C) of liver.

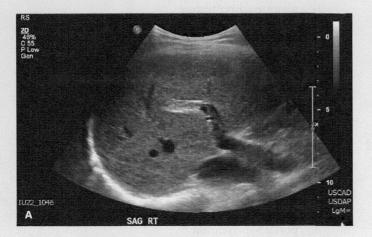

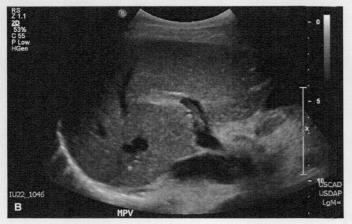

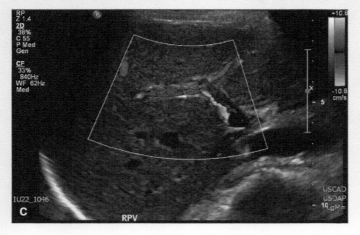

6-1. Which of the following abnormal findings are shown in the images?

A. thrombosis of main portal vein

B. multiple liver masses

C. dilated intrahepatic and extrahepatic bile ducts

D. none of the above

6-2. Which of the following are possible causes of portal vein thrombosis?

A. extension of hepatic tumor into the portal vein

B. hematologic disorder

C. GI inflammatory disorders

D. all of the above

6-3. What is the clinical importance of portal vein thrombosis?

A. hepatic transplantation cannot occur

B. increased risk of metastatic spread

C. may be "bland"; not related to tumor

D. must be removed by catheter technique

CASE 7

History: 19-year-old with left-lower-quadrant pain. Sagittal gray scale and color Doppler sonography of (A) the left kidney and (B) bladder.

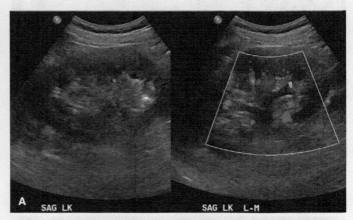

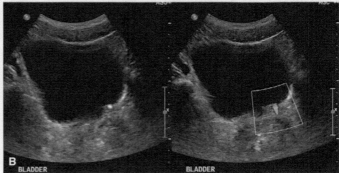

7-1. Which of the following are true statements concerning this sonogram?

A. There is a nonobstructing stone in the left kidney.

B. There is a stone at the left ureterovesicular junction.

C. Both A and B are true.

D. Neither A nor B is true.

7-2. Which of the following are true statements concerning the "twinkle" sign?

    A. It can overestimate size of stone.

    B. It can underestimate size of stone.

    C. It is only found with certain stones.

    D. It does not occur secondarily to vascular calcification.

7-3. Though not shown here, the presence of a ureteral jet indicates which of the following findings?

    A. no ureteric obstruction

    B. urinary sediment within the bladder

    C. cannot represent urine since all fluids are hypoechoic

    D. none of the above

CASE 8

History: 30-year-old woman with RUQ pain. Sagittal (A) and transverse (B) gray scale and (C) color Doppler sonogram of the gallbladder.

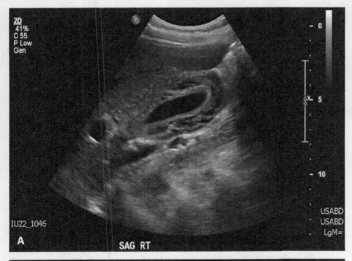

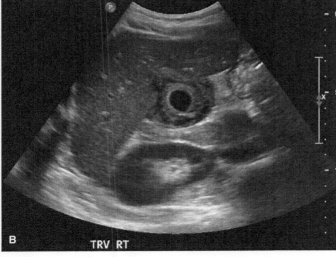

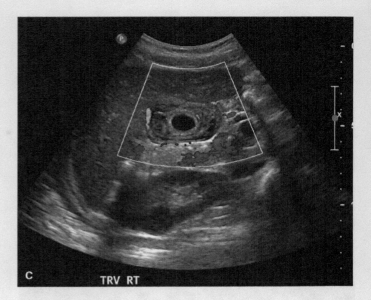

8-1. Which of the following are true statements concerning this sonogram?

    A. There is severe edema of the gallbladder wall.

    B. There are multiple calculi within the lumen.

    C. There is no diffuse cholesterosis of the wall.

    D. There is focal thickening of the wall.

8-2. Which of the following are diagnostic possibilities?

    A. cardiac causes

    B. metastatic involvement

    C. hepatitis

    D. all of the above

8-3. Which of the following is true if the patient experiences pain when the transducer is over the gallbladder?

    A. There must be acute cholecystitis.

    B. This is referred to as Murphy's sign.

    C. You must stop with the examination.

    D. None of the above are true.

CASE 18

Multiple gray scale and color Doppler sonograms of the left kidney.

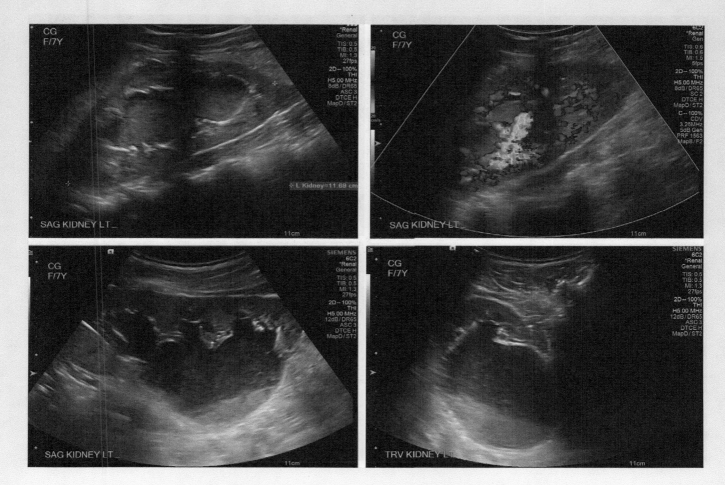

18-1. The abnormal finding is

- A. multiple calculi
- B. dilated collecting system containing low-level echoes
- C. multiple renal masses
- D. renal vein thrombosis

18-2. The most likely diagnosis is

- A. duplicated collecting system
- B. renal cell carcinoma
- C. renal cell thrombosis
- D. severe suppurative pyelonephritis

CASE 19

Multiple gray scale and color Doppler sonogram of the kidneys.

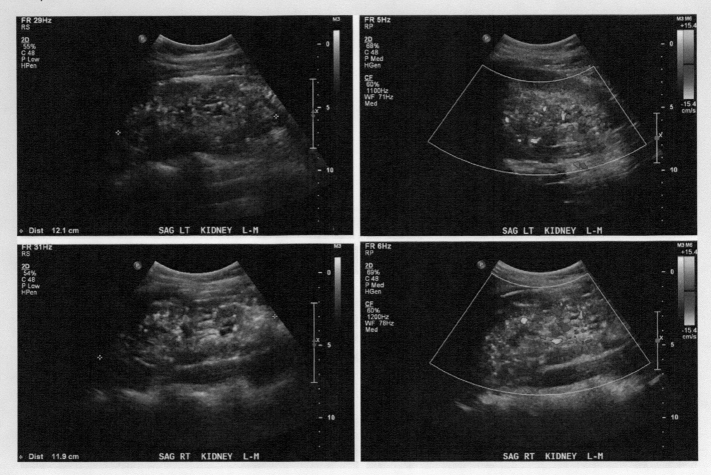

19-1. What is the most abnormal finding?

    A. echogenic medullae with multiple small stones (nephrolithiasis)

    B. hydronephrosis of the right kidney

    C. hydronephrosis of the left kidney

    D. duplex collecting system

19-2. The most likely diagnosis is

    A. autosomal recessive polycystic kidney

    B. medullary sponge kidney

    C. polycystic kidneys

    D. normal

Case Studies Answer Sheet

Case 1

1-1. D
1-2. B
1-3. A

There is both intra- and extrahepatic bile duct dilatation. The color Doppler sonogram shows the multiple tubular structures to be dilated with intra- and extrahepatic bile ducts. The transverse midline image shows a hypoechoic mass in the pancreatic head.

Case 2

2-1. A
2-2. C
2-3. A

This is typical of FNH. These lesions typically have a central vessel. CT or magnetic resonance imaging (MRI) can confirm the diagnosis. FNH is a benign tumor of the liver.

Case 3

3-1. B
3-2. C
3-3. C

This is an example of a diffusely irregular liver texture due to hepatitis. The common bile duct is of normal caliber.

Case 4

4-1. B
4-2. D
4-3. A

There is an hypoechoic mass that shows peripheral "cloud"-like arterial enhancement on arterial-phase CT consistent with the diagnosis of a hemangioma.

Case 5

5-1. A
5-2. A
5-3. C

There is a reverse flow in the portal vein secondary to portal hypertension. There is diffuse fatty change in the liver, which has a variety of causes including rejection, hepatitis, and vascular insult.

Case 6

6-1. A
6-2. D
6-3. A

Portal vein thrombosis may be associated with extension of tumor into the portal vein or "bland" due to hypercoagulability of blood or associated with GI inflammatory disease. If present, hepatic transplantation cannot occur since this requires anastomosis of recipient portal vein to donor portal vein.

Case 7

7-1. C
7-2. A
7-3. D

This patient has a nonobstructing stone in the left kidney and one at the distal ureter. The "twinkle" is created on color Doppler due to reverberation within the stone and thus can overestimate its true size. The presence of a ureteral jet is seen even when there is near occlusion of the ureter by the stone.

Case 8

8-1. A
8-2. D
8-3. B

There is marked thickening of the gallbladder wall, which is a nonspecific finding. If there is localized pain when scanning directly over the gallbladder ("Murphy's sign"), acute cholecystitis may be present.

Case 9

9-1. A
9-2. A
9-3. A

Color Doppler and spectral Doppler are important in establishing flow within a TIPS shunt. Normal velocities range from 50 to 150 cm/s and may vary depending on respiration.

Case 10

10-1. A
10-2. C
10-3. C

There is a thickened loop of bowel in the right lower quadrant. Although this could also be seen in appendicitis, this was an intussuscepted Meckel's diverticulum.

Case 11

11-1. C
11-2. D
11-3. A

This is an example of chronic lymphocytic thyroiditis. There is diffuse irregularity of the mid and lower portion of the right lobe. Biopsy is not indicated.

Case 12

12-1. B
12-2. C
12-3. A

This patient has appendicitis. The appendix is hyperemic on color Doppler and contrasted CT.

Case 13

13-1. A
13-2. A

This is an example of portal venous thrombosis associated with a pancreatic head mass.

Case 14

14-1. A
14-2. B

This is an hepatic mass found to be HCC.

Case 15

15-1. B
15-2. B

These are multiple hepatic adenomas. These images demonstrate smooth border, which suggest transgenicity.

Case 16

16-1. A
16-2. B
16-3. A

This is a stenotic liver. The liver is more echogenic when compared to the right kidney. Shear wave elastography (SWE) valves over 1.37 m/s indicate mild fibrosis.

Case 17

17-1. A
17-2. B

This is mildly dilated upper pole collecting system.

Case 18

18-1. B
18-2. C

This is pyonephrosis within a hydronephrosis renal pelvis.

Case 19

19-1. A
19.2. B

This is medullary sponge kidney with nephrothiasis.

References

1. Rumack CM, Wilson SR, Charboneau JW, Levine D. *Diagnostic Ultrasound*. 4th ed. Mosby; 2011.

2. Hagen-Ansert SL. *Textbook of Diagnostic Ultrasonography*. 6th ed. St. Louis: CV Mosby; 2006.

3. *Dorland's Illustrated Medical Dictionary*. 30th ed. Philadelphia: WB Saunders; 2003.

4. *NCER National Certification Examination Review*. Dallas: Society of Diagnostic Medical Sonography; 2009.

5. Mc Gaham JP, Goldberg BB. *Diagnostic Ultrasound: A logical Approach*. Philadelphia: Lippincott-Raven; 1998.

6. Gill K. *Abdominal Ultrasound A Practitioner's Guide*. Philadelphia: WB Saunders; 2001.

7. Kawamura DM. *Diagnostic Medical Sonography: A Guide to Clinical Practice: Abdomen and Superficial Structures*. 2nd ed. Philadelphia: Lippincott; 1997.

8. Curry RA, Tempkin BB. *Sonography: Introduction to Normal Structure and Function*. 3rd ed. Saunders; 2011.

9. Krebs CA, Giyanani VL, Eisenberg RL. *Ultrasound Atlas of Disease Processes*. Norwalk: Appleton & Lange; 1993.

10. Kremnau F. *Sonography: Principles and Instruments*. 8th ed. Saunders; 2011.

11. Criner GJ, Alonzo GE. *Critical Care Guide: Text and Review*. New York: Springer-Verlag; 2002.

12. Mc Catehey KD. *Clinical Laboratory Medicine*. 2nd ed. Philadelphia: Lippincott-Williams & Wilkins; 2002.

Answers and Explanations

1. **(A)** The most common location of a spermatocele is the head of the epididymis. A spermatocele is a retention cyst that may occur following vasectomy, scrotal surgery, or epididymitis.

2. **(D)** Torsion is more common in children or teenage boys. It is a weakening in the attachment of the mesentery from the spermatic cord to the testicle. Clinically, the patient presents with sudden extreme pain in the scrotum. Treatment must occur within 5 or 6 hours of onset to save the testicle. The sonographic appearance varies according to the length of time that diagnosis is made. Acute torsion occurs within the first 24 hours. In the early stages, there is a decrease in the arterial flow to the testis. An enlarged epididymis and an enlarged hypoechoic testis are imaged. There may be thickening of the scrotal skin or the formation of a hydrocele.

3. **(B)** In patients with uncomplicated acute epididymitis, there will be enlargement of the epididymal head or the entire epididymis. The epididymis has a decrease in echogenicity, and there may be increased blood flow with a reactive hydrocele.

4. **(C)** The head of the epididymis is located superior to the testes. The rest of the epididymis courses along the posterior margin of the testicle inferiorly.

5. **(C)** The seminal vesicles are reservoirs for sperm and are located posterior to the urinary bladder.

6. **(A)** A seminoma is a solid malignant mass of the testicles that is usually unilateral and appears hypoechoic on a sonographic examination.

7. **(B)** Thyroiditis appears sonographically as a diffuse enlargement of the thyroid with a decrease in echogenicity.

8. **(D)** Pheochromocytoma is a benign adrenal tumor of the medulla. It secretes both epinephrine and norepinephrine.

9. **(A)** The image is of a testicular tumor. The epididymis is enlarged in cases of testicular torsion and epididymitis. In cases of varicocele, there will be enlarged vessels, and a spermatocele produces a sonolucent lesion usually in the region near the head of the epididymis. The epididymis is normal on the image.

10. **(D)** Lymphadenopathy, leukemia, or acute scrotal pain may be a presenting symptom associated with a testicular tumor.

11. **(D)** The left renal vein.

12. **(A)** The testicle may have anechoic areas, and the epididymis has a complex appearance. Associated findings include an enlarged epididymis and a reactive hydrocele. Spectral Doppler and color Doppler are used to evaluate whether the torsion is complete or incomplete. In cases of complete torsion, there will be no blood flow to the affected testicle.

13. **(D)** Normal testicles have a homogeneous appearance. When performing color Doppler, the setting should be set as low as possible on the unaffected side and be compared with the affected side. Cryptorchidism is an undescended testicle; orchiectomy is removal of the testicle; and epididymitis is inflammation of the scrotum.

14. **(B)** This sonogram demonstrates dilated vessels near the head of the epididymis.

15. **(A)** A varicocele appears as tortuous vessels near the head of the epididymis, mostly occurring on the left. The reason varicoceles occur more on the left side is that the left testicular vein courses into the left renal vein, whereas the right testicular vein drains into the right spermatic vein.

16. **(D)** An extratesticular cyst is documented on the sonogram. This is consistent with a spermatocele, which is a cyst in the epididymis containing spermatozoa. An epididymis cyst would have the same sonographic appearance. A varicocele (enlargement of the veins of the spermatic cord) is also extratesticular, but it is located on the posterior surface, more common of the left; and sonographically, it has a tubular shape. Seminoma is a malignant germ cell tumor within the testicle.

17. **(B)** Normal head of the epididymis.

18. **(B)** The arrow is pointing to the seminal vesicle, which is posterior to the bladder and superior to the prostate.

19. **(D)** Varicocele is an enlargement of the veins of the pampiniform plexus, which course along the posterior aspect of the testicle and is more prominent on the left testicle. Venous dilatation occurs with an increase of pressure either by having the patient perform a Valsalva maneuver or by having the patient stand. Spermatocele and epididymal cysts are found in the epididymis. Cryptorchidism is another name for undescended testes. Mediastinum testis is found within the testis and connects the rete testis with the epididymis.

20. **(D)** The two lobes of the thyroid are connected by the isthmus, which is anterior to the trachea. The common carotid is located lateral to the thyroid and the sternothyroid muscle is anterolateral to the thyroid.

21. **(A)** A patient with a parathyroid adenoma may present with hypercalcemia and low serum levels of phosphate.

22. **(B)** Posterior urethral valve is the most common cause of urethral obstruction in boys. The valves located in the posterior urethra obstruct the urethra. Dilatation of the urethra, hydroureter, and hydronephrosis may occur secondary to the obstruction.

Case Studies Answer Sheet

Case 1

1-1. A
1-2. B
1-3. B

This is a well-circumscribed hypoechoic area with decreased flow. This can occur as a sequela of infarction or tumor. The sonographer should scan an area of concern and endeavor an abnormality. This is a case of dilated rete testes, a normal variant in older men.

Case 2

2-1. D
2-2. A
2-3. A

This testicle contains a well-circumscribed hypoechoic, hypovascular area in the upper pole that is hypovascular. Though hypovascular, this could have a similar appearance to a testicular tumor such as a seminoma; this represented testicular infarction to lifting weights.

Case 3

3-1. C
3-2. D
3-3. D

This is an enlarged and distorted lymph node. This can be associated with metastatic spread of follicular papillary cancer or can be "reactive" due to inflammation.

Case 4

4-1. B
4-2. A
4-3. B

This is a large papillary thyroid cancer containing numerous vessels. A FNA could be performed safely.

Case 5

5-1. B
5-2. D
5-3. B

There is an ill-defined group of hypervascular nodules in the upper pole. FNA would be indicated for further evaluation.

Case 6

6-1. C
6-2. D
6-3. A

This sonogram shows a parathyroid mass inferior to the left lobe.

Case 7

7-1. B
7-2. C
7-3. A

This is a typical thyroglossal duct cyst. They are usually found in the midline and can contain some low-level echoes.

Case 8

8-1. A
8-2. D
8-3. C

This is a solid nodule that was found to represent a metastatic lesion to the thyroid.

Case 9

9-1. A
9-2. C
9-3. A

9: Ultrasound images A, B, and C are examples of chronic lymphocytic thyroid. It is also known as Hashimoto's thyroiditis. The thyroid gland is often diffusely enlarged with punctate hypoechoic foci echotexture. This study demonstrates hyperemic phase. The diagnosis can be confirmed by assessing serum thyroid peroxidase antibodies.

Case 10

10-1. C
10-2. B
10-3. D

This is a parathyroid adenoma. It is posterior to the right lobe of the thyroid. Serum calcium levels would be elevated.

Case 11

11-1. B
11-2. A
11-3. A

This is an example of recurrent thyroid cancer. This is usually associated with elevate thyroglobulin.

References

1. Reading CC, Charboneau JW, Hay ID, Sebo TJ. Sonography of thyroid nodules—A "classic pattern" diagnostic approach. *Ultrasound Q.* 2005;21(3).

2. Rumack CM, Wilson SR, Charboneau JW, Levine D. *Diagnostic Ultrasound.* 4th ed. Mosby; 2011.

3. Hagen-Ansert SL. *Textbook of Diagnostic Ultrasonography.* 6th ed. St. Louis, MO: CV Mosby; 2006.

4. Gill K. *Abdominal Ultrasound: A Practitioner's Guide.* Philadelphia, PA: WB Saunders; 2001.

5. Kawamura DM. *Diagnostic Medical Sonography: A Guide to Clinical Practice: Abdomen and Superficial Structures.* 2nd ed. Philadelphia, PA: Lippincott; 1997.

6

Transrectal Prostate Sonography

Dunstan Abraham

Study Guide

The prostate is a heterogeneous, oval-shaped organ that surrounds the proximal urethra. In the adult, the normal gland measures approximately 3.8 cm (cephalocaudal) by 3 cm (anteroposterior) by 4 cm (transverse).[1] It normally weighs about 20 g, but it can be slightly larger in men older than 40 years. The prostate is composed of glandular and fibromuscular tissue and is located in the retroperitoneum between the floor of the urinary bladder and the urogenital diaphragm (Fig. 6–1). The base of the prostate, its superior margin, abuts the inferior aspect of the urinary bladder, while the apex is adherent to the urogenital diaphragm. The gland is bounded anteriorly by prostatic fat and fascia, laterally by the obturator internus and levator ani muscles, and posteriorly by areolar tissue and Denonvilliers' fascia, which separates it from the rectum.

The **seminal vesicles** are two sac-like lateral structures that outpouch from the vas deferens and are situated on the posterior-superior aspect of the prostate between the bladder and the rectum. The seminal vesicles join the vas deferens to form the **ejaculatory ducts,** which then enter the base of the prostate to join the urethra at the verumontanum. The **verumontanum** is a midpoint region between the prostatic base and apex and surrounds the urethra. The size and fluid content of the seminal vesicles are variable.

The **prostatic urethra** courses through the substance of the gland and is divided into a proximal and a distal segment. The proximal segment extends from the neck of the bladder to the base of the verumontanum; the distal segment begins at this point and extends to the apex of the gland.

Blood supply to the prostate is from the internal iliac arteries, which eventually give rise to urethral and capsular arteries. Venous return is via the prostatic plexus, which drains into the internal iliac vein.[2] The prostate produces seminal fluid, which is essential to the function of the spermatozoa.

NORMAL SECTIONAL ANATOMY

The earlier anatomic descriptions of the prostate divided the gland into five major lobes: **anterior, posterior, media,** and **two laterals**. More recent histological studies, however, have divided the prostate into three glandular zones: the **transitional, central,** and **peripheral zones**. There is also a nonglandular region called the **anterior fibromuscular stroma** (Figs. 6–2A, B).[2]

Transitional Zone

The transitional zone represents about 5% of the glandular prostate and is located in the central region on both sides of the proximal urethra.[2] The ducts of the transitional zone run parallel to the urethra and end in the proximal urethra at the level of the verumontanum.

Central Zone

The central zone constitutes approximately 25% of the prostatic glandular tissue and is located at the base of the gland.[2] It is wedge-like in shape, is oriented horizontally, and surrounds the ejaculatory ducts throughout their course. The zone narrows to an apex at the verumontanum. Ducts of the vas deferens and seminal vesicles come together to form the ejaculatory ducts, which pass through the central zone and join the urethra at the verumontanum.

Peripheral Zone

The peripheral zone constitutes about 70% of the glandular tissue.[2] This zone consists of the posterior, lateral, and apical parts of the prostate and also extends anteriorly. The ducts of the peripheral zone enter the urethra at, and distal to, the verumontanum.

Anterior Fibromuscular Stroma

The anterior fibromuscular stroma is a thick nonglandular sheath of tissue that covers the entire anterior surface of the prostate. This tissue is composed of smooth muscle and fibrous tissue.

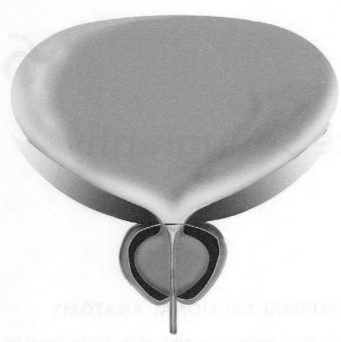

FIGURE 6–1. The base of the prostate, abutting the inferior aspect of the urinary bladder.

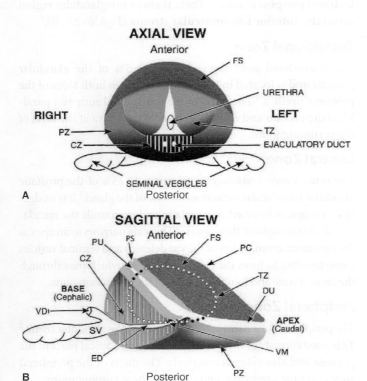

FIGURE 6–2. (**A**) An axial view of normal prostate anatomy: CZ is the central zone, FS is the fibromuscular stroma, TZ is the transition zone, and PZ is the peripheral zone. (**B**) Sagittal view of the normal prostate anatomy: SV is the seminal vesicle, ED is the ejaculatory duct, DU is the distal urethra, PC is the prostatic capsule, VD is the vas deferens, VM is the verumontanum, PU is the proximal urethra, CZ is the central zone, FS is the fibromuscular stroma, TZ is the transition zone, PS is the periurethral stroma, and PZ is the peripheral zone.

INDICATIONS FOR SONOGRAPHY

Patients can be referred for transrectal prostate sonography for various reasons such as the following.[1,2]

- An abnormal digital rectal examination, as indicated by a palpable prostatic nodule or prostate with an asymmetrical size or shape
- Biopsy guidance of sonographically detected abnormal areas
- Clinical evidence of prostate cancer such as an elevated level of prostatic-specific antigen (PSA) or radiographically detected bone metastasis
- Guide treatments for prostate cancer such as radiotherapy and cryotherapy
- Monitoring of a patient's response to therapy
- Inflammation leading to the formation of a prostatic abscess
- Infertility caused by the absence of the seminal vesicles or a bilateral obstruction of the ejaculatory ducts
- Difficulties in voiding caused by an obstruction of the prostatic urethra
- Calculation of prostatic volume prior to surgery

CONTRAINDICATIONS TO PROSTATE BIOPSY

Prostate biopsy may be contraindicated when the following conditions are present.[3]

- Significant coagulopathy
- Painful endorectal conditions (fissures, thrombosed hemorrhoids)
- Severe immunosuppression
- Acute prostatitis

EQUIPMENT AND EXAMINATION TECHNIQUES

Technical innovations have led to the availability of several types of endorectal imaging systems. The original systems were **radial (axial) scanners** that produced transverse-oriented slices of the prostate. Later, **linear array scanners** that imaged the gland in longitudinal sections were introduced. Today, **biplanar endorectal probes** that can produce both longitudinal and transverse sections of the gland are available, thus eliminating the need for two separate probes. The two most common types are "end fire" and "side fire" transducers. The frequency of endorectal probes ranges from 5 to 8 MHz. A guide can be attached directly to the probe allows one to biopsy suspicious prostatic lesions safely and accurately.

Preparation of the patient for endorectal sonography begins with a self-administered enema before the examination. This

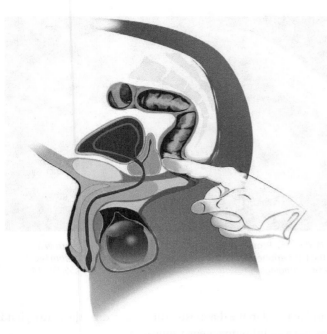

FIGURE 6–3. **Digital rectal examination.** The gloved finger is inserted into the rectum prior to probe insertion. The biopsy can be directed to any abnormal area that is palpated.

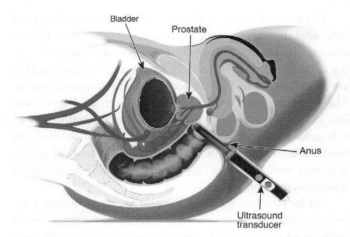

FIGURE 6–4. **Rectal prostate ultrasound.** Diagram shows the transducer inserted into the rectum and its position relative to the prostate gland. Note that the urinary bladder should be empty for the comfort of the patient.

not only eliminates fecal material from the rectum that might adversely affect the quality of the image but also reduces the risk of contamination of the prostate. If biopsy is to be performed, prophylactic antibiotics must be given before the procedure and continued for 24–48 hours afterward.[3]

The patient is generally examined in the left lateral decubitus position. The lithotomy position is sometimes used when other urological procedures are also being performed. The probe is previously sterilized and covered with a condom before insertion. A digital rectal examination is performed to exclude any obstructing lesions or rectal fissures and to correlate the exam with any palpable abnormalities (Fig. 6–3).

Axial scanning begins at the level of the seminal vesicles. The probe is then gradually withdrawn to image the gland sequentially down to the level of the apex.

Sagittal imaging begins in the midline and shows the gland from base to apex with portions of the seminal vesicles. The probe is then rotated clockwise and counterclockwise to demonstrate the right and left sides of the gland (Fig. 6–4).

On color Doppler examination, moderate vascularity from the capsular and the urethral arteries and their branches can be visualized.

NORMAL SONOGRAPHIC ANATOMY

Sonographically, the prostate is a homogeneous gland with low-level echoes. The periurethral glandular tissue that surrounds the proximal urethra is homogeneous and isoechoic. The central zone may be more echogenic than the peripheral zone in the

presence of **corpora amylacea** (calcified deposits). The fibromuscular capsule, located anteriorly, is smooth, hyperechoic, and sharply defined.

In sonography, the terms outer and inner gland are sometimes used to distinguish between the above zones. The outer gland consists of the peripheral and central zones, whereas the inner gland consists of the transitional zone, the inner anterior fibromuscular stroma, and the internal urethral sphincter. The surgical capsule separates the inner gland from the peripheral zone (Fig. 6–5).

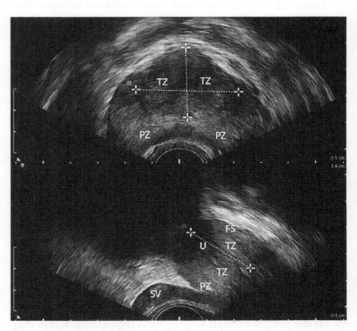

FIGURE 6–5. **The adult prostate.** The top panel represents a transverse view and the bottom a longitudinal view. The transition zone (TZ), peripheral zone (PZ), anterior fibromuscular stroma (FS), seminal vesicle, and urethra (U) are indicated. The calipers are placed on the dimensions of the transition zone. Note the symmetric echogenicity of the left and right sides of the top image. *(Reproduced with permission from Radiology Key https://radiologykey.com/transrectal-ultrasound-of-the-prostate/.)*

The seminal vesicles are visualized as symmetrically paired structures that are slightly less echoic than the prostate. The vas deferens can be depicted as tubular hypoechoic structures joining the seminal vesicles medially. On transverse imaging, they are round or oval and are located between the seminal vesicles. The ejaculatory duct, when empty, can be seen as a hyperechoic line joining the urethra. The empty urethra is identified by its echogenic walls coursing through the prostate. When filled with fluid, the urethra is recognized more easily. The surgical capsule is usually seen as a hypoechoic line but can also be echogenic due to calcification.

On longitudinal sections, the anterior space between the prostate and the seminal vesicles (prostate–seminal vesicle angle) is variable but is the same bilaterally. Similarly, the posterior space between the prostate and the seminal vesicle (or nipple) is symmetrical on both sides.[1]

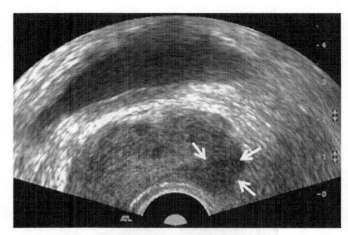

FIGURE 6–6. **Prostate cancer.** A hypoechoic nodule (white arrows) is seen in the left peripheral zone area. *(Reproduced with permission from Lee HJ: Medical imaging of prostate cancer, J Korean Med Assoc 2015;58(1):7-14.)*

PATHOLOGY

Prostatic Carcinoma

It is estimated that in the United States in 2019, there will be 174,650 new cases of prostate cancer and 31,620 prostate cancer mortalities.[4] Men of African American descent and those with a family history of prostate cancer are at higher risk.[2] Although the etiology of prostatic cancer remains unclear, the factors implicated in its causation include age, genetic or racial makeup, hormonal influences, and diet.

Screening tests for prostate cancer include annual digital rectal exam and prostate-specific antigen (PSA) blood test. Regarding prostate screening, The American Urological Association recommends shared decision making for men aged 55–69 who are asymptomatic and at average risk. Outside of this age range, PSA-based screening was not recommended.[5]

Normal PSA is less than 4 ng/mL. Elevated levels can be seen in patients with cancer, benign prostatic hyperplasia (BPH), prostatitis, and following procedures such as cystoscopy, prostate biopsy, and Foley catheter insertion. Artificially reduced levels of PSA are seen in patients taking medication such as Proscar (finasteride), which is used for treatment of BPH.[2]

Anatomic studies have determined that 70% of prostate cancers originate *de novo* in the peripheral zone, 20% originate in the transitional zone, and 10% originate in the central zone.[1] Clinical symptoms include back pain and an obstruction of urinary outflow that may mimic BPH.

Sonographically, prostate cancer varies in echogenicity. However, the most common appearance is a hypoechoic nodule on the peripheral zone (Fig. 6-6). A hypoechoic lesion may also represent benign etiologies such as inflammation, fibrosis, infarction, smooth muscle, BPH, atrophy, and lymphoma.[6]

Hyperechoic cancers can rarely present as focal areas of calcification. Isoechoic cancers are difficult to detect, although secondary signs such as capsular bulging and asymmetry of the gland may aid in the diagnosis. Tumor invading the entire gland may have an inhomogeneous appearance.[2]

Invasion of the tumor into the seminal vesicles can be seen as solid material within this normally fluid-filled structure. Invasion may make the size, shape, and echogenicity of the seminal vesicles asymmetrical in appearance.

Obliteration of the nipple or the prostate–seminal vesicle angle is another diagnostic criterion for invasion by the tumor.[1] However, because the nipple is not imaged consistently, the criterion is of limited usefulness. Doppler ultrasound has not proven to be useful in the diagnosis of prostate cancer. Staging of prostatic cancer with ultrasound is also feasible but is limited by problems of resolution.

Benign Prostatic Hyperplasia and Hypertrophy

Benign prostatic hyperplasia (BPH) affects 80–90% of adult men.[1] Its etiology is believed to be related to hormonal factors. The clinical symptoms of the disease may include decreased flow of urine, difficulty in initiating and terminating urination, nocturia, and urinary retention. BPH originates in the transitional zone and in periurethral glandular tissue.

The sonographic characteristics of hyperplasia nodules are variable. They can be hypoechoic, hyperechoic, or of mixed echogenicity. Enlargement of the central gland by BPH causes lateral displacement of the peripheral zone. The prostatic calculi that are often encountered with BPH are believed to be the result of stasis of prostatic secretions. Corpora amylacea are seen as echogenic foci similar to prostatic calculi. **Benign prostatic hyperplasia** causes the number of cells in the prostate to increase, whereas **benign prostatic hypertrophy** refers to an increase in the size of existing cells. Hyperplasia and hypertrophy often develop concurrently and result in the enlargement of the prostate gland. Transrectal ultrasound is not usually indicated in patients with BPH unless prostate cancer is a clinical concern.

Prostatitis and Prostatic Abscess

Inflammation of the prostate can be the result of acute or chronic bacterial infections or of unknown nonbacterial factors. Clinical symptoms of prostatitis may include fever, pelvic and low back pain, urinary frequency and urgency, and dysuria. Although prostatitis usually involves the peripheral zone in its initial stages, it can originate in any area of the gland.

In acute prostatitis, the main sonographic finding is a hypoechoic gland with anechoic areas that may mimic carcinoma. Another common finding is a hypoechoic halo in the periurethral area. Focal or diffuse increased blood flow may be seen on color or power Doppler. However, increase blood flow is not specific to inflammatory lesions.

In chronic prostatitis, sonographic findings may include focal masses of variable echogenicity, ejaculatory duct calcifications, thickening or irregularity of the prostatic capsule, dilatation of the periprostatic veins, and distention of the seminal vesicles.[2]

A prostatic abscess may develop secondarily to prostatitis. Transrectal sonography may show hypoechoic areas corresponding to liquefaction within the abscess. Sonography can be used to guide aspiration of an abscess if necessary.

Prostatic Utricle Cysts

Prostatic utricle cysts occur as a result of dilatation of the prostatic utricle. On sonography, they are small, anechoic structures located in the midline. They can, however, become large and measure several centimeters in size.

Ejaculatory Duct Cysts

Ejaculatory duct cysts occur secondarily to obstruction or a diverticular of the duct. They contain spermatozoa and are associated with infertility. On sonography, they are seen as anechoic masses within the ejaculatory ducts.

Seminal Vesicle Cysts

Seminal vesicle cysts result from an anomaly of the Wolffian duct. Large, solitary cysts may be associated with renal agenesis. They can also be associated with infertility when they obstruct the seminal vesicle.

Infertility

Patients with azoospermia (no sperm in the ejaculate) can be examined to exclude ejaculatory duct obstruction. This is diagnosed when the seminal vesicle measures more than 1.5 cm in anteroposterior diameter; presence of a dilated ejaculatory duct and a midline cyst. Additional ultrasound findings in infertility may include the following: bilateral absence of the vas deferens; bilateral occlusion of the vas deferens, seminal vesicles, and ejaculatory ducts by calcification or fibrosis; and obstructing cyst of the seminal vesicle, ejaculatory ducts, or prostate.

References

1. Rifkin M. *Ultrasound of the Prostate*. New York: Raven Press; 1988.
2. Toi A, Bree R. The prostate. In: Rumack C, Wilson S, Charboneau W, et al., eds. *Diagnostic Ultrasound*. 3rd ed., Vol. 1. St. Louis, MO: Mosby; 2005.
3. Trabulsi EJ, Halpern EJ, Gomella LG. Ultrasonography and biopsy of the prostate (Chapter 97). In: *Campbell–Walsh Urology*, 10th ed., Vol. 3. Philadelphia, PA: Elsevier; 2012.
4. Siegel RL, Miller KD, Jemal A. Cancer statistics, 2018. *CA Cancer J Clin*. 2018;68(1):7-30.
5. Carter HB, Albertsen PC, Barry MJ, et al. Early detection of prostate cancer: AUA Guidelines. *J Urol*. August 2013;190(2):419-426.
6. Kennedy-Antillon GM. The Prostate gland. In: Kawamura D, Nolan TD, eds. *Diagnostic Medical Sonography (Abdomen and Superficial Structures)*, 4th ed. Philadelphia, PA: Wolters Kluwer; 2018.

Questions

GENERAL INSTRUCTIONS: For each question, select the best answer. Select only one answer for each question unless otherwise specified.

1. Which of the following choices best describes the fibromuscular stroma?

   (A) covers the anterior surface of the prostate
   (B) is the major site of benign prostatic hypertrophy
   (C) is a nonglandular region
   (D) A and C

2. Which of the following is not an indication for transrectal prostate sonography?

   (A) a prostatic abscess
   (B) biopsy guidance of a palpable prostate nodule
   (C) an elevated PSA
   (D) differentiation of a benign from a malignant nodule by imaging

3. Patients having transrectal prostate sonography are commonly examined in which of the following positions?

   (A) left lateral decubitus position
   (B) the erect position
   (C) the Trendelenburg position
   (D) Fowler's position

4. Which of the following statements about the transitional zone is false?

   (A) It is located centrally around the urethra.
   (B) It represents about 5% of the gland.
   (C) It is the primary site of BPH.
   (D) It is the primary site of adenocarcinoma.

5. Which one of the following statements is false?

   (A) The central zone constitutes approximately 25% of the glandular tissue.
   (B) The central zone is located at the apex of the prostate.
   (C) The vas deferens joins the seminal vesicles in the central zone.
   (D) The central zone surrounds the ejaculatory ducts.

6. The peripheral zone accounts for what percentage of the prostatic glandular tissue?

   (A) 50%
   (B) 10%
   (C) 70%
   (D) 1%

7. Which of the following statements about the prostate is false?

   (A) Its apex is located superiorly.
   (B) Its base abuts the urinary bladder.
   (C) It has three zones.
   (D) The urethra runs through the gland.

8. Which of the following is a function of the prostate?

   (A) hormonal secretions
   (B) testosterone production
   (C) secretion of seminal fluid
   (D) spermatozoa production

9. The seminal vesicles join which of the following to form the ejaculatory duct?

   (A) the Denonvilliers' duct
   (B) the vas deferens
   (C) the verumontanum
   (D) the urethra

10. The ejaculatory duct joins which of the following structures at the verumontanum?

    (A) vas deferens
    (B) efferent ducts
    (C) epididymis
    (D) urethra

11. The seminal vesicles are located on which surface of the prostate?

    (A) the anterior-inferior surface
    (B) the posterior-inferior surface
    (C) the posterior-superior surface
    (D) the inferior-lateral surface

12. Which of the following statements about prostatic cancer is *not* true?

    (A) It originates mainly in the central zone.

    (B) It is commonly a hypoechoic lesion.

    (C) Its associated factors include genetic and hormonal influence.

    (D) Clinical presentation may include urinary obstruction.

13. Which of the following is commonly included in the sonographic features of acute prostatitis?

    (A) a hypoechoic gland with anechoic areas

    (B) a hypoechoic nodule on the peripheral zone

    (C) unilateral enlargement of the seminal vesicle

    (D) a midline anechoic mass

14. BPH originates in which of the following areas of the prostate?

    (A) the fibromuscular stroma

    (B) the peripheral zone

    (C) the ejaculatory ducts

    (D) the transitional zone

15. Which of the following statements is true about corpora amylacea?

    (A) They are part of the anterior fibromuscular capsule.

    (B) They are calcified deposits in the prostate.

    (C) They appear hypoechoic on endorectal ultrasound.

    (D) They are never seen on endorectal ultrasound.

16. Which of the following is *not* a common sonographic characteristic of prostatic cancer?

    (A) a hypoechoic nodule in the peripheral zone

    (B) distortion of the capsule

    (C) obliteration of the "nipple"

    (D) marked compression of the prostatic urethra

17. A transrectal examination of the prostate should begin with which of the following?

    (A) transverse scanning

    (B) longitudinal scanning

    (C) views of the seminal vesicles

    (D) a digital rectal examination

18. Which of the following best describes prostate cancer?

    (A) echogenic

    (B) anechoic

    (C) hypoechoic

    (D) sonographically variable

19. Which of the following best describes the verumontanum?

    (A) a midpoint region between the base and apex of the prostate

    (B) a congenital abnormality of the prostate

    (C) part of the peripheral zone

    (D) part of the seminal vesicle

20. An elevated PSA may commonly indicate all of the following *except*

    (A) prostatic inflammation

    (B) prostatic cancer

    (C) BPH

    (D) obstruction of the seminal vesicle

21. Which of the following narrows to an apex at the verumontanum?

    (A) the central zone

    (B) the peripheral zone

    (C) the transitional zone

    (D) the fibromuscular stroma

22. What does the normal adult prostate weigh?

    (A) 10 g

    (B) 20 g

    (C) 30 g

    (D) 40 g

23. Which of the following statements about the seminal vesicles is incorrect?

    (A) Their absence does not usually affect fertility.

    (B) They are joined by the vas deferens.

    (C) They are normally less echoic than the prostate.

    (D) Their sizes varies.

24. **Fig. 6–7 represents a longitudinal scan taken to the right of midline. Which of the following structures is indicated by the arrow?**

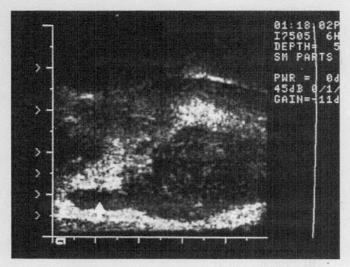

FIGURE 6–7. Longitudinal scan to the right of midline.

   (A) the proximal urethra
   (B) a seminal vesicle
   (C) the verumontanum
   (D) the ejaculatory duct

25. **Fig. 6–8 represents a transverse scan. Which of the following structures are the arrows pointing to?**

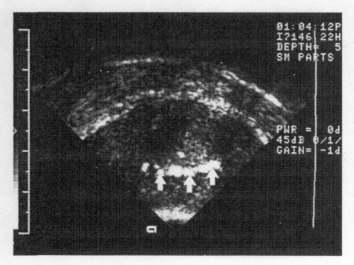

FIGURE 6–8. Transverse scan of the prostate.

   (A) a tumor in the peripheral zone
   (B) prostatitis involving the periurethral areas
   (C) central gland calcification
   (D) distortion of the prostatic capsule

26. **Fig. 6–9 represents a longitudinal scan of a 60-year-old patient presenting with urinary frequency. He was referred for a transrectal prostate sonography examination. What area is outlined by the white arrow?**

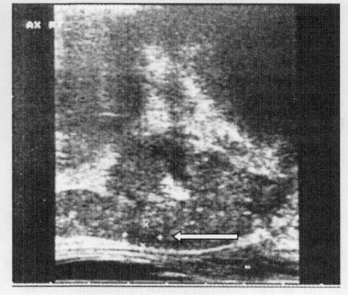

FIGURE 6–9. Longitudinal scan of the prostate.

   (A) obliteration of the "prostate-seminal vesicle angle"
   (B) a hypoechoic mass in the central zone
   (C) a tumor in the peripheral zone
   (D) bulging of the prostatic capsule

27. Fig. 6–10 represents a longitudinal scan. What region is indicated by the white arrow?

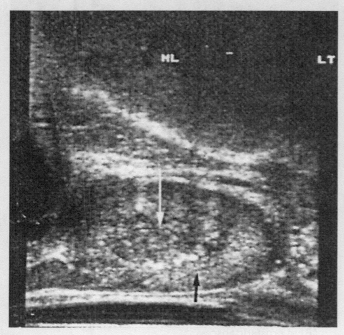

FIGURE 6–10. Longitudinal scan of the prostate.

(A) the fibromuscular stroma
(B) the seminal vesicle
(C) the peripheral zone
(D) the central zone

28. Fig. 6–10 represents a longitudinal scan. What region is indicated by the black arrow?

(A) the peripheral zone
(B) the central zone
(C) the prostatic capsule
(D) the vas deferens

29. Fig. 6–11 represents a longitudinal scan of a patient presenting with a history of infertility. The white arrow most likely indicates which of the following findings?

(A) benign prostatic hypertrophy
(B) a cyst in the ejaculatory duct
(C) extension of a tumor into the nipple region
(D) central gland disease

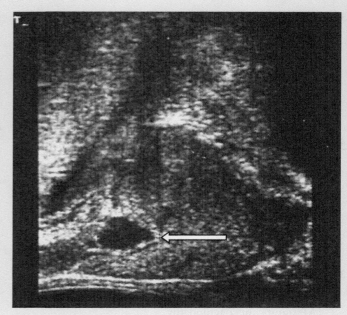

FIGURE 6–11. The white arrow most likely indicates which of the following findings.

30. Which of the following is true about prostatic utricle cysts?

(A) They are located in the midline.
(B) They are located laterally.
(C) They are within the seminal vesicle.
(D) Their location is variable.

31. What type of cyst contains spermatozoa and are associated with fertility.

(A) prostatic utricle cyst
(B) ejaculatory duct cyst
(C) seminal vesicle cyst
(D) all of the above

32. Which of the following is associated with renal agenesis?

(A) prostatic utricle cyst
(B) ejaculatory duct cyst
(C) seminal vesicle cyst
(D) chronic prostatitis

33. **Clinical findings with prostatitis may include all of the following except:**

    (A) fever

    (B) pelvic pain

    (C) prostatic nodule on digital rectal examination

    (D) dysuria

34. **Enlargement of the central gland by benign prosthetic hypertrophy (BPH) may cause:**

    (A) lateral displacement of the peripheral zone

    (B) enlargement of the peripheral zone

    (C) Increase color Doppler

    (D) enlargement of the surgical capsule

35. **Contraindications for prostate biopsy may include all of the following *except*:**

    (A) significant coagulopathy

    (B) painful endorectal conditions (fissures, thrombosed hemorrhoids)

    (C) severe immunosuppression

    (D) prostate size greater than 50 g

36. **The most likely diagnosis in Fig. 6–12A is:**

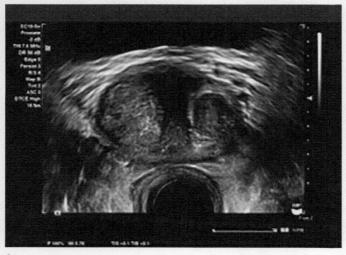

A

FIGURE 6–12A. Transverse scan of the prostate. *(©2019 Siemens Medical Solutions USA, Inc. All Rights Reserved. Clinic images provided courtesy of Siemens Medical Solutions USA, Inc.)*

    (A) peripheral zone nodule

    (B) BPH nodule

    (C) tumor in the anterior fibromuscular stroma

    (D) normal prostate

37. **What does the red arrow points to in Fig. 6–12B?**

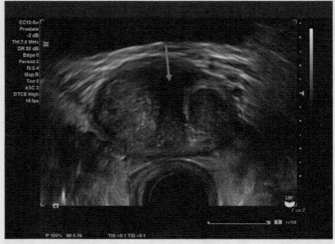

B

FIGURE 6–12B. Transverse scan of the prostate. *(©2019 Siemens Medical Solutions USA, Inc. All Rights Reserved. Clinic images provided courtesy of Siemens Medical Solutions USA, Inc.)*

    (A) fluid within the central gland

    (B) a prostatic abscess

    (C) shadowing from calcifications

    (D) fluid in the urethra

38. **Clinical signs and symptoms in patients with the above finding in (Fig. 6–13) may likely include all of the following *except*:**

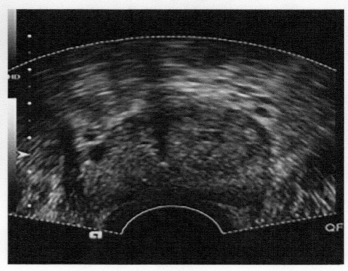

FIGURE 6–13. Longitudinal scan of the prostate. *(©2019 Siemens Medical Solutions USA, Inc. All Rights Reserved. Clinic images provided courtesy of Siemens Medical Solutions USA, Inc.)*

    (A) post void dribbling

    (B) nocturia

    (C) straining to void

    (D) fever and pyuria

Answers and Explanations

1. **(D)** Both A and C. The fibromuscular stroma is a nonglandular region that covers the anterior surface of the prostate. Therefore, both A and C are correct.

2. **(D)** Differentiation of a benign from a malignant nodule by imaging. Ultrasound cannot make a specific diagnosis of prostatic diseases. Biopsy is required to establish the diagnosis.

3. **(A)** The left lateral decubitus. Patients who are having transrectal prostate sonography are usually examined in the left lateral decubitus position.

4. **(D)** It is the primary site of adenocarcinoma. The transitional zone is located on both sides of the proximal urethra and represents 5% of the gland. It also is the primary site of BPH.

5. **(B)** The central zone is located at the apex of the prostate. The central zone is a triangular structure located at the base of the prostate with its apex at the verumontanum.

6. **(C)** 70%. The peripheral zone constitutes more than two-thirds of prostatic glandular tissue.

7. **(A)** Its apex is located inferiorly and the base of the prostate is located superiorly.

8. **(C)** Secretion of seminal fluid. The prostate discharges this fluid into the urethra to enhance the motility of sperm.

9. **(B)** The vas deferens. The seminal vesicles join the vas deferens to form the ejaculatory duct, which passes through the central zone.

10. **(D)** Urethra. The ejaculatory duct empties into the urethra at the verumontanum.

11. **(C)** The posterior-superior surface.

12. **(A)** It originates mainly in the central zone. Seventy percent of prostatic cancers originate *de novo* in the peripheral zone.

13. **(A)** A hypoechoic gland with anechoic areas.

14. **(D)** The transitional zone.

15. **(B)** They are calcified deposits in the prostate.

16. **(D)** Marked compression of the prostatic urethra. Early prostatic cancer can present as hypoechoic lesions on the peripheral zone. They can break through the prostatic capsule causing distortion, or they can invade the seminal vesicles.

17. **(D)** A digital rectal examination. This examination should be done before the probe is inserted to exclude obstructing lesions and to correlate the imaging study with the digital rectal exam.

18. **(D)** Sonographically variable. Prostate cancer can be hypoechoic, hyperechoic, or isoechoic.

19. **(A)** A midpoint region between the base and apex of the prostate.

20. **(D)** Obstruction of the seminal vesicle. An elevated PSA may be indicated in prostate cancer, prostatitis, or BPH.

21. **(A)** The central zone.

22. **(B)** The normal postpubescent prostate weighs approximately 20 g.

23. **(A)** Their absence does not usually affect fertility. In rare cases, infertility can be caused by absence of the seminal vesicles or by an obstruction in the ejaculatory ducts.

24. **(B)** A seminal vesicle. The structure demonstrated in Fig. 6–1B is the right seminal vesicle, that joins the vas deferens (not shown) to form the ejaculatory duct.

25. **(C)** Central gland calcification. Fig. 6–4 shows bright echoes representing prostatic calcification, which can be solitary or can occur in clusters.

26. **(C)** A tumor in the peripheral zone. The hypoechoic mass seen on the peripheral zone in Fig. 6–4 is characteristic of prostatic cancer.

27. **(D)** The central zone. The zone (white arrow) in Fig. 6–10 is clearly demarcated from the peripheral zone (black arrow) by a curved band of echoes.

28. **(A)** The peripheral zone.

29. **(B)** A cyst in the ejaculatory duct. The cystic structure shown in Fig. 6–7 is clearly located within the ejaculatory duct.

30. **(A)** They are located in the midline

31. **(B)** Ejaculatory duct cyst

32. **(C)** Seminal vesicle cyst

33. **(C)** Prostatic nodule on digital rectal examination. Prostate nodule in digital rectal exam may indicate prostate cancer.

34. **(A)** Lateral displacement of the peripheral zone

35. **(D)** Prostate size greater than 50 g.

36. **(B)** BPH nodule. Note that the large nodule seen is located in the inner gland and not the peripheral zone.

37. **(C)** Shadowing from calcifications

38. **(D)** Fever and pyuria. The image shows BPH which can have signs and symptoms as listed in choices A–C.

that the tip of the transducer probe is in the right lateral fornix. To image the left ovary, the sonographer moves the handle toward the patient's right thigh so that the tip of the probe is in the left lateral fornix. Although the ovaries can be depicted from almost any parauterine position, they are usually depicted either lateral to the uterus or in the cul-de-sac. Unlike transabdominal sonography, which allows the simultaneous imaging of both ovaries relatively often, TVS can best image only one ovary at a time. Sonographically, the appearance of the ovaries varies with patient age, stage in menstrual cycle, pregnancy status, and body habitus. In reproductive years, the ovaries may be identified by follicles surrounding the outer edge of the ovaries. Immature follicles are small (<3–5 mm), smooth, thin walled, and anechoic with good sound through transmission. Follicles will increase in size through the cycle with multiple follicles visible at days 5–7. At days 8–12, one or more dominant follicles (>10 mm) will begin to emerge. The dominant follicle reaches a mean diameter of 18–20 mm with a hypoechoic rim. After the ovum is released, bleeding may occur within the follicle, causing it to appear echogenic. The follicular cyst becomes a corpus luteal cyst with thick walls and appears anechoic to hypoechoic. The corpus luteum will retain fluid for 4–5 days and measures approximately 2–3 cm. The corpus luteal cyst has a rich blood supply. Color-flow Doppler will reveal a ring of color around the periphery corresponding to the visualized wall. If no pregnancy occurs, the corpus luteal cyst will gradually atrophy. If pregnancy occurs, the corpus luteal cyst will remain and gradually regress by 12–14 weeks.[2] The follicular cyst and corpus luteal cysts are all functional (physiologic) cysts of the ovary.[1] In postmenopausal women, it is more difficult to identify the ovaries because of the absence of follicles and atrophy of the ovaries.[3,5] In patients who have had a hysterectomy, the ovaries can be difficult to depict because of the air-filled bowel occupying the space left by the removal of the uterus.

Fallopian Tubes

The fallopian tubes originate at the lateral aspect of the uterus, known as the cornua. Fallopian tubes vary in length from 7 to 12 cm. Each Fallopian tube is divided into five subdivisions: (1) interstitial, (2) isthmus, (3) ampulla, (4) infundibulum, and (5) fimbriae.[1] The interstitial portion of the tube sonographically appears as a fine echogenic line extending from the endometrial canal and traveling through the myometrium to cornua of the uterus.[7] The isthmus tubae is the narrowest portion of the tube and is located adjacent to the interstitial segment at the uterine cornua. The tube continues laterally and widens to form the ampulla. The infundibulum is the most lateral portion of the tube and opens to the peritoneum at the fimbria.[1] The purpose of the fallopian tube is to aid in fertilization and to transport the ova from the ovary to the uterus. The normal fallopian tubes are difficult to identify by transabdominal or TVS unless they are surrounded by fluid or filled with fluid.[5]

Ligaments

The uterus is loosely suspended in the center of the pelvic cavity by

- Round ligaments
- Uterosacral ligaments
- Cardinal ligaments

Although the uterus is suspended by ligaments, it has freedom of movement. During pregnancy, or in the presence of a uterine mass, the uterus moves upward, and during uterine prolapse, it moves downward. The upper portion of the uterus is supported by a series of ligaments. The cardinal ligaments or transverse cervical ligaments originate from the cervix and uterine corpus and insert on a broad portion of the lateral pelvic wall and sacrum. At the distal portion, this ligament is called the uterosacral ligament. This ligament anchors the cervix and is responsible for the uterine orientation.[1]

The two round ligaments originate from the uterine cornua and are located in a fold of the peritoneum and terminate in the upper portion of the labia majora.[1] This ligament is responsible for the anterior tilt of the uterus and aids in stabilizing the fundus of the uterus.

There are two ligaments that are not true ligaments, but are folds of the peritoneum. The first is the suspensory ligament. It arises from the pelvic sidewall and contains ovarian vessels. It aids in supporting both the fallopian tube and ovary within the broad ligament.[7] The broad ligament is also a double fold of the peritoneum. It fans over the adnexa and divides the anterior and posterior portions of the pelvis.[1] It does very little to actually support the uterus. The broad ligament is not usually seen on ultrasound except in cases of pelvic ascites or ruptured cyst or hemoperitoneum.[8]

Muscles

A series of different muscle bundles pass through the female pelvis. Some of these muscles are easily visualized by sonography and can often be confused for adnexal structures. The most commonly visualized muscle is the iliopsoas muscle. On sagittal views, it appears as a paired long hypoechoic stripe with echogenic linear lines. On transverse images, however, it appears ovoid and is visualized lateral and anterior to the iliac crests.[1] The iliopsoas muscle descends until it attaches on the lesser trochanter of the femur. This can often be confused for an ovary until the sagittal view is obtained. The pelvic muscles can be identified sonographically by their appearance. The muscles appear hypoechoic and exhibit linear internal echoes. The borders of the muscles are echogenic representing the fascia.[3,4] The rectus abdominis muscle is located in the anterior abdominal wall and extends from the xiphoid process to the symphysis pubis. The obturator internus muscles are bilateral muscles lining the lateral margin of the true pelvis; they lie lateral to the ovaries. The levator ani muscle is a hammock-like muscle that extends from the body of the pubis and ischial spine to the coccyx.

Bladder and Ureters

The urinary bladder is a thick-walled distendable muscle that lies anterior to the uterus. It is fixed in position inferiorly at the symphysis pubis. This lower region is described as the trigone, defined by the orifices of the two ureters and a urethra. The bladder is thicker and more rigid here than at any other location.[1] The ureter originates at the renal pelvis and descends anterior to the internal iliac artery and posterior to the ovary. The ureter travels from posterior to anterior and closely follows the uterine artery in its inferior portion. It then passes anteromedially to enter the trigone of the bladder.[1] During a transabdominal sonographic examination of the pelvis, the urinary bladder must be distended for a variety of reasons. This is because (1) the urine-filled bladder pushes the bowel cephalad out of the true pelvic cavity, (2) it pushes the uterus cephalad away from the symphysis pubis, (3) it permits rapid anatomic orientation, (4) it provides a low-attenuation pathway to which ultrasound can propagate, and (5) it helps to elevate the head of the fetus for easy measurements. Whereas a distended bladder is an extremely important prerequisite for a transabdominal study, an empty bladder is the most important prerequisite for a transvaginal study. The failure to fill the bladder adequately for transabdominal studies can result in serious diagnostic errors. On the other hand, an overdistended bladder can also result in errors. Sonographically, the position and shape of the uterus have an effect on the urinary bladder. If the uterus is anteverted, the normally distended bladder has a mild indentation on its posterocephalad region. If the uterus is surgically removed or absent, the bladder has a different contour. Therefore, bladder contour depends on the shape and position of its surrounding structures. When the bladder is being filled, urine can be observed entering the bladder on real-time and has been referred to as the "ureteral jets."[2] The jets begin at the ureteral orifices and flow toward the center of the bladder (Fig. 7–17). Bladder diverticula may be acquired or congenital. Acquired diverticula result more commonly from bladder outlet obstruction. Congenital diverticula are located near the ureteral orifice and are known as Hutch diverticula.[3,5] Sonographically, bladder diverticula appear as outpouching sacs from the bladder wall with an opening in one end of the sac that communicates with the bladder.

Uterine Pathology

The most common uterine tumors are fibroids (also known as leiomyoma, myoma, and fibromyoma). They are present in 25% of the female population and occur at approximately 30–35 years of age, with a higher percentage in the African American population and becoming more prevalent with advancing female age. Fibroids are thought to be estrogen stimulated, so they tend to increase in size during pregnancy and decrease in size after menopause. Fibroids are classified according to their location on the uterus (Fig. 7–18). If the fibroid is confined in the myometrium, it is called intramural. If is located in the uterine cavity, it is called submucosal, and if projecting from the peritoneal surface, it is called subserosal. Often, they are found on pelvic examination without the patient having symptoms. When symptoms do occur, they can include abnormal bleeding, abdominal pressure, increased urinary frequency, and increased abdominal girth. The malignant form of the leiomyoma, a leiomyosarcoma, though rare, is believed to arise from a preexisting fibroid.[2,3,5] Leiomyosarcoma accounts for about 1.3% of uterine malignancies.[3] On ultrasound it appears similar to the leiomyoma and can be extremely difficult to diagnose preoperatively. Rapid accelerated growth may be the only clinical indication of a possible malignant process.[3,5] Fibroids has variable sonographic appearance:

- Inhomogeneous uterine texture
- Enlarged, irregular-shaped uterus
- Calcifications with distal acoustic shadowing

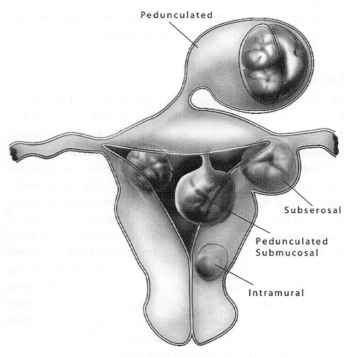

FIGURE 7–18. Diagram demonstrating various locations of fibroids.

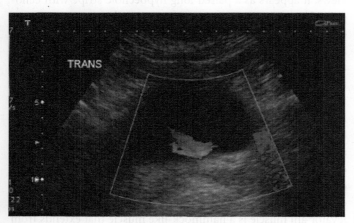

FIGURE 7–17. Transverse sonogram of the urinary bladder with color Doppler demonstrating ureteral jet.

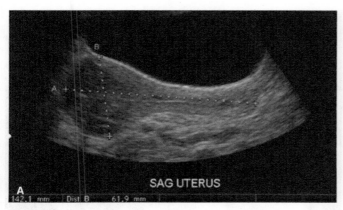

FIGURE 7–19A. Transabdominal sagittal sonogram of an enlarged uterus with fundal myoma.

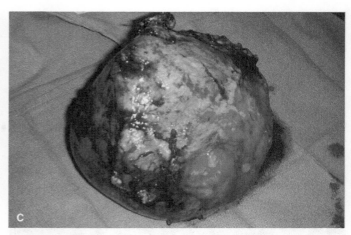

FIGURE 7–19C. Gross pathologic findings of the uterus with fibroids.

- Solid mass on the uterus that cannot be separated from the uterus
- Displacement of the endometrium
- Diffuse uterine enlargement

Fig. 7–19A shows an enlarged uterus with inhomogeneous echotexture. Fig. 7–19B demonstrates an intramural fibroid in the fundus of the uterus. Fig. 7–19C shows gross pathologic findings of the uterus with multiple fibroids.

Degeneration and necrosis of fibroid tissue can produce irregular cystic spaces within the uterine parenchyma[2]. Fibroids are the most common cause of uterine enlargement in the nonpregnant female. When the uterus is enlarged greater than 14 cm in length, the kidneys should be scanned for hydronephrosis. A large fibroid uterus may compress the ureter as it enters the pelvis, resulting in obstruction in flow of urine. Fibroids in the uterine cavity can on some occasions cause heavy vaginal bleeding resulting in acute anemia.

Adenomyosis is defined as an infiltration of endometrial implants into the myometrium greater than 2 mm. *Adenomyosis* occurs in multiparous women who experience prolong, heavy menstruation, and pain during intercourse (dyspareunia). Other symptoms may include menorrhagia, dysmenorrhea, and pelvic tenderness.[9] Sonographically, the uterus is large with small cysts visible in the inner myometrium. Often the myometrium of the uterus will appear inhomogeneous, similar to a fibroid, but distinct borders cannot be identified.[3,5]

Hematocolpos is an accumulation of blood within the vagina. This condition is typically the result from a imperforate hymen or transverse vaginal septum.[3] On ultrasound, the vaginal cavity is distended with hypoechoic echoes and possible fluid/fluid levels, representing retained blood. Because the vagina can be distended to the same size of the uterine fundus, it may have an hourglass appearance.

Hematometra is an accumulation of blood within the uterine cavity secondary to atrophy of the endocervical canal or cervical stenosis. Sonographically, hematometra appears as marked distention of the uterus. Table 7–1 defines the terminology used to describe abnormal vaginal bleeding.

Ovarian Cyst

Benign cystic masses of the ovaries tend to be smooth walled, well-defined, and anechoic with increased posterior acoustic enhancement (Fig. 7–20). The normal ovaries in reproductive-age women have multiple follicles of various sizes (mature and immature). These follicles serve as anatomic sonographic markers to identify the ovaries. A follicular cyst occurs when a mature follicle fails to ovulate. The size of these follicles depends on the menstrual cycle.[3] The mature follicle measures approximately 20–25 mm.[3] A follicular cyst is a functional cyst. The three most common functional cysts of the ovaries are (1) follicular cysts, (2) corpus luteal cysts, and (3) theca-luteal cysts.[1,7,8]

TABLE 7–1 • Abnormal Bleeding Terminology

Menorrhagia—prolonged bleeding occurring at the time of a menstrual period, either in duration or volume

Metrorrhagia—uterine bleeding occurring at irregular intervals

Metromenorrhagia—excessive and prolonged bleeding occurring at irregular, frequent intervals

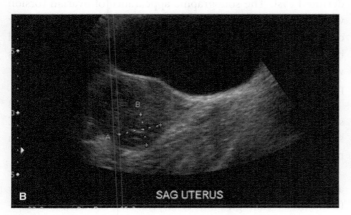

FIGURE 7–19B. Transabdominal sagittal sonogram of a fundal myoma.

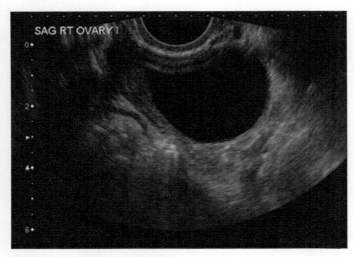

FIGURE 7–20. Right ovarian cyst.

Sonographers should be aware of the normal cyclic changes of the ovaries and their normal multiple sonographic appearances. Fig. 7–21 shows normal ovaries with a follicular cyst.

TVS is an accurate means of evaluating the ovaries and adnexal structures for the presence or absence of a pelvic mass. Pelvic masses can be characterized according to their location (organ of origin) and internal consistency (cystic, solid, mixed, septated, multiloculated). Such physiologic cysts as the corpus luteum cyst can be characterized as arising from within or around the ovary, whereas such extraovarian masses as endometriomas appear outside the ovary.

Cystic masses must be scrutinized with TVS for the intactness of their walls and the presence of any papillary excrescence. Internal structures such as septate or solid areas need to be shown in a minimum of two imaging planes.

Polycystic ovarian disease is an endocrinologic disorder characterized by excessive ovarian androgen production, which has spectrums of clinical manifestations[9]:

- Anovulation
- Amenorrhea

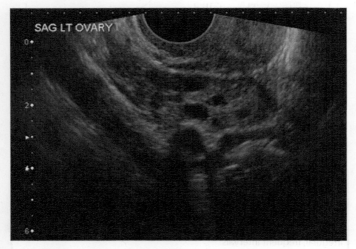

FIGURE 7–21. Left ovary with follicles.

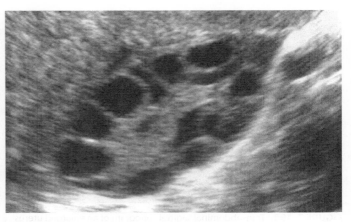

FIGURE 7–22. Polycystic ovary.

- Type 2 diabetes
- Obesity
- Acne
- Hirsutism
- Infertility

Polycystic ovaries are sonographically characterized by bilateral enlarged ovaries with an increased number of small immature follicles ranging in size from 3 to 5 mm and there are usually more than twelve on each ovary (Fig. 7–22). Patients with polycystic ovarian syndrome (PCOS) are at increased risk for infertility and endometrial cancer. The increase risk of endometrial cancer is due to the increased levels of estrogen and abnormally low progesterone.[9]

Ovarian Torsion

Ovarian torsion refers to the twisting of the ovary and its vessels resulting in occlusion of its blood supply. The twisting of the ovary with the vascular pedicle on its axis results in arterial, venous, and lymphatic obstruction causing necrosis of the ovary.[3,5] Approximately 95% of cases are associated with an adnexal mass. The right adnexa are more commonly involved due to the sigmoid colon occupying the left lower quadrant.[3,5,9] The most common mass associated with ovarian torsion is a dermoid cyst. The sonographic appearance of ovarian torsion will depend on whether the torsion is partial, intermittent, or complete. This type of mass is sonographically characterized by hyperechogenic areas, fluid/fluid layering, and calcifications within the mass. CDS is important in the evaluation of suspected torsion (Table 7–2).

Fig. 7–23A shows a left ovary and ovarian mass. Fig. 7–23B shows color and spectral Doppler with no flow. Fig. 7–23C shows gross pathologic findings of a necrotic ovary and ovarian mass surgically removed after an ovarian torsion.

Malignant ovarian disease has a peak incidence between the ages of 55 and 59 years. Other risk factors include family history (maternal or sibling), number of years of ovulation, and environmental (Tables 7–3, 7–4, and 7–5).[2]

| TABLE 7–2 • Doppler Findings for Ovarian Torsion |||
Doppler Study	Findings	Sonographic Findings
No venous or arterial Doppler flow	Complete obstruction	Torsion
No venous flow but arterial flow is present	Partial obstruction	Partial torsion
Venous and arterial flow are present	No obstruction	Decreased chances of torsion

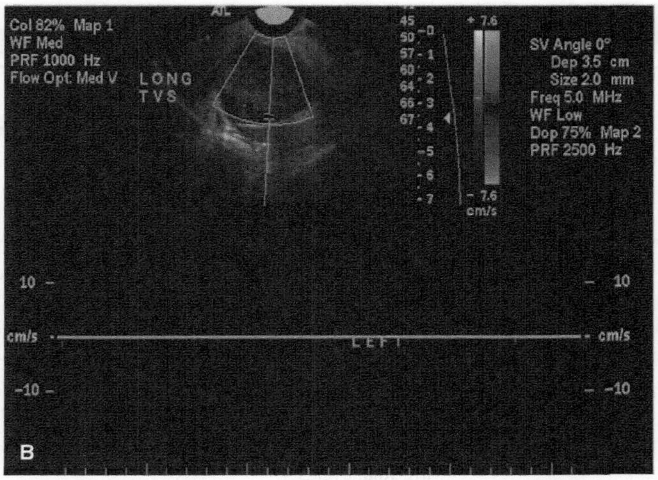

FIGURE 7–23B. Spectral and color Doppler with absence of flow.

OBSTETRICS

Pregnancy Test

Human Chorionic Gonadotropin (hCG). is a glycoprotein synthezed by the syncytiotrophoblastic cells of the trophoblast.[4,8] The hCG is composed of two dissimilar subunits: alpha and beta. The antibodies against the beta subunit are used specifically to measure hCG.[6] The quantitative β-hCG can be used to help establish the diagnosis of ectopic pregnancy, gestational trophoblastic disease, or abnormal pregnancy.

During the first trimester of pregnancy, the serum β-hCG normally doubles every 48 hours (2 days) or increases at least 66% every 48 hours before 8 weeks of gestation. In approximately 80% of ectopic pregnancy, of serum β-hCG has abnormal doubling (low doubling time, remain the same [plateau], or decrease slightly). However, 10% of ectopic pregnancies may have a normal doubling in 48 hours but may eventually drop or plateau.[7] A constant decreasing serial quantitative serum β-hCG in the first trimester is indicative of an abnormal or failed pregnancy, regardless of the pregnancy location.

The serum levels for twins are usually twice as high as those for singleton pregnancies, and patients with a benign mole have higher levels than women with a normal pregnancy. Those with an invasive mole have higher ratios than those with noninvasive moles, and those with choriocarcinoma have even higher levels than those with invasive moles.[7]

There are various methods of reporting quantitative β-hCG. Some laboratories report serum quantitative β-hCG results in terms of First International Reference Preparation (1st IRP), whereas others report the results in terms of Second International Standard (2nd IS). The most current is the Forth International Standard (4th IS).

Rapid Qualitative Pregnancy Test. This small kit used for detection of hCG in urine or serum is readily available for immediate hospital or office use and is now available over the counter for private use. β-hCG is a hormone that is normally produced by the trophoblast and present in the serum and urine

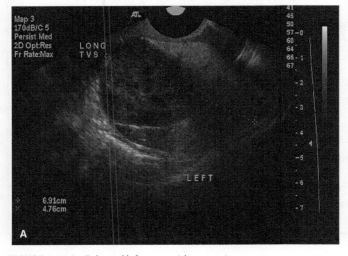

FIGURE 7–23A. Enlarged left ovary with an ovarian mass.

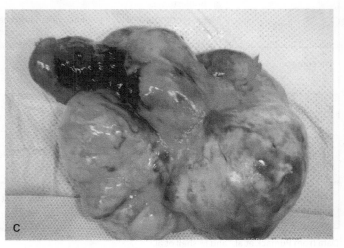

FIGURE 7–23C. Gross pathologic ovarian torsion.

TABLE 7–3 • Ovarian Cystic Masses

Mass	Clinical Findings	Sonographic Findings
Corpus luteum cyst	Associated with pregnancy	Unilocular: may contain low-level internal echoes; may appear as multiseptated cystic mass; normally regress after 14th week of pregnancy
Theca lutein cyst	Represents an exaggerated response to increased hCG Can be associated with ovarian hyperstimulation, molar pregnancy, chorioadenoma destruens, and choriocarcinoma	Bilateral enlarged ovaries; multiple small multilocular cysts
Polycystic ovaries (Stein–Leventhal syndrome)	A buildup of immature follicles with a thick outer covering preventing ovulation Associated with hirsutism, increased testosterone levels, irregular cycles	Bilaterally enlarged ovaries; multiple small cysts, appearing as "string of pearls"
Ovarian remnant syndrome	Residual ovarian tissue after oophorectomy	Can produce cysts, neoplasms; may cause symptoms; common with endometriosis and adhesions
Ovarian torsion	May be caused by a large cyst or tumor causing rotation of the ovary Dermoid cyst	In early phase, will have an enlarged ovary with intraovarian venous flow, but absent intraovarian arterial flow. In late stages, it will appear as a cystic or complex mass with thick walls and absent blood flow.

Data from Rumack et al.[3] and Mishell et al.[10]

TABLE 7–4 • Ovarian Solid Tumors

Mass	Clinical Findings	Sonographic Findings
Dysgerminoma	Uncommon malignant germ cell tumor. Occurs in second and third decades of life. One of the most common neoplasms in pregnancy. Historically similar to seminoma.	Predominately solid with hypoechoic internal echoes. Can grow rapidly.
Fibroma	Occurs in fifth and sixth decades. Part of stromal family, along with the other differentials: thecoma, granulosa cell, androblastoma. Meigs' syndrome a triad of benign ovarian fibroma, ascites, and pleural effusion	Hypoechoic to echogenic with mixed heterogeneous pattern Solid ovarian mass with ascites and pleural effusion
Thecoma	84% occur postmenopausally	Similar sonographic features as in fibroma. Unilocular
Granulosa cell	95% occur postmenopausally	Similar sonographic features as in fibroma; small tumors are solid; large tumors are complex
Androblastoma (Sertoli–Leydig cell)	Occurs in second and third decades. May cause elevated testosterone and hirsutism.	Similar sonographic features as in fibroma.
Transitional cell (Brenner)	Occurs from fourth through eighth decades. Most are benign. Symptoms: abnormal uterine bleeding.	Small, hypoechoic tumors. Larger tumors are at greater risk for malignancy.

Data from Rumack et al.[3] and Mishell et al.[10]

TABLE 7–5 • Complex Ovarian Tumors

Mass	Clinical Findings	Sonographic Findings
Endometriosis	Ectopic endometrial tissue that may bleed during menses. Cysts are called endometriomas or chocolate cysts because of blood in the cysts. Symptoms: pain during menses and infertility.	Single or multiple cystic adnexal masses with thick walls and low-level internal echoes. Small echogenic lesions posterior to the uterus.
Benign cystic teratoma (dermoid)	Most common benign germ cell tumor. Composed of all three germ cell layers. Varies in composition with fat, bone, hair, skin, and teeth. More common in reproductive years.	Fluid–fluid levels. Distal acoustic shadow. Calcifications. Tip-of-the iceberg sign (no through sound transmission).
Serous cystadenoma	Benign. Usually unilateral. Accounts for 25% of benign ovarian tumors. Occurs in fourth and fifth decades.	Large cystic mass with thin-walled internal septations.
Serous cystadenocarcinoma	Accounts for 50% of malignant ovarian tumors in fourth through sixth decades.	Large, multilocular with papillary projections. Ascites is common.
Mucinous cystadenoma	Largest ovarian tumor. Accounts for 25% of benign ovarian tumors. Occurs in third through fifth decades.	Large cystic mass with thick-walled septations. May have debris layering due to thick internal components.
Mucinous cystadenocarcinoma	Malignant. Accounts for 5–10% of malignant ovarian tumors.	Papillary projections are not as common as with serous cystadenocarcinoma. Associated with ascites.
Endometrioid tumor	80% are malignant. Occurs in fifth through sixth decades. Arises from endometriosis.	Cystic mass with papillary projections. Can occasionally be solid.
Clear cell tumor	Invasive carcinoma occurring in fifth and sixth decades.	Complex, predominately cystic mass.
Tubo-ovarian abscess	Infectious process within the tubes and ovaries.	Fluid–fluid levels with hydrosalpinx. May be seen as complex or cystic mass with low-level echoes, irregular borders and internal septations.

Data from Rumack et al.[3] and Mishell et al.[10]

of a pregnant woman. This rapid kit is an excellent marker on qualitative confirmation of pregnancy while awaiting the result of the more accurate quantitative serum β-hCG. The kit uses a color-coded result in a small result window, as the sample contains a detectable amount of hCG in 1–5 minutes. A minus (−) result in the result window means not pregnant or below the range of hCG sensitivity. A plus (+) in the result window indicates pregnancy or was recently pregnant. The first morning urine usually has a higher level of hCG present.

The urine pregnancy test is negative if less than 20 mIU/mL and serum β-hCG is negative less than 5 mIU/mL Both urine and serum can detect hCG as early as 7–10 days postconception. A false-negative result can occur with a urine sample that is too diluted. Therefore, to avoid a false-negative result, the test should be performed before high volume of fluid ingestion for sonography or high volume of intravenous fluid hydration. The test can also be false-negative if the sensitivity of the detectable hCG levels is below 20 mIU/mL. Fertility drugs containing hCG, such as Pergonal can alter the result.[7,9]

Serum Beta-hCG Correlation with Ultrasound

The level of serum β-hCG to which a gestational sac should be seen on ultrasound was formally called the discriminatory zone and was used for years to correlate with the ultrasound findings. The most current establish recommendation, β-hCG levels at which an intrauterine gestational sac can be seen with transvaginal ultrasound is now 3000 mIU/mL.[3,7]. This change is now called "threshold values" and was instituted because of variable levels of quantitative β-hCG.[3,5,6]. However, the current level to which a gestational sac should be seen on ultrasound is expected to decrease as the technology advances. If the gestational sac is not seen at this level, the pregnancy may be either abnormal, failed, or ectopic. However, a repeated level may be needed to confirm. On some rare occasions, the serum β-hCG may be positive without evidence of pregnancy or disease; this is known as phantom β-hCG or false-positive hCG test.[4] Antibodies generated in the body against other human antibodies may bind both human and animal antibodies (heterophilic antibodies). These may interfere with hCG tests, by causing phantom hCG or false-positive hCG results. Surgery and chemotherapy are sometimes performed for ectopic pregnancy, solely on the basis of phantom or false-positive hCG test data.[4] The interfering antibodies are present in serum but not urine samples. Phantom hCG can be confirmed by the demonstration of loss of the hCG in the urine samples.[4]

The Progesterone Level

Progesterone levels normally increase with gestational age. However, when an ectopic pregnancy is present, the corpus luteum does not secrete as much progesterone as occurs in normal pregnancy. Therefore, the concentration of the serum progesterone is usually lower in ectopic pregnancies. A value of 25 ng/mL or more is, 98% of the time, associated with a normal IUP, whereas a value less than 5 ng/mL identifies a nonviable pregnancy, regardless of its location.[10]

The combination of serum β-hCG, progesterone level, and TVS has resulted in great improvement in the diagnosis and management of ectopic pregnancy over the last 15–20 years.

ECTOPIC PREGNANCY

Any pregnancy outside the endometrial cavity is called ectopic pregnancy (Fig. 7–24). Pregnancy can be in the uterus and classified as an ectopic pregnancy, for example, cervical pregnancy, or pregnancy in the cesarean section surgical scar. The incidence of this type of pregnancy has increased, but the rate of death from ectopic pregnancy has declined. This decrease is the result of earlier diagnosis.[3] Most ectopic pregnancies occur in the fallopian tube, approximately 90%. They account for approximately 12% of all maternal deaths.[1,6] They can occur in any anatomic segments of the fallopian tube but occur more frequently in the ampullary region. Other, less common sites for ectopic implantation are the uterine cervix, ovaries, and abdomen. If the pregnancy is in the abdomen with advanced

gestational age, transabdominal scans should be performed first, and if necessary, transvaginal scans should be performed also. Abdominal pregnancy is the only form of ectopic pregnancy that can go to term. The incidence of live-birth after an abdominal pregnancy is very rare. On occasion, the placenta in an abdominal pregnancy may be adherent to bowel and blood vessels; removal could result in massive hemorrhage. In such cases, the placenta is left *in situ* and ultimately resorbs.[7,10]

Pseudogestational sac is intrauterine fluid seen in the present of ectopic pregnancy, and can in some occasion mimic an early intrauterine gestational sac[5,6,7] The differentiation between the gestational sac at 5–6 weeks and the pseudogestational sac is as follows:

Gestational sac	Pseudogestational sac (intrauterine fluid)
Yolk sac	No yolk sac
Embryo	No embryo
Double decidual sac sign	No double decidual sac sign (Single decidual layer)
Highly echogenic ring-choriodecidua	Thin wall
Grows 1 mm/day[3]	No daily increment in size
Lacunar structures with Doppler flow	No lacunar structures
Peritrophoblastic flow	No peritrophoblastic flow

A coexistent IUP and ectopic pregnancy, known as heterotopic, can occur especially in patient undergoing ovulation induction from in vitro fertilization (IVF). It was first reported at a rate of 1 in 30,000, then 1 in 16,000, and most currently 1 in 3900.[1,7] This increase in heterotopic pregnancies may be attributable to increased ovulation induction.[3,7] Twin ectopic pregnancy in the same fallopian tube can also occur (Fig. 7–25). On rare occasions, an ectopic pregnancy can

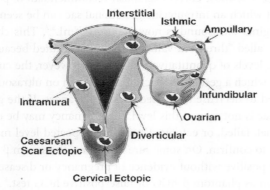

FIGURE 7–24. Diagram demonstrating various location of ectopic pregnancy.

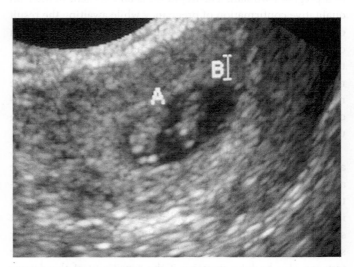

FIGURE 7–25. Transvaginal sonogram with twin ectopic pregnancy in the same fallopian tube.

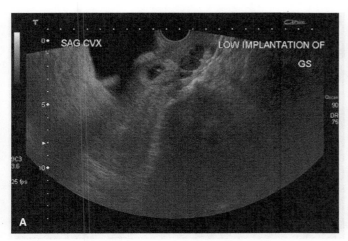

FIGURE 7–26A. Transvaginal sagittal sonogram with an ectopic pregnancy in the cesarean section scar.

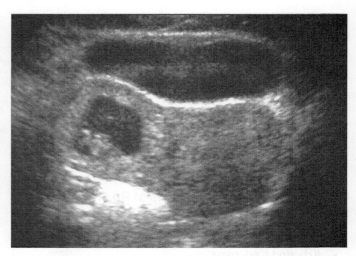

FIGURE 7–27. Transabdominal transverse scan with right cornual ectopic pregnancy.

also occur in a previous cesarean section scar (Fig. 7–26A). This patient had multiple previous cesarean sections and presented with vaginal bleeding in pregnancy. Color illustration of a cesarean section scar ectopic located intramural at the level of the isthmus uteri and above the internal os (Fig. 7–26B). Women with multiple C-sections are at increased risk for placenta previa, placenta accrete, and C-section scar ectopic.[3,5] Cesarean section scar ectopic pregnancy can be differentiated from cervical ectopic by its location. The cause for C-section ectopic is myometrial fistula within the C-section or a wedge defect.[3,6] Cervical ectopic is within the endocervical canal, whereas C-section sac ectopic is in the myometrium close to the maternal bladder at the level above the internal os

of the cervix. Another type of ectopic is called cornual pregnancy. The former definition for cornual ectopic is a pregnancy in one of the two horns of bicornuate uterus. The term intertarsal pregnancy is an ectopic pregnancy in the interstitial segment of the fallopian tube and historically both terms has been used interchangeably for years as a misnomer. Intertarsal ectopic pregnancies, which is often misdiagnosed clinically and sonographically for multiple reasons. Its location allows clinical symptoms and rupture to occur late, approximately 12–16 weeks, and sonographically this type of ectopic pregnancy can be misinterpreted as an IUP with an eccentric implantation.

Interstitial ectopic pregnancy has a higher mortality when compared to other forms of ectopic pregnancies due to larger blood vessels at the implantation site and late rupture. Fig. 7–27 demonstrates a right interstitial ectopic pregnancy.

Risk Factors for Ectopic Pregnancy

- Salpingitis from chlamydial infection or PID
- Previous ectopic pregnancy
- Previous operations on the fallopian tube, bilateral tubal ligation, or tuboplasty surgery
- Cigarette smoking affects the ciliary action in the nasopharynx, respiratory tract, and fallopian tubes[10]

Ultrasound Cause for Misdiagnosis

- Scanning away from the point of pain
- Erasing an image, you do not recognize
- Failure to follow standard protocol
- Inappropriate gain setting
- Inappropriate angle of incidence
- Incorrect annotation
- Failure to call for someone with more experience
- Ultrasound equipment not calibrated

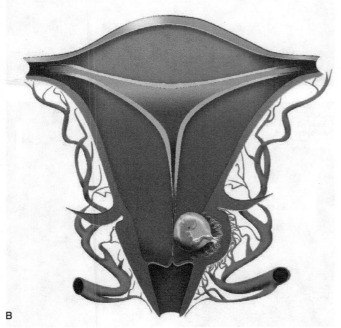

FIGURE 7–26B. Illustration of the uterus with an ectopic pregnancy in the region of cesarean scar.

Clinical Signs and Symptoms of Unruptured Ectopic Pregnancy

- Unilateral pelvic pain, which increases in severity with time
- Vaginal spotting or bleeding
- Amenorrhea
- Adnexal mass
- Positive pregnancy test
- Nausea and vomiting

Clinical Signs and Symptoms of Ruptured Ectopic Pregnancy

- Generalized abdominal pain
- Rebound tenderness
- Cervical motion tenderness
- Bilateral adnexal tenderness
- Right shoulder pain
- Tachycardia and hypotension
- Decreased hematocrit
- Syncope
- Tachypnea

UNRUPTURED ECTOPIC PREGNANCY

Ectopic pregnancy should be suspected when there is no intrauterine gestational sac and the serum β-hCG is at a level in which a pregnancy should be seen (values 1500–3000 mIU/mL).[6] The sonographic appearance of ectopic pregnancy primarily depends on whether the pregnancy is ruptured, unruptured, its location, and size. The sonographic equipment, the frequency of the transvaginal transducer, and the skills of the operator play important roles. Advanced ultrasound equipment in the hands of a skilled operator can sometimes depict an ectopic pregnancy before the patient begins to have clinical symptoms. Early depiction of ectopic pregnancy before a tubal rupture occurs is imperative to avoid the potential risk of massive blood loss and tubal damage. However, some patients delay seeking medical treatment when the symptoms start, arriving at the emergency department after rupture.

The sonographic appearance of an unruptured ectopic pregnancy is an adnexal ring-like mass with increased color flow around its periphery. The center of this adnexal ring is anechoic, and its periphery echogenic, resembling a doughnut. It is imperative for the sonographer to identify and depict the ovary on the side of the adnexal ring. A hemorrhagic corpus luteum cyst could mimic this finding. Rarely, an extrauterine gestational sac is seen with a live embryo. Fig. 7–28 depicts a live ectopic pregnancy in the posterior cul-de-sac.

Fig. 7–29A is a sagittal view demonstrating the uterine cavity free of any IUP. Fig. 7–29B is of the same patient in a transverse view with an extrauterine gestational sac with an embryo.

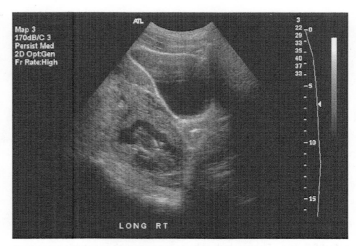

FIGURE 7–28. Transabdominal sagittal scan with ectopic pregnancy in the posterior cul-de-sac.

RUPTURED ECTOPIC PREGNANCY

An ectopic pregnancy in the fallopian tube grows in linear and circumference fashion.[7] The growth occurs more linear than circumferentially due to less resistance to growth in the long axis of the tube. This gives the ectopic pregnancy a sausage-shape appearance (Fig. 7–30). Rupture of the fallopian tube is due to maximum stretching of the tube with ischemia and

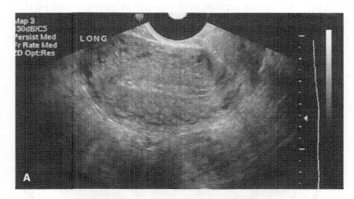

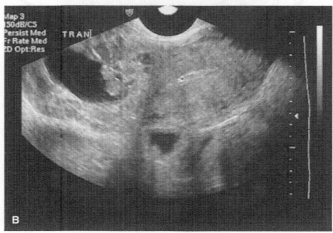

FIGURE 7–29. (A) Transvaginal sagittal scan of the uterus, free of any intrauterine pregnancy (IUP). (B) Transvaginal coronal scan with a right unruptured ectopic pregnancy.

hypoechoic to anechoic. Placental abruption is one of the leading causes of perinatal mortality and accounts for 15–20% of all perinatal deaths.[1] It can be associated with maternal vascular disease, hypertension, abdominal trauma, cocaine abuse, cigarette smoking, advanced maternal age, and unexplained increased MSAFP.[1]

Placenta accreta is the abnormal adherence of placental tissue to the uterus. It is divided into (1) placenta accreta placental attachment to the myometrium without invasion, (2) placenta increta—invasion of the placenta into the myometrium, and (3) placenta percreta—invasion of the placenta through the uterus and often invasion into the bladder or rectum. Risk factors include uterine scarring from cesarean sections and advanced maternal age.[1] Implantation sites at risk are uterine scars, submucous fibroid, lower uterine segment, rudimentary horn, and uterine cornua. With placenta accreta, the normal hypoechoic 1–2 cm myometrial band is absent or thinned (<2 mm) with loss of placental/myometrial interface.[5,10] There may be large hypoechoic to anechoic spaces in the placenta, termed "Swiss cheese appearance." Placental vascularity is also increased.[5] Doppler ultrasound is used to aid in the sonographic diagnosis.

Chorioangioma is the most common benign tumor of the placenta. It is a vascular malformation arising from the chorionic tissue that appears as a well-defined, hypoechoic mass near the chorionic surface and often near the cord insertion site.[3] Color and pulsed Doppler will confirm the increased vascularity of this lesion.

The umbilical cord consists of two arteries and one vein. The vein enters the fetus and drains into the ductus venosum and left portal vein in the liver. The umbilical vein carries oxygenated blood. The umbilical arteries, carrying deoxygenated blood, are seen coursing laterally around the bladder as they leave the fetal body. The vessels in the cord are surrounded by Wharton's jelly for protection. The umbilical cord normally inserts into the central portion of the placenta. It can, however, insert eccentrically or near the membranes. It can also be a velamentous insertion when it inserts into the membranes and courses through the membrane to the placenta.[3,5] Both of these insertions can play a part in placental insufficiency and fetal growth. Occasionally, only one artery will be present resulting in a two-vessel umbilical cord. It may be associated with other abnormalities and could possibly affect fetal growth, although not common. CDS can help identify absence of the umbilical artery, as well as nuchal cord and cord knots.[5]

Fetal Head, Neck, and Spine

Neural Tube Defect. This is a spectrum of malformations of the neural tube, including (1) anencephaly, (2) spina bifida, and (3) cephalocele. Folic acid taken daily before and during pregnancy is known to reduce the risk of neural tube defect.[1]

Anencephaly. This is the most severe form of neural tube defect. It is characterized by absence of the upper portion of the cranial vault and underlying cerebral hemispheres. The fetal face and brainstem are normally present in anencephaly. It may be diagnosed as early as 12 weeks by TVS and is associated with a markedly increased MSAFP, polyhydramnios, spinal defects, and bulging of the fetal orbits, giving the fetus a frog-like appearance.[10]

Spina Bifida. This is a defect in the lateral processes of the vertebrae allowing the spinal canal to be exposed, which in turn disrupts the muscle and skin covering. Herniation can be limited to meninges (meningocele) or involve the neural tissue as well (myelomeningocele). The most common sites of spina bifida are lumbar, lumbosacral, and thoracolumbar. Cranial findings associated with spina bifida are (1) "banana sign," consistently present with a defect (99%), and (2) "lemon sign." The banana sign is the displacement of the cerebrum inferiorly and the cisterna magna is usually obliterated. On the transverse view, the cerebellum resembles a banana instead of its characteristic view. The lemon sign includes bilateral depression of the frontal bone and gives the sonographic impression of a "lemon"-shaped head (Figs. 7–42A and B). Spina bifida is often associated with increased MSAFP, ventriculomegaly, and clubfeet.[1,3,10]

Cephalocele. This is a protrusion of the cranial contents through a bony defect in the skull. An encephalocele contains brain tissue. The majority are occipital (75%).[3,19] They often cause blockage of cerebrospinal fluid and ventriculomegaly results. Very large defects may be associated with microcephaly. Both types have a poor prognosis.[3,10]

Ventriculomegaly. The anatomy of the ventricular system is imperative in order to recognize the normal and abnormal sonographic appearance (Figs. 7–43A and B). This is enlargement of the lateral ventricles, more than 10 mm in the atrial diameter. In the absence of a spinal defect, pronounced ventriculomegaly (>15 mm) is most commonly associated with an obstruction of the ventricular system. In order of occurrence, these obstructions are aqueductal stenosis, communicating hydrocephalus, and Dandy–Walker malformation. Congenital hydrocephaly is an X-linked abnormality with only males affected and females being carriers. If there is a strong family history, DNA testing is available.[3,10] Ventriculomegaly is often associated with other abnormalities.

Dandy–Walker Malformation. This consists of a splaying of the cerebellar vermis, dilated fourth ventricle, increased cisterna magna (>10 mm), and ventriculomegaly. It can be associated with chromosomal abnormalities and is frequently associated with such other cranial midline defects as agenesis of the corpus callosum. It is often associated with other system abnormalities as well.[3]

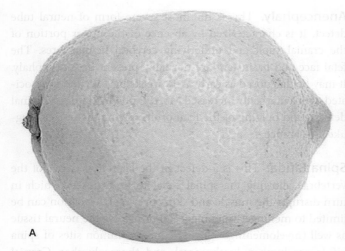
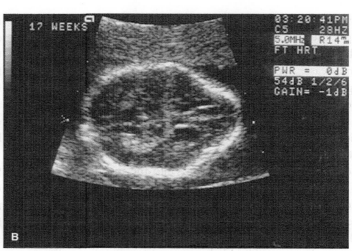

FIGURE 7–42. (A) Lemon. (B) Sonogram of a "lemon"-shaped head.

Holoprosencephaly. This is a group of midline defects resulting from incomplete cleavage of the prosencephalon. The three major varieties are (1) alobar—single rudimentary ventricle, absent cerebral falx, fused thalamus, absent third ventricle. Facial findings may range from cyclopia to severe hypotelorism. A medial cleft lip/palate is common. A proboscis may replace the nose or the nose may be very flattened; (2) semilobar—the cerebral hemispheres are partially separated posteriorly, with partial separation of the lateral ventricles. Both alobar and semilobar holoprosencephaly are associated with microcephaly; (3) lobar—almost complete separation of cerebellum and ventricles except for the fused anterior horns of the lateral ventricles. Other sonographic findings are absent cavum septum pellucidum. Facial findings are less severe than those found with alobar or semilobar holoprosencephaly.[3]

Cystic Hygroma. This most often occurs at the posterior neck. A hygroma is a sac filled with lymphatic fluid caused by an obstruction of the lymphatic system. It may be multiloculated or contain a midline septum and is often associated with Turner's syndrome or Down's syndrome.[10]

Fig. 7–44A shows a longitudinal sonogram of fetal neck with cystic hygroma. Fig. 7–44B shows a transverse sonogram of the same case demonstrating multiple septations in the mass.

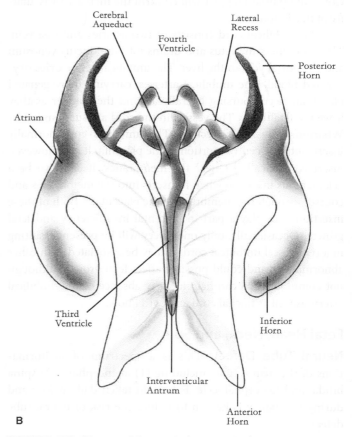

FIGURE 7–43A. Diagram of the ventricular system in the lateral view.

FIGURE 7–43B. Diagram of the ventricular system in the superior view.

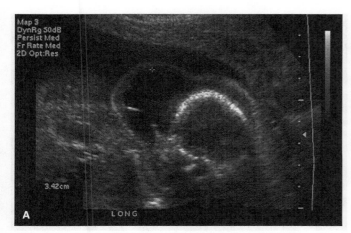

FIGURE 7–44A. Longitudinal sonogram of the fetus with cystic hygroma in the posterior region of the fetal neck.

Choroid Plexus Cyst. This is a cyst in the choroid plexus of the lateral ventricles. With other sonographic findings, it may be associated with trisomy 18 or 21. Alone, many investigators consider this a normal anatomic variant.[3,10]

Iniencephaly. This is a defect in the occiput involving the foramen magnum characterized by marked retroflexion of the fetal head and frequently shortened spine. This is a rare finding and has a strong association with other abnormalities.[3]

Agenesis of the Corpus Callosum. The corpus callosum begins to develop at 12 weeks of gestation and its development is complete at approximately 20 weeks.[10] This abnormality cannot be diagnosed until after 18 weeks of gestation. Findings to aid in diagnosis include (1) absence of the cavum septum pellucidum, (2) enlargement of the posterior horn of the lateral ventricle, (3) extremely narrow frontal horns, and (4) enlargement and upward displacement of the third ventricle. Agenesis of the corpus callosum has a strong association with other abnormalities.[3,10]

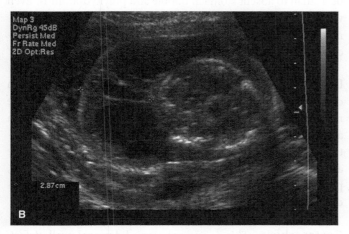

FIGURE 7–44B. Transverse sonogram of the same case demonstrating the multiple septations in the mass.

Hydranencephaly. This is a severe destructive process, believed to result from occlusion of the internal carotid arteries. The cerebral cortex is replaced by fluid, causing macrocephaly. The thalamus, brainstem, and cerebellum are spared.[3,10]

Vein of Galen Aneurysm. This is an arteriovenous malformation in vein of Galen located posterior to the third ventricle in the midline. Color and pulsed Doppler will demonstrate high-velocity arterial and venous blood flow. This is associated with congestive heart failure and hydrops.[10]

Cleft Lip/Palate. Isolated cleft lip and/or palate is the most common congenital facial anomaly. Lateral cleft lip is commonly isolated. Medial cleft lip is associated with chromosomal abnormalities.[10]

Heart

Atrial/Ventricular Septal Defect. This is a congenital malformation of the septum that appears as an opening between the chambers. It is the most common cardiac defect, accounting for 26% of defects.[10]

Atrioventricular Canal Defect. This is also known as atrioventricular septal defect, or endocardial cushion defect. A complete defect has a single ventricle, a single atrium, and a single atrioventricular valve. This appearance may vary with partial defects of the atrial or ventricular septums. This is the most common cardiac defect in trisomy 21.[3,10]

Hypoplastic Left Heart Syndrome. This is hypoplasia of the left ventricle, atrium, mitral valve, and aortic outflow. The right side of the heart will be enlarged.[3] The appearance may vary with different degrees of severity.

Coarctation of the Aorta. This is a narrowed segment of aorta along the aortic arch. It is difficult to see the narrowing but may present as a milder form of hypoplastic left heart syndrome later in pregnancy. Pulsed Doppler studies may also show a decrease in blood flow in the proximal portion of the aorta.[3]

Tetralogy of Fallot. This presents with the following defects: (1) ventricular septal defect, (2) overriding aorta, (3) pulmonary stenosis or atresia, and (4) right ventricular hypertrophy. It has a strong association with chromosomal abnormalities.[5,10]

Ebstein's Anomaly. This is the inferior displacement of the tricuspid valve. The right atrium is enlarged, and the valve, which is commonly abnormal, may appear thick and irregular in motion. Tricuspid valve regurgitation is often appreciated.[10]

Double Outlet Right Ventricle. The pulmonary artery and aorta both originate from the right ventricle, giving the appearance of the great vessels running parallel. Often a ventricular septal defect is present.[10]

Transposition of the Great Vessels. The aorta arises from the right ventricle, and the pulmonary artery arises from the left ventricle. The great vessels appear parallel on ultrasound. The pulmonary bifurcation and brachiocephalic vessels must be identified to correctly diagnosis this entity. Atrial septal defect and ventricular septal defect are often present.[3,5,10]

Truncus Arteriosus. This is a single large ventricular outflow tract overriding a ventricular septal defect. Right ventricular outflow tract will not be visualized, and pulmonary artery branches as well as aortic branches will be seen arising from the truncus.[10]

Rhabdomyoma. This is the most common intracardiac tumor. It can be multiple and appears as an echogenic mass located anywhere within the cardiac system. It is not visualized less than 22 weeks and has a strong association with tuberous sclerosis.[10]

Supraventricular Tachycardia. The fetal heartbeat is more than 200 bpm. Both supraventricular tachycardia and atrial flutter can lead to cardiac failure because of increased cardiac output.[10]

Thorax

Congenital Diaphragmatic Hernia. This is a congenital defect in the diaphragm allowing abdominal contents to herniate into the thorax. It may be left sided (75–90%), right sided (10%), or bilateral (<5%). Sonographically, (1) the fetal heart may be deviated, (2) stomach or bowel may be visualized in the thorax, (3) the area adjacent to the heart may appear inhomogeneous, and (4) polyhydramnios may be present. The intrathoracic abdominal contents can cause pulmonary hypoplasia, a significant factor in the high perinatal mortality (50–80%) of this disorder. If the liver is intrathoracic, congenital diaphragmatic hernia has a poorer prognosis (43% survival) versus an intra-abdominal liver (80% survival). Associated anomalies (15–45%) and chromosomal abnormalities (5–15%) will also affect perinatal survival.[3,10]

Congenital Cystic Adenomatoid Malformation. This is the most frequently identified mass in the fetal chest. It is typically unilateral and has three types: (1) type I, macrocystic—multiple large cysts measuring 2–10 cm; (2) type II—multiple medium-sized cysts less than 2 cm; and (3) type III, microcystic—sonographically appearing as a solid, homogenous echogenic lung mass. Many congenital cystic adenomatoid malformations (CCAMs) spontaneously regress in size during the third trimester. Prognosis is dependent on size, degree of mediastinal shift, and presence or absence of hydrops and polyhydramnios. Types I and II typically have a better prognosis.[10]

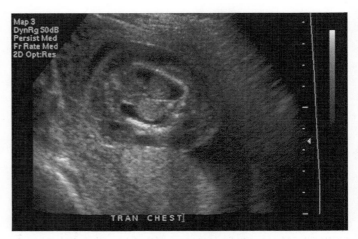

FIGURE 7–45. Transverse sonogram of a fetus with bilateral pleural effusions.

Pulmonary Sequestration. This is a solid, nonfunctioning mass of lung tissue that lacks communication with the tracheobronchial tree. It has its own blood supply commonly arising directly from the aorta and is fed by a single vessel. The majority are visualized as well circumscribed masses in the left lower lung base. They may cause mediastinal shift and hydrops. Ten percent can be found below the diaphragm and should be considered with any suprarenal mass in the left abdomen. Approximately 50–75% of sequestrations regress spontaneously.[10]

Pleural Effusion. This is an abnormal accumulation of fluid in the pleural lining of the fetal thorax. The etiologies are hydrops fetalis, chromosomal, and fetal infection. Fig. 7–45 shows a transverse sonogram of the fetal thorax with bilateral pleural effusions.

Gastrointestinal

Esophageal Atresia. This is an incomplete formation of the esophagus. There are five types of atresia, with 90% of those having a tracheoesophageal fistula that communicates with the fetal stomach. Sonographically, the exam may be normal or there may be a small to absent stomach bubble and polyhydramnios. Even with a stomach bubble visualized, this must be considered normal with unexplained polyhydramnios. This has a strong association with other anomalies and chromosomal abnormalities.[10]

Duodenal Atresia. This is a partial to complete obstruction caused by the failure of recanalization of the duodenum. It is the most common perinatal intestinal obstruction. The stomach and duodenum fill with fluid proximal to the site of the obstruction creating the classic "double-bubble" sign. Fifty percent are associated with other findings, including growth restriction, polyhydramnios, gastrointestinal, and cardiac anomalies. Duodenal atresia has a strong association with trisomy 21.[3,10]

Gastroschisis. This is an anterior abdominal wall defect, most commonly to the right side of the umbilicus, which allows herniation of abdominal contents into the amniotic cavity. The most common finding is free-floating bowel in the amniotic fluid, but stomach and bladder may also herniate into the amniotic fluid. Exposure to amniotic fluid and compression at an abdominal wall can lead to dilation and edema of the bowel. Overall, this has a good prognosis and does not have a strong association with chromosomal defects or other anomalies. It is associated with an elevated MSAFP.[3]

Omphalocele. This is a midline defect in the anterior abdominal wall with herniation of abdominal contents into the base of the umbilical cord. The mass is covered by a membrane and may not always have an elevated MSAFP, or may not elevate the MSAFP as significantly as gastroschisis. The umbilical cord can be seen inserting into the abdominal mass. Omphaloceles commonly contain liver but may contain other abdominal organs such as bowel. They have a strong association with other anomalies (50–80%), particularly cardiac, as well as chromosomal abnormalities (40–60%). If the omphalocele is small and contains only small bowel, the risk of aneuploidy increases.[2]

Pentalogy of Cantrell. This is an extensive defect of the thoraco-abdominal wall characterized by (1) ectopia cordis, (2) omphalocele, (3) ventricular septal defect, (4) defect of the sternum, and (5) diaphragmatic hernia. This anomaly is sonographically distinctive because of an omphalocele and ectopia cordis. There are many other associated craniofacial abnormalities, and it is often associated with chromosomal abnormalities.[3,10]

Beckwith–Wiedemann Syndrome. This is a group of disorders, including omphalocele, macroglossia, organomegaly, hypoglycemia, and hemihypertrophy.[10]

Cloacal Exstrophy. This is an association of anomalies, including omphalocele, herniated, fluid-filled structure inferior to omphalocele in place of urinary bladder, imperforate anus, and neural tube defect. This defect has a marked increased MSAFP.[10]

Meconium Ileus. This is the third most common cause of neonatal bowel obstruction. Sonographic findings include echogenic small bowel, dilated fluid-filled loops of bowel, and echogenic dilated bowel. It has a strong association with cystic fibrosis. If the internal diameter of the small bowel is more than 7 mm, it is suggestive of obstruction.[1,3]

Meconium Peritonitis. This is a reaction to bowel perforation. Meconium causes a peritoneal reaction that forms a membrane, which seals the perforation and may be seen as a thick-walled cyst. Other findings are ascites and meconium calcifications.[1,3,10]

Limb–Body Wall Complex (LBWC). This is a complex set of abnormalities caused by failure of the anterior abdominal wall to close. Findings include complete body wall defects, absence of umbilical cord, severe scoliosis, and lower limb abnormalities. Abnormalities are widespread and appearance may be a mass of tissue with few distinctive features.[3,10]

Amniotic Band Syndrome. Rupture of the amnion early in pregnancy resulting in formation of amniotic strands that stick and entangle fetal parts resulting in amputation of digits, arms, and legs. Fetal movement restriction due to amniotic bands is helpful for the sonographic diagnosis.[3,10]

Hydrops. There are two types: (1) nonimmune—accumulation of fluid in body cavities (pleural, pericardial, and peritoneal) and soft tissue. There are many causes for this entity, but major causes are cardiac failure, anemia, arteriovenous shunts, mediastinal compression, metabolic diseases, fetal infections, fetal tumors, congenital fetal defects, and chromosomal and placental anomalies; (2) immune—sonographic findings are the same. These are caused by maternal antibodies destroying fetal red blood cells (RBCs), which ultimately leads to erythroblastosis fetalis or congestive heart failure.[2]

Figs. 7–46A, B, and C are sonograms demonstrating fetal hydrops, bilateral pleural effusions, and polyhydramnios, respectively.

Ascites. This is free fluid within the abdominal cavity. It may be part of the hydrops complex or isolated because of bowel perforation or bladder perforation.

Situs Inversus Totalis. This is complete thoracic and abdominal organ reversal. Partial situs involves the abdominal organs only. Often associated with polysplenia and congenital heart defects.[2]

Abdominal Cyst. The differential for an isolated abdominal cyst not related to the GI or GU tract includes ovarian cyst, mesenteric cyst, omental cyst, or urachal cyst as the most common listings.

Genitourinary

Ureteropelvic Junction Obstruction. This is an obstruction at the junction of the renal pelvis and ureter. It is the most common cause of hydronephrosis. A complete obstruction will lead to massive hydronephrosis eventually causing dysplasia.

Obstruction. This is an obstruction at the junction of the ureter and bladder. Sonographic findings include mild hydronephrosis and hydroureter. Often associated with duplicated renal anomalies, including the ureter. The abnormal ureter commonly has a stenotic opening into the bladder and forms an ureterocele, which appears as a cystic structure within or adjacent to the bladder.

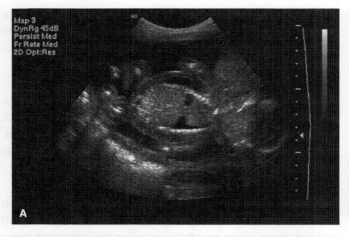

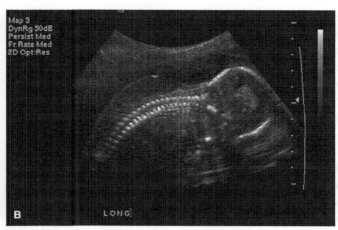

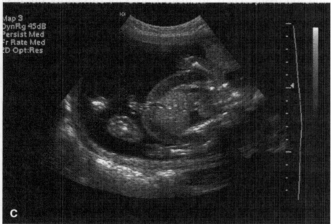

FIGURE 7–46. (A, B, C) Sonograms demonstrating fetal hydrops, bilateral effusions, and polyhydramnios.

Posterior Urethral Valve Bladder Outlet Obstruction. This is an obstruction of the posterior urethral valves. Overwhelming found in males, the bladder is massively dilated with hydroureters and hydronephrosis. The massive hydronephrosis may lead to atrophy of the kidneys. Anhydramnios is present with complete obstruction. On ultrasound, the bladder has the characteristic "keyhole" appearance as urine fills the proximal urethra. The abdominal wall becomes overly distended, which results in prune belly syndrome (abnormal development of abdominal musculature leading to a lax abdominal wall in newborns). The lack of amniotic fluid causes Potter facies (flattened facies, low set ears) and flexion contractures of the extremities. Pulmonary hypoplasia, caused by anhydramnios, is the primary cause of neonatal death in this syndrome.

Renal Agenesis. Diagnosis is made by the following findings: anhydramnios to severe oligohydramnios, nonvisualized bladder, and absent kidneys without evidence of renal blood flow. The adrenal glands appear flattened and elongated, which may aid in the diagnosis.

Multicystic Dysplastic Kidney. This is an obstruction in the first trimester that leads to atretic kidneys and formation of randomly positioned and varying sized cysts in the parenchyma of the kidney. The parenchyma is usually increased in echogenicity as well.

Autosomal Dominant Polycystic Kidney Disease. There must be one affected parent for this disorder to occur. Findings are not always seen in pregnancy and if so, typically do not appear until third trimester. Kidneys may appear enlarged and echogenic with multiple large cysts.

Autosomal Recessive Polycystic Kidney Disease. This is also known as infantile polycystic kidney disease. Multiple microscopic cysts give the appearance of very large, echogenic kidneys with decreased AFV after 20 weeks. Findings may be normal less than 20 weeks.

Congenital Mesoblastic Nephroma. This is a rare renal tumor that sonographically appears as a large, solid, well-circumscribed, highly vascular mass. The increased vascularity can cause cardiac overload and polyhydramnios.

Neuroblastoma. This malignant tumor is commonly found in the adrenal gland. Sonographically, it appears as an echogenic, heterogeneous, suprarenal mass.[19,20]

Skeletal

Limb shortening may be described as (1) rhizomelic—shortening of the proximal limb, (2) mesomelic—shortening of the forearm bones or lower leg bones, (3) micromelia—shortening of all portions of the limbs, both severe and mild. There are many types of short-limb syndromes, and the more common lethal and nonlethal varieties are discussed in this review.

Short-limb syndromes are considered lethal if the thoracic circumference is less than fifth percentile for the gestational age, suggesting pulmonary hypoplasia. Other findings are (1) severe micromelia, less than four standard deviations of mean, and (2) identification of such specific features as severe fractures.

Lethal

Thanatophoric Dysplasia. This is the most common skeletal dysplasia and is uniformly lethal.

Findings are the following:

- Cranium—macrocrania, hydrocephaly, frontal bossing, cloverleaf-shaped skull, depressed nasal bridge
- Thorax—severely hypoplastic giving the "bell-shaped" appearance, short ribs
- Bones—severe rhizomelia with bowing ("telephone receiver"); hypomineralization; spinal column appears narrow; polyhydramnios

Achondrogenesis—Type I, Most Severe. This exhibits severe micromelia, protruding abdomen, poor skull, and vertebral ossification. Type II, accounts for 80%.

- Cranium—macrocrania
- Thorax—shortened trunk
- Bones—severe micromelia with bowing and decreased mineralization

Osteogenesis Imperfecta (OI) Type II—Lethal. OI type II is subcategorized into three types, but all three are discussed in general terms for this text.

- Thorax—bell shaped, with small thorax; ribs have multiple fractures, may appear thin and flared
- Bones—micromelia; may see fractures or bones may appear thickened, irregular, and bowed because of fractures folding on themselves
- Decreased fetal movement and polyhydramnios

Nonlethal

Heterozygous Achondroplasia. This is the most common form of genetic skeletal dysplasia. It may not always be identified before less than 27 weeks.

- Cranium—increased HC, frontal bossing, depressed nasal bridge
- Bones—mild to moderate rhizomelic shortening, "trident" hand

Osteogenesis Imperfecta—Types I, III, IV

- Type I—may not identify less than 24 weeks; mild micromelia and bowing; may see isolated fractures
- Type III—will show lagging long-bone growth early with mild-to-moderate shortening and bowing
- Type IV—similar to type I

Asphyxiating Thoracic Dysplasia (Jeune Thoracic Dystrophy)

- Thorax—may appear bell shaped
- Bones—mild-to-moderate micromelia (rhizomelic) with possible bowing, possible polydactyly polyhydramnios.[2]

MULTIPLE GESTATIONS

Multiple pregnancies account for 3.3% of live births. Dizygotic, or fraternal, twins occur when two separate ova are fertilized. Monozygotic, or identical, twins occur when a single ovum divide. Seventy-five percent of twins are dizygotic, and 25% are monozygotic. The frequency of monozygotic twinning is constant and occurs in 1:250 births. Dizygotic twinning varies widely and is dependent on race, maternal age, parity (increased risk with increased parity), maternal family history, and infertility medication.[1,10]

It is very important to determine the number of chorionic and amniotic sacs in twin pregnancies. The best and most accurate time to assess this is in the first trimester. All dizygotic twins are dichorionic, diamniotic. Monozygotic twins, on the other hand, may have a variety of presentations depending on the day the zygote divides.[3]

Day of Division	Appearance
<4 days	Dichorionic/diamniotic, same gender, occurs 24% of time
4–8 days	Monochorionic, diamniotic, occurs 75% of time
8–12 days	Monochorionic, monoamniotic, 1%
>13 days	Conjoined, monochorionic, monoamniotic

Sonography cannot distinguish between dizygotic and monozygotic twins unless they are different genders. There are sonographic clues to aid in the identification of chorionicity and amniocity.

First-trimester sonographic findings are the following:

Dichorionic—sacs will be divided by a thick echogenic rim, counting the sacs determines the chorionicity.

Monochorionic—will appear similar to a single gestation with a thick echogenic gestational sac surrounding both fetuses.

Diamniotic—each sac will have its own yolk sac (> 8 weeks). The amniotic sac is very thin and can be difficult to identify in the first trimester.[3]

Second trimester—Dichorionic findings:

1) Different gender

2) Two separate placentas

3) Twin peak sign—triangular projection of chorion into dividing membrane appears as a "peak" on ultrasound; strong predictor less than 28 weeks

4) Thickness of membrane—thick membrane, more than 1 mm, is suggestive of dichorionicity. This finding is more accurate less than 26 weeks but is still a weak predictor.[2]

Twin pregnancies carry a four to six times higher perinatal mortality, and a two times higher morbidity rate for a variety of reasons. The most common complication of twins is preterm labor. Other complications are growth restriction, anomalies (two to three times more than a singleton), and such maternal conditions as hypertension and preeclampsia.[3,4]

Twin Abnormalities

Twin-to-Twin Transfusion Syndrome (TTTS). This condition can occur with monochorionic twins. Arteriovenous communications within the placenta can result in TTTS. One fetus will have blood shunted away and is labeled the donor, while the other fetus will receive the shunted blood and is labeled the recipient. This syndrome presents with a series of sonographic findings related to the shunting of blood. The donor twin is commonly growth restricted with a discordance between the twins of more than 20%. There is often oligohydramnios with the donor and polyhydramnios with the recipient. The donor fetus will appear "stuck" in the sac. This appearance is characteristic of TTTS. The donor will become hypovolemic and anemic. Umbilical cord Doppler images often show an increased systolic/diastolic ratio, demonstrating the increased resistance in the umbilical cord. The recipient will become larger, hypervolemic, and plethoric. Hydrops may occur as the fetus enters into congestive heart failure. The ventricular walls of the heart may thicken, and the contractility of the heart may be decreased as the heart failure becomes worse. As the blood flow increases to the recipient, the S/D ratio decreases, and the overall blood velocity is high. Both fetuses are at a significantly increased risk for intrauterine and perinatal mortality.[1,]

Monoamniotic Twins. This entity carries a 50% mortality risk because of cord entanglement that obstructs blood flow to the fetus. Sonographically, color Doppler may be helpful to look for a mass of cord with areas of increased velocity, suggesting stenotic flow.

Conjoined Twins. This is rare. Most conjoined twins are born prematurely, and 40% are stillborn. The most common presentation is fusion of the anterior wall. They may share organs, and those organs can often have abnormalities. Polyhydramnios is present 50% of the time. The most common types are thoraco-omphalopagus (conjoined chest and abdomen), thoracopagus (conjoined chest), and omphalopagus (conjoined abdomen). They account for 56% of the types of conjoined twins.[1,3]

Acardiac Twin. This is rare. All cases have an arterial-to-arterial shunt and a venous-to-venous shunt allowing for perfusion of the acardiac twin.[20] The acardiac twin either has a rudimentary heart or is completely acardiac. It has a poorly underdeveloped upper body with a small or absent cranium and brain. If it does develop, there are often significant abnormalities. The lungs and abdominal organs may also be abnormal or absent. The lower extremities are slightly more developed.[1] The normal, or pump twin is at a great risk for congestive heart failure, which will present on ultrasound as polyhydramnios and fetal hydrops. Chromosomes have been reported to be abnormal in up to 50% of the cases. Doppler can verify the reversed flow in the umbilical cord of the acardiac twin.[3]

CHROMOSOMAL ABNORMALITIES AND TESTING

Trisomy 21. This is the most common chromosome disorder. Trisomy 21 occurs when there are three copies of chromosome 21. The Down's syndrome frequency increases with advanced maternal age. At this time, the only definitive test to determine Down's syndrome is amniocentesis. Noninvasive testing includes blood tests and ultrasound.[1]

First-trimester screening combines biochemistry markers, maternal age (MA), and fetal nuchal translucency. Nuchal translucency is a measurement made at the back of the fetal neck on the CRL image. It is applicable from 11 to 14 weeks. The nuchal translucency increases with gestational age and normal tables are available for comparison; however, any measurement less than 3 mm is normal. Screening for Down's syndrome by maternal age and nuchal translucency has been shown to identify 80% of fetuses with Down's syndrome (with a 5% false-positive rate). Other chromosomal defects (trisomy 18, 13, triploidy, and Turner's syndrome), cardiac defects, skeletal dysplasia's, and genetic syndromes can also present with increased nuchal translucency.[3,19,20]

For the nuchal translucency to be accurate, very strict rules should be followed. The fetus is measured in the sagittal plane, the same used for the CRL. Careful consideration should be taken to bisect the fetus exactly in the midline, evidenced by the umbilical cord insertion. The image should be magnified so that the fetus occupies at least three-fourths of the image. The imager should be able to distinguish between the fetal skin and the amnion, both appearing as a thin membrane. This is accomplished by waiting for the fetus to spontaneously move away from the amnion. The first caliper should be placed so that the horizontal bar of the caliper is on the outside edge of the inner membrane in the nuchal region. The second caliper should be placed so that the horizontal bar is on the inside edge of the fetal skin. The placement of the caliper is very important

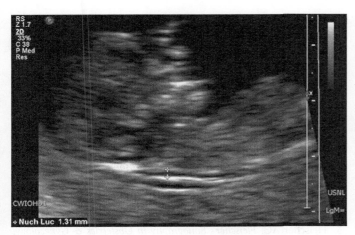

FIGURE 7–47. Fetus with electronic calipers measuring the nuchal translucency.

for the predictability and accuracy of the nuchal translucency. Great care should be taken to achieve the correct image and caliper placement (Fig. 7–47).[2,3,5]

First-trimester biochemistry includes the analysis of hCG and PAPP-A (pregnancy-associated plasma protein A).[6] The higher the hCG and the lower the PAPP-A, the higher the trisomy 21 risk. The detection rate of trisomy 21, combining MA, nuchal translucency, and biochemistry is 90%, with a 5% false-positive rate.[10]

Second-trimester ultrasound markers can be divided into major and minor findings. Major findings warrant offering invasive testing alone; whereas, minor markers require two or more findings to warrant offering invasive testing. Major sonographic markers include increased nuchal skinfold (>6 mm), cardiac defect, diaphragmatic hernia, omphalocele, facial cleft, and atresia (esophageal or duodenal).[3,10] Minor markers include abnormal ratio of observed/expected femur and humeral lengths, hypoplasia of midphalanx of fifth digit, echogenic foci of the heart, pyelectasis, echogenic bowel, sandal gap toe, choroid plexus cysts, small ears, and, most recently, nasal bone.[6,10]

Second-trimester biochemistry or maternal serum AFP3 (MSAFP3) consists of hCG, AFP, and estriol. A risk of trisomy 21 is calculated based on these values. The risk increases with a higher hCG, lower AFP, and lower estriol. Combining the ultrasound with the biochemistry markers will detect approximately 60% of trisomy 21 fetuses.[10]

Trisomy 18. In this disorder, there are three copies of chromosome 18. Ninety-five percent are an intrauterine demise or stillborn.[10] It is commonly, but not always, associated with multiple defects. Sonographically, these major findings may be seen with trisomy 18; growth restriction, increased nuchal translucency, neural tube defect, strawberry-shaped head, choroid plexus cysts, ACC, enlarged cisterna magnum, decreased extremity lengths, cardiac defects, diaphragmatic hernia, esophageal atresia, omphalocele, and renal agenesis. Minor ultrasound findings include clenched hands, echogenic

bowel, rocker-bottom feet, micrognathia, and single umbilical artery.[6,20] MSAFP3 shows all three markers decreased.[10]

Trisomy 13. In this disorder, there is an extra copy of chromosome 13. It may be associated with multiple abnormalities; however, the most common sonographic findings are holoprosencephaly (including the facial spectrums), cardiac defects, postaxial polydactyly, echogenic or polycystic kidneys, omphalocele, and microcephaly.[1,10]

Triploidy. In this disorder, there are three complete sets of chromosomes. If paternally derived, the typical finding is a large placenta with multiple cystic areas (partial mole). If maternally derived, multiple findings include severe IUGR with an abnormally large head and small abdomen, hypertelorism, micrognathia, ventriculomegaly, cardiac defects, neural tube defect, holoprosencephaly, Dandy–Walker malformation, cystic hygroma, renal anomalies, clubbed feet, single umbilical artery, and oligohydramnios.[1,10]

Sex Chromosome Abnormalities. The main sex chromosome abnormalities are Turner's syndrome, 47, XXX; 47, XXY; and 47, XYY.[20] Sonographically, Turner's syndrome findings are cystic hygroma, lymphangiectasia, cardiac defects, renal abnormalities, and hydrops.[1,10] The other sex chromosome abnormalities do not typically have prenatal sonographic findings.

INVASIVE TESTING

Amniocentesis. This is an invasive procedure in which a needle is inserted into the amniotic cavity and amniotic fluid is withdrawn. The amniotic fluid is typically assessed for karyotype, levels of amniotic fluid bilirubin associated with Rh disease, amniotic fluid alpha-fetoprotein, acetylcholinesterase for spinal defects, infection, fetal lung maturity, and specific DNA studies. Our institution quotes a 1:300 risk of miscarriage with amniocentesis based on the national average. The standard amniocentesis is offered after 14 weeks.

Fluorescence *In Situ* Hybridization (FISH). This is currently an adjunct to amniocentesis. It is considered experimental at this time, so all findings from this test must be confirmed by amniocentesis results. "Tags," or markers, that attach to certain chromosomes (currently testing 13, 18, 21, X, and Y) fluorescence. This allows the geneticist to count the chromosomes for extra or deleted chromosomes. Results are available in 24–48 hours.[10]

Early amniocentesis is performed the same as amniocentesis but during the 11th to 14th weeks of gestation. It has been associated with many problems. The loss rate is higher, 1:100, and is technically more difficult to perform because of the lack of fusion of the amnion and chorion. The unfused membranes are difficult to penetrate and often cause the need for multiple sticks, which in turn, increases the loss risk. Early amniocentesis has also been associated with talipes equinovarus.[10]

Chorionic Villus Sampling (CVS).

This is a procedure in which a catheter is inserted into the placenta and chorionic villi are aspirated for karyotyping. This procedure may be done transabdominally or transvaginally, depending on placental location. CVS is performed between 10 and 12 weeks and results are obtained in 3–8 days versus 10–14 days for amniocentesis. CVS does not test for amniotic fluid alpha-fetoprotein and cannot rule out spinal defects. Although the loss rate is slightly higher than amniocentesis, the CVS loss rate is comparable to early amniocentesis. CVS performed less than 10 weeks has an association with severe limb defects and is not typically performed at that time.[2,6,10]

Percutaneous Umbilical Blood Sampling (PUBS).

This is similar to an amniocentesis except that the needle is advanced through the amniotic fluid to the cord insertion site into the placenta. The needle is then inserted into the base of the umbilical cord. CDS can aid in locating the umbilical cord insertion into the placenta.[5] This procedure has a higher loss rate, 1–2%, and is technically more difficult to perform. It allows for rapid karyotyping (48–72 hours). PUBS most common application is with Rh isoimmunization testing. The fetal blood is tested for the amount of bilirubin pigment and allows the perinatologist to perform a blood transfusion if necessary.[1]

References

1. Cunningham GF, Leveno K, Bloom S, et al. *Williams Obstetrics.* 25th ed. New York, NY McGraw Hill; 2018.

2. Fleischer AC. Eugene C, Manning J, et al. *Sonography in Obstetrics and Gynecology: Principles and Practice.* 8th ed. . New York, NY: McGraw Hill; 2017.

3. Rumack CM, Levine D. *Diagnostic Ultrasound.* 5th ed. St. Louis, MO: Elsevier Mosby; 2018.

4. Callen PW. *Ultrasonography in Obstetrics and Gynecology.* 6th ed. Philadelphia, PA: Sanders, Elsevier; 2017.

5. Fleischer AC. *Fleischer's Sonography in Obstetrics & Gynecology: Textbook and Teaching Cases.* 8th ed. New York, NY: McGraw Hill; 2016.

6. Abramowicz J. *First-Trimester Ultrasound: A Comprehensive Guide.* New York, NY: Springer; 2016.

7. Lobo R, Gershenson D, Lentz G. *Comprehensive Gynecology.* 7th ed. St. Louis, MO: Elsevier Mosby; 2018.

8. Rizzo D. *Fundamentals of Anatomy and Physiology.* 4th ed. Boston, MA: Delmar Cengage Learning; 2015.

9. Hagen-Ansert SL. *Textbook of Diagnostic Ultrasonography.* 8th ed. New York, NY: Elsevier Health Sciences; 2017.

10. Creasy RK, Resnik R. *Maternal-Fetal Medicine: Principles and Practice.* 8th ed. Philadelphia, PA: WB Saunders Company; 2018.

Questions

GENERAL INSTRUCTIONS: For each question, select the best answer. Select only one answer for each question unless otherwise specified.

1. The sonographic finding in Fig. 7–48 is

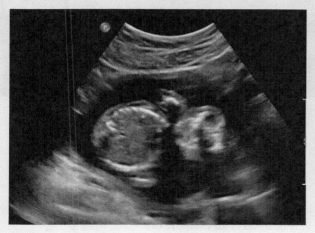

FIGURE 7–48.

(A) acephaly
(B) cleft lip
(C) anencephaly
(D) hypertelorism

2. Fig. 7–49 demonstrates

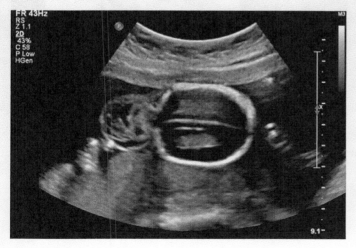

FIGURE 7–49.

(A) omphalocele
(B) encephalocele
(C) cystic hygroma
(D) arachnoid cyst

3. The sonographic finding in Fig. 7–50 includes

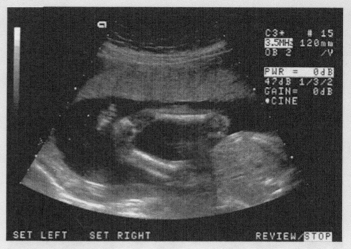

FIGURE 7–50.

(A) equinovarus
(B) micromelia
(C) bilateral femoral hypoplastic
(D) all of the above

4. The sonogram of the fetal head in Fig. 7–51 demonstrates

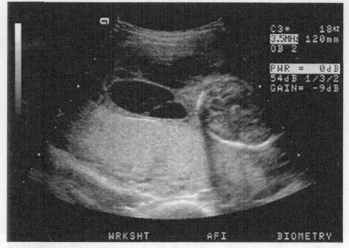

FIGURE 7–51.

(A) cystic hygroma
(B) spina bifida
(C) encephalocele
(D) scalp edema

5. **Fig. 7–51 is a sonographic marker for**

   (A) Turner's syndrome

   (B) Potter's syndrome

   (C) trisomy 18

   (D) fetal infection

6. **The most likely diagnosis for Fig. 7–52 includes**

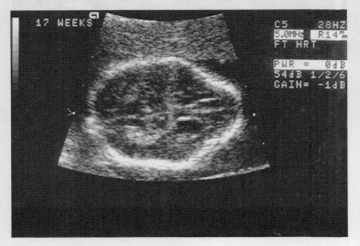

FIGURE 7–52.

   (A) spalding's sign

   (B) Down's syndrome

   (C) "lemon"-shaped skull

   (D) hydrocephaly

7. **The sonographic finding in Fig. 7–53 is**

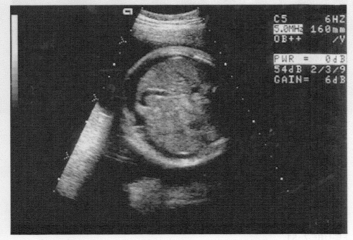

FIGURE 7–53.

   (A) fetal abdominal ascites

   (B) scalp edema

   (C) Spalding's sign

   (D) nonimmune hydrops

8. **Fig. 7–54 demonstrates**

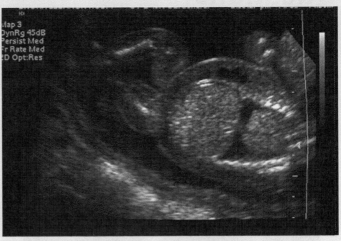

FIGURE 7–54.

   (A) bilateral pleural effusions and edema

   (B) cystic hygroma and scalp edema

   (C) increased nuchal sonolucency and fetal ascites

   (D) encephalocele

9. **Fig. 7–55 is an example of**

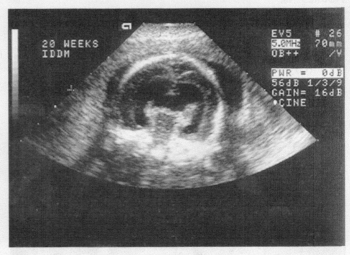

FIGURE 7–55.

   (A) sonographic artifact

   (B) severe ventriculomegaly

   (C) holoprosencephaly

   (D) scalp edema

10. **Which of the following sonographic findings is not associated with trisomy 18?**

   (A) IUGR

   (B) clenched hands

   (C) holoprosencephaly

   (D) cystic hygroma

11. **Paternally derived triploidy has the following sonographic markers**

    (A) complete mole

    (B) severe asymmetrical intrauterine growth retardation

    (C) large placenta with multiple cystic areas

    (D) oligohydramnios

12. **Which of the following sonographic findings are seen in maternally derived triploidy?**

    (A) complete mole

    (B) severe asymmetrical IUGR

    (C) large placenta with multiple cystic areas

    (D) polyhydramnios

13. **Oligohydramnios is most likely associated with which one of the following?**

    (A) Potter's syndrome

    (B) duodenal atresia

    (C) hydrocephalus

    (D) maternal diabetes

14. **Which one of the following is within the normal range of the fetal heart rate when documented on M-mode at 6 weeks gestation?**

    (A) 40–80 beats per minutes

    (B) 80–100 beats per minutes

    (C) 112–136 beats per minutes

    (D) 136–200 beats per minutes

15. **A 60-year-old woman with primary adenocarcinoma of the stomach now presents with a large complex right ovarian mass and ascites. What is the most likely diagnosis?**

    (A) neurofibromatosis

    (B) Sertoli–Leydig tumor

    (C) Krukenberg's tumor

    (D) Meigs' syndrome

16. **A 25-year-old patient presents for ultrasound with a history of hyperemesis gravidarum and preeclampsia. Fig. 7–56 is a sonogram of the uterus that demonstrates which of the following?**

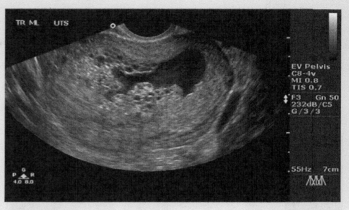

FIGURE 7–56.

    (A) blighted ovum

    (B) leiomyosarcoma

    (C) missed abortion

    (D) hydatidiform mole

17. **When the sole of the foot is visualized in the same anatomical plane as the tibia and fibula, what is this finding most likely to be?**

    (A) talipes

    (B) dwarfism

    (C) polydactyly

    (D) osteogenesis imperfecta

18. **What is the most common twin zygosity?**

    (A) conjoined twins

    (B) monochorionic/diamniotic

    (C) dichorionic/diamniotic

    (D) monochorionic/monoamniotic

19. **Which of the following best describes the "twin peak" sign?**

    (A) double decidua

    (B) a triangular projection of chorion into the dividing membrane

    (C) tip of iceberg

    (D) bright band

20. Which of the following statements about conjoined twins is *not* true?

    (A) 60% are born alive.

    (B) 56% of conjoined twins are fused on the ventral wall.

    (C) Polyhydramnios is commonly present.

    (D) The largest risk of fetal demise is because of cord entanglement.

21. Which of the following best describes the uterine position shown in Fig. 7–57?

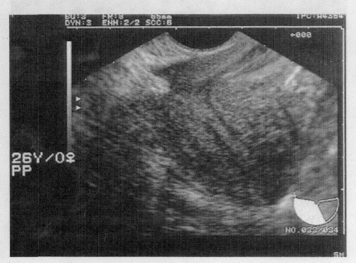

FIGURE 7–57.

    (A) retroverted

    (B) retroflexed

    (C) anteverted

    (D) anteflexed

22. What is the most reliable indicator for fetal demise in the second and third trimester?

    (A) absence of cardiac motion

    (B) polyhydramnios

    (C) mother stating, she has not detected any fetal movement

    (D) the sonographic presence of fetal scalp edema, ascites and hydrops

23. Fluid in the endometrial cavity in a postmenopausal patient may be associated with which of the following?

    (A) cervical stenosis

    (B) vaginal atrophy

    (C) endometriosis

    (D) adenomyosis

24. Which one of the following signs/symptoms is usually not associated with placenta abruption?

    (A) bloody amniotic fluid

    (B) painless bright red blood

    (C) sudden onset of pain and increase uterine tone

    (D) fetal distress

25. Which of the following is not a midline structure?

    (A) cavum septum pellucidum

    (B) third ventricle

    (C) foramen of Monro

    (D) hippocampus

26. Which of the following is the most common short limb syndrome?

    (A) achondrogenesis

    (B) thanatophoric dysplasia

    (C) osteogenesis imperfecta

    (D) Jeune thoracic dystrophy

27. What sonographic findings would be identified in a fetus with heterozygous achondroplasia?

    (A) hydrocephaly

    (B) frontal bossing

    (C) "bell-shaped" thorax

    (D) none of the above

28. Fig. 7–58 is a transverse plane of view through the uterus. What do the two-echogenic lines represent?

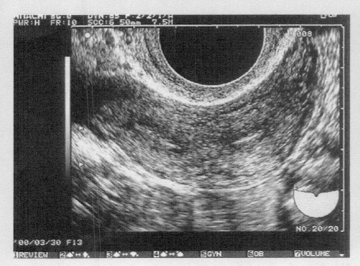

FIGURE 7–58.

(A) the interstitial portion of the fallopian tube

(B) two endometrial linings of a septate uterus

(C) single endometrial lining

(D) two endometrial linings of a bicornuate uterus

29. Fig. 7–59 demonstrates what fetal anomaly?

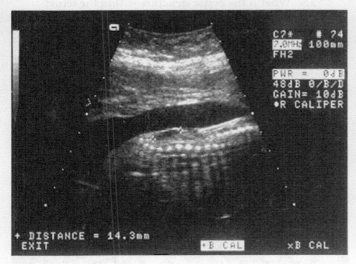

FIGURE 7–59.

(A) sacral agenesis

(B) meningocele

(C) myelomeningocele

(D) sacrococcygeal teratoma

30. Fig. 7–60 is a sonographic example of which of the following?

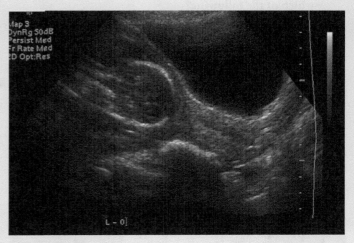

FIGURE 7–60.

(A) placenta accreta

(B) placental abruption

(C) marginal placenta previa

(D) normal findings

31. Fig. 7–61 is a transverse plane of view in the fetal nuchal region. Which of the following is the sonographic finding?

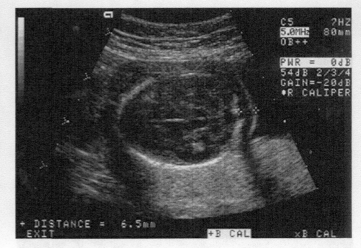

FIGURE 7–61.

(A) cystic hygroma

(B) increased nuchal skin fold

(C) fetal scalp edema

(D) increased nuchal translucency

129. **What does the term LGA refer to?**

(A) a fetus weighing >4000 g

(B) fetus >90%

(C) a clinical assessment of an increased fundal height

(D) polyhydramnios

130. **A macrosomic fetus is at risk for which of the following?**

(A) shoulder dystocia

(B) increased perinatal morality

(C) prolonged labor

(D) all of the above

131. **Which of the following is usually not a cause of oligohydramnios?**

(A) cystic hygroma

(B) IUGR

(C) post maturity

(D) premature rupture of the membranes (PROM)

132. **An increased fundal height may be caused by which of the following?**

(A) macrosomic fetus

(B) polyhydramnios

(C) pregnancy with fundal fibroids

(D) all of the above

133. **IUGR is**

(A) estimated fetal weight (EFW) below10% for a given gestational age

(B) decreased AFV

(C) increased umbilical cord size

(D) abnormal growth ratios

134. **An increased HC/AC is a suggestion of**

(A) late onset of IUGR

(B) brain sparing effort

(C) placental insufficiency

(D) anasarca

135. **Causes of asymmetric IUGR include**

(A) fetal infection

(B) chromosomal abnormality

(C) placental insufficiency

(D) all of the above

136. **Which of the following is the most sensitive indicator for assessment of IUGR?**

(A) BPD to OFD ratio

(B) FL to AC ratio

(C) HC to AC ratio

(D) AC

137. **Doppler testing of vessels that may aid in the diagnosis of IUGR is**

(A) umbilical cord

(B) straight sinus

(C) celiac axis

(D) jugular vein

138. **Doppler sampling of the maternal uterine artery <26 weeks shows a diastolic notch. This notch is indicative of**

(A) IUGR

(B) maternal hypertension

(C) normal

(D) none of the above

139. **In Fig. 7–81, what is the most likely diagnosis in this midline transabdominal pelvic sonogram in a 16-year-old gravida 0 para 0 patient?**

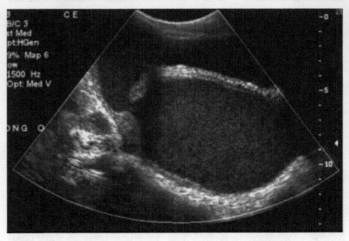

FIGURE 7–81.

(A) hydrometra

(B) hematometra

(C) Dermoid cyst

(D) hematometrocolpos

140. When a patient being treated for infertility demonstrated bilaterally enlarged multicystic ovaries and ascites, the diagnosis of ovarian hyperstimulation syndrome (OHSS) was made. Patients who are at risk of developing OHSS are

   (A) patients on Clomid or Pergonal

   (B) patients with Stein–Leventhal syndrome

   (C) patients with a history of OHSS

   (D) all of the above

141. In Fig. 7–82, the endovaginal image was taken at the level of the uterine corpus. The patient is a 55-year-old woman on HRT. Which of the following should not be included in the differential diagnosis?

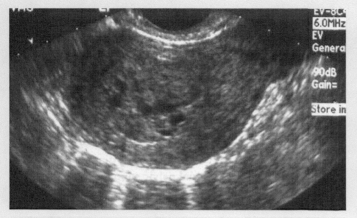

FIGURE 7–82.

   (A) endometrial hyperplasia

   (B) endometrial carcinoma

   (C) endometriosis

   (D) multiple endometrial polyp

142. In Fig. 7–83, what is the arrow pointing to?

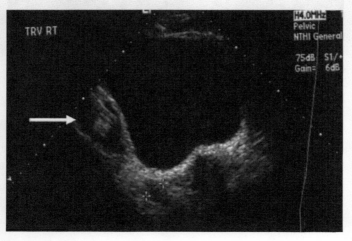

FIGURE 7–83.

   (A) iliopsoas muscle

   (B) right ovary

   (C) bowel mass

   (D) piriformis muscle

143. A pseudogestational sac will normally demonstrate

   (A) a secondary yolk sac within the pseudogestational sac

   (B) high-amplitude chorio-decidua

   (C) anechoic center with a thin ring

   (D) a dead embryo

144. In Fig. 7–84, the endovaginal image of a 32-year-old woman with abnormal vaginal bleeding is most suggestive of which of the diagnoses?

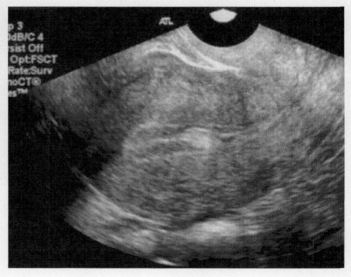

FIGURE 7–84.

   (A) endometrioma

   (B) adenomyosis

   (C) endometrial polyp

   (D) endometrial cyst

145. In Fig. 7–85, this 25-year-old patient presents with a history of chronic pelvic pain especially during menses, back pain, and dyspareunia. What is the most likely diagnosis?

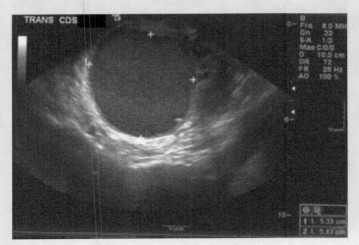

FIGURE 7–85.

(A) Brenner's tumor
(B) fibroma
(C) thecoma
(D) endometrioma

146. Fig. 7–86 is of a 38-year-old black female patient who presented with an enlarged palpated uterus, pain, and abnormal vaginal bleeding. What is the most likely diagnosis?

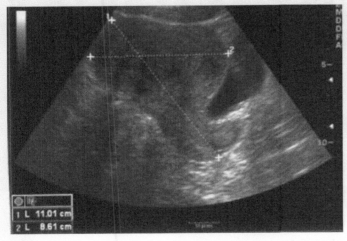

FIGURE 7–86.

(A) cervical myoms
(B) subserosal myoma
(C) submucosal myoma
(D) pedunculated fibroid

147. Fig. 7–87 is an endovaginal sonogram of the right adnexa of a 24-year-old patient that presented with an acute onset of pelvic pain. What does this most likely represent?

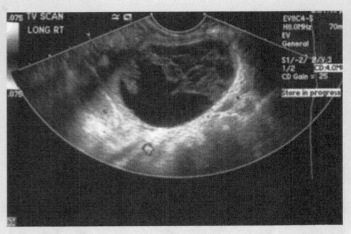

FIGURE 7–87.

(A) hemorrhagic cyst
(B) hyperstimulated ovarian syndrome
(C) endometrioma
(D) serous cystadenocarcinoma

148. Fig. 7–88 is suggestive of which of the following diagnoses?

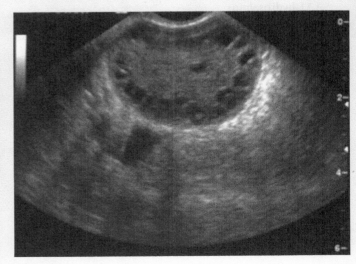

FIGURE 7–88.

(A) normal appearing ovary
(B) corpus luteal cyst
(C) cystadenoma
(D) polycystic ovary

149. The patient described in the previous question may present with any of the following *except*

   (A) ovarian agenesis
   (B) obesity
   (C) infertility
   (D) hirsutism

150. A 35-year-old patient presented with vaginal discharge and pelvic tenderness. The clinical information together with the endovaginal sonogram in Fig. 7–89 is most suggestive of which of the following diagnoses?

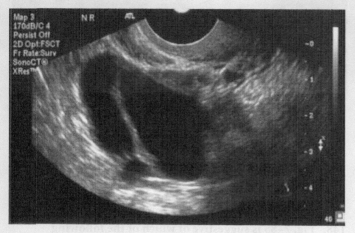

FIGURE 7–89.

   (A) hydrosalpinx
   (B) endometrioma
   (C) ascites
   (D) dermoid

151. A 29-year-old patient presented with menorrhagia and dysmenorrhea. On physical examination an enlarged uterus was palpated. The sonogram Fig. 7–90 is suggestive of which of the following diagnoses?

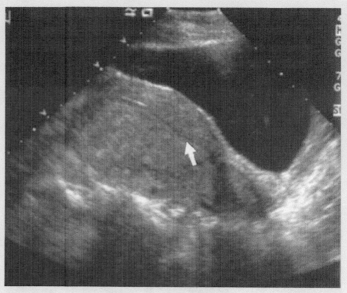

FIGURE 7–90.

   (A) a myomatous uterus
   (B) adenomyosis
   (C) endometriosis
   (D) hematometra

152. In Fig. 7–91, This endovaginal sonogram of a postmenopausal female being treated with tamoxifen for breast cancer is suggestive of which of the following diagnoses?

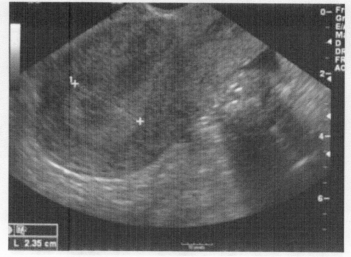

FIGURE 7–91.

   (A) endometrial hyperplasia
   (B) normal endometrium
   (C) adenomyosis hematometra
   (D) endometriosis

153. In Fig. 7–92, what is the name of this fluid-filled structure seen in this sonogram?

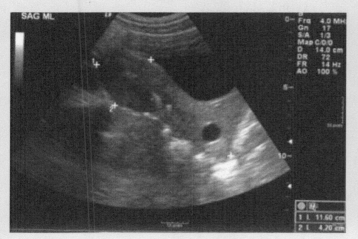

FIGURE 7–92.

(A) intrauterine gestational sac

(B) Nabothian cyst

(C) Bartholin's cyst

(D) cervical myoma

154. The endovaginal sonogram in Fig. 7–93 of a 28-year-old patient with a history of chlamydia, pelvic pain, and fever. Serum β-hCG is negative. This sonogram is suggestive of which of the following diagnoses?

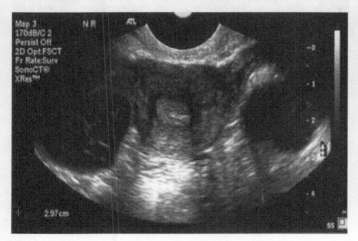

FIGURE 7–93.

(A) bilaterally enlarged ovaries

(B) right corpus luteal cyst

(C) bilateral dermoids

(D) TOAs

155. The uterus in Fig. 7–94 is poorly visualized. What can be done to improve the visualization of the uterus?

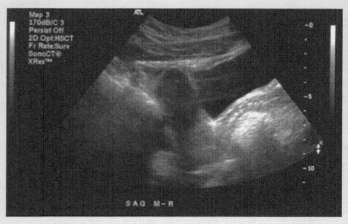

FIGURE 7–94.

(A) have the patient post void

(B) increase the far gain

(C) change transducers focal zone

(D) distend the urinary bladder more

156. In Fig. 7–95, the echoes on the anterior aspect of the urinary bladder are an example of which artifact normally seen?

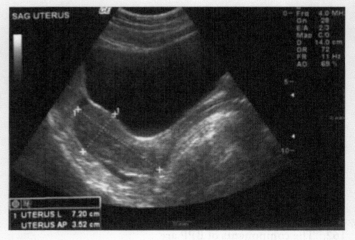

FIGURE 7–95.

(A) edge

(B) enhancement

(C) attenuation

(D) reverberation

157. **Which of the following is not an ectopic pregnancy?**

    (A) pregnancy *in situ*

    (B) abdominal pregnancy

    (C) pregnancy in the cesarean scar

    (D) extrauterine pregnancy

158. **The one of the following best describe the discriminatory zone**

    (A) the hCG level at which the embryo should be visualize

    (B) the hCG level at which the gestational sac should be visualize

    (C) the area between the decidua parietalis and decidua capsularis

    (D) an unfair proliferation within a small region of biological tissue

159. **Which of the is not one of the variables in BPP?**

    (A) umbilical artery Doppler evaluation

    (B) amniotic fluid assessment

    (C) placenta grading

    (D) fetal tone

160. **Which of the following is a known association with fetal macrosomia?**

    (A) maternal cigarette smoking

    (B) maternal hypertension

    (C) maternal alcohol abuse

    (D) maternal diabetes

161. **The pathological condition characterized by a solid ovarian tumor, right pleural effusions, and ascites is**

    (A) Meigs syndrome

    (B) dysgerminoma

    (C) Stein–Leventhal syndrome

    (D) mucinous cystadenoma

162. **The components of BPP are**

    (A) fetal breathing, Doppler, NST, gross body movement, and AFV

    (B) placental grading, NST, gross body movement, and AFV

    (C) NST, Doppler, gross body movement, AFV, and fetal flexion/extension

    (D) AFV, gross body movement, fetal flexion/extension, fetal breathing, and NST

163. **Fetal breathing must last how long to be counted in the BPP?**

    (A) 20 seconds

    (B) 30 seconds

    (C) 1 minute

    (D) 2 minutes

164. **In a normal fetus, if the middle cerebral artery were sampled, one would expect to find which of the following?**

    (A) an increased S/D ratio

    (B) a decreased S/D ratio

    (C) retrograde flow

    (D) absent flow

165. **A 27-year-old female presented to the emergency department complaining of heavy vaginal bleeding and pain in pregnancy. What is the finding in the sonogram in Fig. 7–96?**

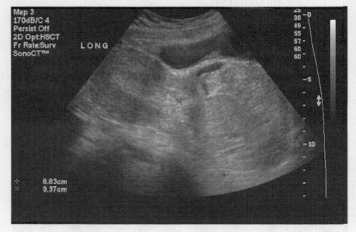

FIGURE 7–96.

    (A) ruptured ectopic pregnancy

    (B) fundal fibroid uterus

    (C) unruptured ectopic pregnancy

    (D) cervical phase of an impending abortion

166. **The fetus starts swallowing the amniotic fluid at what gestational age in pregnancy?**

    (A) 8 weeks

    (B) 12 weeks

    (C) 20 weeks

    (D) 33 weeks

167. Which of the following is not a cause for PID but has been implicated in male infertility?

    (A) chlamydia
    (B) actinomycetes
    (C) gonorrhea
    (D) genital herpes

168. Which one of the following is not part of the adnexa?

    (A) nabothian cyst
    (B) fimbria
    (C) follicular cyst
    (D) broad ligaments

169. Using the single-pocket technique for assessment of amniotic fluid, oligohydramnios is suggested when the amniotic fluid is?

    (A) a single pocket of 2 cm
    (B) a single pocket of 20 cm
    (C) a single pocket of 5 cm
    (D) a single pocket of 8 cm

170. In the AFI method of measuring four quadrants, when is the diagnosis of oligohydramnios made?

    (A) When the amniotic volume is less than 300 mL
    (B) When the amniotic volume is less than 200 mL
    (C) When the AFI is less than the 10th percentile
    (D) When the AFI is less than the 2.5th percentile

171. Which of the following are nonspecific signs of fetal death: (1) echoes in the amniotic fluid, (2) the absence of the falx cerebri, (3) a decrease in the biparietal diameter (BPD) measurements, (4) a double contour of the fetal head (sonographic halo sign), (5) no fetal heart motion?

    (A) both 3 and 4
    (B) only 4
    (C) only 1, 2, 3, and 4
    (D) only 5

172. How long after fetal death can scalp edema be first seen?

    (A) 2–3 days
    (B) 5–10 days
    (C) 10–20 days
    (D) 20–30 days

173. The term decidua denotes the transformed endometrium of pregnancy. What are the different regions of the decidua?

    (A) two regions called decidua basalis and chorionic villi
    (B) one region called decidual reaction
    (C) three regions called decidua basalis, decidua parietalis, and decidua capsularis
    (D) three regions called endoderm, mesoderm, and ectoderm

174. Which of the following cannot be included in the category of cystic masses of the vagina?

    (A) Gartner's duct cyst
    (B) Nabothian cyst
    (C) hematocolpos
    (D) Bartholin cyst

175. What are the functions of the secondary yolk sac?

    (A) nutrients for the embryo
    (B) hematopoiesis
    (C) contributing to the development of the reproductive system
    (D) all of the above

176. In about 2% of adults, the yolk sac persists as a diverticulum of the ileum. What is this known as?

    (A) Michael's diverticulum
    (B) Meckel's diverticulum
    (C) Turner's diverticulum
    (D) Smith's diverticulum

177. The location of the yolk sac is

    (A) with the stomach of the embryo
    (B) inside the amniotic sac
    (C) in the chorionic cavity between the amnion and the chorion
    (D) outside the chorionic cavity between the chorion and the endometrial wall

178. On TVS, the yolk sac is visible as early as how many weeks?

    (A) 4 weeks
    (B) 5 weeks
    (C) 6 weeks
    (D) 7 weeks

179. Patau syndrome is the result of that type of chromosomal abnormality

    (A) trisomy 13
    (B) trisomy 18
    (C) trisomy 21
    (D) trisomy 22

180. Which of the following is not a sonographic findings suggestive finding of Down's syndrome?

    (A) increase nuchal fold
    (B) increased nuchal translucency
    (C) absent nasal bone
    (D) intramembranous ossification

181. The most common cause for postpartum hemorrhage is

    (A) uterine atony
    (B) placenta previa
    (C) placenta abruption
    (D) prior caesarean section or uterine rupture

182. High level of FSH levels >50 IU/mL and amenorrhea is suggestive of

    (A) polycystic ovaries
    (B) ectopic pregnancy
    (C) hydatidiform mole
    (D) menopause

183. Which of the following is not a complication associated with oligohydramnios?

    (A) PROM
    (B) IUGR
    (C) postdate pregnancy (>42 weeks)
    (D) urethral stenosis

184. The umbilical cord S/D ratio normally

    (A) increases throughout the pregnancy
    (B) decreases throughout the pregnancy
    (C) remains the same throughout pregnancy
    (D) is controlled by the fetal cerebellum

185. Placental insufficiency is indirectly monitored by

    (A) an increasing umbilical cord S/D ratio
    (B) a decreasing umbilical cord S/D ratio
    (C) Doppler of placental intervillous spaces
    (D) Doppler of maternal arcuate arteries

186. The terminology vasa previa best describes

    (A) premature separation of the placenta
    (B) placenta touching the internal os
    (C) placenta crossing the internal os
    (D) placenta vessels crossing the internal os

187. What is the primary cause of third-trimester painless vaginal bleeding?

    (A) placenta previa
    (B) ruptured ovarian cyst
    (C) placentomegaly
    (D) placenta abruption

188. Which of the following is true concerning pseudogestational sac?

    (A) It is located in the ampullary segment of the fallopian tube.
    (B) It is located in the uterine cavity.
    (C) It has two layers of decidua called double decidual sign.
    (D) Its growth rate is approximately 1 mm per day.

189. Which of the following statements is not true concerning the yolk sac?

    (A) The yolk sac contains amniotic fluid.
    (B) The yolk sac shrinks as pregnancy advances.
    (C) The yolk sac plays a role in blood development and transfer of nutrients.
    (D) The yolk sac is attached to the body stalk and located between the amnion and chorion.

190. The vessels of the normal umbilical cord consist of

    (A) two arteries, one vein
    (B) two veins, one artery
    (C) one artery, one iliac vein, and the iliac artery
    (D) one artery, one vein

191. The term "neural tube defect" refers to

    (A) spinal defect
    (B) open tube defect
    (C) anencephaly
    (D) all of the above

192. **Myelomeningocele refers to**

(A) neural tube defect characterized by absent of the cerebellum

(B) protrusion of meninges and neural tissue though a defect

(C) fat tumor and meninges at the lumbar region

(D) meninges and brain herniate through a defect in the calvarium

193. **What is the estimated gestational age for a CRL of 28 mm?**

(A) 9.3 weeks

(B) 6.5 weeks

(C) 5.5 weeks

(D) 12 weeks

194. **The "lemon" sign of the fetal cranium in diagnosing spina bifida refers to**

(A) the narrowing of the vertebral process at the area of the defect

(B) lemon shape of the cerebellum

(C) the appearance of the cerebellum in the presence of a spinal defect

(D) the appearance of the fetal skull in the presence of a spinal defect

195. **The "banana" sign of the fetal cranium in diagnosing spina bifida refers to**

(A) banana shape of the fetal skull bones

(B) the overall appearance of the fetal spine in the presence of a defect

(C) the appearance of the cerebellum in the presence of a spinal defect

(D) the appearance of the fetal skull in the presence of a spinal defect

196. **The "banana" sign is present with spinal defects**

(A) 50% of the time

(B) 75% of the time

(C) 85% of the time

(D) 95% of the time

197. **Which of the following is true about the "lemon" sign and neural tube defects?**

(A) The "lemon" sign is not as accurate as the "banana" sign.

(B) The "lemon" sign may be present in the normal fetus in the third trimester.

(C) The "lemon" sign can be artificially produced at the level of the ventricles.

(D) All of the above statements are true.

198. **The diagnosis of placenta previa is most accurately made**

(A) transabdominally with a full maternal bladder

(B) transabdominally with an empty maternal bladder

(C) transrectally

(D) transvaginally

199. **The definition of "low lying placenta" in the third trimester is**

(A) placental edge greater than 3 cm from the internal os

(B) placental edge less than 2 cm from the internal os

(C) placental edge less than 3 cm from the internal os

(D) placental edge in lower uterine segment

200. **The rotation of the heart in the fetal chest should be**

(A) 45° with apex pointed to the right

(B) 45° with apex pointed to the left

(C) 60° with apex pointed to the right

(D) the heart should not be rotated in fetal chest

201. **The fetal heart is horizontal in the chest because of**

(A) large spleen

(B) flat diaphragm

(C) large liver

(D) large bowel

202. **The type of hydrops defined as absence of a detectable circulating antibody against RBCs in the mother is**

(A) immune

(B) nonimmune

(C) erythroblastosis fetalis

(D) isoimmunization fetalis

203. **What percentage of cephaloceles are occipital?**

(A) 50

(B) 60

(C) 75

(D) 99

204. The diagnosis of ventriculomegaly may be made when the ventricle measures

  (A) greater than 10 mm in the atrium of the occipital horn

  (B) greater than 10 cm in the posterior horn

  (C) when the third ventricle may be visualized

  (D) when the choroid does not touch the medial wall of the lateral ventricle

205. A patient state she was given a medication called RhoGAM after she had vaginal spotting in pregnancy. This was most likely due to

  (A) ectopic pregnancy

  (B) prevention of neural tube defect

  (C) Rh-negative status of the mother

  (D) pelvic infection

206. Congenital hydrocephalus is

  (A) genetically linked affecting both male and females

  (B) able to be detected in both male and females by DNA testing

  (C) expressed in males only

  (D) not detected in the DNA testing

207. Intracranial calcifications and microcephaly of the fetus are associated with

  (A) Dandy–Walker cyst

  (B) vein of Galen aneurysm

  (C) gestational diabetes

  (D) TORCH infections

208. Which of the following is a type of ectopic pregnancy that when ruptured is less likely to have internal hemorrhage?

  (A) cervical ectopic

  (B) cornual ectopic

  (C) abdominal ectopic

  (D) ampullary ectopic

209. A 29-year-old female presented to the emergency department with painless vaginal bleeding. The serum β-hCG taken was 3500 mIU/mL. What is the finding in the transvaginal sonograms shown in Figs. 7–97A and B?

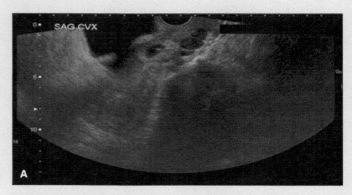

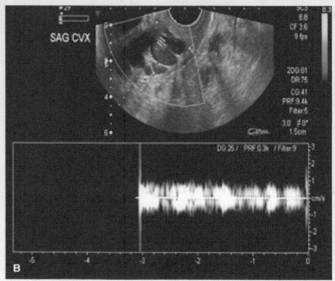

FIGURE 7–97.

  (A) caesarean section scar ectopic

  (B) pseudogestational sac

  (C) abdominal pregnancy

  (D) cornual pregnancy

210. What does the arrow in the sonogram shown in Fig. 7–98 point to?

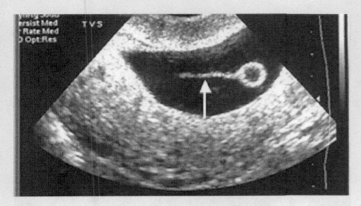

FIGURE 7–98.

(A) yolk sac

(B) Wharton's duct

(C) chorion

(D) vitelline duct

211. Fig 7–99 is a transvaginal sonogram after placement of an intrauterine device (IUD). What does this image demonstrate?

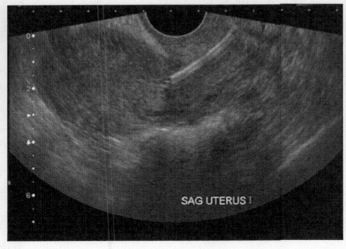

FIGURE 7–99.

(A) IUD *in situ*

(B) IUD in the cervix

(C) IUD in the vagina

(D) essure birth control in the left tube

212. The cisterna magna is considered increased when

(A) The measurement is greater than 5 mm.

(B) The cerebellum may be seen outlined by fluid.

(C) The cerebellar vermis is splayed.

(D) The measurement is greater than 11 mm.

213. Findings on ultrasound include an increased cisterna magna, agenesis of the cerebellar vermis with communication to the fourth ventricle and ventriculomegaly. What is the most likely diagnosis?

(A) Dandy–Walker malformation

(B) Dandy–Walker malformation variant

(C) arachnoid cyst

(D) communicating hydrocephaly

214. Findings on ultrasound include hydrocephaly, an enlarged cisterna magna, and an intact cerebellar vermis elevated by a cyst in the posterior fossa. What is the most likely diagnosis?

(A) Dandy–Walker malformation

(B) Dandy–Walker malformation variant

(C) arachnoid cyst

(D) communicating hydrocephaly

215. What other findings are associated with Dandy–Walker malformation?

(A) holoprosencephaly

(B) facial clefting

(C) cardiac defects

(D) all of the above

216. A patient who presented for pelvic ultrasound informs you that she has secondary infertility and is currently on a medication to stimulate ovulation induction. This drug is most likely

(A) folic acid

(B) clomiphene citrate

(C) methotrexate

(D) Lupron

217. Complications associated with Dandy–Walker malformation include

(A) chromosomal abnormalities

(B) subnormal intelligence after birth

(C) increased neonatal death

(D) all of the above

218. The most common cause of hypotelorism is

(A) Dandy–Walker malformation

(B) Arnold–Chiari type II

(C) Goldenhar syndrome

(D) holoprosencephaly

219. Cyclopia, hypotelorism, proboscis, cebocephaly, and cleft lip/palate are

    (A) abnormal intracranial findings
    (B) abnormal facial findings
    (C) associated with hydrocephaly
    (D) all of the above

220. The most common chromosomal abnormality associated with holoprosencephaly is

    (A) trisomy 21
    (B) trisomy 18
    (C) trisomy 13
    (D) Turner's syndrome

221. The most common cause of hypertelorism is

    (A) anterior cephalocele
    (B) holoprosencephaly
    (C) hydranencephaly
    (D) craniosynostosis

222. Teratomas in pregnancy are located in

    (A) the sacrococcygeal region
    (B) cervical
    (C) lumbar
    (D) all of the above

223. Maternal Graves' disease and Hashimoto thyroiditis may cause what finding in the fetus?

    (A) fetal ascites
    (B) fetal goiter
    (C) oligohydramnios
    (D) there is no effect on the fetus

224. The most common cause of macroglossia is

    (A) micrognathia
    (B) trisomy 18
    (C) Beckwith–Wiedemann syndrome
    (D) obstruction of the fetal airway

225. The arrow is pointing to what anatomical structure Fig. 7–100.

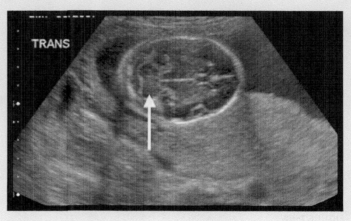

FIGURE 7–100.

    (A) cerebrum
    (B) cerebellum
    (C) cisterna magna
    (D) cerebral peduncle

226. Macroglossia is present how often in Beckwith–Wiedemann syndrome?

    (A) 15% of the time
    (B) 25% of the time
    (C) 50% of the time
    (D) 97% of the time

227. What is the most common type of isolated cleft lip/palate?

    (A) unilateral cleft lip
    (B) unilateral cleft lip and palate
    (C) bilateral cleft lip
    (D) bilateral cleft lip and palate

228. The arrow in Fig. 7–101 is pointing to what anatomic structure?

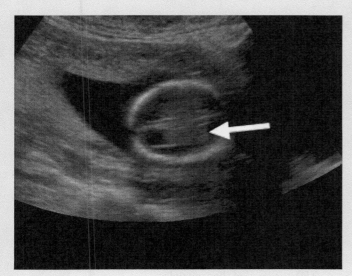

FIGURE 7–101.

(A) falx cerebri

(B) choroid plexus

(C) cavum septum pellucidum

(D) third ventricle

229. A medial cleft lip has a strong association with what abnormality?

(A) hydrocephaly

(B) Turner's syndrome

(C) holoprosencephaly

(D) hydranencephaly

230. Micrognathia may be associated with which of the following syndromes?

(A) Pierre Robin syndrome

(B) trisomy 18

(C) campomelic dysplasia

(D) all of the above

231. A 32-year-old female is complaining of lower abdominal cramping and vaginal bleeding with clots. Her serum β-hCG 2 days ago was 5200 mIU/mL and a repeated serum β-hCG taken 48 hours after the first β-hCG is now 1200 mIU/mL. Figs. 7–102A and B are her sonograms. What are the most likely findings?

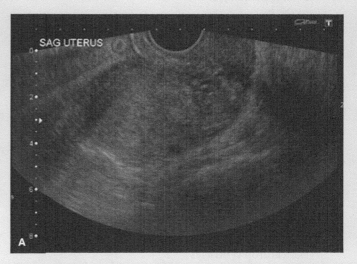

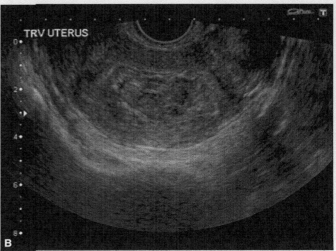

FIGURE 7–102.

(A) ruptured ectopic pregnancy

(B) unruptured ectopic pregnancy

(C) hydatidiform mole

(D) incomplete abortion

232. If a fetal nasal bone is not visualized, which of the following should one look for?

(A) increase nuchal fold

(B) protruding tongue

(C) cardiac defects

(D) all of the above

233. **Which of the following is true in reference to focal myometrial contraction?**

    (A) It is physiologic.

    (B) It increases the risk of spontaneous abortion.

    (C) It increases the risk of premature labor.

    (D) It is pathologic.

234. **Agenesis of the corpus callosum is difficult to diagnosed by ultrasound before**

    (A) 10 weeks

    (B) 14 weeks

    (C) 18 weeks

    (D) 28 weeks

235. **In 90% of cases with agenesis of the corpus callosum, what other sonographic finding is present?**

    (A) polyhydramnios

    (B) omphalocele

    (C) polydactyly

    (D) teardrop ventricles

236. **Absent cerebral cortex is found in what cranial abnormality?**

    (A) holoprosencephaly

    (B) hydrocephaly

    (C) hydranencephaly

    (D) agenesis of the corpus callosum

237. **Microcephaly is defined as**

    (A) HC greater than 10 SD of mean

    (B) HC less than or equal to 3 SD of mean

    (C) 2-week lag in HC

    (D) none of the above

238. **A fetus presents with an anechoic midline lesion in the brain, fetal hydrops, and congestive heart failure. What is the most likely diagnosis for the lesion?**

    (A) agenesis of the corpus callosum

    (B) dilation of the third ventricle

    (C) arachnoid cyst

    (D) atrioventricular malformation

239. **Choroid plexus cysts, when found with other associated abnormalities, have a strong association with which of the following conditions?**

    (A) Noonan's syndrome

    (B) trisomy 18

    (C) trisomy 13

    (D) X-linked hydrocephaly

240. **Which of the following is not a known cause for ectopic pregnancy**

    (A) cigarette smoking

    (B) sterilization by bilateral tubal ligation

    (C) chlamydia trachomatis

    (D) herpes genitals

241. **The nuchal skin fold in the second trimester should be measured at what level?**

    (A) the level of the cerebral peduncle

    (B) the same image as the circle of Willis, falx cerebri, and 4th ventricle

    (C) the level of the cavum septi pellucidi, cerebellum, and cisterna magna

    (D) the level of the ventricles

242. **Where are the ovaries normally located?**

    (A) fallopian tubes

    (B) pouch of Douglas

    (C) Morrison's pouch

    (D) ovarian fossa

243. **Abnormal accumulation of intraperitoneal fluid that becomes trapped by adhesions in a patient with a history of previous surgery is most likely caused by which of the following?**

    (A) inclusion cyst

    (B) ovarian torsion

    (C) dermoid cyst

    (D) follicular cyst

244. **If the cephalic index is greater than 85, it is an indication of what condition?**

    (A) brachycephaly

    (B) dolichocephaly

    (C) microcephaly

    (D) macrocephaly

245. **If the cephalic index is less than 75, it is an indication of what condition?**

    (A) brachycephaly

    (B) dolichocephaly

    (C) microcephaly

    (D) macrocephaly

246. When a sonographic procedure is to be performed that requires a needle insertion. The sonographer should use which one of the following types of gel?

(A) warm ultrasound gel

(B) sterile gel

(C) hypoallergenic gel

(D) transmission gel only

247. Which one of the following lubricants should *not* be used on latex probe covers?

(A) hypoallergenic gel

(B) coupling gel

(C) water-based gel

(D) oil-based products

248. Dolichocephaly is often associated with what conditions?

(A) breech fetus

(B) oligohydramnios

(C) LGA fetus

(D) cephalic fetus

249. Brachycephaly is associated with what conditions?

(A) trisomy 21

(B) normal variant

(C) myelomeningocele

(D) all of the above

250. Which of the following is responsible for the production of hCG?

(A) syncytiotrophoblastic

(B) cytotrophoblast

(C) yolk sac and yolk stalk

(D) zygote

251. Which of the follow produce estrogen and progesterone?

(A) uterus

(B) ovaries

(C) pituitary gland

(D) yolk sac

252. FSH and LH is produced by

(A) pituitary gland

(B) ovaries

(C) uterus

(D) trophoblast

253. If performing a BPD measurement and the midline echo is continuous and unbroken, this would indicate what about the scanning plane?

(A) normal

(B) too high

(C) too low

(D) correct

254. Which of the following is true regarding the fluid within a cystic hygroma?

(A) serous fluid

(B) amniotic fluid

(C) ascites

(D) lymphatic fluid

255. Cystic hygromas are caused by which of the following?

(A) obstruction of the lymph system at the level of the jugular veins

(B) obstruction of the lymph system at the level of the iliac veins

(C) obstruction of the venous system at the level of the jugular veins

(D) carotid artery obstruction

256. Which of the following is *not* true of hydatidiform mole?

(A) preeclampsia before 24 weeks of gestation

(B) may have a clinical symptoms of hyperemesis gravidarum

(C) patient may show signs of toxemia or hyperthyroidism

(D) the uterus is frequently smaller for dates

257. Eighty percent of cystic hygromas occur in what region?

(A) the axilla

(B) the mediastinum

(C) the cervical region

(D) the lumbar region

258. Cystic hygromas are associated with which of the following?

(A) Potter's syndrome

(B) Beckwith–Wiedemann syndrome

(C) oligohydramnios

(D) Turner's syndrome

259. Which of the following best describes the sonographic appearance of molar pregnancy?

(A) "snowstorm"

(B) vesicular sonographic texture

(C) Swiss cheese appearance

(D) honeycomb

Questions 260–269: Match the structures in Fig. 7–103 with the list of terms in Column B.

Early Pregnancy

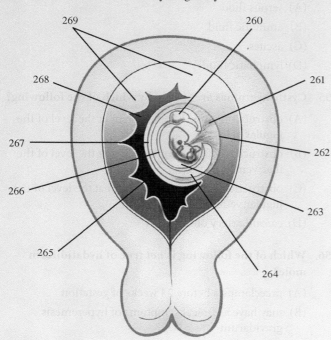

FIGURE 7–103.

COLUMN A	COLUMN B
260. _____	(A) amnion
261. _____	(B) chorion
262. _____	(C) decidua parietalis (vera)
263. _____	(D) decidua capsularis
264. _____	(E) yolk sac
265. _____	(F) amniotic cavity
266. _____	(G) uterine cavity
267. _____	(H) chorionic cavity
268. _____	(I) chorionic villi
269. _____	(J) decidua basalis

Questions 270–272: Match the structures in Fig. 7–104 with the list of terms in Column B.

Fibroids

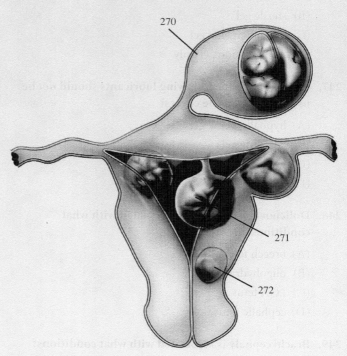

FIGURE 7–104.

COLUMN A	COLUMN B
270. _____	(A) submucous
271. _____	(B) pedunculated
272. _____	(C) intracavitary

Questions 273–281: Match the structures in Fig. 7–105 with the list of terms in Column B.

Ventricular System

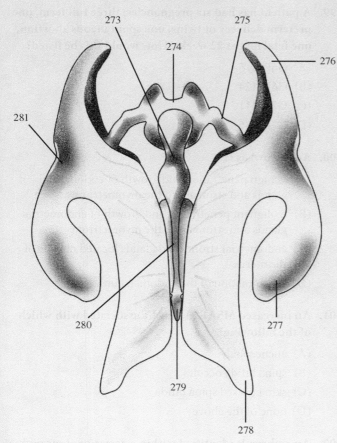

FIGURE 7–105.

COLUMN A	COLUMN B
273. _____	(A) third ventricle
274. _____	(B) atrium
275. _____	(C) inferior horn
276. _____	(D) posterior horn
277. _____	(E) interventricular antrum
278. _____	(F) cerebral aqueduct
279. _____	(G) lateral recess
280. _____	(H) anterior horn
281. _____	(I) third ventricle

282. **The fetal shunt between the left and right atria is**

(A) ductus venosum

(B) ductus arteriosus

(C) foramen ovale

(D) pulmonary ductus

283. **The fetal shunt connecting the transverse aortic trunk and the main pulmonary trunk is**

(A) ductus venosum

(B) ductus arteriosus

(C) foramen ovale

(D) pulmonary ductus

284. **Hydranencephaly is thought to result from**

(A) chromosomal abnormalities

(B) a vascular accident of the jugular veins

(C) a vascular accident of the internal carotid arteries

(D) calcification of the circle of Willis

285. **The differential diagnosis for hydranencephaly may be**

(A) semilobar holoprosencephaly

(B) arachnoid cyst

(C) severe hydrocephaly

(D) none of the above

286. **Hemivertebrae may be identified on sonogram**

(A) as a narrowing of the individual vertebrae in the coronal plane of view

(B) as a narrowing of the individual vertebrae in the sagittal plane of view

(C) as a narrowing of the individual vertebrae in the axial plane of view

(D) all of the above

287. **The downward displacement of the cerebellar vermis, the fourth ventricle, and medulla oblongata through the foramen magna is termed**

(A) "lemon" sign

(B) Dandy–Walker malformation

(C) arachnoid cyst

(D) Arnold–Chiari malformation

288. **Large encephaloceles may be associated with**

(A) hydranencephaly

(B) hypotelorism

(C) microcephaly

(D) macrocephaly

457. Overdistension of the urinary bladder may cause

(A) anterior placenta to appear previa

(B) closure of an incompetent cervix

(C) distortion or closure of the gestational sac

(D) all of the above

458. Ovulation is assumed to occurs

(A) during intercourse

(B) on the 7th day of the menstrual cycle

(C) on the 14th day of the menstrual cycle

(D) on the 2nd day of the menstrual cycle

Questions 459–467: Match the terms in Column A to the correct description in Column B.

COLUMN A

459. Gravida _____

460. Multipara _____

461. Nullipara _____

462. Primipara _____

463. Nulligravida _____

464. Primigravida _____

465. Multigravida _____

466. Para _____

467. Trimester _____

COLUMN B

(A) a woman who has given birth two or more times

(B) one who has never been pregnant

(C) a woman who is pregnant

(D) a woman who has never given birth to a viable infant

(E) pregnant for the first time

(F) one who has been pregnant several times

(G) the number of pregnancies that have continued to viability

(H) a woman who has given birth one time to a viable infant

(I) a 3-month period during gestation

468. Puerperium refers to the period

(A) surrounding conception time

(B) after death

(C) 6–8 weeks before delivery

(D) beginning with the expulsion of the placenta

469. The one of the findings is not clinical or a sonographic associated with PCOS

(A) infertility and obesity

(B) endometrial cancer

(C) hirsutism and acne

(D) ectopic pregnancy

470. Which of the following components of the ultrasound system exposes a patient to greater potential risk?

(A) a cracked transducer face

(B) a transducer cable that is wet with ultrasound gel

(C) a hot TV monitor

(D) ultrasound equipment that need calibration

471. Which of the following structures is most likely not seen in a postpartum pelvic sonogram?

(A) uterus

(B) endometrial echo

(C) vagina

(D) ovaries

472. Approximately what level is the fundus of the gravid uterus at 20 weeks of gestation?

(A) umbilicus

(B) xiphoid process

(C) half way between the umbilicus and the symphysis pubic

(D) at the level of the symphysis pubic

473. Which one of the following is not a common complication during the postpartum period?

(A) hemorrhage

(B) thromboembolism

(C) infection

(D) placenta previa

474. Which of the following is a least likely cause for abdominal and pelvic ascites?

(A) heart failure

(B) nephrotic syndrome

(C) pancreatitis

(D) fibroid uterus

475. What percentage of fetuses is in the breech presentation at term?

(A) 25%

(B) 50%

(C) 75%

(D) 5%

476. Which of the following characteristic is most suspicious of malignant ascites?

(A) free intraperitoneal fluid in paracolic gutters and Morison's pouch

(B) loculated fluid with loops of bowel adherent and fixed to the abdominal wall

(C) free echogenic fluid in the peritoneal cavity with floating bowel loops

(D) anechoic free fluid in the in the gravity-dependent position of the abdomen

477. The abbreviation VBAC refers to

(A) vaginal blockage and closure

(B) vaginal blockage after cesarean

(C) vaginal birth after cesarean

(D) vaginal bacteria at cesarean

478. Which of the following anatomical sites is where the normal implantation of pregnancy occurs?

(A) ampullary region of the fallopian tube

(B) endometrial cavity

(C) myometrium

(D) ovaries

Questions 479–484: Match the terms in Column A to the correct description in Column B.

COLUMN A

COLUMN B

479. placenta previa _____

(A) abnormal adherence of part or all of the placenta to the uterine wall

480. placenta accreta _____

(B) premature separation of the placenta after 20 weeks of gestation

481. placenta succenturiate _____

(C) accessory lobe of placenta

482. abruptio placentae _____

(D) implantation of the placenta in the lower uterine segment

483. placenta increta _____

(E) abnormal adherence of part or all of the placenta in which the chorionic villi invade the myometrium

484. placenta percreta _____

(F) abnormal adherence of part or all of the placenta in which chorionic villi invade the uterine wall

485. The chorion frondosum progressively develops to become

(A) fetal component of the placenta

(B) maternal component of the placenta

(C) the amniotic cavity

(D) the yolk sac and stalk

486. The decidua basalis progressively develops to become

(A) fetal component of the placenta

(B) maternal component of the placenta

(C) the amniotic cavity

(D) the yolk sac and stalk

487. Which of the following choices is true about HELLP syndrome?

(A) abbreviation for hemolysis elevated liver enzymes, and low platelets

(B) abbreviation for hemivertebrae elevated liver enzymes, and low-lying placenta

(C) treated similar to severe preeclampsia

(D) Doppler may help in assessing HELLP syndrome

488. A large fibroid uterus is seen on the ultrasound. The sonographer should scan what organ?

(A) kidneys

(B) liver

(C) posterior cul-de-sac

(D) pancreas

489. What is the primary infection that causes varicella-zoster virus (VZV)?

(A) 5ths disease

(B) chicken pox

(C) human papilloma virus (HPV)

(D) herpes simplex (HSV)

490. What is the most common congenital intrauterine viral infection?

(A) toxoplasmosis

(B) HIV

(C) parvovirus

(D) cytomegalovirus

491. Which of the following statements about the secondary yolk sac is false?

(A) located in amniotic cavity

(B) disappears at approximately 12 weeks of gestation

(C) is depicted before the embryo is seen

(D) contains vitelline fluid

492. What is the most common cause for hematocolpos?

(A) bicornuate uterus

(B) endometritis

(C) PID

(D) imperforate hymen

493. Sampling of the middle cerebral artery is helpful in determining

(A) IUGR and related complications

(B) prediction of fetal anemia

(C) the need for a fetal transfusion

(D) all of the above

494. Which of the following statements regarding leiomyoma is *false*?

(A) calcifies and attenuates the ultrasound beam

(B) may mimic a myometrial contraction

(C) normally increases in size after menopause

(D) distorts the endometrial cavity

495. A 24-year-old presents for an ultrasound with a markedly elevated serum β-hCG. Her sonogram demonstrates multiple small anechoic spaces about 3–5 mm in the uterine cavity. What is this finding most likely to be?

(A) Nabothian cyst

(B) missed abortion

(C) pseudogestational sac

(D) hydropic villi

496. Which of the following statements about stromal tumors is false?

(A) All have a similar sonographic appearance and cannot be differentiated from one another.

(B) solid, hypoechoic ovarian tumors.

(C) types include: fibromas, thecomas, Sertoli–Leydig cell tumors.

(D) types include: fibromas, thecomas, and Brenner tumors.

497. Endometrioma may appear sonographically similar to

(A) BCT

(B) polycystic ovaries

(C) hemorrhagic cyst

(D) hydrosalpinx

498. Hydrosalpinx may be differentiated from a multicystic ovarian mass on sonogram by

(A) following the cystic spaces to ensure that they all communicate

(B) using color Doppler to follow the ovarian artery to the ovary

(C) having the patient roll to lengthen out the fallopian tube

(D) the two cannot be differentiated

499. An anechoic, smooth-walled cyst is identified in a patient who has had a hysterectomy/oophorectomy. Which of the following should be included in the differential diagnosis?

(A) inclusion cyst

(B) ovarian remnant cyst

(C) mesonephric cyst

(D) all of the above

500. The hydatid cyst of Morgagni is

(A) a complex ovarian mass

(B) an hydatidiform mole cyst

(C) para-tubal cyst

(D) a hydatid cyst of the ovaries

501. The formula for determining ovarian volume is

(A) D1 × D2 × D3 × 0.523

(B) D1 + D2 + D3 × 3.14

(C) D1 × D2 × D3 × 3.14

(D) D1 + D2 × 100

502. The image in Fig. 7–109 represents

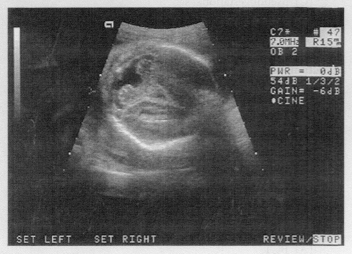

FIGURE 7–109.

(A) arachnoid cyst

(B) choroid plexus cyst

(C) "banana" sign

(D) Dandy–Walker malformation

503. Fig. 7–110 demonstrates a

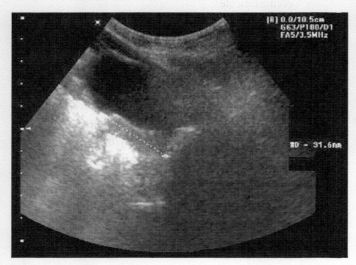

FIGURE 7–110.

(A) normal adult uterus

(B) multiparous uterus

(C) prepubertal uterus

(D) nulliparous uterus

504. Fig. 7–111 is of a 19-year-old patient referred for a sonogram because a right adnexal mass was palpated. What is the most likely diagnosis?

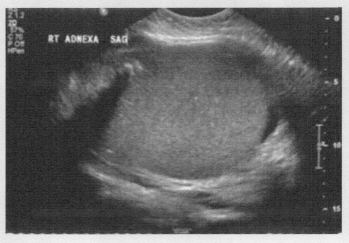

FIGURE 7–111.

(A) cystadenoma

(B) fibroma

(C) cystic teratoma

(D) endometrioma

505. In Fig. 7–112, what are the arrows pointing to?

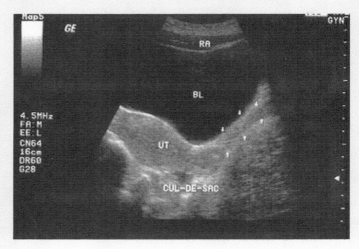

FIGURE 7–112.

(A) cervix

(B) broad ligament

(C) obturator internus muscle

(D) vagina

506. In Fig. 7–113, the markers are placed on the endocervical canal; what do the markers represent?

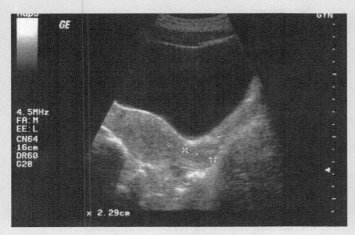

FIGURE 7–113.

(A) isthmus to corpus

(B) anterior cul-de-sac and internal os

(C) internal os to external os

(D) the vaginal fornixes

Questions 507–510. Match the structures numbered in Fig. 7–114 with the list of terms in Column B.

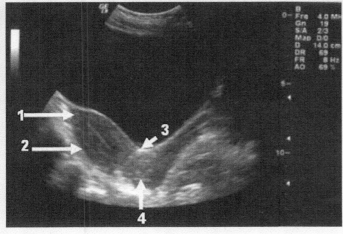

FIGURE 7–114.

507. Arrow no. 1 is pointing to _____   (A) cervix

508. Arrow no. 2 is pointing to _____   (B) fundus

509. Arrow no. 3 is pointing to _____   (C) corpus

510. Arrow no. 4 is pointing to _____   (D) isthmus

(E) endometrium

511. In Fig. 7–115, identify the potential space that is marked by the asterisk.

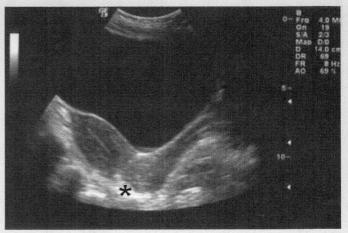

FIGURE 7–115.

(A) space of Retzius

(B) pouch of Douglas

(C) anterior cul-de-sac

(D) Morrison's pouch

512. Female infertility may be caused by which of the following?

(A) uterine synechiae

(B) PCOS

(C) Asherman's syndrome

(D) all of the above

569. **A 32 years old presented to Labor and Delivery at 24 weeks gestation with complain of leaking fluid. She states her baby is moving normally and denies any fever or chills. A biophysical physical profile (BPP) was done with a score of 8/8. Her AFI was 13 cm which was normal. At what week of gestation does the AFI peak?**

    (A) 24 weeks

    (B) 34 weeks

    (C) 36 weeks

    (D) 37 weeks

570. **What is the presumptive cause for single umbilical artery?**

    (A) Thrombotic atrophy

    (B) Omphalocele

    (C) Prune belly syndrome

    (D) Cord knot

571. **Human fertilization usually occurs in the ampulla region of the fallopian tube. This is the result of union of an egg and sperm which is known as**

    (A) gestational sac

    (B) Blastocyst

    (C) Zygote

    (D) Morula

Answers and Explanations

1. **(C)** The fetal calvarium is absent superior to the prominent obits (frog eyes). This finding is consistent with anencephaly. Anencephaly is a defect of the central nervous system in which the cerebrum and cerebellum are absent but the hindbrain is present. Acephaly is a complete absent of the fetal head.

2. **(B)** The image shows a defect in the posterior cranial vault. Because brain tissue is herniated through the defect, this would be an occipital encephalocele. This fetus also demonstrates microcephaly caused by the large defect.

3. **(A)** Equinovarus, or clubfoot, may be isolated or associated with other defects, most commonly neural tube defects.

4. **(A)** The image represents a cystic hygroma. The multiple septations seen are characteristic of second-trimester cystic hygroma. The intact cranium differentiates it from an encephalocele.

5. **(A)** Seventy-five percent of fetuses with cystic hygromas have a chromosomal abnormality, most commonly Turner's syndrome. Less frequent association is fetal hydrops and Down's syndrome.

6. **(C)** The image is an example of a "lemon"-shaped skull. It is most commonly associated with spinal defects, but can be present with encephaloceles and in normal fetuses 1–2% of the time.

7. **(A)** Abdominal ascites outlines the abdominal viscera. Ascites associated with meconium peritonitis may have particles of debris within it, and echogenic foci are often present in the fetal liver. Nonimmune hydrops must have two fluid collections or one fluid collection with anasarca.

8. **(A)** Bilateral pleural effusions and edema.

9. **(C)** Alobar holoprosencephaly is characterized by a single ventricle, single choroid, and fused thalamus.

10. **(D)** Cystic hygroma is associated with Turner's syndrome, not trisomy 18 (Edwards' syndrome) which is associated with overlapping of the fingers.

11. **(C)** Paternally derived triploid is associated with a relatively normally grown fetus that has a proportionate head size. The placenta is large with multiple cystic spaces resembling a molar pregnancy. This accounts for 90% of triploidy.

12. **(B)** Maternally derived triploidy is associated with a small placenta. The fetus has severe asymmetric growth restriction and oligohydramnios.

13. **(A)** Potter's syndrome is associated with renal agenesis, oligohydramnios, pulmonary hypoplasia, and malformation of the hands and feet. Oligohydramnios is associated with renal agenesis, IUGR, PROM, and postmaturity.

14. **(C)** The embryo cardiac activity can be seen at 6 weeks gestation and on some occasion at 5 and half weeks with higher-frequency transducers. The embryo heart rate at 6 weeks range from 112 to 136 bpm, which increases to a rate of 140 to 160 bpm at 9 weeks. A heart rate of less than 80 bpm is associated with pregnancy failure.

15. **(C)** Krukenberg's tumor is a malignant tumor of the ovary that metastasizes from a primary in the gastrointestinal tract. Meigs' syndrome is a benign tumor of the ovaries associated with ascites and pleural effusion.

16. **(D)** Hydatidiform mole. This sonogram demonstrates multiple tiny cystic spaces representing vesicles. This gives a sonographic appearance of honeycomb, swiss cheese, or snowstorm appearance, which is characteristic of hydatidiform mole. However, snowstorm was the first sonographic description of H-mole and it is the most common acceptable term used today.

17. **(A)** Talipes equinovarus or clubfoot is a developmental deformity in which the foot is inverted and planter flexed so that the metatarsal long axis is in the same plane as the tibia and fibula. The deformity affects the muscles and tendons of the foot. Clubfoot can also occur from restriction of movement due to oligohydramnios.

18. **(C)** Seventy-five percent of twins are dizygotic.

19. **(B)** The twin peak is formed when the placental tissue migrates between the chorionic layers. This is 94–100% predictive of dizygotic twins.

20. **(D)** Forty percent of conjoined twins are born stillborn. Fifty-six percent of conjoined twins are thoracoomphalopagus, thoracopagus, and omphalopagus. Polyhydramnios is present 50% of the time. Commonly, there is one umbilical cord that may have an abnormal number of vessels and is shared by the conjoined fetuses.

21. **(A)** Ninety percent of the time, the uterus tilts forward in anteverted position, meaning the uterus forms a 90-degree angle with the posterior vaginal wall. The uterus, however, may be in any of the following positions:

    • Anteverted: The uterus tilts forward with a 90-degree angle to the posterior vaginal wall.

    • Anteflexed: The uterine corpus is flexed anteriorly on the cervix, forming a sharp angle at the cervix.

    • Retroverted: The uterus tilts backward without a sharp angle between the corpus and cervix.

    • Retroflexed: The uterine corpus is flexed posteriorly on the cervix, forming a sharp angle at the cervix.

    This sonogram demonstrates a retroverted uterus.

22. **(A)** Absence of cardiac motion.

23. **(A)** Fluid in the endometrial cavity in a postmenopausal patient may be associated with cervical stenosis or malignancy.

24. **(B)** Painless bright red blood is associated with placenta previa.

25. **(D)** The hippocampus is a horseshoe-shaped paired structure located in the left and right brain hemisphere. It is not a midline structure.

26. **(B)** The occurrence rate for thanatophoric dysplasia is 1/6000–1/17,000 births. Sonographic findings are polyhydramnios, severe rhizomelia, and micromelia with bowing. The thorax is bell-shaped, and the cranium is cloverleaf-shaped with hydrocephaly and frontal bossing.

27. **(B)** Heterozygous achondroplasia accounts for 80% of achondroplasias. It is the most common form of genetic skeletal dysplasia. It is often not identified before 26–27 weeks and associated with frontal bossing of the fetal head.

28. **(B)** The outline of a septate uterus is relatively normal and contains two endometrial cavities separated by a thin fibrous septum. A bicornuate uterus contains two endometrial cavities, but there is a deep indentation on the fundal contour.

29. **(B)** A meningocele is a spina bifida with herniation of the meninges only.

30. **(D)** Normal cephalic presentation, with the fetal head close to the internal os of the cervix. The placenta is not identified in this image.

31. **(B)** This is an image of an increased nuchal skinfold (>6 mm). Nuchal fold measurements are obtained between 15 and 20 weeks' gestation. Nuchal translucency is performed between 11 and 14 weeks gestation. Both nuchal fold and nuchal translucency are used for screening Down's syndrome.

32. **(D)** This sonogram demonstrates an intrauterine contraceptive devices (IUD) that is eccentric in position.

33. **(C)** The image represents a BCT. A differential for this mass could be an endometrioma. *(Table 7–5)*

34. **(D)** Normal left ovary with iliac vessels.

35. **(A)** The cystic structure in the posterior aspect of the embryonic head represents the rhombencephalon. It is a normal structure seen between 7 and 9 weeks which later forms the fourth ventricle.

36. **(D)** Subserosal fibroid.

37. **(D)** The serum β-hCG normally decreases significantly after a dilation and curettage (D&C). An increase after the procedure is highly suggestive of an ectopic pregnancy. This image after a D&C is a transabdominal sagittal sonogram with a left unruptured ectopic pregnancy next to the left ovary.

38. **(A)** Serous cystadenomas are the most common ovarian neoplasm accounting for 20–25% of all benign ovarian neoplasms. They usually present as large, thin-walled, unilocular cystic masses that may contain thin echogenic septations.

39. **(C)** Hydrops fetalis is an accumulation of fluid in body cavities and soft tissue. This image shows cystic hygroma with body anasarca.

40. **(D)** The abnormality is spina bifida of the lumbar spine. The differential may include a sacrococcygeal teratoma based on the image alone; however, this fetus had a positive lemon/banana sign.

41. **(C)** The image is an increased nuchal translucency. It has an 80% positive predictive value for trisomy 21. If combined with the first trimester biochemistry, it has a 90% positive predictive value for trisomy 21.

42. **(D)** An increased nuchal translucency is associated with specific chromosomal abnormalities (Trisomy 18 and 21), cardiac defects, and structural defects.

43. **(B)** The dilation of the proximal urethra gives the fetal bladder the classic "keyhole" appearance associated with posterior urethral valve obstruction.

44. **(D)** Tetralogy of Fallot is comprised of a VSD, overriding aorta, pulmonary stenosis, and right ventricular hypertrophy. The hypertrophy is not always present, particularly in the early to midsecond trimester. This image shows the VSD and overriding aorta.

45. **(D)** The stomach is located posterior to the fetal heart, which is deviated to the right side of the chest. The solid appearance on the left side of the thorax is consistent with the liver.

46. **(D)** This image demonstrates a displaced and irregular shape cerebellum, which is curved like a banana and known as the "banana sign." It is characterized by the inferior displacement of the cerebellum and has a strong association with spinal defects and Arnold–Chiari malformation.

47. **(B)** The image is an example of an omphalocele. Atypically, the bowel is herniated instead of the liver. Notice the membrane around the bowel and the umbilical cord inserting into the membrane.

48. **(D)** The image is consistent with enlarged kidneys. Dysplastic kidneys would have multiple cysts. Infantile polycystic kidney disease is associated with large kidneys; however, they are echogenic and oligohydramnios is present.

49. **(B)** The tongue can be seen protruding from the mouth, consistent with macroglossia. The chin, forehead, and profile are normal.

50. **(C)** Beckwith–Wiedemann syndrome is a group of disorders including omphalocele, macroglossia, organomegaly, and hemihypertrophy.

51. **(A)** Multicystic, dysplastic kidneys have multiple cysts of various sizes. The cysts occur randomly and do not follow any pattern, as with dilated renal pyramids. The parenchyma is usually echogenic.

52. **(C)** It has a variable prevalence, with Native American being the highest at 3.6/1000 births.

53. **(D)** Three-dimensional imaging of the internal organs is termed volume imaging. Three-dimensional images of surface structures, such as the fetal face, is surface rendering.

54. **(B)** There is a limitation on what can be visualized by the human eye using medical imaging. A 7–10 MHz transvaginal transducer can depict a 5 mm gestational sac as early as 4 weeks.

55. **(B)** Fetal echocardiogram can be done earlier than 18 weeks, but is dependent on maternal habitus. After 24 weeks, the fetal bones become denser and more calcified and begin to limit the sonographic windows that allow visualization of the cardiac structures.

56. **(A)** Three-dimensional imaging of surface structures, such as the fetal face, is termed surface rendering.

57. **(B)** Although duodenal atresia has been detected in the first trimester, the classic "double bubble" sign is not usually present until the late second and early third trimesters.

58. **(D)** When an increased in alpha fetoprotein (AFP) is unexplained, it is thought to be because of an increased placental transfer of AFP. The placental dysfunction can occur with various placental abnormalities that may be associated with certain third-trimester complications. The most common cause for elevated AFP levels is inaccurate dating of pregnancy. Other high of AFP are associated with neural tube defect such as spina bifida. and anencephaly which are well known and understood.

59. **(B)** Cloacal exstrophy is characterized by an abdominal wall defect inferior to the umbilical cord insertion with exstrophy of a cloacal sac and a neural tube defect. It is associated with a markedly increased MSAFP. Amniotic sheets and congenital diaphragmatic hernia do not increase MSAFP. Smith–Lemli–Opitz syndrome is associated with a low level of maternal uE3 and normal MSAFP.

60. **(C)** If AFP (<0.6 MoM), uE3 (<0.5 MoM), and hCG (<0.3 MoM) are all decreased, the triple screen will show an increased risk for trisomy 18.

61. **(D)** Pulmonary hypoplasia can be assumed by the small thoracic circumference and anhydramnios, but underdeveloped fetal lungs are not visible by sonography.

62. **(A)** Vein of Galen aneurysm is an AV malformation located posterior to the third ventricle in the midline of the brain.

63. **(A)** Truncus arteriosus consists of one outflow tract overriding a VSD. The right ventricular outflow tract is absent. Differential diagnosis includes tetralogy of Fallot with pulmonary atresia. Identifying the pulmonary arteries branching from the main trunk would differentiate the defect.

64. **(D)** The most predictive sonographic findings are the overriding aorta and VSD. If the VSD is perimembranous, it will not appear on the four-chamber view. The right ventricle may appear larger than the left, but this is not a consistent finding and is dependent of the degree of pulmonary stenosis. Differential diagnosis would include truncus arteriosus.

65. **(A)** CCAM is divided into three subsets: macro, medium, and microcystic. Survival rate combines all types and sizes and is 75–80%. Studies have shown that CCAM regresses 55–69% of the time.

66. **(C)** Congenital diaphragmatic hernia is left sided 75–90% of the time. Prognosis is poor, particularly if the liver is herniated into the chest. Five to fifteen percent of congenital diaphragmatic hernias are associated with chromosomal abnormalities, commonly trisomy 18.

67. **(D)** Ninety percent of esophageal atresia have a tracheoesophageal fistula. This allows amniotic fluid to reach the stomach, but at a slower rate. The stomach will be visualized, but may be smaller than usual. Polyhydramnios occurs in the mid to late second trimester. The VACTERL complex is vertebral anomalies, anal atresia, cardiac abnormalities, tracheoesophageal atresia, renal anomalies, and limb anomalies. At least three of the anomalies listed must be present to diagnosis the VACTERL condition.

68. **(A)** Trisomy 21 is associated with a decreased MSAFP and an increased hCG.

69. **(C)** The uterosacral ligament is the distal portion of the cardinal ligament. It anchors the cervix and is responsible for uterine orientation.

70. **(B)** Both the suspensory and broad ligaments are folds of peritoneum.

71. **(A)** The piriformis muscles lie more posteriorly and are ovoid and symmetrical.

72. **(A)** The most dependent portion is the pouch of Douglas, or the posterior cul-de-sac. It is located posterior to the cervix and anterior to the rectum.

73. **(C)** The posterior cul-de-sac (pouch of Douglas) is located posterior to the uterus. The anterior cul-de-sac (vesicouterine pouch) is located anterior to the uterus. The prevesical space (retropubic space) is anterior to the

bladder. They form the peritoneal spaces of the pelvic cavity.

74. **(D)** Transvaginal probes need to be pre-cleaned with soap and water as well as soaked in a disinfecting solution and covered by a disposable probe cover. The probes should be cleaned after each examination.

75. **(D)** An invasive mole and a hydatidiform mole are excessive trophoblastic proliferation. Unlike the hydatidiform mole, chorioadenoma destruens is malignant and invades into the myometrium.

76. **(C)** Paternally derived trisomy 13 presents with a large placenta sometimes termed a partial mole. Less commonly, a dizygotic pregnancy may occur. One fetus result from normal fertilization of one egg and a complete molar pregnancy results from the fertilization of the other egg. In those cases, it is possible for the hydatidiform mole to advance to choriocarcinoma.

77. **(C)** The ovum enters the fallopian tube at the fimbriated ends. It courses to the ampulla where fertilization occurs 24–36 hours after ovulation.

78. **(B)** Methotrexate (MTX) is a folic acid antagonist used as a medical treatment for a unruptured ectopic pregnancy. The recommended candidates for medical treatment are hemodynamically stable, hCG of less than 5000 mIU/mL, no fetal cardiac activity, and the ectopic mass size should be less than 4 cm. The is the current recommendation at the time of writing. Previously the recommended was a serum β-hCG of less than 10,000 mIU/mL.

79. **(D)** This patient most likely had a ruptured ectopic pregnancy. Medical treatment is the first option if the patient is hemodynamically stable and with an unruptured pregnancy. However, this patient stated that she had a syncope episode followed by a salpingectomy in which case a ruptured ectopic pregnancy is most-likely.

80. **(B)** Intrauterine fetal demise (IUFD) is defined as an absence of fetal heart tones after 20 weeks. A blighted ovum does not have an embryo (anembryonic pregnancy). Missed abortion is a demise embryo that has not aborted in the first trimester. A fetus can be in a resting mode without movement but demonstrate a fetal heart tone.

81. **(D)** Dysgerminoma is a malignant tumor.

82. **(A)** Dermoid cysts are more common in younger women and they have a variable sonographic appearance ranging from completely anechoic to hyperechoic.

83. **(A)** Normal adult ovarian size is 3 × 2 × 2 cm.

84. **(B)** The earliest and first sonographic finding suggesting an IUP is a gestational sac with a yolk sac; however, as the pregnancy advance in gestational age, the fetal pole becomes the second most reliable indicator an IUP. An ectopic pregnancies can present with a pseudo-sac resembling a gestational; however, it does not have a yolk sac or trophoblastic rind.

85. **(B)** The detection rate is 65%, but may vary among patients depending on the maternal habitus, fetal position, AFV, ultrasound scanner, and expertise of the sonographer and physician.

86. **(D)** The detection rate is 85%, but may vary among patients depending on the maternal habitus, fetal position, AFV, ultrasound scanner, and expertise of the sonographer and physician.

87. **(D)** Distal acoustic shadowing is associated with a solid mass.

88. **(C)** Theca lutein cysts are present in 18–37% of hydatidiform moles.

89. **(A)** The CRL is the most accurate because fetal growth is very uniform and is rarely affected by pathological disorders. The LMP is based on human memory and also on the assumption that ovulation occurs on day14 after the first day of menstruation. The CRL is more accurate than LMP, BPD, AC, and FL.

90. **(A)** Fetal growth in the first trimester is very uniform, thus allowing for accurate dating if the total of three CRL measurements are taking and then averaged. *(Table 7–6)*

91. **(B)** Fetal growth is starting to show variation and multiple parameters are used to calculate the EDC. Both of these factors allow for an increased range of error. *(Table 7–6)*

92. **(C)** Fetal growth is showing a moderate amount of variation, which allows for an increasing range of error. *(Table 7–6)*

93. **(D)** Fetal growth has a large amount of variation in the third trimester and obtaining the images for EFW can be challenging depending on fetal position and size. This allows for the largest range of error in the pregnancy. *(Table 7–6)*

94. **(B)** The hCG doubles in approximately 48 hours until 10 weeks or a minimum of 66% in 48 hours.

95. **(A)** Twin pregnancy is associated with an elevated hCG.

96. **(D)** The internal component of an endometrioma is typically blood from bleeding ectopic endometrial tissue during menstruation. Differential diagnosis may include a dermoid tumor; however, most women tend to be asymptomatic with dermoids. *(Table 7–5)*

97. **(C)** Nagele's rule is (1) identify the LMP, (2) add 7 days, (3) subtract 3 months, and (4) add 1 year.

98. **(D)** Krukenberg tumor is a metastatic adenocarcinoma of the ovary. The stomach is the primary site in most cases. The mass is usually bilateral.

drug and used for other medical conditions such as ectopic pregnancy and rheumatoid arthritis.

368. **(B)** This condition will cause immune hydrops in the fetus.

369. **(C)** A blighted ovum is also known as anembryonic pregnancy. Sonographically, this is a large gestational sac that does not contain a yolk sac or an embryo. A missed abortion is defined as a dead embryo. Both blighted ovum and missed abortion are fail pregnancies. The difference is a blighted ovum is without an embryo and missed abortion is with an embryo but does not have heart activity.

370. **(D)** Findings of heart failure include pericardial effusions, decreased contractility, increased ventricular thickness, abnormal umbilical cord, and middle cerebral artery Doppler.

371. **(D)** Fetal hydrops is defined as two sites of fluid accumulation or one site of fluid accumulation and fetal ascites.

372. **(A)** The cardiac ventricular walls will thicken and contractility decreases. This causes the cardiac output to decrease. This may lead to acidosis, increased hematocrit, and increased neonatal morbidity.

373. **(A)** The list of causes for nonimmune hydrops fetalis (NIHF) is more than 120 conditions, some of which are rare. Major causes are cardiac arrhythmias and tumors, abnormal chromosomes, cardiac failure, anemia, arteriovenous shunts, mediastinal compression, metabolic disease, fetal infection, fetal tumors, congenital fetal defects, and placental defects.

374. **(A)** *In situ* is defined as follows: in the correct place or position. The correct placement of an IUD is in the uterine cavity, and the IUD string is placed in the vagina. The IUD string cannot be seen on ultrasound. Eccentric denotes "away from the center" and is a descriptive term for an IUD not in the correct position. Today's IUDs are made of flexible plastic with or without copper. When *in situ*, the IUD sonographically appears as high-amplitude linear echoes with a distal acoustic shadow.

375. **(A)** Fitz–Hugh–Curtis syndrome is inflammation of the liver capsule and diaphragm secondary to bacterial spread, from the pelvis to the right upper quadrant. These findings are seen in cases of PID.

376. **(D)** Partial situs inversus, divided into asplenia and polysplenia, has a 40% incidence of anomalies. They include complex heart disease, absent gallbladder, interrupted inferior vena cava with an azygous venous return, and splenic abnormalities.

377. **(B)** A UPJ obstruction is an obstruction at the junction of the ureter and renal pelvis. Therefore, the fetal urine is obstructed within the kidney causing hydronephrosis, but not hydroureter. As long as the contralateral kidney is functioning normally, the amniotic fluid should remain normal.

378. **(A)** A UVJ obstruction is an obstruction at the junction of the ureter and fetal bladder. It is associated with ureter anomalies, such as duplication and abnormal insertion sites. There is often an ureterocele caused by the abnormal insertion of the ureter. Hydroureter and mild hydronephrosis are commonly present.

379. **(D)** The ureters are about 1–2 mm in diameter and not normally visible on ultrasound.

380. **(C)** The trigone is located at the inferior portion of the posterior bladder wall.

381. **(D)** Spontaneous abortion is characterized by lower abdominal cramping and vaginal bleeding due to uterine contraction. When the abortion is complete, the contractions and vaginal bleeding stop. The serum β-hCG will usually decrease greater than half in 48 hours. Sonographically, the uterus will be free of any retain products.

382. **(A)** Complete PUV obstruction does not allow for any fetal urination; therefore, severe oligohydramnios occurs.

383. **(A)** Potter's facies is characterized by low set ears, flat nose and chin. Potters syndrome is predominately a male disorder and is associated with bilateral renal agenesis, oligohydramnios, and clubfoot. Small mouth with protruding tongue and small ears is facial features of Down's syndrome.

384. **(D)** The primary cause of neonatal death in PUV syndrome is pulmonary hypoplasia, although the other entities are also serious complications.

385. **(C)** In cases of renal agenesis, particularly after 16 weeks, anhydramnios is present.

386. **(D)** A normal fetal bladder should empty every 30–45 minutes.

387. **(C)** Ovarian torsion can cause internal bleeding but not related to vaginal bleeding. All the others given choices are associated with abnormal vaginal bleeding. Hyperthyroidism and hypothyroidism can also cause abnormal vaginal bleeding.

388. **(D)** Three pairs of kidneys form in successive stages: pronephros, mesonephros, and metanephros, with metanephros remaining as the functioning kidney.

389. **(B)** The urinary system develops closely with the uterine development. Twenty to thirty percent of patients with uterine anomalies also have renal ectopia or agenesis.

390. **(B)** Multicystic dysplastic kidney disease is caused by a first trimester obstruction. The kidney is nonfunctioning with ureteral atresia.

391. **(A)** In cases of a unilateral nonfunctioning kidney, the contralateral kidney will often enlarge to compensate. The unilateral kidney usually provides enough function to be sufficient for the individual.

392. **(B)** The risk to the fetus in an autosomal dominant disease with one parent affected is 50%.

393. **(B)** Autosomal dominant polycystic kidney disease does not typically cause renal disease prenatally therefore the amniotic fluid is normal. The kidneys may appear large and echogenic. Autosomal recessive polycystic kidney disease does affect renal function and is associated with oligohydramnios. Meckel's syndrome is associated with encephaloceles and post-axial polydactyly.

394. **(B)** Although kidneys grow throughout gestation, the ratio of kidneys to abdomen remains constant at 0.27–0.30.

395. **(C)** Unless the kidney is echogenic or obstructed, the anechoic cysts in the periphery represent normal renal pyramids.

396. **(B)** Fetal urine production begins at 12 weeks, but the fetal kidneys do not produce the majority of the fetal urine until 16 weeks.

397. **(B)** Ectopic pregnancy is defined as any pregnancy outside of the endometrial cavity. Although approximately 95% of ectopic pregnancies occur in the fallopian tube, it can occur in other locations such as the abdomen and ovaries. Ectopic pregnancy can occur in the uterus such as a cervical or a hysterotomy scar from a previous cesarean section. Extrauterine pregnancy occur outside of the uterus.

398. **(D)** Although this is somewhat debated, many sources quote a number from 4 to 6 mm as the upper limit of normal in the second trimester.

399. **(B)** Grade 0—no dilation.

400. **(C)** Grade I—renal pelvic dilation with or without infundibula visible.

401. **(E)** Grade II—renal pelvic dilation with calices visible.

402. **(A)** Grade III—renal pelvis and calices dilated.

403. **(D)** Grade IV—renal pelvis and calices dilated with parenchymal thinning.

404. **(C)** Because of its vascularity, the fetus may experience heart failure and polyhydramnios. On ultrasound, a congenital mesoblastic nephroma will resemble a Wilms' tumor.

405. **(A)** A neuroblastoma appears as a suprarenal mass and should be considered when a mass is identified superior to the kidney. Nephroblastoma (Wilms' tumor) is a malignant renal tumor that affects children.

406. **(C)** Nephroblastoma, also known as Wilm's tumor, is a malignant renal tumor that sonographically appears similar to a mesoblastic nephroma.

407–409. **(B)** Rectus abdominis. **(A)** Obturator internus. **(C)** Piriformis. In a transverse plane, the rectus abdominis muscles appear as low-level hypoechoic echoes on the most midline anterior portion of the abdominal-pelvic wall. The obturator internus muscles are posterior and medial to the iliopsoas muscles and appear as thin, bilinear, low-level echoes on the posterolateral aspect of the urinary bladder. The piriformis muscles are bilateral hypoechoic structures seen posterior to the uterus and anterior to the sacrum.

410. **(D)** The levator ani muscles make up the pelvic diaphragm and are easily visualized in a transabdominal transverse plane. These bilateral muscles appear hypoechoic and are seen medial to the obturator internus muscles and posterior to the cervix and vagina.

411. **(C)** A change in head shape, such as brachycephaly or dolichocephaly, affects accurate measurement in predicting gestational age. The degree to which fetal head shape affects BPD can be estimated with the formula: $CI = BPD/OFD \times 100$.

412. **(A)** Ovarian tumors account for 50–81% of torsion. Hyperstimulated ovaries produce large cysts that may get a torsion but less common than ovarian tumors.

413. **(A)** The ovary has a dual blood supply: the ovarian and uterine arteries. The ovarian arteries originate from the aorta just below the renal vessels, with each coursing into the retroperitoneal space. It enters the broad ligament and then enters through the hilum of the ovary. The left ovarian vein drains into the left renal vein. The right ovarian vein connects directly into the inferior vena cava. The uterine artery arises from the anterior division of the hypogastric (internal iliac artery).

414. **(B)** Hyperstimulated ovaries produce large cysts that may be torsed, as well as cause fullness and nausea to the patient. Rarely, more severe complications can occur because of the shift in fluid resulting in ascites and effusions.

415. **(B)** The presentation of ovarian torsion varies, depending on the duration and degree of vascular compromise. Ovarian torsion is twisting of the ovary and its vessels resulting in occlusion of its blood supply. Approximately 95% of cases are associated with an adnexal mass. Although torsion of a normal ovary can occur, this is more frequent in children than adults. Doppler ultrasound is very helpful in confirming the presence of blood flow. However, on rare occasions, ultrasound may demonstrate bilateral flow in a patient who has an ovarian torsion. This is due to twisting and untwisting of the ovary. The clinical symptoms of unilateral pain with nausea and vomiting are usually present even in a false-positive sonogram. Ovarian torsion does not occur if the ovaries and fallopian tubes are removed.

416. **(A)** Endometrial cancer is one of the most common gynecologic malignancies, after cervical cancer. Postmenopausal bleeding is an early sign. Abdominal/pelvic ascites, intra-abdominal mass, and pelvic pain are late signs. Most cancers are painless in early stages.

417. **(B)** Fibroids are estrogen dependent and commonly increase in pregnancy and decrease postmenopausally. The only sonographic difference between a leiomyoma and a leiomyosarcoma is a rapid increase in growth.

418. **(A)** On sonography, a leiomyoma and a leiomyosarcoma appear the same. Clinically, the only difference is a rapid increase in growth in postmenopausal women.

419. **(C)** The fetal lung is isoechoic to the fetal liver in the second trimester.

420. **(A)** Although the lung increases in echogenicity throughout the pregnancy, researchers have not been able to correlate the increase with lung maturity.

421. **(D)** Visualization of the femoral epiphyseal plate is seen on fetuses with a gestational age greater than 33 weeks with 95% accuracy.

422. **(A)** Polydactyly may be isolated or occur as part of a syndrome. The extra digit may have a bone or may be soft tissue only. Postaxial refers to the ulnar aspect of the hand.

423. **(B)** Cephalad.

424. **(B)** Discordance in dichorionic/diamniotic twins is more acceptable because of their different genetic makeup, provided that the smaller twin is not less than the 10th percentile in EFW. In monochorionic twins, EFW should be concordant and not differ by more than 20%.

425. **(A)** Supine hypotensive syndrome is due to obstruction by the gravid uterus on the inferior vena cava, resulting in decreased venous return to the heart. The patient should be turned on the left side and the symptoms will disappear. Sitting up will also help.

426. **(C)** Twin fetal discordance is determined by subtracting the largest twin from the smallest twin and dividing by the largest twin. This number is multiplied by 100 to determine the percentage.

427. **(D)** Frank breech is described as the buttocks descending first with the thighs and legs extending upward along the anterior fetal trunk.

428. **(C)** Complete breech is described as the buttocks descending first with the knees flexed, and the fetus sitting cross-legged.

429. **(A)** A footling breech is when one or both feet are prolapsed into the lower uterine segment.

430. **(B)** Ectopic pregnancy in the interstitial (cornual) region of the fallopian tube increases the risk for maternal mobility or mortality. This is due to its location giving the ectopic more room to grow. It ruptures at a larger size with a close proximity to the uterine artery, making this type of ectopic most potentially life-threatening.

431. **(B)** XY karyotype indicates a male fetus. XX karyotype indicates a female fetus. Down's syndrome is labeled 47, +21, and Turner's syndrome in labeled 45X.

432. **(D)** HIPAA, is a federal law, which forbid health care workers from giving out patient information without consent, even to other family members. Sonographers must comply with this legislation. If the sonographer is not compliant, he or she can face up to $250,000 in fines and/or jail time up to 10 years.

433. **(C)** The fetus (regardless of the body part), as well as the sac, closest to the internal os is labeled fetus A.

434. **(A)** The fetus would be lying on its right side, with left side closest to the maternal abdominal wall.

435. **(A)** The fetus would be laying on its right side, with the left side closest to the maternal abdominal wall.

436. **(A)** The fetus would be laying on its right side, with the left side closest to the maternal abdominal wall.

437. **(C)** Placental lakes are areas of fibrin under the chorion, on the fetal side of the placenta. They carry no clinical significance.

438. **(A)** Hypertension and maternal smoking can cause the placenta to undergo early maturation. Smoking can cause an increase in calcifications in the placenta. Unfortunately, placenta maturation has not proved to be a reliable tool in assessing placental function or fetal well-being.

439. **(D)** Triploidy from the paternal component, presents with a large cystic placenta.

440. **(D)** Maternal hypertension can cause a restrictive flow in the uterine vessels, which in turn, may decrease the placental perfusion.

441. **(D)** Gestational diabetes mellitus is a cause for macrosomia because of the increased maternal blood sugars.

442. **(B)** Although it is important to make sure the exam room and the transducer are sterilized prior to any procedure. The informed consent is most imperative prior to the procedure. An informed consent is an agreement by the patient to undergo a specific medical intervention. This agreement includes risks, benefits, and alternatives to the procedure. The form should be signed by the patient and physician and include a witness. The patient must be of legal age and mentally competent.

443. **(A)** Caudal regression syndrome is associated with IDDM in up to 16% of the cases. It is thought to occur with poor glucose control in the first trimester. Findings include sacral agenesis, spinal, and lower limb abnormalities, femoral hypoplasia, gastrointestinal and genitourinary abnormalities.

444. **(B)** Adult tissue is more tolerant of temperature increases than embryo tissue or ossifying fetal bones.

445. **(A)** Duplex pulse Doppler studies (pulse-wave Doppler with real time) are of significantly higher output intensities than power Doppler or fetal Doppler monitor.

446. **(D)** The phenotype for Turner's syndrome is 45X, indicating only one single X, or female, chromosome.

447. (A) The ALARA principle (as low as reasonably achievable) employs keeping the power output as low as possible and increasing the receiver gain in order to change the quality of the image. This principle also employs reducing the scanning time in order to minimize the patient's ultrasound exposure.

448. (D) Caudal regression syndrome and cardiac defects are first-trimester insults and a risk of occurrence increases with increasing blood sugar levels in the first trimester. Shoulder dystocia can occur with delivery of macrosomic fetuses.

449. (A) Depending on the fetal gestational age, lung maturity amniocentesis may be performed to assure lung maturation before delivery. In cases of complete PROM, often there is not an adequate sample of amniotic fluid available for maturity testing.

450. (D) Although an increased AFV is associated with macrosomia, it is not a direct assessment of macrosomia.

451. (D) CVS and PUBS may be performed provided the placenta or umbilical cord is accessible. If the fetal bladder is full, as in cases of PUV syndrome, fetal urine may be tested for karyotype.

452. (D) Amniocentesis is a prenatal test to analyze the amniotic fluid. It can be used to detect multiple potential abnormalities such as Down's syndrome, cystic fibrosis, sickle cell disease, neural tube defects, and fetal lungs maturity. It also can be used to test the level of fetal bilirubin, infection, and for a limited number of short-limb syndromes. However, amniocentesis is not useful in detecting cleft palate or cleft lips.

453. (C) Hypertension can affect the vascular bed of the placenta resulting in intrauterine growth restriction (IUGR).

454. (A) Excessive maternal smoking has been linked to accelerated maturation of the placenta. It is not predictive, however, in actual placenta perfusion to the fetus.

455. (C) BBOW, bulging bag of water, refers to the amniotic membrane bulging into the vagina.

456. (D) PROM, premature rupture of membranes, is the rupture of membranes before 37 weeks.

457. (D) All of the above. Overdistension of the urinary bladder can result in serious diagnostic error. Overdistension of the urinary bladder may result in closure of an incompetent cervix due to bladder compression on the cervix; placenta previa caused by bladder compression on the lower uterine segment; closure of the gestational sac caused by bladder compression that causes both sides of the sac walls to meet resulting in a loss of the anechoic center or a change in sac shape (distortion); nonvisualization of the internal iliac vein because of displacement.

458. (C) Ovulation occurs approximately 14 days after the first day of the LMP.

459. (C) Gravida is a woman who is pregnant.

460. (A) Multipara is a woman who has given birth two or more times.

461. (D) Nullipara is a woman who has never given birth to a viable infant.

462. (H) Primipara is woman who has given birth one time to a viable infant, regardless of whether the child was living at birth and regardless of whether the birth was single or multiple.

463. (B) Nulligravida is a woman who has never been pregnant.

464. (E) Primigravida is a woman who is pregnant for the first time.

465. (F) Multigravida is a woman who has been pregnant several times.

466. (G) Para is the number of pregnancies that have continued to viability.

467. (I) Trimester is a 3-month period during gestation.

468. (D) The puerperium period begins with the expulsion of the placenta and continues until maternal physiology and anatomy return to a pre-pregnancy level, approximately 6–8 weeks.

469. (D) Ectopic pregnancy.

470. (A) When the transducer is in direct contact with the patient, it exposes the patient to the greatest risk of electrical shock from a cracked transducer. Water and metals are conductors of electricity.

471. (D) The ovaries are least likely to be seen on a postpartum pelvic sonogram. This may be because of extrapelvic position of the ovaries caused by the large uterus.

472. (A) At approximately 20–22 weeks of gestation, the fundus of the gravid uterus is at the level of the umbilicus, and at 12 weeks of gestation, it is at the symphysis pubic. This is known as fundal height.

473. (D) Hemorrhage, thromboembolism, and infection are the most common complications during the postpartum period. Placenta previa is an antepartum complication.

474. (D) Ascites is an abnormal accumulation of fluid in the abdominal (peritoneal) cavity. There are multiple causes: heart failure, nephrotic syndrome pancreatitis, cancer alcoholic hepatitis, and tuberculosis. Fibroid uterus is a benign tumor and generally does not cause ascites.

475. (D) 25% of fetuses are breech at 28 weeks, 7% at 32 weeks, and 3–5% at term.

476. (B) Malignant ascites is characterized by loculated intraperitoneal fluid collection with loops of bowel adherent to the abdominal wall.

477. (C) VBAC is a commonly used abbreviation for vaginal birth after cesarean section.

478. **(B)** The normal anatomical site for implantation of pregnancy is the endometrial (uterine) cavity, and the normal location for fertilization of the ovum is the ampullary region of the fallopian tube.

479. **(D)** Placenta previa is the implantation of the placenta in the lower uterine segment.

480. **(A)** Placenta accreta is the abnormal adherence of part or the all of placenta to the uterine wall.

481. **(C)** Placenta succenturiata is an accessory lobe of placenta.

482. **(B)** Abruptio placentae is the premature separation of the placenta after 20 weeks of gestation.

483. **(E)** Placenta increta is the abnormal adherence of part or all of the placenta in which the chorionic villi invade the myometrium.

484. **(F)** Placenta percreta is the abnormal adherence of part or all of the placenta in which the chorionic villi invade the uterine wall.

485. **(A)** The fetal component of the placenta.

486. **(B)** The maternal component of the placenta.

487. **(A)** Sonographic fetal HELLP findings include IUGR, oligohydramnios, and possible signs of fetal distress (poor BPP, abnormal UC Doppler's, for example). Clinically, HELLP is an acronym for hemolysis, elevated liver enzyme, and low platelet count. It is a variant of pre-eclampsia but can occur on its own.

488. **(A)** The kidneys should be scanned to look for hydronephrosis. An enlarged fibroid greater than 14 cm in size can compress the distal ureter and cause hydronephrosis. These findings can also be due to the gravid uterus in pregnancy. A pseudohydronephrosis can occur with over-distended urinary bladder but disappears after post-void.

489. **(B)** The primary infection that cause VZV results from chicken pox. Herpes zoster, also known as shingles results from reactivation of VZV.

490. **(D)** Cytomegalovirus (CMV) is the most common intra-uterine congenital fetal viral infection. The maternal risk of transmission to the fetus is 40–50%, regardless of gestational age.

491. **(A)** The secondary yolk sac is located in the chorionic cavity (extraembryonic coelom). The primitive yolk sac is not seen on ultrasound. The yolk sac contains vitelline fluid and has many functions including transfer of nutrients and development of blood (hematopoiesis). At approximately 12 weeks, the amnion and chorion begin to fuse and the yolk is no longer seen.

492. **(D)** Hematocolpos is blood in the vagina and is caused more commonly by imperforate hymen. Cervical stenosis is an acquired condition with obstruction at the cervical os, which can also result in hematometra but is less

common. Hematometrocolpos is blood in the vagina and uterus.

493. **(D)** In the case of IUGR, the fetus will direct more blood flow to the brain. This will lower the PI and S/D ratio of the middle cerebral artery (MCA). More recently, multiple studies have been conducted showing that the peak velocity of the MCA is a good predictor of fetal anemia. The peak velocity is measured and plotted of a curve to determine whether the fetus is in need of a fetal blood transfusion because of fetal anemia.

494. **(C)** Leiomyomas (fibroids) are benign tumors of the muscle of the uterus, which are stimulated by estrogen. After menopause, the fibroid normally decreased in size due to the decrease in estrogen. An increase in size of fibroids after menopause is suggestive of leiomyosarcoma.

495. **(D)** Multiple fluid-filled spaces in the uterine cavity with markedly elevated serum β-hCG are highly suggestive of hydatidiform mole, which is characterized by hydropic villi. The most common cyst associated with hydatidiform mole is theca lutein cyst, which is located on the ovary. Corpus lutein cyst is associated with an IUP. Pseudogestational sac is associated with an ectopic pregnancy.

496. **(D)** Sex cord-stromal tumors include fibroma, thecoma, granulosa cell, and androblastoma (Sertoli–Leydig cell). They appear hypoechoic to echogenic with a mixed heterogeneous pattern and appear similar to each other on ultrasound.

497. **(C)** Endometriomas have a variety of sonographic appearances. Hemorrhagic cyst and ovarian abscesses is known to mimic its appearances.

498. **(A)** A hydrosalpinx may initially look like a cystic mass with septations. On closer examination, the septations are not complete. The sonographer is able to follow the connection of the cystic spaces. This assumes that the structure is tubular and communicates as with hydrosalpinx.

499. **(D)** A paraovarian, or mesonephric cyst originates from the mesonephric duct. A paraovarian cyst may form, regardless of uterine or ovarian status. Ovarian tissue does occasionally remain after an oophorectomy, especially if adhesions were present. The remaining ovarian tissue can still function and produce a cyst. It is called ovarian remnant syndrome and should be considered with any cystic mass identified in a post-oophorectomy patient. Peritoneal inclusion cyst is sometimes seen after oophorectomy due to fluid trapped between the adhesions.

500. **(C)** Hydatid cyst of Morgagni also known as a paratubal cyst is the most common paramesonephric cyst. It measures 2–10 mm and appears similar to ovarian cysts.

501. **(A)** D1 × D2 × D3 × 0.523.

502. **(D)** The image is a Dandy–Walker malformation. The cerebellum is splayed, and the vermis is absent. There is communication with the fourth ventricle.

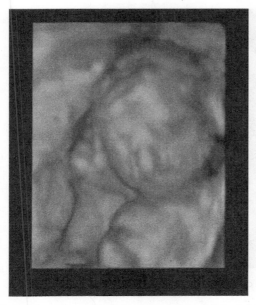

FIGURE 8–11. Three-dimensional sonogram showing bilateral cleft palate.

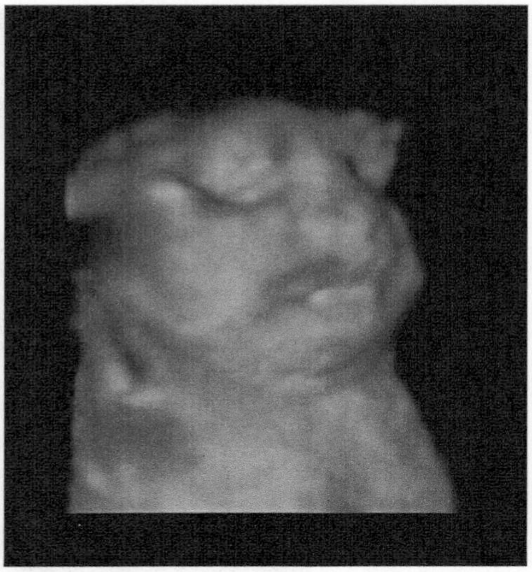

FIGURE 8–13. Three-dimensional sonogram of anencephalic fetus.

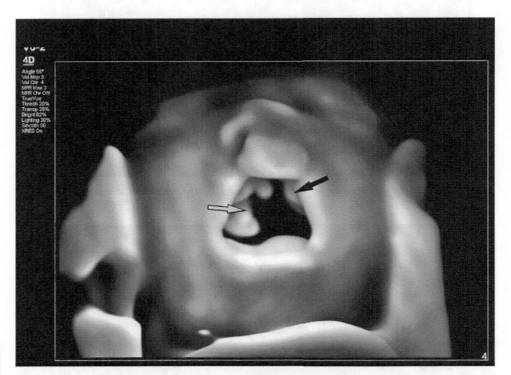

FIGURE 8–12. TrueView 3D showing cleft lip (yellow arrow) and palate (black arrow).

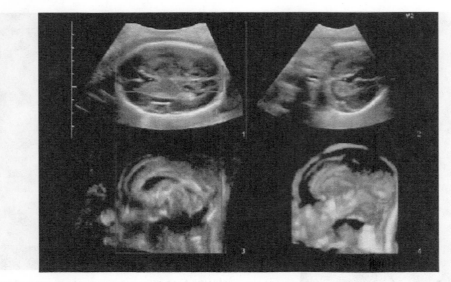

FIGURE 8–14. Multiplanar image and 3D reconstruction of the brain of a fetus at 25 weeks' gestation. The corpus callosum is clearly depicted on the volumetric image (4).

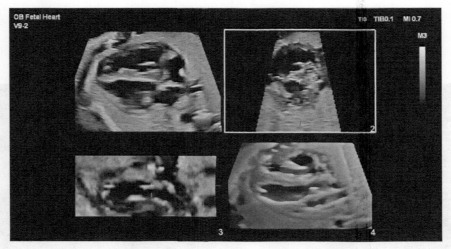

FIGURE 8–15. Spatial temporal image correlation (STIC) of normal fetal ventricles/atria and outflow tracts.

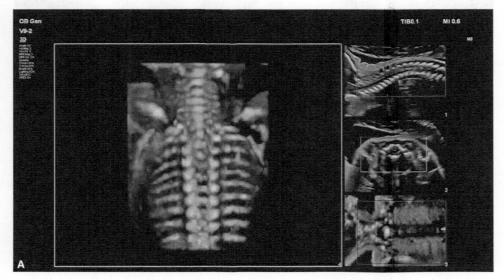

FIGURE 8–16A. 3D US of normal spine. **(A)** cervical, thoracic; **(B)** lumbar, sacral.

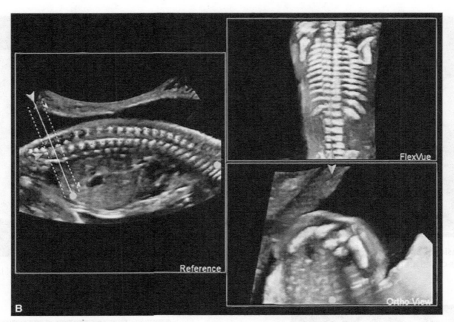

FIGURE 8–16B. (Continued)

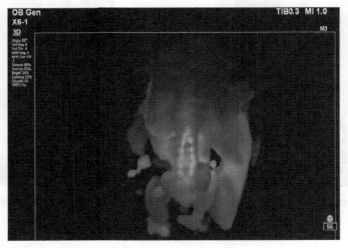

FIGURE 8–17. Multiplanar 3D of normal lower lumbar and sacral spine.

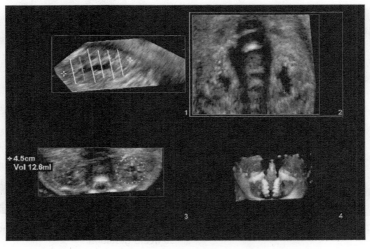

FIGURE 8–18. Multiplanar reconstructed image of normal kidneys.

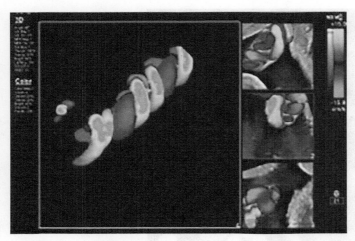

FIGURE 8–19. Three-dimensional sonogram of normal umbilical cord showing two (paired) arteries coiled around umbilical vein.

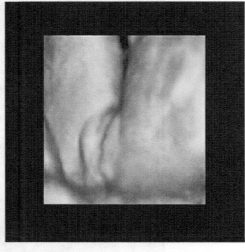

FIGURE 8–22. Three-dimensional sonogram of labia majora of a female fetus at 30 weeks' gestation.

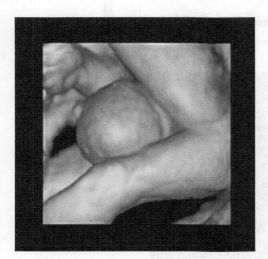

FIGURE 8–20. Three-dimensional sonogram of a fetus 26 weeks' gestation with a large omphalocele.

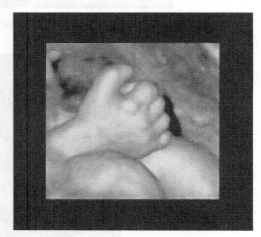

FIGURE 8–23. Three-dimensional sonogram of hand of a fetus at 29 weeks' gestation.

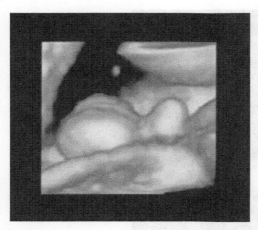

FIGURE 8–21. Three-dimensional sonogram of the scrotum and penis of a fetus at 31 weeks' gestation.

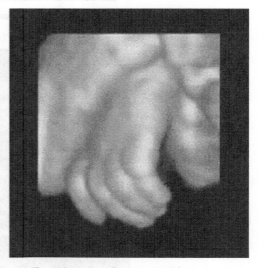

FIGURE 8–24. Three-dimensional sonogram of fingers of a fetus at 30 weeks' gestation.

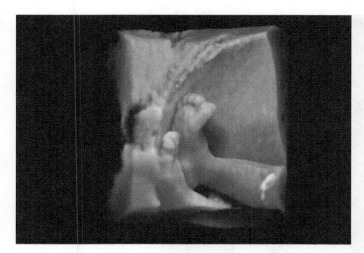

FIGURE 8–25. Three-dimensional sonogram of fetal feet and toes

Three-dimensional sonography is particularly useful in the evaluation of the fetal heart. This is due to the ability to depict selected scan planes that may not be obtainable on 2D. The heart volume can be obtained with special software that affords spatial temporal image correlation (STIC). This technique allows for systematic evaluation of cardiac structures regardless of fetal position.

Three-dimensional sonography may be useful in depicting complete anomalies involving an abnormal abdominal wall such as omphalocele or internal disruptions such as congenital diaphragmatic hernia. Using 3D, the actual volume of the remaining lungs of a fetus with congenital diaphragmatic hernia can be estimated.

Other applications of 3D in obstetrics include evaluation of placental vascular bed or umbilical cord insertion or coiling anomalies. Umbilical cord knots and nuchal cords are readily depicted on 3D.

Three-dimensional color Doppler sonography can provide the arrangement of intraplacental vessels as well as focal areas of retroplacental hemorrhage. Three-dimensional sonography can depict abnormal umbilical cord placental insertion such as velamentous cord insertions onto the membrane rather than the placental surface chorionic plate.

Other applications may include using 3D sonography to depict ectopic pregnancies and their spatial relationship to the ovary, as well as to assess internal organ malformations. As 3D sonography is used more, sonographers will undoubtedly discover new and expanded clinical applications of this technique.

GYNECOLOGIC 3D SONOGRAPHY

Three-dimensional sonography has many clinical applications in gynecologic disorders (Figs. 8–27 through 8–38). As in obstetrical 3D, gynecologic 3D affords depiction of the uterus and ovaries in any selectable scan plane, including those not readily obtained with 2D. These include improved depiction of endometrial masses such as polyps or submucosal fibroids, improved localization and calculation of changes in fibroid volume, enhanced depiction of tubal masses, intrauterine device localization, and uterine malformations. Three-dimensional depiction of tumor morphology and vascularity within ovarian masses has important implications in distinguishing benign from malignant masses.

Three-dimensional sonography affords depiction of the configuration of the uterine fundus. With a septate uterus, the fundal contour is smooth, whereas with bicornuate and didelphys, a sharp cleft is seen. The relative length of the septum can be shown.

Fibroids have a peripheral rim of vascularity and this is seen readily with 3D color Doppler sonography. Any collaterals such as those arising from the ovarian vessels can be seen. Marked changes in the vascularity fibroids such as that occurring post-uterine artery embolization can be documented accurately with 3D sonography.

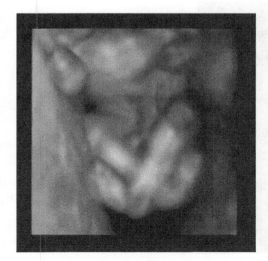

FIGURE 8–26. Three-dimensional sonogram showing bilateral club feet.

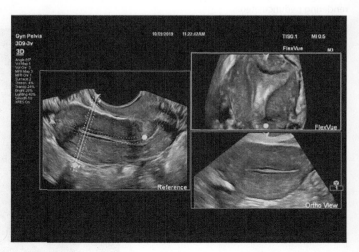

FIGURE 8–27. Composite images of 3D TVS of uterus using Flex View. (left half) Long axis of uterus showing curved imaging plane and level for coronal (top right) and short axis (bottom right) images of the endometrium.

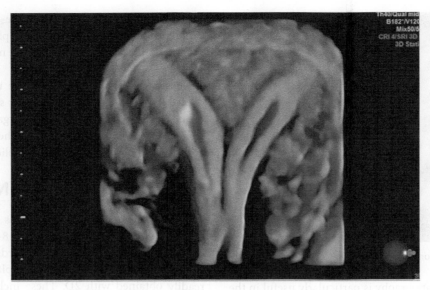

FIGURE 8–28. Three-dimensional sonogram of a septate uterus.

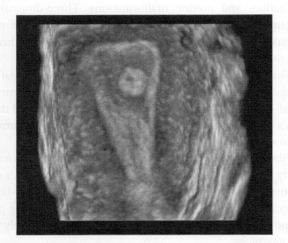

FIGURE 8–29. Endometrial polyp as shown in coronal plane 3D surface rendering pedunculated.

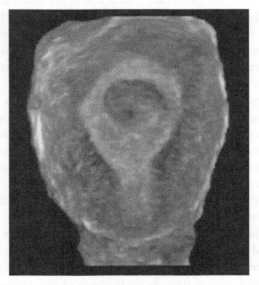

FIGURE 8–30. Submucosal fibroid that is intraluminal as depicted in coronal 3D.

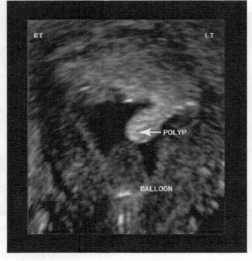

FIGURE 8–31. Three-dimensional surface-rendered image obtained during sonohysterography showing polyp (arrow). *(Reproduced with permission from Philips Healthcare.)*

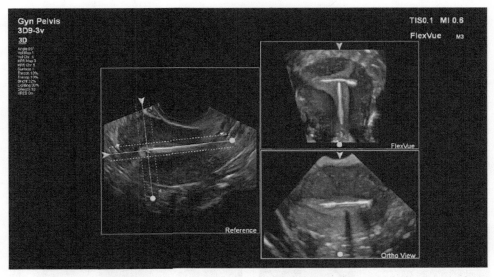

FIGURE 8–32. Multiplanar image showing centrally located intrauterine contraceptive device.

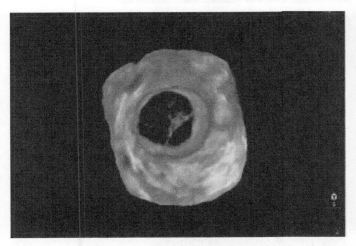

FIGURE 8–33. Three-dimensional image of ovarian cyst containing fibrin strands.

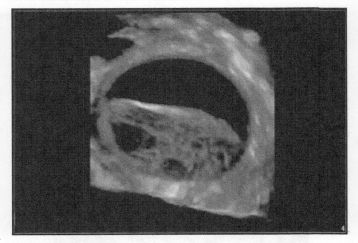

FIGURE 8–34. Three-dimensional image of hemorrhagic ovarian mass containing formed clot.

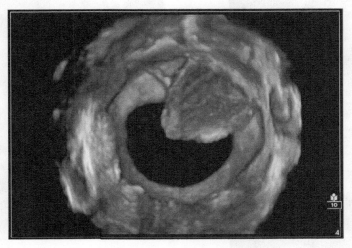

FIGURE 8–35. Three-dimensional image of ovarian tumor containing a papillary excrescence.

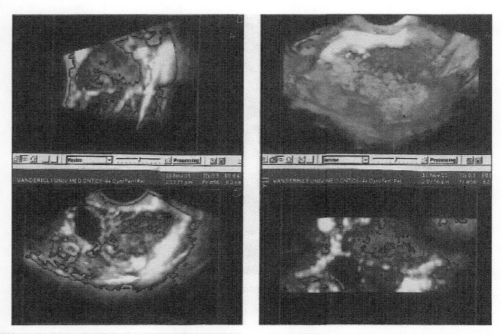

FIGURE 8–36. Three-dimensional images of ovarian cancer showing clusters of abnormal vessels (top right) in area of papillary excrescence.

Because of its ability to display in the coronal plane, 3D sonography is accurate in depicting intraluminal masses such as polyps or fibroids. The exact extent of the fibroid relative to surrounding myometrium can be depicted with 3D. Similarly, the location of the arms, shaft, and string of an intrauterine contraceptive device (IUCD) within the endometrium is readily depicted with 3D sonography. Embedded arms within the myometrium can be detected. Three-dimensional sonography obtained in the transverse plane of the uterus fundus is also useful in identifying tubal masses since their origins can be traced to the cornual area of the uterus.

Three-dimensional sonography can depict focal wall irregularities within mostly cystic adnexal lesions. Three-dimensional color Doppler sonography can depict vessel density and

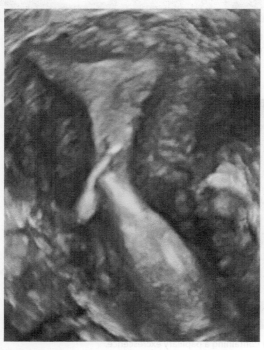

FIGURE 8–37. Embedded arm of malpositioned IUD.

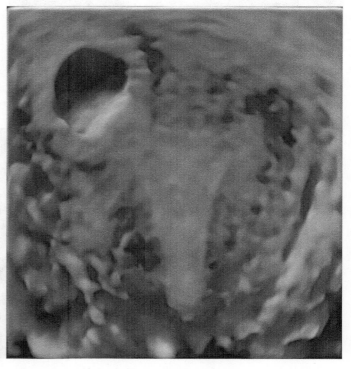

FIGURES 8–38. Three-dimensional images of the uterus showing an interstitial ectopic pregnancy.

branching pattern. The vessels within a tumor typically are clustered and show differences in their caliber.

VOLUMETRIC SONOGRAPHY

Acquisition of large sample volumes affords later evaluation of organs in selected scan planes. Some advocate that volumetric acquisition in obstetrics and gynecology can expedite the examinations, making them quicker to obtain and complete.[3] Additional time is needed to obtain the required scan plans from the 3D volume set.

FUTURE APPLICATIONS

It is clear that 3D sonography has a role in the evaluation of certain obstetric and gynecologic disorders. Live 3D or "4D" can depict fetal behavior and also will have many applications for guided procedures.[4] Undoubtedly, future applications of this technique will evolve within its greater use.[5-8]

References

1. Merz E. *3D Ultrasound in Obstetrics/Gynecology.* New York: Lippincott Publishers; 1998.

2. Fleischer AC, Black AS, Grippo RJ, Pham T. 3D pelvic sonography: current use and potential applications. *J Women's Imaging.* 2003; 5(2):52-59.

3. Benacerraf BR. Tomographic sonography of the fetus: is it accurate enough to be a frontline screen for fetal malformation? *J Ultrasound Med.* 2006;25:687-689.

4. Goncalves LF, Espinoza J, Kusanovic JP, et al. Applications of 2-dimensional matrix array for 3- and 4-dimensional examination of the fetus: a pictorial essay. *J Ultrasound Med.* 2006;25:745-755.

5. Goncalves LF, Nien JK, Espinoza J, et al. What does 2-dimensional imaging add to 3- and 4-dimensional obstetric ultrasonography? *J Ultrasound Med.* 2006;25:691-699.

6. Abu-Rustum R. *A Practical Guide to 3D Ultrasound.* New York: CRC Press; 2015.

7. Fleischer AC. *Fleischer's Sonography in Ob/Gyn.* 8th ed. New York: McGraw Hill; 2018:p1202.

8. Samson C. Volumetric sonography. In: *Fleischer's Sonography in Ob/Gyn.* New York: McGraw Hill; 2018:1351.

9

Fetal Echocardiography

Teresa M. Bieker

Study Guide

INTRODUCTION

Congenital heart disease is a leading cause of infant mortality, with a reported incidence of approximately 1 in 100 live births.[1] However, these numbers are based on live-born infants and, therefore, probably underestimate the true incidence in the fetus.[2] Early fetal loss and stillbirths are often the result of complex cardiac defects or chromosomal defects, which have an associated heart defect. For this reason, the incidence of congenital heart disease in the fetus has been reported to be as much as five times that found in live-born children[1] (Table 9–1).

In utero diagnosis of congenital heart disease allows a variety of treatment options to be considered, including delivery at an appropriate facility, termination, and in some cases, *in utero* therapy.[3] Conversely, a normal fetal echocardiogram in the setting of an increased risk factor provides reassurance for both the patient and the physician.

INSTRUMENTATION AND TECHNIQUE

The American Institute of Ultrasound in Medicine (AIUM) Technical Bulletin on the performance of a basic fetal cardiac ultrasound recommends that a four-chamber view and both the right and the left ventricular outflow tracts be obtained on all obstetrical ultrasound exams.[4] Evaluation of a four-chamber view alone may substantially decrease the detection rate of some major cardiac malformations.

When risk factors increase the likelihood of congenital heart disease, a formal and more detailed fetal echocardiogram should be performed.

Various reports advocate evaluation of the fetal heart at different gestational ages[5]; however, the AIUM Technical Bulletin recommends that fetal echocardiographic exams be performed between 18 and 22 weeks of gestation.[4] During this period, optimum image quality and, therefore, diagnostic accuracy are achieved. It should be borne in mind that even at 18 weeks of gestation, the fetal heart is a very small structure. Before this age, many cardiac structures may be too small to evaluate accurately.[6] Recent advances in ultrasound have led to first-trimester screening of the fetal heart. Cardiac position, as well as a four-chamber view and outflow tracts, can be evaluated by a transabdominal or endovaginal approach. Obtaining these views, however, is dependent on fetal size and position.[7] In addition, cardiac lesions such as coarctation of the aorta and hypoplastic left heart syndrome (HLHS) may be progressive lesions.[8,9] Therefore, scanning the fetus too early in gestation may result in a false-negative diagnosis.

Later in gestation, the echocardiographic exam may be hindered by increased attenuation from the fetal skull, ribs, spine, and limbs, as well as decreased amniotic fluid as pregnancy progresses.[6]

Equipment

Fetal echocardiography requires the use of high-resolution ultrasound equipment.[10] Preferred transducer frequencies usually range from 5 to 7 MHz, depending on gestational age, maternal body habitus, and the amount of amniotic fluid present. Equipment utilized for fetal echocardiography should have M-mode and pulsed Doppler capabilities to provide physiologic assessment, as well as color Doppler capabilities to assess spatial and directional information. All of these modalities are vital to performing a complete and accurate examination.

Indications

A family history of congenital heart disease is the most common indication to perform a fetal echocardiogram. Recurrence risk for fetuses varies depending on the type of lesion and their relationship to the affected relative.

TABLE 9–1 • Frequency of Congenital Heart Lesions Among Affected Abortuses and Stillborn Infants

Defect	Frequency (%)
Ventricular septal defect	35.7
Coarctation of the aorta	8.9
Atrial septal defect	8.2
Atrioventricular septal defect	6.7
Tetralogy of Fallot	6.2
Single ventricle	4.8
Truncus arteriosus	4.8
Hypoplastic left heart	4.6
Complete transposition of the great arteries	4.3
Double outlet right ventricle	2.4
Hypoplastic right heart	1.7
Single atrium	1.2
Pulmonic stenosis	0.7
Aortic stenosis	0.5
Miscellaneous	10.6

Modified with permission from Hoffman JI. Incidence of congenital heart disease: II. Prenatal incidence, *Pediatr Cardiol.* Jul-Aug 1995;16(4):155-165.

TABLE 9–2 • Recurrence Risk in Siblings for any Congenital Heart Defect

Defect	Suggested Risk (%)	
	If One Sibling Affected	If Two Siblings Affected
Aortic stenosis	2	6
Atrial septal defect	2.5	8
Atrioventricular canal	3	10
Coarctation of the aorta	2	6
Ebstein anomaly	1	3
Endocardial fibroelastosis	4	12
Hypoplastic left heart	2	6
Pulmonary atresia	1	3
Pulmonary stenosis	2	6
Tetralogy of Fallot	2.5	8
Transposition	1.5	5
Tricuspid atresia	1	3
Truncus arteriosus	1	3
Ventricular septal defect	3	10

Adapted with permission from Nora JJ, Fraser FC, Bear J, et al. Medical Genetics: Principles and Practice, 4th ed. Philadelphia, PA: Lea & Febiger; 1994.

The risk of congenital heart disease for a fetus with an affected sibling is approximately 2–4%.[11,12] If two or more siblings are affected, this risk increases to approximately 10% (Table 9–2). When the mother of the fetus has a congenital heart abnormality, the recurrence risk is also approximately 10–12%.[12] An affected father carries a lower risk (Table 9–3).[11,12]

Exposure to known cardiac teratogens also increases the risk of having a fetus with a cardiac defect.[13] The list of substances considered teratogenic is extensive.[14] Specific occurrence risk varies with length and type of exposure, as well as the specific substance involved.

Chromosomal abnormalities have been reported to occur in 13% of live-born infants with a congenital heart defect.[15,16] The incidence of abnormal karyotype in the fetus with a congenital heart abnormality is approximately 35%.[2,17] Fetuses with an increased nuchal translucency during a first-trimester ultrasound also have an increased risk for congenital heart defects.[18]

The specific type and occurrence risk of a congenital heart defect vary depending on the chromosomal abnormality. Trisomy 21 is associated with a 40–50% occurrence of congenital heart disease,[15] whereas in trisomies 13 and 18, the association is almost 100%.[19] As with teratogenic agents, the list of abnormal karyotypes and syndromes associated with cardiac defects is extensive.[14]

Several maternal conditions may also carry an inherent risk to the fetus. Congenital heart disease is increased fivefold among infants of diabetic mothers,[17] whereas phenylketonuria has a reported risk of 12–16%.[20]

TABLE 9–3 • Suggested Offspring Recurrence Risk for Congenital Heart Defects Given One Affected Parent		
	Suggested Risk (%)	
Defect	**Father Affected**	**Mother Affected**
Aortic stenosis	3	13–18
Atrial septal defect	1.5	4–4.5
Atrioventricular canal	1	14
Coarctation of the aorta	2	4
Pulmonary stenosis	2	4–6.5
Tetralogy of Fallot	1.5	2.5
Ventricular septal defect	2	6–10

Adapted with permission from Nora JJ, Fraser FC, Bear J, et al. Medical Genetics: Principles and Practice, 4th ed. Philadelphia, PA: Lea & Febiger; 1994.

TABLE 9–4 • Incidence of Associated Congenital Heart Defects Occurring with Extracardiac Malformations in Infants	
System or Lesion	**Frequency of CHD (%)**
Central nervous system	
Hydrocephalus	4.5–14.8
Dandy–Walker malformation	2.5–4.3
Agenesis of the corpus callosum	14.9
Meckel–Gruber syndrome	13.8
Gastrointestinal	
Tracheoesophageal fistula	14.7–39.2
Duodenal atresia	17.1
Jejunal atresia	5.2
Anorectal anomalies	22
Imperforate anus	11.7
Ventral wall	
Omphalocele	19.5–32
Gastroschisis	0–7.7
Diaphragmatic hernia	9.6–22.9
Genitourinary	
Renal agenesis (bilateral)	42.8
Renal agenesis (unilateral)	16.9
Horseshoe kidney	38.8
Renal dysplasia	5.4
Ureteral obstruction	2.1

Modified with permission from Copel JA, Pilu G, Kleinman CS. Congenital heart disease and extracardiac anomalies: associations and indications for fetal echocardiography. *Am J Obstet Gynecol* 1986 May;154(5):1121-1132.

Complete heart block in the fetus is associated with maternal collagen vascular disease (systemic lupus erythematosus). In these patients, circulating antinuclear antibodies of the SSA or SSB types damage the developing conduction tissue.[21]

Maternal infections such as human parvovirus and cytomegalovirus also have a reported association with cardiac defects in the fetus.[22]

Another indication for performing a fetal echocardiogram is the presence of extracardiac anomalies in a fetus.[23] The overall incidence of extracardiac malformations in children identified as having a congenital heart abnormality ranges from 25% to 45% (Table 9–4).[23] Cardiac abnormalities such as atrioventricular septal defects (AVSDs) are associated with extracardiac defects in more than 50% of cases, while atrial septal defects (ASDs), ventricular septal defects (VSDs), tetralogy of Fallot, and cardiac malpositions are associated with extracardiac malformations in about 30% of cases.[23]

A suspected structural or rhythm abnormality seen in the fetal heart on a routine obstetrical examination should also warrant a formal fetal echocardiogram to rule out an underlying structural abnormality or, in some cases, to implement *in utero* therapy.

Nonimmune hydrops fetalis is also an indication for fetal echocardiography. In some cases, it may reflect structural heart disease, while in others, it is the result of a dysrhythmia.[21] Finally, massive polyhydramnios is a recognized indication for fetal echocardiography.[21] An increase in amniotic fluid may be the result of congestive heart failure, but it is more likely related to associated defects in the fetus, such as those that cause difficulty

in swallowing or compression of the esophagus. Although there are several predisposing indications to perform a fetal echocardiogram, up to 90% of congenital heart disease occurs in unselected "normal" obstetric patients.[1] Therefore, routine obstetric scanning should identify the majority of fetuses with cardiac lesions that will need a formal fetal echocardiogram.

Position

A fetal echocardiographic exam should always begin by determining fetal position. Unlike a pediatric or adult patient, the fetus cannot be placed in a standard position, nor can the heart be evaluated consistently from routine angles. Although the fetus may move throughout the exam, establishing basic position will allow the examiner to identify various cardiac structures more quickly.[6] Once fetal position is determined, the location and orientation of the heart should be established. In a cross-sectional transverse view of the fetal chest, the correct orientation for the fetal heart is with the apex pointing to the left and the bulk of the heart occupying the left chest. The normal angle of the fetal heart, relative to midline is 45 ± 20°.[24] The left atrium should be located closest to the fetal spine and the right ventricle nearest to the anterior chest wall. This normal orientation is termed *levocardia*.

The normal fetal heart should occupy approximately one-third of the fetal thorax.[25] Fetal cardiac size can be calculated by measuring the diameter or the circumference of the heart and comparing it to the diameter or circumference of the fetal chest, respectively. When calculating this ratio, both measurements must be obtained from the same image.

Scanning Technique

The first view to obtain when beginning a fetal echocardiographic examination is the four-chamber view.[14] There are two different four-chamber views: apical four-chamber and subcostal four-chamber views. The apical four-chamber view is obtained in a transverse view of the fetal chest, with the transducer imaging the fetal heart from either the anterior or the posterior aspect.

In the apical four-chamber view, all four cardiac chambers can be visualized (Fig. 9–1). In addition, color or pulsed Doppler interrogation of the mitral and tricuspid valves can be performed. Doppler should be performed on the atrial side of the valves to assess for valvular insufficiency, whereas Doppler distal to the valves should be done to evaluate for stenosis or atresia. The two superior pulmonary veins should also be identified entering the left atrium from this projection. The two inferior pulmonary veins are usually not visualized on a fetal echocardiogram.

The apical four-chamber view is not optimal for evaluating the interventricular septum (IVS). In this view, the angle of incidence of the sound beam is parallel to the IVS and may result in

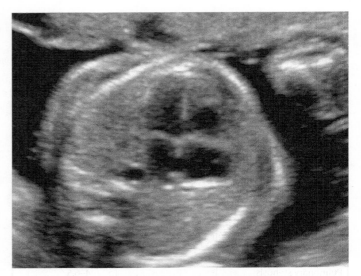

FIGURE 9–2. Apical four-chamber view showing a "pseudo" interventricular septal defect, caused by the septum being parallel to the sound beam.

an artifactual dropout of echoes at the level of the membranous portion, simulating a "pseudo" septal defect (Fig. 9–2).[26]

By sliding the transducer cephalad from an apical four-chamber view, the aorta and pulmonary artery should be visualized side by side (Fig. 9–3). This confirms that both are present and normally of equal size.

The subcostal four-chamber view is obtained by imaging the fetal chest in a transverse projection from the anterior chest wall and angling the transducer slightly cephalad (Fig. 9–4). This view also allows identification and comparison of both atria and ventricles. It is ideal for obtaining M-mode measurements of the ventricles and IVS by placing an M-mode cursor perpendicular to the septum at the level of the atrioventricular valves (Fig. 9–5).

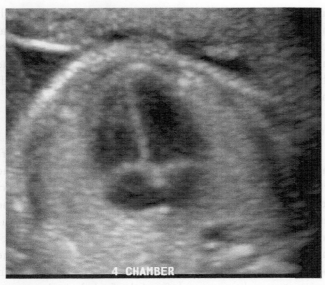

FIGURE 9–1. Apical four-chamber view showing the interventricular and interatrial septae parallel to the ultrasound beam.

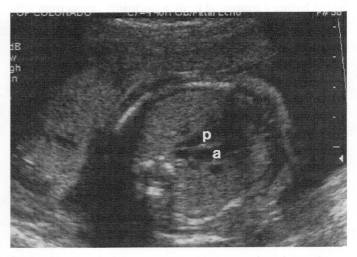

FIGURE 9–3. Three-vessel view. The aorta (a) and pulmonary artery (p) can be seen as two parallel structures by angling the transducer cephalad from the apical four-chamber view. The superior vena cava is seen in cross section. This view allows you to confirm that both great vessels are present and are of similar size.

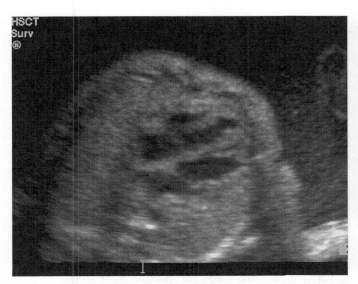

FIGURE 9–4. Subcostal four-chamber view with the interventricular and interatrial septae perpendicular to the sound beam.

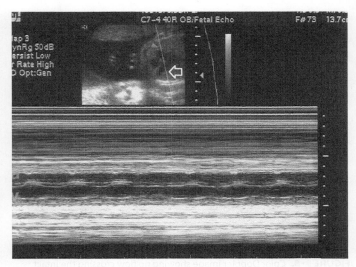

FIGURE 9–6. M-mode tracing through the right atrial (a, arrowhead) and left ventricular (v, open arrow) wall simultaneously to assess the response of each in the setting of a dysrhythmia.

Atrial measurements can be obtained by moving the M-mode cursor through both atria. The subcostal four-chamber view is also preferable for evaluating a fetal dysrhythmia by placing the M-mode cursor through an atrial wall and a ventricular wall simultaneously (Fig. 9–6). This allows visualization of the timing of dysrhythmic events and may aid in making a definitive diagnosis.

Either pulsed Doppler or color Doppler can be used to evaluate the foramen ovale in the subcostal projection. Documentation of flow from the right atrium to the left atrium by either modality rules out restriction of the foraminal flap (Fig. 9–7). It is also valuable in assessing altered flow direction secondary to a structural defect. A spectral Doppler tracing will display normal foraminal flow as being twice the fetal heart rate.

The IVS is best evaluated in the subcostal four-chamber view since the ultrasound beam is perpendicular to the intraventricular septum. Color Doppler is the best means of achieving this because it allows a large area to be evaluated simultaneously (Fig. 9–8). Pulsed Doppler may not detect flow across a septal defect if the sample volume is not precisely located.

Larger VSDs may be detected with gray scale imaging alone; however, many remain undetected by any means. Even when a VSD is present, the pressures in the fetal heart are such that no flow may be appreciated across the IVS.

Obtaining a subcostal four-chamber view is critical in performing a complete fetal echocardiogram. By angling the transducer systematically toward the fetal right shoulder from this view, most of the remaining fetal heart views are obtained.

A slight angulation from the subcostal four-chamber view toward the fetal right shoulder will result in visualization of a long-axis view of the proximal aorta. In this view, continuity of the anterior wall of the aorta with the IVS and the posterior wall

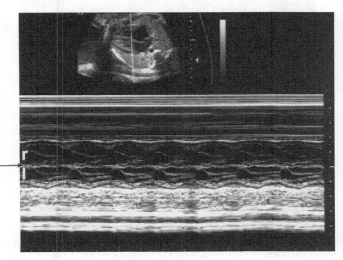

FIGURE 9–5. M-mode tracing of the right (r) and left (l) ventricles at the level of the atrioventricular valves. Arrowhead = interventricular septum (IVS).

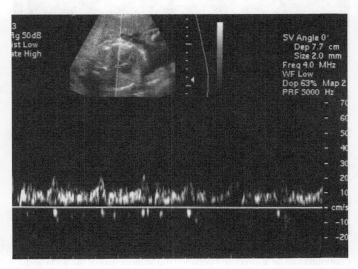

FIGURE 9–7. Pulsed Doppler tracing of the foramen ovale documenting flow from the right atrium into the left atrium.

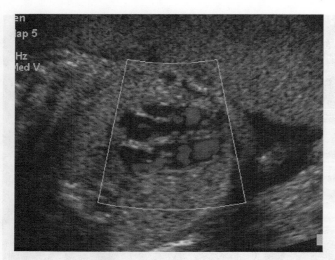

FIGURE 9–8. Color Doppler image showing no flow crossing the intact interventricular septum.

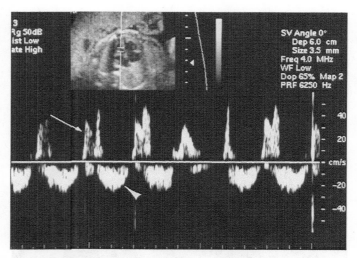

FIGURE 9–10. Pulsed Doppler tracing showing the mitral valve inflow (arrow) simultaneously with the aortic valve (arrowhead) outflow.

with the anterior leaflet of the mitral valve can be determined (Fig. 9–9). The aortic valve can be interrogated with pulsed Doppler in this view, both proximally looking for aortic insufficiency, and distally to detect stenosis or atresia.

The long-axis view of the aorta also provides another means of evaluating a dysrhythmia. By utilizing a wide sample gate and placing the pulsed Doppler cursor between the mitral and aortic valves, both left ventricular inflow and outflow can be evaluated simultaneously (Fig. 9–10). The inflow through the mitral valve will reflect rhythm disturbances occurring in the atria; whereas, the left ventricular outflow through the aorta reflects the ventricular response. Being able to visualize both events simultaneously may help in differentiating the type of dysrhythmia present.

The right ventricular outflow tract is visualized next by rotating the transducer further in the direction of the fetal right

shoulder. In the normal fetus, this view demonstrates the pulmonary artery coursing cephalad, leftward, and posteriorly from the right ventricle (Fig. 9–11). The course of the pulmonary artery should cross the aorta in the normal fetus. In other words, by angling the transducer from the long-axis view of the aorta to the long-axis view of the pulmonary, the great vessels should "crisscross" directions if they are correctly oriented. Color or pulsed Doppler is again used in this projection to evaluate the valve proximally for pulmonic insufficiency and distally for pulmonic stenosis or atresia.

A further rightward rotation of the transducer will result in a sagittal view of the fetal thorax and thus a short-axis view through the ventricles (Fig. 9–12). The echogenic moderator band should be apparent near the apex to help in identifying the right ventricle.

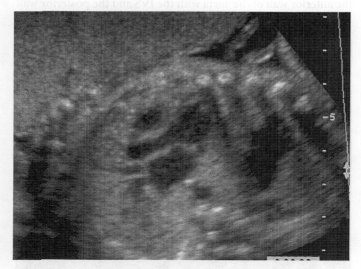

FIGURE 9–9. Long-axis view of the aorta arising from the left ventricle. Continuity can be appreciated between the anterior wall of the aorta and the interventricular septum, and the posterior wall of the aorta with the anterior leaflet of the mitral valve.

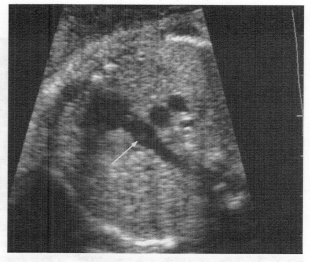

FIGURE 9–11. Continuous angulation of the transducer toward the fetal right shoulder from the long-axis view of the aorta, resulting in a long-axis view of the pulmonary artery (arrow) arising from the right ventricle. This is the three-vessel view.

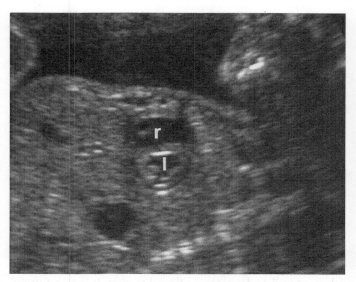

FIGURE 9–12. Sagittal view of the fetus, showing a short-axis view of the right (r) and left (l) ventricles.

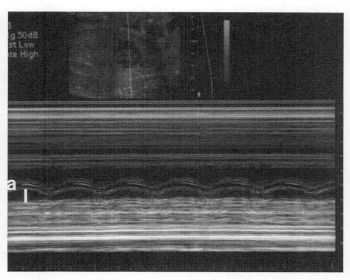

FIGURE 9–14. Simultaneous M-mode through the aorta (a) and the left atrium (l) is a useful means of assessing a dysrhythmia.

The short-axis view of the ventricles is useful for obtaining measurements of the ventricular free walls and IVS, as well as chamber size. Color Doppler should be used in this view to again evaluate the IVS for defects. With the color Doppler activated, the ventricles should be scanned from the apex to the level of the atrioventricular valves. If color is seen crossing the septum, pulsed Doppler can be used to confirm a septal defect.

From the short-axis view of the ventricles, a short-axis view of the great vessels can be obtained by angling the transducer slightly toward the fetal left shoulder (Fig. 9–13). In this view,

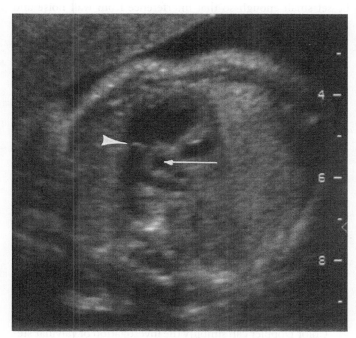

FIGURE 9–13. Angulation toward the fetus's left shoulder from the short-axis view of the ventricles (Fig. 9–12), resulting in a short-axis view of the great vessels. The pulmonary artery (arrowhead) can be seen normally draping over the aorta (arrow).

the aorta appears as a circular structure with the pulmonary artery draping over it. The aortic, pulmonic, and tricuspid valves are usually well visualized in this projection. The main pulmonary artery can often be seen bifurcating into the ductus arteriosus and the right pulmonary artery. This view provides a reasonable angle from which the pulmonary and tricuspid valves can be interrogated with pulsed Doppler for insufficiency or stenosis or atresia. The great vessels can also be evaluated for size discrepancy in the short-axis view.

Simultaneous M-mode through the aorta and left atrium is another useful method for evaluating fetal dysrhythmias (Fig. 9–14). The atrial contraction will be depicted in atrial wall movement, while the ventricular response is reflected in the motion of the aortic valve.

In the normal heart, the short-axis view of the great vessels confirms the perpendicular relationship of the aorta to the pulmonary artery, thereby excluding such defects as complete or *d*-transposition of the great arteries or truncus arteriosus.

The aortic arch view is obtained from a sagittal plane of the fetal torso, with the transducer angled from the left shoulder to the right hemithorax. The aortic arch can be differentiated from the flatter, broader, more caudally located ductal arch by identifying the three brachiocephalic vessels arising from its superior aspect (Fig. 9–15). The aortic arch has been described as having a rounded "candy cane" appearance.[25]

Pulsed Doppler should be used to evaluate the arch from the aortic valve to the descending aorta, looking for areas of increased or decreased velocities. Of particular importance is the section of the arch between the origin of the left subclavian artery and the insertion of the ductus arteriosus, as this is where most *in utero* coarctations occur. It should be borne in mind, however, that diagnosis of coarctation of the aorta is extremely difficult, and a coarctation may be present even in the setting of a normal appearing aortic arch, with normal velocities. When

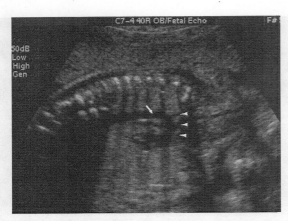

FIGURE 9–15. Sagittal view of the aortic arch (arrow) with the three brachiocephalic vessels (arrowheads) arising from it.

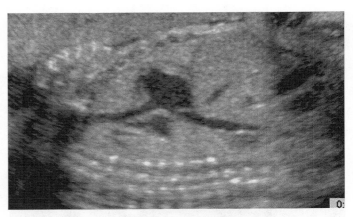

FIGURE 9–17. Right atrial inflow view showing the inferior vena cava and the superior vena cava entering the right atrium.

evaluating the aortic arch, it is also important to remember to confirm a left-sided location of the descending aorta.

The ductal arch view is obtained by returning to a more anteroposterior axis of the thorax. It is often helpful to image the short-axis view of the great vessels and then angle the transducer slightly until the pulmonary artery/ductus arteriosus confluence connects with the descending aorta (Fig. 9–16). The ductal arch has a flatter appearance than the aortic arch. It is often referred to as having a "hockey stick" appearance.[25] The ductal arch is composed the pulmonary artery, ductus arteriosus, and the descending aorta.

The final view that should be obtained is the right atrial inflow view, allowing visualization of the inferior and superior vena cavae. This is achieved by sliding the transducer rightward from the aortic arch while remaining in a sagittal plane of the fetus (Fig. 9–17).

Pulsed Doppler

Pulsed Doppler substantially enhances the ability to detect cardiac malformations *in utero*. It is an effective means of quantitating flow velocity in the cardiac vessels and across the heart

valves, as well as determining flow direction. It is also a useful adjunct in differentiating dysrhythmias.[21] In a standard fetal echocardiogram, pulsed Doppler should be used to evaluate all four cardiac valves, both proximal and distal to the valve. Pulsed Doppler interrogation of the foramen ovale should be done to document the presence of flow into the left atrium. The ductus arteriosus and aortic arch should also be interrogated to document the presence and normality of flow. In addition, pulsed Doppler of the pulmonary veins can be used to confirm their presence and course into the left atrium.

Technical factors to consider include attempting to place the Doppler cursor in the area of interest at an angle as close to 0° as possible by using transducer angulation and the angle correction capabilities of the equipment used. The sample gate should be set small enough so that interference from wall noise and transmitted flow from adjoining vessels or valves can be minimized. Wall filter should be set to eliminate unnecessary noise without losing essential low flow information, and velocity scale should be set to record maximum velocities accurately.

Color Doppler

Color Doppler also plays an essential role in fetal echocardiography by providing a more efficient and expedient means of assessing normal and abnormal flow patterns in the fetal heart. Color Doppler supplies information on the presence or absence of flow, flow direction, and flow patterns. By superimposing color over the gray-scale image, morphologic and hemodynamic information can be assessed simultaneously.

Color Doppler allows visualization of flow in entire structures, such as the aortic arch, thus making it much more time efficient than pulsed Doppler. This efficiency is also prudent when imaging a fetus because color Doppler imaging produces lower peak intensities than pulsed Doppler.

Color Doppler can simplify the investigation of valvular stenosis or insufficiency, again, by sampling a large area and identifying areas of turbulence or flow reversal. In some cases, color may aid in visualizing such cardiac structures as the outflow

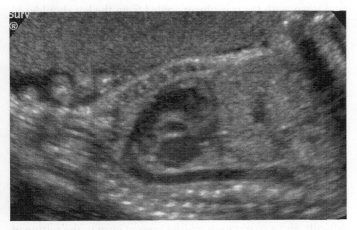

FIGURE 9–16. Sagittal view of the ductal arch with a flatter appearance than the aortic arch.

tracts, which may be difficult to see with gray-scale imaging alone. Also, it may occasionally lead to detection of an abnormality not obvious on the gray-scale image, such as valvular stenosis, small VSDs, and flow reversal within the aortic and ductal arches.

Equipment used for fetal echocardiography should have specific fetal cardiac capabilities utilizing higher pulse repetition frequencies, which allow color imaging at a frame rate fast enough to evaluate the rapid fetal heart rate. Using a narrow color field or reducing the image depth, when possible, may be necessary to maintain an adequate frame rate.

It is important to remember that color Doppler will only provide mean velocity information; therefore, pulsed Doppler is a necessary adjunct to color Doppler to provide quantitative information regarding peak velocities.

Power Doppler

Power Doppler, in general, may hold several advantages over color Doppler such as increased sensitivity, lack of aliasing, and direction independence. In the fetal heart, however, flow direction and maximum velocities are essential in making an accurate diagnosis. Therefore, power Doppler is typically not useful except for establishing the presence of blood flow.

M-Mode

Although M-mode echocardiography is not routinely necessary in fetal echocardiographic examinations, it is essential to differentiate some dysrhythmias.[27] By placing the M-mode cursor through both an atrial and ventricular wall or structure simultaneously, the response of both structures can be visualized, aiding in identifying the type of dysrhythmia. M-mode can also be used to acquire measurements of chamber size and wall thickness; however, it is not absolutely necessary because these measurements can also be obtained from two-dimensional (2D) images.

M-mode is also helpful in evaluating contractility in heart abnormalities, which may affect wall motion, such as cardiomyopathies, and is a quick and accurate method of measuring fetal heart rate.

Three- and Four-Dimensional Ultrasound

The advances in three-dimensional (3D) and four-dimensional (4D) ultrasound have recently been applied to evaluate the fetal heart.

Two-dimensional imaging of the fetal heart remains the gold standard; however, there are advantages to 3D volume imaging. By obtaining a volume set of the fetal heart, a third scan plane is obtained. This may be advantageous when a fetus is in a difficult position.[28,29]

Several 3D/4D techniques have been applied to scan the fetal heart. The most common include spatiotemporal image correlation (STIC) and multiplanar reconstruction.

STIC: The transducer performs a sweep and a volume set is acquired. The images are then correlated with the fetal heart rate and a complete cardiac cycle is produced.[28,29]

Multiplanar reconstruction: A volume set is obtained and all three image planes are displayed on the screen. The sonographer or physician can then manipulate each plane as needed to obtain a surface rendering in a fourth image.[28,29]

ANATOMY AND PHYSIOLOGY

Several important structural and physiologic differences exist between the fetal and adult cardiovascular systems.[14] Unlike the adult, fetal oxygen and carbon dioxide exchange takes place in the placenta. For oxygenated blood to reach the systemic circulation and deoxygenated blood to return to the placenta for oxygenation, the fetal cardiovascular system contains several shunts not present in the adult.

In utero, oxygenated blood travels from the placenta to the fetus via the umbilical vein. After entering the fetus, the majority of this blood travels through the ductus venosus, bypassing the liver, and entering the inferior vena cava (IVC). The remainder of this oxygenated blood enters the liver and mixes with the portal circulation.

After entering the IVC, this oxygenated blood mixes with deoxygenated blood returning from the lower extremities of the fetus. It then enters the right atrium. As it enters the right atrium, the majority of blood is shunted across the foramen ovale into the left atrium. A smaller amount of blood mixes with the desaturated blood returning from the fetal head and upper extremities. This blood travels into the right atrium and into the pulmonary artery. Resistance to blood flow is high *in utero*; therefore, the majority of the blood that enters the pulmonary artery passes directly into the descending aorta via the ductus arteriosus.

The blood that was shunted through the foramen ovale into the left atrium mixes with a small amount of desaturated blood returned from the lungs by way of the pulmonary veins. This blood then enters the left ventricle and then the aorta. As this blood travels through the aortic arch, a majority passes through the head and neck vessels to supply the fetal head and upper extremities. The remainder continues down the descending aorta, mixes with blood from the ductus arteriosus, and flows out of the fetus by way of the umbilical arteries to the placenta.

The three shunts present *in utero*, the ductus venosus, the foramen ovale, and the ductus arteriosus, all normally close after birth. The ductus arteriosus closes almost immediately after birth. This results in increased pressure within the left atrium which combined with decreased pressure in the right atrium causes the foramen ovale to close. Complete fusion of the foramen ovale is usually complete by 1 year of age. The umbilical arteries also close immediately after birth. This leads to closure of the ductus venosus.

CONGENITAL CARDIAC ABNORMALITIES

Ventricular Septal Defect

The pooled reported frequency of congenital heart lesions among affected abortuses and stillborn infants shows that ventricular septal defect (VSD) is the most common type of heart defect found (see Table 9–1).[14]

In children, VSDs account for 20–57% of cases of congenital heart defects.[2] Unfortunately, it is also one the most commonly missed defects *in utero*. The sonographic diagnosis of a VSD is based on identifying an interruption in the ventricular septum. This area of dropout may be bordered by a hyperechoic specular reflector, representing the blunted edge of the intact portion of the septum (Fig. 9–18A). The subcostal four-chamber view is often the most useful view in detecting a VSD.

VSDs are classified into membranous and muscular defects. Membranous VSDs occur at the base of heart, near the valves. Membranous VSDs are the most common type and usually occur in isolation. Muscular VSDs are located in the muscular septum, at the apex of the heart. Muscular VSDs are divided into four types: inlet, outlet, trabecular, and apical defects. They are typically multiple and are characterized by their location.[14]

VSDs vary in size and may be singular or multiple. Obviously, smaller defects are more difficult to recognize *in utero*. In addition, spontaneous closure of a VSD may occur during later gestation. Therefore, a defect that was present earlier in pregnancy may not be present when reevaluated.

Pulsed and color Doppler are useful in making the diagnosis of a VSD. In fact, some small defects that are virtually unseen by 2D alone may be visualized with the utilization of color (Fig. 9–18B). However, it should be borne in mind that because

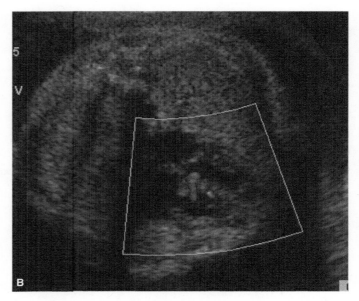

FIGURE 9–18B. Subcostal, four-chamber view of a small membranous ventricular septal defect shown by color Doppler.

of the near equal pressures of the right and left ventricles *in utero*, flow across a small VSD may not be appreciated by either color or pulsed Doppler.

Atrial Septal Defect

Atrial septal defects (ASDs) account for approximately 6.7% of congenital heart disease in live-born infants.[30] Overall, ASDs are twice as common in females as in males. It is difficult to make the diagnosis of ASD *in utero* because of the normal atrial shunt, the foramen ovale, which allows blood flow from the right atrium to the left atrium in the fetus. Most *in utero* ASDs are best visualized in the subcostal four-chamber view (Fig. 9–19).

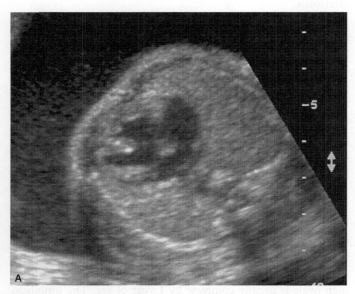

FIGURE 9–18A. Subcostal, four-chamber view showing an anechoic area in the membranous portion of the interventricular septum representing a ventricular septal defect.

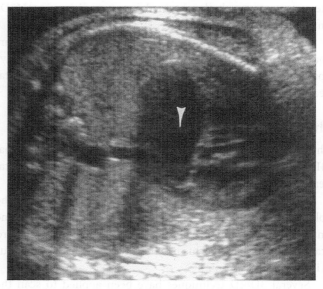

FIGURE 9–19. Subcostal, four-chamber view showing an anechoic area (arrowhead) in the interatrial septum representing an atrial septal defect.

An ostium secundum ASD would appear as a larger than expected area of dropout in the vicinity of the foramen ovale. An ostium primum ASD would result in the absence of the lower portion of the atrial septum, just above the atrioventricular valves. As with VSDs, color Doppler may be a useful adjunct in making the diagnosis.

Atrioventricular Septal Defect

Atrioventricular septal defect (AVSD) refers to a constellation of cardiac malformations that include abnormal development of the interatrial septum, the IVS, and the atrioventricular (mitral and tricuspid) valves. It is also referred to as an atrioventricular canal defect or endocardial cushion defect. Approximately 30% of AVSDs in the fetus are associated with polysplenia.[3] Of these, most are accompanied by complete heart block. Chromosomal abnormalities, especially Down's syndrome, are associated in up to 78% of cases.[3] When an AVSD is present without complete heart block, it is more likely to be associated with abnormal chromosomes.

A complete AVSD can usually be appreciated from either a subcostal or an apical four-chamber view (Fig. 9–20A). The endocardial cushion is absent, creating a wide opening within the center of the heart (Fig. 9–20B). The continuity between the interatrial and interventricular septa and the atrioventricular valves is lost. Instead of identifying separate mitral and tricuspid valves, one single multileaflet valve is seen.

A partial form of AVSD occurs less frequently. With this, two atrioventricular valves are present; however, their leaflet formation is always abnormal. This may be difficult to appreciate by ultrasound, with the presence of an atrial and a VSD being the only clue that an abnormality is present. In a partial AVSD, the apical four-chamber view is useful in demonstrating

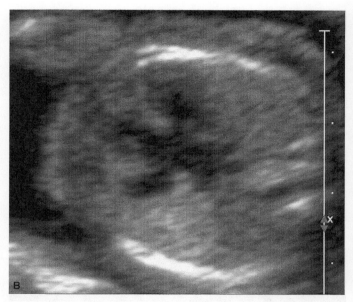

FIGURE 9–20B. Apical four-chamber view in the same fetus. The valve is open showing the large endocardial cushion defect.

the abnormal insertion level of the atrioventricular valves. In the normal heart, the tricuspid valve has a more apical insertion than the mitral valve. When a partial AVSD is present, the two atrioventricular valves appear to insert at the same level.[5]

Additional echocardiographic views of the heart such as a short-axis view and long-axis views of the aorta and pulmonary artery may be useful in defining the extent of the AVSD, as well as identifying associated cardiac malformations.

Hypoplastic Left Heart Syndrome

Hypoplastic left heart syndrome (HLHS) refers to a group of structural abnormalities affecting the left side of the heart. Its hallmark is a small left ventricle, which can be accompanied by aortic atresia, a hypoplastic ascending aorta, an atretic or hypoplastic mitral valve, and a small left atrium (Fig. 9–21).[4] HLHS results from decreased blood flow into or out of the left ventricle. This lack of blood flow results in the underdevelopment of the left ventricle.[6] Sonographically, a very small left ventricle is usually seen. This is apparent in either a four-chamber view or a short-axis view of the ventricles.

When a small left ventricle is identified, accompanying abnormalities of the mitral and aortic valves must be determined. With valve atresia or hypoplasia, the valve orifice will appear smaller than normal for gestational age. Color and pulsed Doppler will demonstrate a lack of blood flow through the valve. The aorta itself will also appear small or atretic. In some cases, the walls of the aorta will appear more hyperechoic than expected. Blood flow through the ascending aorta may be absent or reversed. Reversal of flow represents blood flowing through the ductus arteriosus and then retrograde through the ascending aorta.

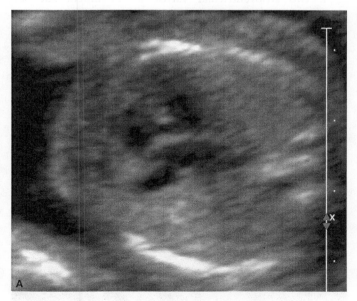

FIGURE 9–20A. Apical four-chamber view in a fetus with an atrioventricular septal defect. A singular atrioventricular valve can be seen closing within a ventricular and atrial septal defect.

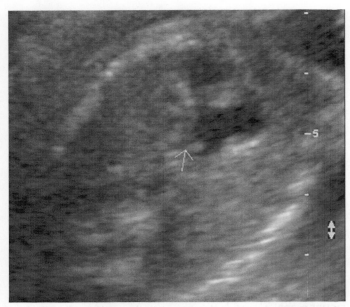

FIGURE 9–21. Apical four-chamber view in a fetus with hypoplastic left heart syndrome. The left heart (arrow) is nearly obliterated, whereas the right ventricle and right atrium are enlarged.

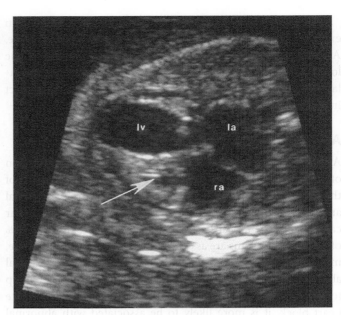

FIGURE 9–22. Subcostal, four-chamber view in a fetus with hypoplastic right heart syndrome. The right ventricle (arrow) is nearly obliterated, whereas the right atrium (ra), left atrium (la), and left ventricle (lv) are enlarged.

HLHS has a very poor prognosis, carrying a 25% mortality rate within the first week of life. All untreated infants die within the first 6 weeks. Treatment of this lesion usually involves surgical repair via a two-stage Norwood procedure or heart transplantation.[10]

Hypoplastic Right Heart

Hypoplastic right heart is the result of either pulmonary atresia with intact ventricular septum or tricuspid atresia.[14] As with HLHS, it occurs when normal blood flow into or out of the ventricle is compromised. Sonographic findings include a small right ventricle accompanied by a small or atretic and pulmonary artery and valve. Either an apical or a subcostal four-chamber view is most useful in assessing this abnormality (Fig. 9–22). Color and pulsed Doppler will confirm the absence of blood flow across the pulmonary valve.

In tricuspid atresia, flow will be absent or substantially decreased across the tricuspid valve (Fig. 9–23). The pulmonic valve is usually stenotic, so an increased velocity may be appreciated distal to the valve. If severe stenosis is present, no flow may be detectable, making differentiation from pulmonary atresia difficult. Color Doppler is essential for evaluating the IVS for defects. As stated previously, this should be done in a subcostal four-chamber view.

Both tricuspid atresia and pulmonary atresia with intact ventricular septum are associated with a large left atrium and a dilated, often hypertrophied, left ventricle. The aortic root may be dilated with either entity. This left-sided enlargement is a result of the vast quantity of blood being forced across the foramen ovale because it is unable to enter the right ventricle.[10] Retrograde blood flow within the ductus arteriosus is also

possible because of the increased flow through the aorta and the accompanying decreased or absent flow through the pulmonary artery.

Univentricular Heart

Univentricular heart is defined as the presence of two atrioventricular valves or a common atrioventricular valve emptying into a single ventricle. From either four-chamber view, only three chambers are present, two atria and one large ventricle (Fig. 9–24).

If two atrioventricular valves are identified, but one appears atretic, the most likely diagnosis is tricuspid or mitral atresia, which is usually considered a defect separate from

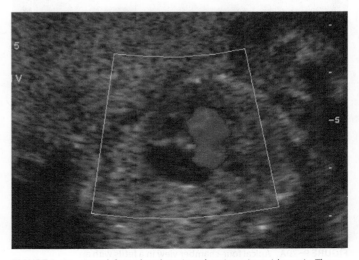

FIGURE 9–23. Apical, four-chamber view showing tricuspid atresia. There is no flow across the echogenic, nonmobile tricuspid valve.

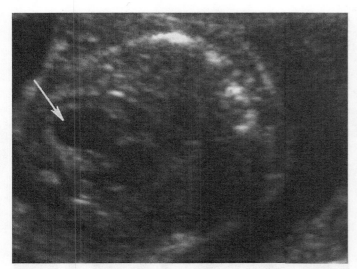

FIGURE 9-24. Subcostal, four-chamber view showing the single ventricle (arrow) present in a univentricular heart.

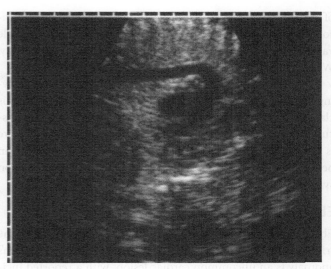

FIGURE 9-25. Sagittal view of the aortic arch showing a normal appearing arch in the setting of a coarctation of the aorta.

a univentricular heart. The aorta and pulmonary artery are almost always transposed in the setting of a univentricular heart. Pulmonary atresia or stenosis is also common. Univentricular heart has been associated with asplenia or polysplenia in 13% of cases.[11]

Coarctation of the Aorta

When the diagnosis of coarctation of the aorta is made *in utero* or in early infancy, it is easily correctable, but if left undetected, the effects can be devastating. Coarctation is a narrowing of the aortic lumen, which results in an obstruction to blood flow. In 98% of cases, this narrowing occurs between the origin of the left subclavian artery and the ductus arteriosus.[12] The severity of a coarctation can range from a slight narrowing of the distal end of the arch to severe hypoplasia of the entire arch.

Intuitively, the *in utero* diagnosis of a coarctation seems straightforward. It is, however, extremely difficult. Subtle changes associated with coarctation, such as a narrowing of the aortic arch, may not be appreciated, even when the arch is well visualized (Fig. 9-25). This may be caused by the physiologic shunts present in the fetal heart, allowing for the severity of the narrowing not to present until after birth.

These shunts may also explain why Doppler velocities may not be affected in the presence of a coarctation. Interestingly, one of the most reliable signs of a coarctation *in utero* to be reported is a right ventricular dimension greater than that expected for a gestational age (Fig. 9-26). Pulmonary artery size may also be increased.[13]

This finding may be subtle; therefore, measurements of the ventricles and great vessels should always be performed in the fetus at risk for coarctation such as those with Turner's syndrome (XO) or a prior family history of left heart anomalies. It is also important to remember that coarctation of the aorta is often a progressive lesion, with the distal arch becoming more

hypoplastic as pregnancy advances. Reversal of blood flow through the foramen ovale is often, but not always, present with a coarctation.

Aortic and Pulmonic Stenosis

Congenital aortic stenosis is an obstruction of the left ventricular outflow tract. Aortic stenosis is classified into three types: valvular, subvalvular, and supravalvular stenosis. Sixty to 70%

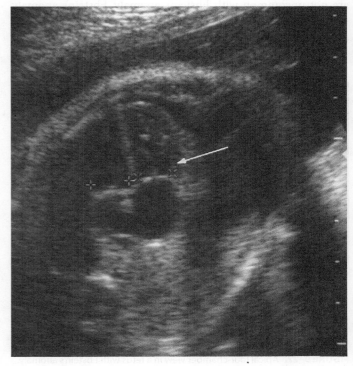

FIGURE 9-26. Apical four-chamber view in a fetus with coarctation of the aorta. The only clue in this case was a right ventricle (arrow) that was slightly larger than expected for gestational age.

of patients with aortic stenosis have valvular stenosis. On ultrasound, aortic stenosis may appear as a thickened or immobile valve. Flow distal to the aortic valve is increased in velocity. With severe stenosis, no flow or reversed flow may be seen.[14]

Congenital pulmonic stenosis is an obstruction or narrowing of the right ventricular outflow tract. Pulmonary stenosis is classified as obstructive or valvular. A thickened valve or muscular ring may be seen by ultrasound. By pulsed Doppler, there is increased velocity distal to the valve. Pulmonic stenosis can been found in the recipient twin of twin-to-twin transfusion syndrome.[14,31]

Ebstein's Anomaly

Ebstein's anomaly is defined as the inferior displacement of the tricuspid valve leaflets from their normal location. Ebstein's anomaly is an uncommon cardiac lesion, with a reported incidence of 1 in 20,000 live births.[15] It has often been associated with maternal lithium use; however, more recent data have shown this association to be substantially less than previously reported.[16]

The sonographic diagnosis of Ebstein's anomaly is usually straightforward. Apical displacement of the tricuspid valve leaflets is readily apparent from either four-chamber view (Fig. 9–27). This results in "atrialization" of the right ventricle, which, along with the tricuspid insufficiency that is almost always present, causes an often massively enlarged right atrium. This is turn, causes the axis of the heart to be severely levocardic, giving the heart a very horizontal position within the fetal chest. Pulmonary atresia or stenosis, as well as dysrhythmias are not uncommon with Ebstein's anomaly. Ebstein's anomaly frequently causes *in utero* cardiac dysfunction, resulting in cardiomegaly and hydrops fetalis.

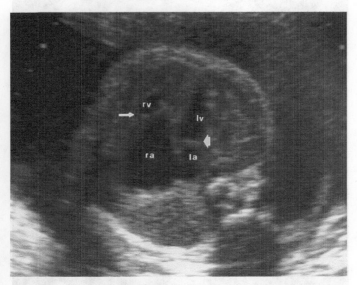

FIGURE 9–27. Apical four-chamber view in a fetus with Ebstein's anomaly. The tricuspid valve (arrow) is displaced apically, causing atrialization of the right atrium (ra) and a small right ventricle (rv). la = left atrium, lv = left ventricle.

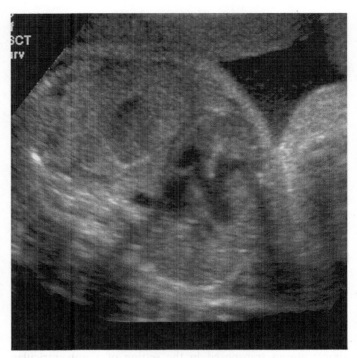

FIGURE 9–28. Apical view of the heart in a fetus with tetralogy of Fallot showing the aorta overriding a ventricular septal defect.

Tetralogy of Fallot

Tetralogy of Fallot consists of four classic structural defects: a VSD, aortic override of the VSD, pulmonary stenosis, and right ventricular hypertrophy.[14] Because of the normal shunts present in the fetus, the right ventricular hypertrophy may not occur *in utero*. To diagnose this malformation *in utero*, an aortic root overriding the IVS must be identified (Fig. 9–28). It is often not possible to make this diagnosis solely from a four-chamber view, either apical or subcostal. The VSD may be seen on the four-chamber view; however, color Doppler should be used to confirm that the defect is real and not artifactual. A slight angulation of the transducer toward the fetus' right shoulder from a subcostal four-chamber view, or cephalad from an apical four-chamber view should allow the overriding aorta to be appreciated. Dilatation of the aortic root is usually present in later gestation.[17]

Once an overriding aorta has been observed, the diagnosis of tetralogy of Fallot relies on the evaluation of the right ventricular outflow tract. This is usually best accomplished in either a long-axis view of the pulmonary artery or a short-axis view of the great vessels. The pulmonary artery will appear small, often so much so that it cannot be identified. Pulsed Doppler interrogation of the pulmonic valve may show a greatly increased velocity, indicative of stenosis, or absence of flow in the setting of severe stenosis or atresia. Retrograde flow through the ductus arteriosus may also be present. Making an accurate diagnosis of tetralogy of Fallot relies on identifying the pulmonary artery. If a pulmonary artery cannot be visualized, the differential diagnosis would include pulmonary atresia with a VSD. If there is no main pulmonary artery arising from the right ventricle but smaller pulmonary artery branches are seen arising from the overriding aorta, the diagnosis is truncus arteriosus.

When the diagnosis of tetralogy of Fallot is established, the laterality of the aortic arch should be determined because approximately 25% of cases are associated with a right-sided aortic arch.[19]

Truncus Arteriosus

Truncus arteriosus is rare. It is an embryological failure that results in a single great vessel arising from the heart.[14] The systemic, pulmonary, and coronary circulations are all supplied by this single great vessel. Sonographically, truncus arteriosus appears very similar to tetralogy of Fallot. A VSD is present, and the singular great vessel overrides the defect, similar to the aorta in tetralogy of Fallot (Fig. 9–29). The difference is that the pulmonary artery arises from this great vessel, not the right ventricle. Depending on the type of truncal defect present, the number and position of the pulmonary arteries on the great vessel will vary.[32]

The *in utero* diagnosis of truncus arteriosus may be challenging. The definitive diagnosis can be made only if the origin of the pulmonary artery can be identified arising from the large, single great vessel. Because of the inherent technical factors associated with fetal echocardiography, this may be difficult.

As with tetralogy of Fallot, identification of the overriding great vessel is usually accomplished with slight angulation from either the apical or the subcostal four-chamber view. Several views, including long- and short-axis views of the right outflow tract, must be obtained to confirm the absence of a pulmonary artery. Evaluation of the aortic arch is also important. A right-sided arch has been reported in 15–30% of cases. Interruption of the aortic arch has also been associated with truncus arteriosus.[32]

Complete Transposition of the Great Arteries

Eighty percent of fetuses with transposition of the great arteries have complete or *d*-transposition.[20] In this setting, the connections between the atria and ventricles are normal, meaning that the right atrium connects through the tricuspid valve to the right ventricle, and the left atrium connects through the mitral valve to the left ventricle. However, the aorta arises from the right ventricle, and the pulmonary artery arises from the left ventricle. This results in two parallel circulations that will only allow mixing of venous and arterial blood through the ductus arteriosus, interatrial, or interventricular connections.

The four-chamber views are often normal in the presence of complete transposition. The diagnosis is made by identifying the aorta arising from the right ventricle and connecting to the aortic arch and descending aorta, and identifying the pulmonary artery arising from the left ventricle and then branching into the left and right pulmonary arteries. From a long-axis view of the great vessels, the aorta and pulmonary artery will appear to run in a parallel fashion (Fig. 9–30). The short-axis view, at the level of the great vessels, is also useful in making this diagnosis. In this view, both the pulmonary artery and aorta appear as circular structures adjacent to each other, instead of their normal relationship of the pulmonary artery draping over the aorta. A VSD is present in 20% of cases, so color Doppler should be used to assess the IVS thoroughly.[21]

Congenitally Corrected Transposition of the Great Arteries

Congenitally corrected or *l*-transposition of the great arteries comprises the remaining 20% of transposition cases.[20] In corrected transposition, the great vessels arise from the correct sides; however, the left and right ventricles and the left and right atrioventricular valves are transposed. In other words, the right atrium is connected to the left ventricle, and the left atrium is

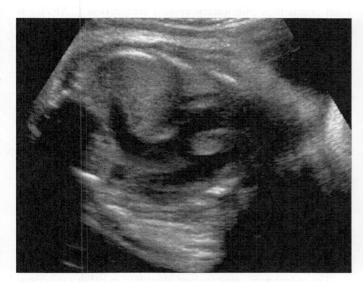

FIGURE 9–29. Subcostal view of the heart in a fetus with truncus arteriosus showing a single truncal vessel overriding a ventricular septal defect.

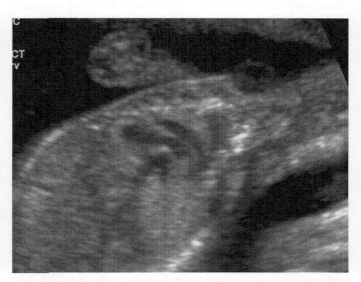

FIGURE 9–30. Complete transposition of the great arteries. The aorta and pulmonary arteries are running parallel.

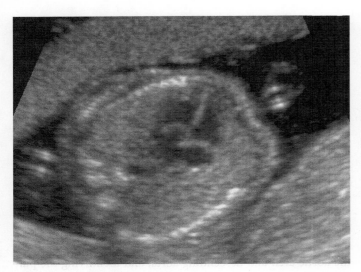

FIGURE 9–31. Corrected transposition of the great arteries. Note how the tricuspid valve is slightly superior to the mitral valve. In the normal heart, the tricuspid valve is more apical.

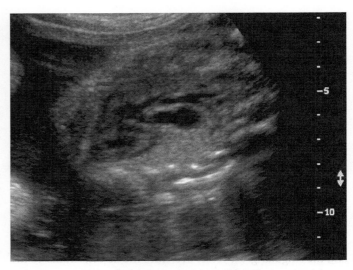

FIGURE 9–32. Double outlet right ventricle in a fetus. The aorta and the pulmonary artery are both arising from the right ventricle.

connected to the right ventricle. The aorta then arises from the left-sided right ventricle, and the pulmonary artery arises from the right-sided left ventricle. Blood circulation in this abnormality is in series, as it is in the normal heart; therefore, surgical correction is not required unless associated cardiac anomalies are present.

Sonographic identification of this abnormality can be subtle. Correct identification of the cardiac chambers is crucial in making this diagnosis. In the normal heart, the tricuspid valve insertion is slightly more apical than the mitral valve (Fig. 9–31). The right ventricle also has a prominent moderator band near the apex that is usually seen on fetal echocardiography. If these findings appear to be left sided, the diagnosis of corrected transposition should be considered. As with complete transposition, the great vessels exit the heart in a more parallel relationship than seen in the normal heart. This may be appreciated on a short-axis view of the great vessels but is far more subtle than in complete transposition. It is not uncommon to miss the diagnosis of corrected transposition *in utero*, particularly when no other cardiac defects are present.

VSDs have been reported in about 50% of patients with corrected transposition. Pulmonic stenosis and abnormalities of the mitral and tricuspid valves are also common.[20]

Double-Outlet Right Ventricle

Double-outlet right ventricle (DORV) is a condition in which more than 50% of both the aortic root and the main pulmonary artery arise from the right ventricle. A VSD is almost always present.[22]

This, again, is one of many cardiac defects easily missed when only a four-chamber view is obtained. The long-axis views of the aorta and pulmonary artery are most useful in identifying both great vessels as arising from the right ventricle (Fig. 9–32). In DORV, the most common relationship of the great vessels is side by side, with the aorta right and lateral to the pulmonary artery. When this occurs, the normal perpendicular course of the great vessels is lost. As with transposition of the great arteries, they will appear parallel to each other. Differentiating DORV from transposition relies on identifying both great vessels as arising from the right ventricle. This can be challenging *in utero*. As with all congenital cardiac abnormalities, the surgical intervention depends heavily on the presence or absence of other cardiac anomalies. Therefore, a thorough interrogation of the fetal heart must be undertaken.

Double outlet left ventricle, in which both the aortic root and the main pulmonary artery arise from the left ventricle, has also been reported, but it is exceedingly rare.[23]

Total Anomalous Pulmonary Venous Connection

Total anomalous pulmonary venous connection (TAPVC) is an anomaly in which all of the pulmonary veins drain either directly into the right atrium or into channels that terminate in the right atrium.[24] In the normal heart, venous return is to the left atrium. TAPVC is rare and, as with many other congenital cardiac anomalies, is a difficult diagnosis to make in the fetus.

The diagnosis relies on the inability to identify any pulmonary veins entering the left atrium and the identification of all four pulmonary veins entering the right atrium or abnormally converging and entering the superior vena cava, IVC, portal vein, or ductus venosus.

If any pulmonary veins are seen entering the left atrium, or if all pulmonary veins are not seen entering an ectopic structure, the diagnosis of TAPVC is excluded. Partial anomalous pulmonary venous connection may be present in this setting, but cannot be definitively ascertained *in utero*.

The pulmonary veins are best identified in either a subcostal or an apical four-chamber view. Usually only the two superior

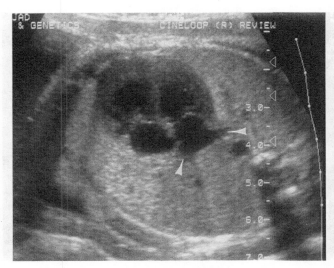

FIGURE 9–33. Apical four-chamber view showing the two normal superior pulmonary veins appropriately entering the left atrium.

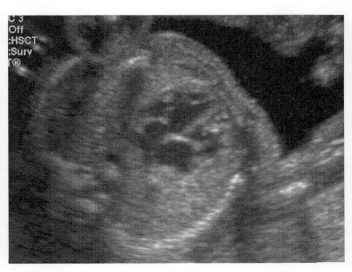

FIGURE 9–35. Four-chamber view showing mesocardia, with the apex of the heart pointing midline.

veins are identified *in utero* (Fig. 9–33), adding to the difficulty of making this diagnosis. Enlargement of the right ventricle and pulmonary artery may be secondary signs of TAPVC.[24]

When enlargement of these structures is present and the normal pulmonary veins cannot be identified as they drain into the left atrium, the possibility of TAPVC should be entertained. Using color Doppler to identify an abnormal convergence of veins posterior to the right atrium may also be useful.

Cardiac Axis and Position

As stated previously, determining cardiac axis and position is one of the first steps in performing a fetal echocardiogram. Abnormal cardiac axis or position may be an important clue that a structural defect is present.[14]

Normal cardiac axis is termed levocardia, meaning the apex of the heart points to the left side of the fetal chest. Even if a heart is levocardic, if its axis is > 45 ± 20° to the left, an abnormality may be present. Cardiac anomalies that result in severe levocardia are usually those that cause an enlarged right atrium, such as Ebstein's anomaly (Fig. 9–34). It is thought that this enlargement causes the heart to shift and lie more horizontally. Mesocardia occurs when the apex of the heart points midline. Mesocardia is uncommon but has been associated with transposition of the great vessels[14] (Fig. 9–35).

The terms *dextrocardia* or *dextroversion* refer to the apex of the heart pointing abnormally to the right (Fig. 9–36). Isolated dextrocardia is associated with a structural cardiac abnormality in 95% of cases.[14] Dextrocardia associated with abdominal

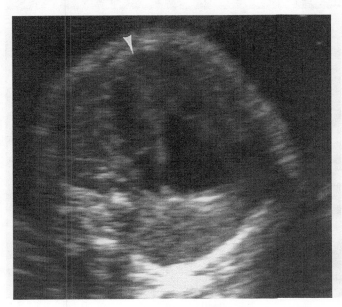

FIGURE 9–34. Severe levocardia in a fetus with Ebstein's anomaly. The apex of the heart (arrowhead) is angled too far to the left chest.

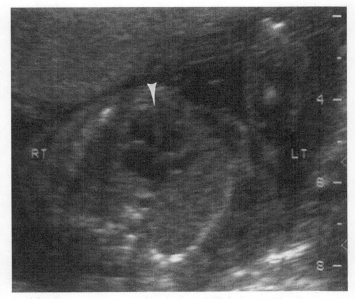

FIGURE 9–36. Dextrocardia of the fetal heart. The apex of the heart (arrowhead) is pointing incorrectly to the right chest.

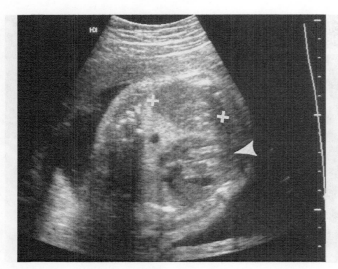

FIGURE 9–37. Dextroposition of the fetal heart. The apex of the heart (arrowhead) is pointing correctly to the left chest; however, the entire heart is being displaced into the right chest by the mass in the left chest (calipers).

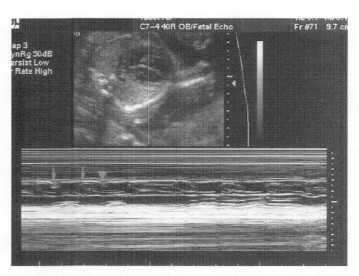

FIGURE 9–38. M-mode tracing of premature atrial contractions in a fetus. Normally spaced atrial beats (arrows) can be seen followed by a premature beat (arrowhead).

situs abnormalities carries a lower risk. Dextroposition is present when the apex of the heart points normally to the left side of the fetal chest, but the heart itself is positioned in the right chest (Fig. 9–37).

When dextroposition is present, two possibilities should be considered. Either the heart is being displaced to the right by a left-sided thoracic defect such as a diaphragmatic hernia or a cystic adenomatoid malformation, or the heart is filling a potential space in the right thorax. This may be indicative of an absent or hypoplastic right lung.

Whenever a fetal echocardiogram is performed, special attention should be paid to identifying cardiac axis and position. Any deviation from normal may be indicative of an underlying intra- or extracardiac defect.

Dysrhythmias

The normal fetal heart rate is regular and between 100 and 180 beats/min. A dysrhythmia is present if the fetal heart rate is noted to be abnormally fast, slow, or irregular. Dysrhythmias are detected in approximately 1% of fetuses.[30]

Most dysrhythmias are benign; however, in a small number of cases, they may be life threatening. M-mode is the most useful method of assessing the type of dysrhythmia present. As stated previously, the M-mode cursor should be placed simultaneously through a structure in the fetal heart that represents an atrial beat (atria wall or atrioventricular valve) and the ventricular response (ventricle wall or semilunar valve).

Premature atrial contractions (PACs) are the most common dysrhythmia encountered in the fetus (Fig. 9–38).[14] They have been associated with a redundant foraminal flap, as well as maternal use of caffeine, cigarettes, or alcohol.[33] Rarely, PACs may evolve into a sustained tachycardia; however, most resolve around the time of delivery and seldom present a problem in the newborn. Tachycardias are the second most common

dysrhythmia seen in the fetal population. Tachycardias are classified as:

- Supraventricular tachycardia (SVT)—heart rate of 180–280 beats/min, with atrioventricular concordance (Fig. 9–39)
- Atrial flutter—atrial heart rate of 280–400 beats/min, with variable ventricular response (Fig. 9–40)
- Atrial fibrillation—atrial heart rate of >400 beats/min, with variable ventricular response

Sustained SVT can result in fetal hydrops or death and represents a fetal medical emergency.[34] SVT is associated with structural heart disease in 5–10% of cases.[35]

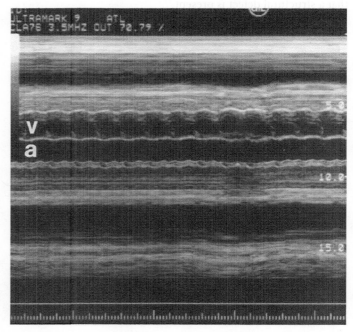

FIGURE 9–39. M-mode tracing of supraventricular tachycardia in a fetus. Both the ventricular (v) and atrial (a) rates were 240 beats/min.

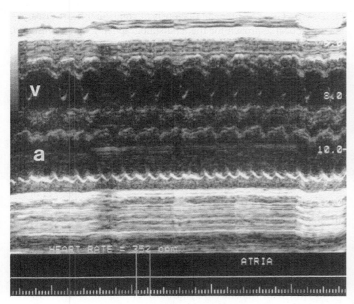

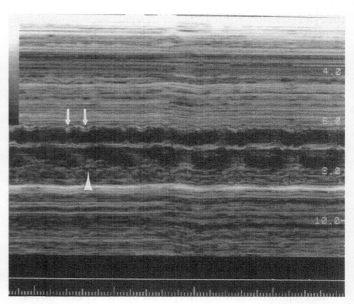

FIGURE 9–40. M-mode tracing of a fetal heart with atrial flutter. The atrial (a) rate was 352 beats/min, while the ventricular (v) rate was 180 beats/min.

FIGURE 9–41. M-mode tracing of a fetal heart with a 2:1 heart block. The atrial rate is 120 beats/min, whereas the ventricular rate is 60 beats/min.

The treatment of SVT *in utero* is difficult. Immediate medical therapy should be implemented if there are signs of fetal compromise. Digoxin has been the initial drug of choice when treating fetal SVT; however, several other medications are available and may be used in place of or in combination with digoxin.

Bradycardia may also be encountered in the fetus. Transient bradycardia is often encountered during the course of an ultrasound examination secondary to pressure from the transducer. The bradycardia is resolved when the transducer is removed. This entity should not be confused with pathologic bradycardias that result in a sustained slow heart rate.

Ninety-six percent of fetuses with sustained bradycardia will have second-or third-degree heart block.[14] Second-degree heart block is commonly referred to as a 2:1 or 3:1, etc., heart block, referring to the fact that the ventricular rate will be a submultiple of the atrial rate. In other words, two atrial contractions will occur for every one ventricular contraction, or three atrial contractions will occur for every one ventricular contraction (Fig. 9–41).

Third-degree, or complete, heart block is present when there is complete dissociation between the atrial and ventricular rates, with the atrial rate being faster. Approximately 50% of fetuses with complete heart block have significant structural heart disease, specifically, AVSDs, corrected transposition of the great arteries, cardiac tumors, or a cardiomyopathy.[14] Complete heart block associated with an AVSD is highly suggestive of polysplenia syndrome.[36] In fetuses with complete heart block without structural defects, there is a high association with maternal connective tissue diseases such as lupus.[37]

Second-and third-degree heart blocks are difficult to treat *in utero*. Increasing fetal heart rate through the maternal administration of sympathomimetic agents and placement of an *in utero* pacemaker have been attempted, but with dismal results.[38] Administration of maternal steroids has also been reported.[39]

The prognosis for fetuses with complete heart block and structural heart disease is poor. In fetuses without structural heart disease, outcome is dependent on the atrial and ventricular rate and the presence of fetal hydrops.

References

1. Hoffman JIE. Incidence of congenital heart disease: II. Prenatal incidence. *Pediatr Cardiol.* 1995;16:155-165.

2. Allan LD, Crawford DC, Anderson RH, et al. Spectrum of congenital heart disease detected echocardiographically in prenatal life. *Br Heart J.* 1985;54:523-526.

3. Allan LD. Fetal cardiology. *Ultrasound Obstet Gynecol.* 1994;4:441-444.

4. AIUM Technical Bulletin: performance of the fetal cardiac ultrasound examination. American Institute of Ultrasound in Medicine. *J Ultrasound Med.* 1998;17:601-607.

5. Dolkart LA, Reimers FT. Transvaginal fetal echocardiography in early pregnancy: normative data. *Am J Obstet Gynecol.* 1991;165:688-691.

6. DeVore GR, Medearis AL, Bear MB. Fetal echocardiography: factors that influence imaging of the fetal heart during the second trimester of pregnancy. *J Ultrasound Med.* 1993;12:659-663.

7. McAuliffe FM, Trines J, Nield LE, et al. Early fetal echocardiography—a reliable prenatal diagnosis tool. *Am J Obstet Gynecol.* 2005;193:1253-1259.

8. Allan LD. Diagnosis of fetal cardiac abnormality. *Br J Hosp Med.* 1988;40:290-293.

9. Fliedner R, Kreiselmaier P, Schwarze A, et al. Development of hypoplastic left heart syndrome after diagnosis of aortic stenosis in the first trimester by early echocardiography. *Ultrasound Obstet Gynecol.* 2006;28:106-109.

24. **(A)** In the fetus, the main pulmonary artery bifurcates into the ductus arteriosus and the right pulmonary artery.

25. **(D)** The aortic arch does not have the appearance of a hockey stick. The ductal arch is flat and broader, much like a hockey stick.

26. **(B)** The majority of coarctations occur just distal to where the ductus arteriosus inserts into the aorta. Aortic valve insufficiency is obtained proximal to the aortic valve. Aortic stenosis occurs at the level of the aortic valve. Pulmonary valve insufficiency would be identified in the right ventricle, proximal to the pulmonary valve.

27. **(C)** The ductal arch has a hockey stick appearance. The pulmonary artery, ductus arteriosus, and the descending aorta comprise the ductal arch.

28. **(C)** The most common indication for a fetal echocardiogram is family history. The risk for a reoccurring heart defect is highest when the mother has a defect (10–12%). The percentages are lower with other family members.

29. **(D)** Suboptimal heart views on a 12-week ultrasound are not an indication for a fetal echocardiogram. At 12 weeks, the fetal heart is small and structures are difficult to visualize. If the heart is suboptimal on an 18- to 20-week ultrasound, a fetal echocardiogram should be performed.

30. **(C)** Peak velocities can only be obtained with pulsed Doppler. Color Doppler, however, can help in determining areas of increased velocity or turbulence.

31. **(D)** M-mode is not useful in determining direction of flow. Color or pulsed Doppler can be used to determine direction.

32. **(B)** In the fetus, oxygenated blood travels from the umbilical veins through the ductus venosus, bypassing the liver. This blood then enters the IVC. The blood that enters the liver mixes with the portal system. Once the fetus is born, the ductus venosus closes and becomes the ligamentum venosum of the liver.

33. **(A)** The pulmonary veins enter the left atrium. Pulsed Doppler is helpful in determining appropriate direction and location of the pulmonary veins.

34. **(D)** The Doppler angle should be as close to zero as possible. With a 90° angle, a Doppler signal cannot be obtained.

35. **(D)** The Doppler gate should be small to avoid interference of other structures and vessels.

36. **(A)** Blood flows from the placenta to the fetus by way of the umbilical vein. The umbilical arteries return blood back to the placenta. The ductus venosum is a shunt that allows blood to bypass the liver. The ductus arteriosus shunts blood from the pulmonary artery to the descending aorta.

37. **(C)** Oxygenated blood flows from the placenta through the umbilical vein. Most of this blood bypasses the liver via the ductus venosum and enters the IVC. Deoxygenated blood from the lower extremities travels up the IVC and mixes with the oxygenated blood. This oxygenated and deoxygenated blood then enters the right atrium.

38. **(D)** The umbilical vein is not considered a shunt. It carries blood from the placenta to the fetus. The ductus venosus allows blood to bypass the liver. It closes shortly after birth and becomes the ligamentum venosum in the liver. The foramen ovale shunts blood from the right atrium to the left atrium. The ductus arteriosus is a shunt between the pulmonary artery and the descending aorta. It also closes shortly after birth and becomes the ligamentum arteriosum. Closure of the ductus arteriosus causes a pressure change in the heart. After birth the pressure is higher in the left side of the heart, causing the foramen ovale to close.

39. **(D)** M-mode is not very useful in identifying a VSD in the fetus. It is useful in determining heart rate and rhythm, chamber size, and wall thickness.

40. **(A)** An AVSD is an abnormal development of the interatrial septum, IVS, and the atrioventricular valves (tricuspid and mitral valves).

41. **(A)** With HLHS, there is a decrease in the blood flow coming in or out of the ventricle. The decrease in flow results in underdevelopment of the ventricle.

42. **(D)** Because HLHS affects the left heart, the mitral and aortic valves can be abnormal.

43. **(A)** With HLHS, the flow through the ascending aorta may be absent or reversed. This is caused by the blood flowing back through the ductus arteriosus into the ascending aorta.

44. **(C)** AVSDs are associated with polysplenia approximately 30% of the time.

45. **(C)** Approximately 78% of AVSDs are associated with Down's syndrome (trisomy 21).

46. **(B)** An isolated VSD has the best prognosis. With Ebstein's anomaly, the displacement of the tricuspid valve can lead to an enlarged right atrium, pulmonary atresia or stenosis, and cardiomegaly. Truncus arteriosus has a poor prognosis when left untreated. When treated, there is still mixing of oxygenated and deoxygenated blood. If a coarctation of the aorta is untreated it can be fatal.

47. **(A)** HLHS has the poorest prognosis. If left untreated, it is uniformly fatal. The poor prognosis is because of the small left heart, hypoplastic mitral valve, and ascending aorta. Hypoplastic right heart syndrome, however, has a better prognosis with a survival rate of approximately 25%. A *mild* aortic stenosis and an isolated ASD are treatable and have a good prognosis.

48. **(B)** With hypoplastic right heart syndrome, the pulmonary artery and valve can be small or atretic. The aorta and pulmonary veins are not affected by hypoplastic right heart syndrome since they are left-sided structures.

49. **(D)** When a valve is stenotic, the velocity will be increased distal to the valve. The sample gate can be placed proximal to the valve to determine valvular regurgitation.

50. **(C)** With the decrease in size and flow through the right side of the heart, there is decreased flow through the pulmonary artery.

51. **(A)** A univentricular heart has two atria and one ventricle. Often, when a univentricular heart is present, there is transposition of the great vessels coming off this one ventricle.

52. **(A)** With a univentricular heart, two atrioventricular valves may be seen. One, however, is usually atretic, indicating tricuspid or mitral atresia. This atresia is not related to the univentricular heart but is considered a separate pathology. Pulmonary stenosis, asplenia, and polysplenia are all associated with a univentricular heart.

53. **(C)** Coarctation is a narrowing of the aorta. Coarctation is often difficult to diagnosis *in utero*.

54. **(D)** Approximately 98% of coarctations occur between the left subclavian artery and the ductus arteriosus.

55. **(B)** Coarctation of the aorta is often difficult to visualize *in utero*. A narrowing of the aorta or increased velocities in the aorta can help confirm the diagnosis. A large right ventricle may be a secondary sign of a coarctation.

56. **(A)** Coarctation of the aorta is most commonly seen with Turner's syndrome.

57. **(C)** Ebstein's anomaly is a right-sided heart anomaly. The tricuspid valve is displaced inferiorly.

58. **(A)** Maternal use of lithium has been associated with Ebstein's anomaly.

59. **(D)** The four criteria for tetralogy of Fallot are a VSD, overriding aorta, pulmonary stenosis, and right ventricular hypertrophy.

60. **(C)** Right ventricular hypertrophy may not be seen *in utero* because of the presence of fetal shunts. An ASD is not a defect associated with tetralogy of Fallot.

61. **(D)** VSDs are present with truncus arteriosus. The single vessel overrides this defect.

62. **(A)** With truncus arteriosus, a single vessel arises from the heart. The pulmonary arteries then branch off this single vessel.

63. **(B)** Congenitally corrected transposition of the great vessels occurs when ventricles are switched. The aorta arises from the left-sided right ventricle and follows the normal course toward the left side. With truncus arteriosus, a right-sided aortic arch is seen in approximately 15–30% of cases. Tetralogy of Fallot has a right side aortic arch in 25% of cases. With situs inversus of the chest, all anatomy above the diaphragm would be transposed.

64. **(B)** Truncus arteriosus and tetralogy of Fallot appear similar sonographically. Both pathologies have a single vessel overriding a VSD. Truncus arteriosus, however, occurs when the pulmonary arteries arise from this single vessel; where with tetralogy of Fallot, the pulmonary artery arises from the right ventricle. A univentricular heart's vessels are often transposed.

65. **(C)** With complete transposition of the great vessels, the great arteries arise from the heart in a parallel fashion; therefore, a normal short-axis view of the great vessels cannot be obtained. A normal four-chamber heart can be identified. This stresses the point of why outflow tracts should always be obtained.

66. **(A)** With complete transposition of the great vessels, the atria, ventricles, and valves are in the appropriate location. The aorta arises from the right ventricle, and the pulmonary artery arises from the left ventricle. This differs from congenitally corrected transposition of the great vessels. With congenitally corrected transposition, the right atrium and left ventricle are connected, and the left atrium and right ventricle are connected. The aorta arises from the left-sided right ventricle, and the pulmonary artery arises from the right-sided left ventricle. Identification of the moderator band in the right ventricle is helpful in the diagnosis of congenitally corrected transposition of the great vessels.

67. **(D)** The moderator band will always be located in the right ventricle. In congenitally corrected transposition of the great vessels, the right ventricle is located on the left side of the chest.

68. **(D)** With congenitally corrected transposition, the right atrium and left ventricle are connected, and the left atrium and right ventricle are connected. The aorta arises from the left-sided right ventricle, and the pulmonary artery arises from the right-sided left ventricle. Identification of the moderator band in the right ventricle is helpful in the diagnosis of congenitally corrected transposition of the great vessels. With complete transposition of the great vessels, the atria, ventricles and valves are in the appropriate location. The aorta arises from the right ventricle, and the pulmonary artery arises from the left ventricle.

69. **(A)** When the long-axis views of the aorta and pulmonary artery are obtained, both great arteries would be visualized arising from the right ventricle. Four-chamber views of the heart will not demonstrate DORV.

70. **(C)** DORV occurs when both great arteries arise from the right ventricle running parallel.

71. **(C)** The pulmonary veins normally drain into the left atrium. When TAPVC is present, all four pulmonary veins will drain into the right atrium, or other venous structures.

72. **(D)** Of the choices listed, HLHS would be the most likely diagnosed *in utero* when only a four-chamber heart view is visualized. All of the other pathologies listed can be diagnosed with careful interrogation of the outflow tracts.

73. **(B)** Severe levocardia is defined as the heart's apex pointing toward the left at an angle greater than the normal

45° ± 20°. Severe levocardia is commonly seen with Ebstein's anomaly, or other cardiac lesions that cause right-sided enlargement.

74. **(C)** Dextrocardia is when the heart is in the right chest, and the apex of the heart is pointed toward the right. Levocardia is the normal position of the heart. Severe levocardia is defined as the heart's apex pointing toward the left at an angle greater than the normal 45° ± 20°. Dextroposition is when the heart's apex points toward the left, but the heart is in the right chest.

75. **(A)** A diaphragmatic hernia and cystic adenomatoid malformation can push the heart into the right chest. Hypoplastic right lung causes a potential space on the right side that the heart can move into. Tricuspid insufficiency will not cause abnormal cardiac axis or position.

76. **(D)** The most common dysrhythmia is Premature atrial contraction (PACs). PACs can be caused by maternal use of caffeine, cigarettes or alcohol, or by a redundant foraminal flap. The majority of PACs resolve by delivery.

77. **(D)** SVT occurs when the fetal heart rate is 180–280 beats/min, and there is also atrial–ventricular concordance. If SVT remains throughout pregnancy, fetal hydrops or death can occur.

78. **(C)** Transducer pressure can lead to bradycardia. When pressure is released, normal rate returns.

79. **(B)** A second-degree heart block of 3:1 occurs when there are three atrial contractions for every one ventricular contraction.

80. **(A)** ASDs, cardiac tumors, and polysplenia are all associated with complete heart block. Chordae tendineae are cord-like tendons that connect the papillary muscles to the tricuspid valve.

10

Breast Sonography

Lawrence E. Mason, Charles S. Odwin, Cara Connolly, and Tamarya L. Hoyt

Study Guide

INTRODUCTION

For many years, breast sonography has been an important tool in the management of breast disorders. In recent years, its role in the workup of breast disorders has become more defined as technical advances has improved in spatial and temporal resolution. It is now required by the American College of Radiology (ACR) that a breast imaging facility offer breast sonography to be considered for accreditation. Due to the potentially harmful effects of ionizing radiation, the role of sonography in breast imaging will continue to evolve as technical advances occur.

EPIDEMIOLOGY OF BREAST CANCER[1]

It is our primary role as sonographers and physicians to provide our best efforts to educate patients on the detection of breast disorders, namely breast cancer. Except for skin cancer, breast cancer is the most common cancer among women. The chance of developing invasive breast cancer at sometime in a woman's life is about one in eight (13% of women).[1] At this time, there are more than 3.8 million breast cancer survivors in the United States. Women living in North America have the highest rate of breast cancer in the world. Ninety-nine percent of breast cancers occur in women with only about 1% in men. However, men carry a higher mortality rate than women due to the delay in seeking treatment.[1] No routine mammographic screening for men and the delay in diagnosis are the contributing factors to why male breast cancers are diagnosed at more advance stages. The risk factors for both men and women are advance age, obesity, and family history of breast cancer.

INDICATIONS FOR BREAST SONOGRAPHY

Breast sonography is used as an adjunct to mammography and physical examination. The most common indications to perform an ultrasound exam are the presence of a palpable mass or discovery of an abnormality on mammography. Ultrasound is useful to determine if a mass is cystic or solid, which helps determine management. Ultrasound guidance for aspirations and biopsies is also an indication. Also, ultrasound is the first imaging study in the evaluation of breast mass in pregnant or lactating women, under the age of 30 and in women following mastectomy with a complaint on the side of the mastectomy.

Indications for breast ultrasound include:

- Identification and characterization of palpable abnormalities
- Identification and characterization of clinical and mammographic findings
- Guidance for procedures
- Follow up a finding from a magnetic resonance imaging (MRI) or other examination of the breast.

EXAMINER QUALIFICATIONS

All examiners performing breast ultrasound examinations, including those assisting physicians with ultrasound guided breast biopsy procedures, are encouraged to meet minimum criteria (Table 10–1).[2]

When breast sonography is performed by an experienced examiner, patients with breast related complaints can be appropriately triaged for clinical follow up, biopsy or referred for surgery as necessary. However, the detection of breast cancer and breast disorders is a daunting task for the inexperienced breast sonographer and the responsibility for the detection of breast disorders does not rest exclusively on the shoulders of the sonographer. The sonographer's primary function is to document anatomic regions of the breast with knowledge of normal anatomy. In fulfilling this role, the sonographer should be able to bring to the attention of the physician areas of interest that require further evaluation. In the majority of cases, a breast sonogram will require correlation of the sonographic findings

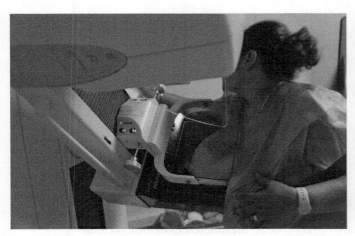

FIGURE 10–25. Breast compression utilized to reduce motion artifact and to reduce breast thickness requiring lower-radiation dose.

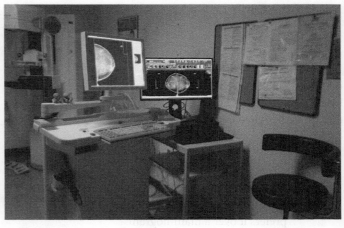

FIGURE 10–27. Film-viewing station.

This can result in false negative and false positive on the mammogram. The mammographic appearance of fatty tissue is radiolucent (dark), and dense breast is radiopaque (white), which can result in difficulty in recognizing some breast tumors that are also white. The mammogram unit is composed of a rotating x-ray tube with a breast compression plate. The patient breast is placed between the compression paddle and compression grid (Fig. 10–25). Breast compression is used to decrease breast thickness and radiation dose to the breast and to prevent movement of the breast during radiographic imaging.[2] Fig. 10–26 shows the components of a mammogram unit. After images are processed, the data are transferred to a

reading station for interpretation (Fig. 10–27). Digital images are stored on picture archiving communication system (PACS).

SUMMARY

Breast sonography is a useful tool in the workup of breast disorders. As operator experience increases, the ability of the sonographer to differentiate subtle abnormalities of the breast will develop. With an understanding of technique and breast anatomy, adherence to the examination requirements and knowledge of the necessary language for appropriate characterization of the findings.

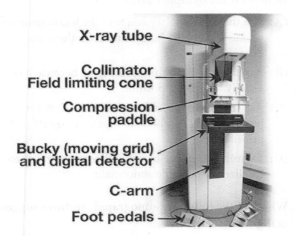

X-ray tube

Collimator
Field limiting cone

Compression
paddle

Bucky (moving grid)
and digital detector

C-arm

Foot pedals

FIGURE 10–26. Components of a mammogram unit.

Questions

GENERAL INSTRUCTIONS: For each question, select the best answer. Select only one answer for each question unless otherwise instructed.

1. Which of the following is *not* an indication for breast ultrasound?

    (A) Guidance for a breast biopsy.

    (B) A patient who had a breast sonogram last year and prefers it over a mammogram.

    (C) An abnormality is palpated by the patient's physician.

    (D) An abnormality is palpated by the patient.

2. Which of the following statements is true regarding focal zone setting in breast sonography?

    (A) The focal zone should be set above the level of the lesion being imaged.

    (B) The focal zone should be set at the level of the lesion being imaged.

    (C) There should only be one focal zone used for maximum image optimization.

    (D) The focal zone placement is not critical in sonographic breast imaging.

3. What breast lesion is an acoustic standoff pad most helpful?

    (A) deep within the breast tissue

    (B) axillary in location

    (C) superficially positioned within the breast

    (D) mobile upon palpation

4. Each breast lesion should be measured in which of the following scan planes?

    (A) radial, antiradial

    (B) radial, transverse

    (C) sagittal, transverse

    (D) longitudinal, antiradial

5. A sonographic exam demonstrating a 2 cm anechoic, circumscribed mass at the 4 o'clock position in the left breast is compared to the patient's mammogram that suggests a 2 cm spiculated mass at the 9 o'clock position. Which of the following should the sonographer do?

    (A) Tell the patient she has a cyst and there is nothing to worry about.

    (B) Tell the patient that the mammogram was a false positive and she should be followed up with sonography for future evaluation of the mass.

    (C) Take images of all abnormalities and tell the patient she may leave and return next year for her follow-up mammogram.

    (D) Discuss the differences in location and characteristics of the masses seen on the mammogram and sonogram with the interpreting physician.

6. Which of the following best describes the thickness of normal skin overlying the breast?

    (A) 2–3 cm

    (B) 1–2 cm

    (C) 5–10 mm

    (D) 2–3 mm

7. While preparing to perform a sonographic exam on a patient who was referred for evaluation of a palpable abnormality, the patient states she cannot feel the area reliably while lying down. Which of the following should the sonographer do?

    (A) Ask the patient to try and find the lesion lying down because this is the best position for the sonographic exam.

    (B) Ask the patient to find it sitting up because it is usually the easiest position.

    (C) Ask the patient to find the lesion in whatever position necessary and attempt to image it from this position.

    (D) Examine the entire breast without attempting to localize the palpable abnormality.

8. Which of the following sonographic features suggests malignancy?

    (A) round

    (B) posterior acoustic enhancement

    (C) spiculated

    (D) circumscribed

9. What minimum frequency in MHz is required for breast sonography?

(A) 2.5 MHz

(B) 7.5 MHz

(C) 10 MHz

(D) 15 MHz

10. In order for a breast mass to be characterized as anechoic, it must

(A) not contain any internal echoes

(B) demonstrate reverberation artefacts at the near-field edge

(C) produce refraction artifacts on the lateral borders

(D) demonstrate reduced echogenicity deep to the mass

11. What is the approximate chance of a woman developing invasive breast cancer in her lifetime?

(A) 1 in 8

(B) 1 in 15

(C) 1 in 40

(D) 1 in 100

12. Positioning to reduce the breast thickness of the upper outer quadrant can be achieved by placing the patient in which of the following positions?

(A) Place the ipsilateral hand behind the head and roll the patient into an ipsilateral posterior oblique position.

(B) Place the contralateral hand behind the head and roll the patient into an ipsilateral posterior oblique position.

(C) Place the ipsilateral hand behind the head and roll the patient into a contralateral posterior oblique position.

(D) Place the contralateral hand behind the head and roll the patient into a contralateral oblique position.

13. Which of the following information is not required documentation for diagnostic sonograms?

(A) laterality (right or left breast)

(B) distance from the nipple

(C) scan plane orientation

(D) patient's last name only

14. Using the length of the transducer's footprint may provide a means to determine what sonographic feature of breast abnormalities?

(A) depth of the lesion

(B) distance of the lesion from the nipple

(C) the transverse diameter of the lesion

(D) the depth at which to place the focal zone for best optimization

15. The utilization of the radial/antiradial scan planes provides the best demonstration of what breast anatomy?

(A) lobes of the glandular tissue

(B) Cooper's ligaments

(C) ductal anatomy of the breast

(D) terminal ductal-lobular units (TDLU)

16. Which two characteristics are most helpful to establish concordance between a lesion seen on ultrasound and mammography?

(A) margins and density

(B) echogenicity and distance from the nipple

(C) margins and echogenicity

(D) size and location

17. The mass in Fig. 10–28 can best be described as

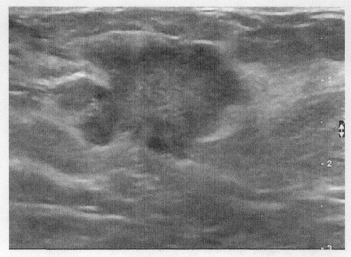

FIGURE 10–28.

(A) irregular

(B) circumscribed

(C) macrolobulated

(D) spiculated

18. The mass in Fig. 10–29 is best described as

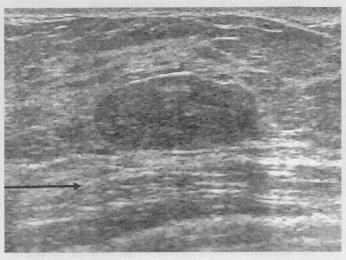

FIGURE 10–29.

(A) round
(B) circumscribed
(C) posteriorly enhancing
(D) spiculated

19. In Fig. 10–29, what structure is the arrow pointing to?

(A) Cooper's ligaments
(B) pectoralis muscle
(C) fibroglandular tissue
(D) skin

20. This image in Fig. 10–30 demonstrates

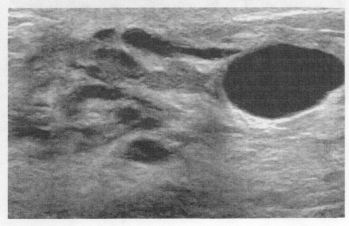

FIGURE 10–30.

(A) dilated ductal anatomy
(B) a simple cyst with breast implant rupture
(C) multiple, irregular cysts
(D) a single cyst with dilated ductal anatomy

21. What abnormal finding is not demonstrated in Fig. 10–31?

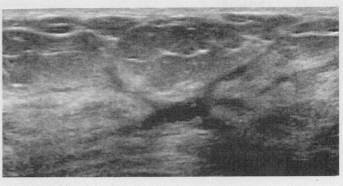

FIGURE 10–31.

(A) architectural distortion
(B) posterior acoustic attenuation
(C) angular margins
(D) calcifications

22. An asymptomatic patient receives a breast sonogram as additional workup. The exam reveals a mass with multiple internal punctuate echogenic foci. What do these foci most likely represent?

(A) calcifications
(B) gas
(C) artifact
(D) fat

23. Sonography is the recommended initial imaging modality for the evaluation of an area of palpable interest in patients younger than what age?

(A) 30
(B) 40
(C) 50
(D) 60

24. Which of the following terms is not an appropriate descriptor of breast lesion shape?

(A) oblong
(B) round
(C) oval
(D) irregular

25. If sonographic scanning in the upper outer quadrant of the breast demonstrates findings suspicious for a tubular structure, which of the following techniques should be used to further evaluate it?

    (A) imaging in an orthogonal plane
    (B) use of Doppler
    (C) adjusting the gray scale
    (D) adjusting the focal zone

26. What type transducer should be used for breast sonography?

    (A) curved
    (B) linear
    (C) vector
    (D) curvilinear

27. Echogenicity of a mass is assessed relative to which of the following structures?

    (A) Cooper's ligaments
    (B) skin
    (C) fat
    (D) muscle

28. The appearance of hazy, echogenic material with posterior acoustic shadowing seen in an augmented breast should raise the suspicion for which of the following?

    (A) malignancy
    (B) scar
    (C) fibrocystic disease
    (D) implant rupture

29. An image from a sonogram performed on a patient referred for evaluation of a palpable abnormality reveals an hypoechoic mass-like area with mixed internal echogenicity seen deep to the pectoralis muscle. What does these findings most-likely represent?

    (A) fibroadenoma
    (B) cyst
    (C) invasive malignancy
    (D) rib

30. Which of the following statements is true regarding a biopsy performed with a vacuum-assisted device?

    (A) Pre-fire and post-fire images should be obtained.
    (B) Pre-fire images only should be obtained.
    (C) Post-fire images only should be obtained.
    (D) Images demonstrating the needle in or adjacent to the mass should be obtained.

31. Which of the following statements is true regarding a breast cyst post-aspiration?

    (A) There is no need to acquire a postaspiration image.
    (B) A postaspiration image should only be obtained if a small amount of fluid remains.
    (C) A postaspiration image should only be obtained if there is question if a solid component is present.
    (D) A postaspiration image should be obtained routinely.

32. During imaging of an area of concern, there is evidence of interruption of the Cooper's ligaments. An irregular hypoechoic region with angular margins and posterior acoustic shadowing is seen, but no mass is visualized. Which of the following is the most appropriate descriptor for this appearance?

    (A) spiculation
    (B) architectural distortion
    (C) dirty shadowing
    (D) normal parenchyma

33. The finding discussed in question 32 is most likely to be seen in which of the following scenarios?

    (A) benign lesions
    (B) postsurgical change
    (C) young, asymptomatic patients
    (D) pregnant patients with a palpable mass

34. What percent of men get breast cancer?

    (A) 1%
    (B) 5%
    (C) 50%
    (D) 90%

35. What is the most common type of breast cancer in men?

    (A) inflammatory breast cancer
    (B) IDC
    (C) triple-negative breast cancer
    (D) invasive lobular carcinoma

36. Which of the following does not increase the chances of breast cancer?

    (A) OCPs
    (B) first-degree relative with genetic mutation
    (C) ionizing radiation exposure
    (D) breast-feeding

37. *BRCA1* and *BRCA2* genetic mutation genes are prevalent in what ethnic population?

(A) Hasidic Jews

(B) Native Americans

(C) Ashkenazi Jews

(D) Afro-American

38. What percent of men with breast cancer have hormone receptors?

(A) 25%

(B) 50%

(C) 75%

(D) 90%

39. A 35-year-old with bilateral palpable nonpainful, mobile mass with popcorn-like calcifications on mammogram is most likely to have

(A) ductal carcinoma in situ

(B) fibroadenoma

(C) papillary carcinoma

(D) invasive lobar carcinoma

40. Which of the following artifacts is not routinely seen on breast ultrasound?

(A) acoustic shadowing

(B) reverberation artefact

(C) slice thickness

(D) flash artefact

41. To avoid nipple shadowing on breast ultrasound, the sonographer should

(A) roll the nipple to the side

(B) place a nipple maker over the nipple

(C) scan perpendicular to the nipple

(D) use a higher-frequency transducer

42. A 40-year-old woman presented to the breast clinic with complain of bilateral breast lump. On bilateral breast examination by her physician, multiple tender breast masses occur at the time of her menstruation. This most likely clinical finding is

(A) ductal carcinoma in situ

(B) fibrocystic disease

(C) fibroadenoma

(D) mastitis

43. What is the most common cause for a bloody nipple discharge?

(A) ductal carcinoma in situ

(B) mastitis

(C) galactorrhea

(D) benign intraductal papilloma

44. The imaging modality that uses an injectable radiopaque contrast into the milk ducts to investigate nipple discharge is called

(A) MRI

(B) galactography

(C) 3D ultrasound

(D) positron emission tomography (PET) scan

45. What is the most common cause for greenish discharge from the nipple?

(A) duct ectasia

(B) fibrocystic disease

(C) ductal carcinoma in situ

(D) benign intraductal papilloma

46. The white arrow in Fig. 10–32 points to

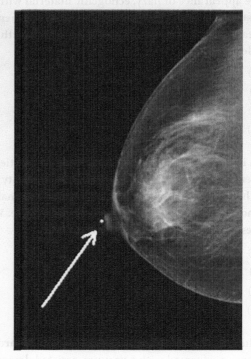

FIGURE 10–32. Mammogram image.

(A) nipple microcalcification

(B) titanium nipple piercing ring

(C) nipple skin tag

(D) nipple marker

47. **The white arrow in Fig. 10–33 points to**

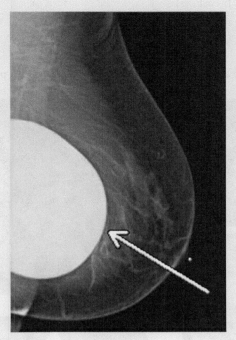

FIGURE 10–33. Mammogram image.

    (A) large breast cyst

    (B) large radiopaque breast cancer

    (C) saline breast implant

    (D) silicone breast implant

48. **A condition that results in male breast enlargement due to hyperplasia of glandular and stroma tissue is called**

    (A) lipoma

    (B) galactorrhea

    (C) invasive lobular carcinoma

    (D) gynecomastia

49. **What type of tissue does the male breast predominately comprise?**

    (A) subcutaneous

    (B) fibrous tissue

    (C) connective tissue

    (D) dense tissue

50. **Which one of the following is not a risk factor for gynecomastia?**

    (A) anabolic steroids

    (B) increased testosterone levels

    (C) Klinefelter's syndrome

    (D) increased estrogen

51. **What is the most common cause for pseudogynecomastia?**

    (A) obesity

    (B) increased serum level of estrogen

    (C) marijuana

    (D) hypothyroidism

52. **Which one of the following best describes the sonographic appearance of gynecomastia?**

    (A) hypoechoic fingerlike structure extending from the nipple to chest wall

    (B) round mass with well-circumscribed margins within the dermis

    (C) solid mass with ill-defined, irregular margins

    (D) multiple microcalcifications with distal acoustic shadow

53. **A 41-year-old G5P2 who presented to the department of radiology for her annual screening mammogram. Breast examination by her private physician prior to her mammogram was normal. What is the finding in this mammogram (Fig. 10–34)?**

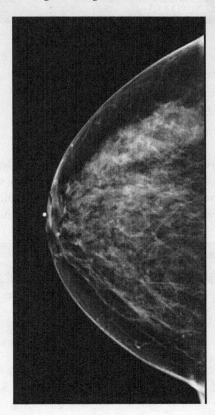

FIGURE 10–34. Mammogram image.

    (A) fibroadenoma

    (B) ductal carcinoma in situ

    (C) dense breast

    (D) galactocele

105. **What is the most common site for sentinel node in metastatic breast cancer?**

    (A) axilla

    (B) areola

    (C) nipple

    (D) internal thoracic

106. **Which of the following is not typical of metastatic lymph node?**

    (A) axilla lymph node less than 10 mm in size ovoid and tender

    (B) internal mammary node 15 mm in size, bulky, and lobulated

    (C) displaced echogenic hilum of the node

    (D) pectoral nodes 12 mm size, irregular in shape with absent of echogenic hilum

107. **A 28-year-old G1P1 with a known history of bilateral silicone augmentation 5 years ago. She presented to the GYN clinic with swelling and discomfort in her right breast. She stated this started after a motorcycle accident 2 months ago. Physical examination of her right breast revealed a significant difference in size and shape when compared to her left breast. Which imaging modality would give more accuracy?**

    (A) breast ultrasound

    (B) mammogram

    (C) MRI

    (D) PET

108. **A 30-year-old had bilateral breast augmentation 2 years ago. She presented to the Department of Radiology for her annual screening mammogram. To get better visualization of her breast tissue, which of the following is best?**

    (A) increaseing the dosage of radiation in order to see more breast tissue

    (B) avoiding breast compression

    (C) using a standoff pad

    (D) implanting displacement views

109. **Which one of the following is not one of the sonographic findings of breast implant rupture?**

    (A) teardrop

    (B) snowstorm

    (C) echodense noise

    (D) dirty shadow

110. **Which of the following is not palpable on physical examination of the breast?**

    (A) lipoma

    (B) breast infarct

    (C) postoperative scarring

    (D) breast implant fibrous capsule

111. **What does BI-RADS with a category score of 4 indicate?**

    (A) Cancer of the breast was previously diagnosed and confirmed by the pathologist.

    (B) Incomplete test and requirement of additional test.

    (C) Mammogram is negative with no evidence of cancer.

    (D) Suspicious of cancer and requirement of a biopsy.

112. **The snowstorm sign seen on breast ultrasound is associated with**

    (A) multiple bright echoes from postsurgical skin retraction

    (B) extracapsular breast implant rupture

    (C) intracapsular breast implant rupture

    (D) breast cancer TRAM reconstruction

113. **What type of breast cancer is associated with breast implant?**

    (A) anaplastic large cell lymphoma (ALCL)

    (B) triple-negative breast cancer

    (C) ductal carcinoma in situ

    (D) inflammatory breast cancer

114. **A 54-year-old postmenopausal presented to the breast clinic complaining of changes on her nipples, with itching and redness. Physical breast examination was done with findings of eczematous patches bilaterally with scaly nipples. A 10-mm mass was palpated on the left subareolar. All the above findings are suggestive of what type of breast condition?**

    (A) galactorrhea

    (B) mammary duct ectasia

    (C) Paget's disease of the breast

    (D) Peau d' orange of the nipple

115. A 35-year-old woman presented to the emergency department with left chest and breast pain after an automobile accident 1 month ago. She was wearing her safety belt at the time of the accident. She also complained of pain when her left arm is elevated. Physical examination of the chest and breasts revealed a painful left cord-like mass under the skin of the left breast. The most likely finding is

    (A) Mondor's disease

    (B) mammary duct ectasia

    (C) hamartoma

    (D) mastitis

116. 25-year-old breast-feeding mother presented to the GYN clinic with complaints of headache, fever, and general malaise. She also complains of pain in her left breast. Physical examination revealed a tender, erythematous, and indurated left breast. What are the expected bacterial and sonographic findings in this case?

    (A) *Klebsiella* and calcifications with eggshell appearance on ultrasound

    (B) *Staphylococcus aureus* and ultrasound skin thickening and prominent lymph channels

    (C) *Actinomycosis israelii* and with taller-than-wide with vertical orientation on ultrasound

    (D) *Bifidobacterium* and ultrasound findings of markedly hypoechoic with distal shadow

117. What is the most common location for invasive ductal carcinoma?

    (A) lower-outer quadrant

    (B) lower-inner quadrant

    (C) upper-outer quadrant

    (D) upper-inner quadrant

118. Which one of the following sonographic signs is characteristic of malignancy?

    (A) eggshell

    (B) taller-than-wider

    (C) popcorn calcifications

    (D) stepladder sign with dirty shadowing

119. Which one of the following is usually not part of the normal protocol for local breast biopsy?

    (A) time-out and local anesthesia

    (B) proper hand hygiene

    (C) informed consent

    (D) prophylactic antibiotic

120. A 17-year-old presented to the emergency room 1 week after an automobile accident. She was the passenger in the front seat and was wearing her seat belt at that time. She was not pregnant at the time. She presented with bruising and tenderness to the right breast and denies any other complaint. Ultrasound of the right breast revealed a heterogeneous mass with smooth margins. What is the most likely diagnosis?

    (A) hematoma

    (B) abscess

    (C) Mondor's disease

    (D) radial scar

121. The arrow in Fig. 10–56 points to

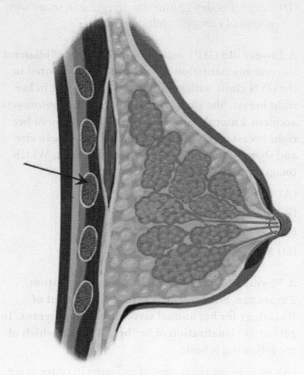

FIGURE 10–56.

    (A) pectoral muscles

    (B) thoracic lymph node

    (C) intracostal muscles

    (D) rib

122. **Tiny bumps on the surface of the areola most likely represent**

(A) folliculitis

(B) areola cyst

(C) pimples

(D) sebaceous glands

123. **A lesion located in in the upper outer quadrant of the left breast would be describe as**

(A) 5 o'clock position

(B) 2 o'clock position

(C) 10 o'clock position

(D) 7 o'clock position

124. **The thick portion of the female breast tissue that extends into the axilla is known as**

(A) deep fascia

(B) Cooper's Ligaments

(C) pectoralis major

(D) tail of Spence

125. **The average adult female breast extends vertically at what thoracic rib levels?**

(A) first to the ninth rib

(B) first to the third rib

(C) second to the sixth rib

(D) third to the eighth rib

126. **A 12-year-old girl was seen in the breast clinic with a congenital absent of one of her breast nipples. This condition is known as**

(A) amastia

(B) athelia

(C) amazia

(D) hypoplasia

127. **The arrow in Fig. 10–57 points to**

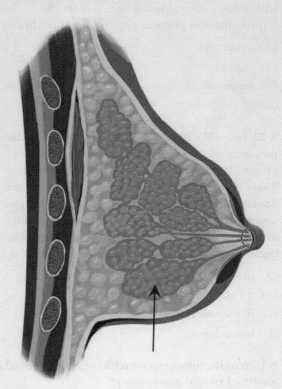

FIGURE 10–57.

(A) Montgomery gland

(B) Cooper's ligaments

(C) subcutaneous fat

(D) lobules

128. **What artery provides blood supply to the breast?**

(A) circumflex

(B) lateral thoracic artery

(C) marginal artery

(D) mesenteric

129. **What anatomical structure within the breast parenchyma decreases as a woman ages?**

(A) nipple

(B) areola

(C) adipose tissue

(D) ligaments

130. **What muscles is located under the subcutaneous tissue beneath the pectoralis major muscle?**

(A) trapezius muscle

(B) pectoralis minor muscle

(C) intercostal muscle

(D) rhomboid muscle

131. **What procedure or procedures is often performed without any clinical indication, just for the improvement of physical appearance of the breast?**

    (A) mammoplasty

    (B) augmentation

    (C) reduction

    (D) all the above

132. **A 22-year-old without any previous medical history presented with a 6-month history of painless progressively enlarged mass on the right breast. There is no history of trauma, fever, or weight loss. Breast examination reveals a 2 cm by 1.5 cm, well-circumscribed, and mobile mass. The mass is not associated with the menstrual cycle and is not fixed to the underlying tissue. What is the most likely diagnosis?**

    (A) mastitis

    (B) intraductal breast carcinoma

    (C) fibrocystic disease

    (D) fibroadenoma

133. **Which of the following structures is not removed in modified radical mastectomy?**

    (A) both breast tissue

    (B) breast skin

    (C) muscles

    (D) lymph node

134. **What structure is seen in the female breast but is absent in the male breast?**

    (A) lobules

    (B) pectoralis muscle

    (C) fatty tissue

    (D) lymph nodes

135. **Which veins give access to metastatic spread of breast cancer to the vertebral bones?**

    (A) intercostal veins

    (B) axillary veins

    (C) varicose veins of the breast

    (D) mesenteric vein

136. **What ligament attaches the mammary gland to the dermis and gives shape and structure to the breast to prevent sagging?**

    (A) pectineal ligament

    (B) suspensory ligament

    (C) capsular ligament

    (D) longitudinal ligament

137. **The right lymphatic duct empties into**

    (A) right thoracic duct

    (B) left subclavian vein

    (C) left subclavian artery

    (D) right subclavian vein

138. **A common congenital condition in which accessory breast is seen in addition to normal breast tissue is known as**

    (A) polymastia

    (B) athelia

    (C) amastia

    (D) polymass

139. **A 28-year-old G2P1 presented to the GYN Clinic for her annual GYN examination. Her sister was diagnosed with breast cancer 2 years ago, which was treated with mastectomy and chemotherapy. After her physician performed a thorough breast examination, a circumscribed, mobile, rubbery, and a nontender mass was palpated in the right breast. The mass is approximately 2 cm in size and not fixed to the underlying tissue. What finding does Fig. 10–58 show in this diagnostic ultrasound of the right breast?**

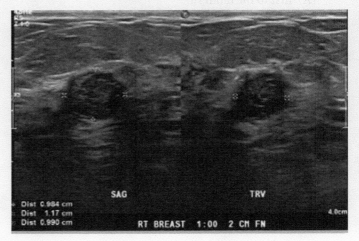

FIGURE 10–58. Sagittal and transverse images of the right breast.

    (A) fibrocystic mass

    (B) seroma

    (C) ductal carcinoma in situ

    (D) fibroadenoma

140. A 42-year-old G4P1 presented to the GYN Clinic complaining of a left painful breast mass that she palpated prior to her menstruation. She denies any history of trauma or fever. After her physician performed a thorough breast examination, a circumscribed, tender, mobile mass was palpated in the left breast at 2 o'clock position. The mass is approximately 10 mm in size and not fixed to the underlying tissue. What finding does Fig. 10–59 show in a diagnostic ultrasound of the left breast?

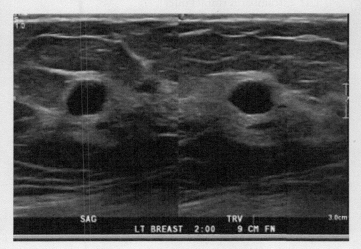

FIGURE 10–59. Sagittal and transverse images of the left breast.

(A) simple breast cyst

(B) lymphoma

(C) fibrocystic disease

(D) fibroadenoma

141. A 22-year-old G0P0 has a family history of genetic mutation *BRCA1*. She presented to the GYN clinic with concern that she may have an inherited breast cancer. There is no history of nipple discharge, dimpling of breast skin, breast pain, or weight loss. Her physician performed a breast examination, which was inconclusive due to large breast size. Her BMI was 35 kg/m². What is the sonographic finding shown in Fig. 10–60A and B?

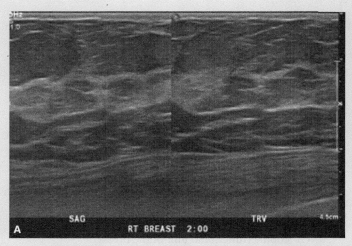

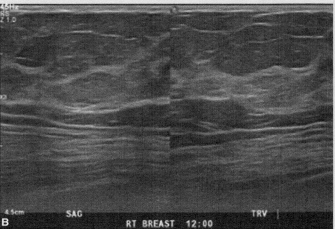

FIGURE 10–60. Sonograms (**A** and **B**) of the right breast.

(A) inflammatory breast cancer

(B) triple-negative breast cancer

(C) invasive ductal carcinoma

(D) no sonographic evidence of malignancy

142. Breast growth and appearance in a male and female prior to puberty are

(A) female breast is larger

(B) virtually identical

(C) male breast is larger due to hormones

(D) male breast nipples are inverted prior to puberty

143. At puberty, the female mammary glands undergo a series normal growth changes called

(A) Tanner stages

(B) precocious puberty

(C) mammary hypertrophy

(D) mammary hyperplasia

26. **(B)** Linear array transducers provide the best resolution and are particularly useful in superficial structures, such as the breast, when a wide field of view is not essential.

27. **(C)** Fat is hypoechoic relative to the mammary/glandular tissue. The gray scale and gain settings should be set to demonstrate fat as the medium level echo and compare all other tissue/findings to its echogenicity.

28. **(D)** Free silicone has the appearance of "dirty shadowing," which is described in this question.

29. **(D)** The ribs and chest wall are the only structures that are typically identified deep to the pectoralis muscle.

30. **(D)** Vacuum-assisted devices do not "fire" when obtaining the specimen.

31. **(D)** This protocol is important to determine and document the completeness of the aspiration.

32. **(B)** Spiculation is used in oncology to describe the margins of a mass when the tissue surrounding the mass is altered and has angular characteristics. Architectural distortion is best used when a mass is not appreciated, but the tissue is similarly altered.

33. **(B)** Architectural distortion is usually seen postsurgically or in association with a malignancy.

34. **(A)** Only about 1% of men get breast cancer. Though men do not normally develop milk-producing breasts, the tissue to male breast can still develop cancer.

35. **(B)** IDC, also called invasive ductal carcinoma, is the most common type of breast cancer in both men and woman. Subareolar is the most common location.

36. **(D)** As women get older, the chances of breast cancer increase, with postmenopausal women having the greatest risk. However, postmenopausal women have better prognosis due to the lack of estrogen. HRT and OCPs increase the chances of breast cancer whereas OCP is known to decrease the chances of ovarian cancer. The incident of breast cancer decreases with breast-feeding.

37. **(C)** The *BRCA1* and *BRCA2* genetic mutation genes are prevalent in the Ashkenazi Jewish population. These types of gene mutation tend to develop in younger women and occur more often in both breasts.

38. **(D)** Approximately 90% of male breast cancers have hormone receptor, which respond much better to therapy.

39. **(B)** Fibroadenoma is a benign tumor in the breast that is commonly found in women younger than 30. The mass is composed of fibroglandular and stromal tissue. The coarse or popcorn-like calcification is the classic description of fibroadenoma seen on mammogram.

40. **(D)** A flash artefact is motion of reflectors that results in Doppler shift, giving a false appearance of blood flow. The types of artefact commonly seen in breast ultrasound are posterior acoustic shadowing, slice thickness, reverberation, grating lobe, and distal acoustic enhancement. Flash is a Doppler artefact not routinely seen in breast ultrasound.

41. **(A)** Nipple shadowing can be reduced by transducer angulation or by rolling the nipple to the side. Nipple markers are lead ball-bearing disposable skin stickers, which is placed on the nipple for mammography. Nipple markers are radiopaque and immediately identify breast nipple location on mammograms. These markers cause distal acoustic shadow on ultrasound and therefore not useful to prevent nipple shadowing.

42. **(B)** Fibrocystic breasts are benign tender mass that are rope-like to palpation that fluctuate in size with the menstrual cycle.

43. **(D)** The most common cause for a bloody nipple discharge is benign intraductal papilloma that is caused by twisting of the papilloma on its stalk.

44. **(B)** Galactography uses an injectable radiopaque contrast into the milk ducts to investigate nipple discharge on mammogram.

45. **(A)** Duct ectasia. When the mammary milk ducts beneath the nipple becomes dilated and filled with fluid due to blocked ducts, this, in turn, produces an inflammatory reaction, which results in greenish nipple discharge.

46. **(D)** Nipple marker. Adhered stickers with BB pellet or small ball-bearing is placed on the nipples to help locate the nipple on mammogram. These nipple markers are normally removed during breast ultrasound as it interferes with contact scanning.

47. **(D)** Intact silicone breast implant. Breast implants are placed in the breast to augment the breast size. They are placed either in front of the pectoral muscle (subglandular) or behind the pectoral muscle (subpectoral). This mammogram demonstrates a normal opaque white oval silicone implant. It is possible to determine the type of implant by mammography. Implant type is distinguished by assessing the density of the fluid. Silicone is denser than saline, and saline implant has filling valve, but silicone implant does not.[4,5] On mammogram images, the saline implant is (gray) and less dense than silicone (white). Both saline and silicone can decrease the ability to reveal breast cancer. On sonographic image, saline and silicone implants have a similar appearance. MRI is more sensitive for implant rupture than mammography and ultrasound.[13]

48. **(D)** Gynecomastia is the most common cause for breast enlargement of the male's breasts due to reduced male hormone testosterone or an increase in female hormone estrogen. Gynecomastia goes away in about 2 years without treatment; however, treatment may be necessary if symptoms persist. Gynecomastia is enlargement of the male breast due to hyperplasia of glandular and stroma tissue.

49. **(A)** The male breast is composed of skin, subcutaneous fat, and atrophic ducts with subcutaneous fat the predominance of the male breast tissue.

50. **(B)** Increased testosterone. The risk factors for gynecomastia are Klinefelter's syndrome, hypothyroidism, increase estrogen, anabolic steroids, and decrease testosterone. Klinefelter's syndrome occurs when a male is born extra X chromosome, resulting in low testosterone, small testicles, and enlarged breasts.[3]

51. **(A)** Obesity. Pseudogynecomastia is male breast enlargement caused by increased fat deposition. Pseudogynecomastia is fatty proliferation without proliferation of gander tissue.[4]

52. **(A)** Hypoechoic fingerlike structure extending from the nipple to chest wall.

53. **(C)** This image demonstrates heterogeneous dense breast that may obscure small masses. There is no mass or suspicious calcification, and there is no mammographic evidence of malignancy. Dense breasts are seen in younger women, and the density can decrease with age.[4]

54. **(B)** This sonogram demonstrates a single 1 cm by 1.2 cm isoechoic circumscribed mass that represents fibroadenoma.

55. **(B)** This targeted ultrasound of the breast a 4 mm by 4 mm breast cyst.

56. **(D)** Mammograms involve compression of the breast. Spot views apply a compression paddle to a smaller area of the breast tissue.

57. **(A)** This mammogram demonstrates almost entirely fatty breast tissue, no calcifications, no mass demonstrated, with no mammographic evidence of malignancy.

58. **(D)** This diagnostic mammogram of the right breast demonstrates a 4 cm by 3 cm high-density mass with microlobulated margins that correlate with the palpable mass found on physical exam. This right breast mass is suggestive of malignancy. The left breast was normal. Ultrasound demonstrated a hypoechoic microcirculated mass with echogenic surrounding also suggestive of malignancy. A core biopsy confirmed invasive ductal right breast carcinoma. Most breast cancer are asymptomatic in the early stages. However, the most common physical findings are nonpainful, irregular, and immobile. Breast cancer on some occasion can be painful.

59. **(C)** Titanium cosmetic nipple barbells. It is customary to remove pierced cosmetic nipple jewelry before having a mammogram or when breast-feeding.

60. **(A)** Mole marker. These types of breast marker provide a more certainty that densities on the mammogram images are raised skin moles and not a mass inside the breast. Moles can be easily seen by inspecting the breast skin before performing the mammograms.

61. **(C)** The TDLU, as the name implies, is the basic functional unit of the breast containing a lobule composed of multiple small secretory ductules connected to an extralobular terminal duct via the intralobular terminal duct. Multiple TDLUs converge into larger collecting ducts that terminate in the nipple.

62. **(D)** Approximately 15–20 lobes converge at the nipple. There are typically fewer openings at the nipple than there are lobes since some of the collecting ducts from each lobe merge before the nipple.

63. **(C)** Fat should appear as medium to light gray in echogenicity. Fibroglandular tissue appears as areas of increased echogenicity (Answer A). Cooper's ligaments, also known as suspensory ligaments, appear as hyperechoic linear structures radiating through the breast tissue to the skin. Fluid (Answer D) is not typically seen in normal breast tissue.

64. **(B)** The skin should measure no more than 2 mm in thickness, except in the periareolar tissues and the inframammary fold, where up to 3 mm of thickness is within normal limits.

65. **(A)** The areolar and retroareolar tissues regularly demonstrate posterior acoustic shadowing that is normal. Because the nipple is a superficial structure with uneven overlying skin, using adequate gel is necessary to displace air. Use of a standoff pad and a high-frequency transducer will optimize visualization of superficial structures (Answers C and D). The focal zone should be adjusted to the depth of the area of interest (Answer A).

66. **(B)** Punctate echogenic foci within a breast mass likely represent microcalcifications. Larger or coarser calcifications, or macrocalcifications, may sometimes produce posterior shadowing. Air (Answer C) produces a "dirty" posterior shadow. While fat and metal may appear hyperechoic, features in this image are not consistent with either.

67. **(D)** The image depicts the dirty shadowing, or "snowstorm" appearance of free silicone that has accumulated within a lymph node. This finding is indicative of a ruptured silicone breast implant/free silicone injection.

68. **(C)** The fifth edition of the BI-RADS atlas describes the following ultrasound characteristics of noncircumscribed masses on ultrasound: indistinct, angular, microlobulated, and spiculated. Lobulated (Answer A) and smooth (Answer B) are distractors. Spiculated would also have been an appropriate answer but was not given as a choice.

69. **(B)** The classic features of a simple cyst are a round, circumscribed mass with posterior acoustic enhancement and no adjacent tissue distortion. Answer C describes a round, anechoic mass, but with posterior shadowing instead of enhancement. Answers A and D are distractors.

70. **(C)** Complicated cysts contain low-level internal echoes or debris that may layer and shift with changes in

patient position. Complex breast cysts (Answer B) are cysts with thick walls, thick septa, intracystic masses, or other discrete solid components. A microcyst cluster is a group of small anechoic structures with thin intervening septations and no solid components.

71. **(C)** Answer A describes Mondor's disease, a superficial thrombophlebitis. Answer B describes the normal appearance of ductal structures in the breast. Answer D describes a galactocele or abscess. Ductal ectasia is enlarged ducts and can be seen in both benign and pathologic processes such as intraductal papilloma and carcinoma.

72. **(B)** The hypoechoic cortex of a lymph node should not measure greater than 3 mm in thickness. A lymph node should also maintain a reniform, or kidney-like, shape. Although this node maintains its fatty (hyperechoic) hilum, the overall shape is rounded and the cortex is too thick.

73. **(D)** Overall measurements of the lymph node, as well as a measurement of the thickness of the cortex, is important to obtain to evaluate the morphology of a lymph node. The thickness of the fatty hilum is not a reliable indicator for pathology and is not typically measured.

74. **(B)** The echogenicity of a mass should be compared to the surrounding background fat and glandular tissue. The shape of a mass (round, oval, or irregular) as well as a descriptor of the margins should be included. If the margins are not circumscribed, they may be characterized as indistinct, angular, microlobulated, or spiculated.

75. **(C)** Fibroadenomas are the most commonly encountered breast mass (Answer B), occurring in women in their 20s and 30s (Answer D). Imaging features of fibroadenomas sometimes overlap that of malignant masses, and biopsy is needed in these cases (Answer A). Recurrence after resection, growth by more than 2 cm in 1 year, or postmenopausal enlargement is suspicious for malignancy.

76. **(D)** A mass may be described as parallel (wider than tall) or antiparallel (taller than wide) to the skin surface. Parallel orientation is suggestive of benignity.

77. **(A)** The ribs appear as a hyperechoic curvilinear line with posterior acoustic shadowing. The ribs are deep to the breast parenchyma and chest wall muscles.

78. **(D)** Use of clock face position helps localize lesions within the breast for reproducible results. The clock face is superimposed on each breast without reorientation, such that the upper inner quadrant of the left breast is the 9–12 o'clock region while the upper inner quadrant of the right breast is in the 0–3 o'clock position.

79. **(A)** The normal aging process typically results in the replacement of glandular tissue with fatty tissue (Answer D). Weight gain and cessation of hormone therapy (Answers B and C) will also increase the ratio of fat to glandular tissue. New hormone therapy (Answer A) is the best answer to explain the changes described.

80. **(D)** The use of radial/antiradial planes correlates to the ductal anatomy of the breast, with the nipple at the center of spoke-wheel-like duct distribution.

81. **(C)** An image should be captured to document the palpable area. Survey of the corresponding quadrant of the breast is also appropriate. Image capture of all four quadrants (Answer A) is indicated for whole breast ultrasound only. Nontargeted imaging of the axilla (Answer B) is not indicated.

82. **(C)** It is the sonographer's responsibility to bring to attention additional findings that may warrant further workup. Therefore, it would be appropriate to document both masses. However, bilateral whole breast ultrasound would not be indicated.

83. **(B)** The post-biopsy ultrasound should include a picture of the biopsy marker that is left in place. The remainder of the answer choices are not indicated.

84. **(A)** The triangle indicates the site of the focal zone, which is the depth of greatest lateral resolution.

85. **(A)** Ultrasound waves interact with tissue in all the above waves except for ionization. Ionization occurs when energy adds or removes an electron from an atom. The energy levels used in ultrasound imaging are not high enough to cause ionization like in general radiography.

86. **(D)** Multiple artifacts exist in ultrasound imaging. When sound waves encounter a strong reflector, in this case the muscle interface, the machine perceives the delayed, reflected waves as being received from a deeper structure, creating a mirror image. Side lobe artifact (Answer A) occurs when there is a strong reflector outside of the central beam, such that the echoes are displayed as if they originated from within the central beam, and can occur within cysts or other fluid collections. Ring-down artefact (Answer B) is a resonance artifact caused by fluid trapped between air bubbles and is seen posterior to a collection of gas. Posterior enhancement (Answer C) is seen as increased, not decreased, echogenicity deep to a cyst.

87. **(C)** Ultrasound machines have manual gain controls. Gain is the measure of strength of the signal displayed as echoes. Gain can be adjusted to amplify the ultrasound signal to evenly depict echoes regardless of depth.

88. **(A)** When the gain is set too low, echoes within hypoechoic masses may not be visualized, and a solid mass may be mistaken for a cyst. A high gain setting will amplify the internal echoes (Answer B). Harmonic imaging can eliminate echoes from within a cyst, so when harmonic imaging is turned off, this will not affect the appearance of the mass (Answer C). Answer D is a distractor.

89. **(C)** Harmonics may be used to reduce incident echoes within cystic structures if scatter is suspected by displaying echoes derived from a second frequency, or harmonic, sound wave. Adjusting the focal zone will adjust the depth of maximum resolution (Answer A). The use of harmonics also reduces side lobe artifact and increases lateral resolution (Answers A and B).[8]

90. **(B)** The use of elastography can highlight the desmoplastic response that may occur around a breast lesion. While not specific for malignancy, desmoplasia is the response of the body to a process by increasing the degree of fibrosis of the surrounding tissue.

91. **(A)** Compression of the breast is done during mammography to reduce tissue thickness. This minimizes the radiation absorption and improves image quality. Mammography generates an average of 20 lb of pressure to breast tissue. Today's implants (fifth-generation breast implants) can withstand 200 lb of pressure before any type of rupture.

92. **(B)** BI-RADS is an acronym for Breast Imaging-Reporting and Data System on mammograms. It uses category scores from 0 to 6.

93. **(D)** The multiple small, painless, bumps seen frequently on the areola are mammary gland, which is also called Montgomery glands (sebaceous gland). These glands secrete oil to help lubricate the areola and nipple during pregnancy and lactation to prevent cracking of the nipple during breast-feeding.

94. **(B)** Duct ectasia, also known as mammary duct ectasia, is a benign breast condition that occurs when milk duct widens and gets clogged with thick green or blue-black sticky nipple discharge.

95. **(C)** The most common location for breast cancer in men is underneath the nipple and subareolar.

96. **(C)** Lipoma is a benign, soft-tissue tumor that is composed of adipose tissue. The sonographic appearance of lipoma is hyperechoic with no posterior acoustic enhancement and more reflective than adjacent subcutaneous fat.

97. **(B)** Breast-feeding lowers the risk of breast cancer. Advance age, HRT, OCPs, obesity, inherited gene mutation, and smoking increase the risk of breast cancer.

98. **(A)** Swiss cheese disease, also known as juvenile papillomatosis, is a rear benign proliferative disease.

99. **(D)** Galactoceles are the most common benign breast lesions during breast-feeding period. This condition is secondary to obstruction of a lactiferous ducts.

100. **(B)** Mastitis is inflammation of mammary glands: Symptoms include tender, warmth, and swollen breast.

101. **(A)** The most common location of breast cancer in men is the ductal and subareolar region.

102. **(D)** Lipoma of the breast is a benign tumor that occurs due to an overgrowth of fat cells (adipose tissue). Lipomas are mostly asymptomatic and sometimes discovered on breast exam or screening mammography. Occasionally lipomas are not always visible on mammogram or ultrasound because fatty breast tissue blend in with fat cells of the lipoma (isoechoic). This finding makes breast lipomas difficult to diagnose. However, when visible on mammogram, it has a radiolucent gray appearance surrounded by a radioopaque capsule. On ultrasound, lipomas demonstrates a mildly hyperechoic mass adjacent to normal fat lobules.

103. **(D)** IDC. The most common breast cancer in men is IDC. This type of cancer is invasive because it begins in the duct and then breaks through the duct wall, eventually invading into the fatty surrounding tissue of the breast.

104. **(B)** Brachytherapy is used to treat early-stage breast cancer that is an alternative to the traditional whole breast radiation. Brachytherapy uses high dose of internal radiation to a smaller area of the breast using a brachytherapy catheter device, which is inserted into the lumpectomy cavity. Cyberknife uses external beam radiation that delivers stereotactic body radiation therapy (robotic radiosurgery) to the target lesion. Cyberknife is now used in treating breast, prostate, brain, and lung cancers.

105. **(A)** Sentinel lymph node is the first lymph node or group of nodes that receive drainage from a tumor with the axilla, the most common site for lymph node metastases. The axilla contains about 15–40 lymph nodes. Breast cancer can spread from the lymphatic system to the bones, lungs, liver, or brain.[1-4]

106. **(A)** The normal lymph node is less than 10 mm in size and nontender. Lymph node can be enlarged >10 mm in size when there is inflammation or in the presence of infection. Infection in the lymph nodes can be painful. Metastatic lymph nodes are painless and enlarged.

107. **(C)** Physical sign of silicone implant rupture is a change in shape and size of the breast. MRI is the most accurate modality for detection of a ruptured implant.

108. **(D)** Implant displacement views are warranted as breast tissue is hidden by implants and can result in a failure to detect breast cancer. When prepectoral breast implant is placed above the pectoralis major chest muscle, it will demonstrate more breast tissue than subpectoral breast implants. All breast MRIs, except of breast implant assessment, require contrast-enhanced imaging.[6]

109. **(A)** Teardrop sign represents an implant rupture on MRI. The sonographic signs of breast implant rupture are stepladder, snowstorm, echodense noise, and dirty shadow.[5-7]

110. **(D)** Fibrous capsule forms around breast implant are undetectable on physical examination.[2]

111. **(D)** Suspicious of cancer that requires a biopsy.

112. **(B)** Extracapsular breast implant rupture. A snowstorm sign represents silicone granulomas droplets mixed with

breast tissue. Intracapsular breast implant rupture gives a stepladder sign on ultrasound.

113. **(A)** ALCL

114. **(C)** Paget's disease of the breast. This disease is a malignant with physical findings of eczematous patches, eroding, and bleeding ulcer of the nipple. It is a rare form of breast cancer that collects under the areola and nipple. Most Paget's disease of the breast is associated with ductal carcinoma in situ.[3–5] Peau d' orange is the dimpling of the skin similar to the texture of an orange rind and associated with inflammatory breast cancer.

115. **(A)** Mondor's disease involves painful thrombophlebitis of the superficial veins of the breast and anterior chest wall. Physical examination finding is a cord-like elongated mass just below the skin. The associated causes are previous central venous catheters, safety belt, resent surgery, or dehydration. On ultrasound, Mondor's disease appears as a tubular anechoic structure. Mondor's disease is self-limited and resolves over 2–12 weeks period.[2]

116. **(B)** *S. aureus* and ultrasound skin thickening, prominent lymph channels, dilated ducts, and edematous breast parenchymal are all associated with mastitis. This patient has the classic symptoms of mastitis; swelling, fever, and tender and erythematous breast, which commonly occurs during lactation. Lactation mastitis is an inflammation of the breast tissue. It is the most common complication of breast-feeding caused by the bacteria *S. aureus* that penetrates the cracked nipple, resulting in blocking of the milk duct.[2] The treatment is antibiotic and the patient should continue breast-feeding.

117. **(C)** The most common location is the upper outer quadrant (43%) and more common in the left breast than the right.

118. **(B)** Taller-than-wider with vertical orientation. Popcorn calcifications in the breast are a classic description for old fibroadenomas seen on mammogram.

119. **(D)** Prophylactic antibiotic. Surgical "time out" is performed for reassurance and accuracy of patient identity, surgical site, and the procedure to be performed. Hand hygiene is standard care prior to any surgical procedure. It reduces the hand microbial count to prevent infection. An informed consent is a written joint agreement with the understanding of the procedure including the risk, benefits, and alternative to the procedure. Prophylactic antibiotic is usually not warranted for local biopsy procedures.

120. **(A)** Hematoma. A three-point seat belt used in automobiles can cause blunt crushing injuries such as hematoma, fat necrosis, and skin blistering. The shoulder belt can cause injury to the left breast in the driver's seat and right breast in the passenger seat. The lap belt should be placed below the pregnant belly and the shoulder belt between the breast.[4]

121. **(D)** Thoracic ribs that are located posterior to the pectoral muscles.

122. **(D)** Sebaceous gland, also known as Montgomery glands, in the areola that surrounds the nipple. This gland makes oily secretions which lubricate the areola. It becomes more pronounced during pregnancy.

123. **(B)** 2 o'clock position. A lesion located in in the upper outer quadrant of the left breast is between 12 and 3 o'clock position.

124. **(D)** Tail of Spence. The tail of Spence is a cone-shape breast tissue that extends from the upper lateral quadrant of the breast to the axilla.

125. **(C)** Second to the sixth rib. Although the size of the female breast varies, the female breast extends from the second to the sixth rib in an adult.

126. **(B)** Athelia. Children born with one or both nipple missing is a congenital condition, known medically as Athelia. The absent of breast tissue with the nipple present is called Amazia.

127. **(D)** A breast lobule is a gland that makes milk.

128. **(B)** The lateral thoracic artery and internal mammary artery provide blood supply to the breast.

129. **(C)** Adipose tissue. As a woman ages, she loses fat tissue in the breast and mammary glands. These changes are due to decrease in the production of estrogen.

130. **(B)** Pectoralis major muscle is a large fan-shape muscle underneath the breast tissue. Beneath the pectoralis major is the pectoralis minor.

131. **(D)** All of the above. The three most common cosmetic surgery of the breast are (1) mammoplasty and (2) augmentation, and breast reduction.

132. **(D)** Fibroadenoma is a benign mass. The symptoms for fibroadenoma are mobile mass, painless, rubbery, and not associated with menstruation.

133. **(C)** Muscles. There are different types of mastectomy: total mastectomy, modified radical mastectomy, radical mastectomy, partial mastectomy, and nipple-sparing mastectomy. Modified radical mastectomy involves removal of both the breast, skin, areola, nipple, and lymph nodes but not the pectoralis muscle.

134. **(A)** Lobules. Anatomically, the male breast is similar to the female breast, except that male breast lacks of Cooper's ligaments and lobules. The lobules in the female breast produce breast milk.

135. **(A)** Breast cancer can spread beyond the breast to nearby lymph nodes and lungs, then to any bone. However, the most common are ribs and spine.[7] The intercostal veins connect with the vertebral veins, which is a common route of metastatic spread of breast cancer to the vertebral bones.

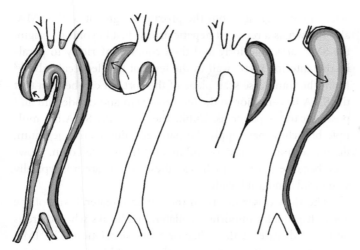

FIGURE 11-10. DeBakey classification of aortic dissection.

Sonographic and Doppler Characteristics. The real-time image will detail the echogenic intima separated from the aortic wall (Fig. 11–11). Color-flow imaging facilitates identification of the true and false lumens. Flow direction may reverse in the false lumen if there is only one tear; however, there may be multiple points of entry and exit and flow patterns may be complex. Doppler spectral waveforms should demonstrate antegrade flow in the true lumen with evidence of spectral broadening. Turbulent flow and elevated velocity are not commonly seen in the true lumen unless the lumen is significantly narrowed. The spectral waveforms in the false lumen may demonstrate increased resistance with low or absent diastolic flow if an outflow channel is not present. Because the false lumen often thromboses, it is important to determine, to the extent possible, whether the aortic branch vessels originate from the true or the false lumen.

Confirmation of aortic dissection is most often achieved with standard contrast arteriography or dynamic contrast or helical CT imaging.

SPLANCHNIC ARTERIES (CELIAC AND MESENTERIC ARTERIES)

Celiac, Common, Hepatic, Splenic, Left Gastric

Anatomy. The celiac artery is the first major branch of the abdominal aorta. It arises from the anterior aortic wall approximately 2 cm below the diaphragm at about the level of the twelfth thoracic vertebra and the first lumbar vertebra. The celiac artery (a.k.a. celiac axis, celiac trunk) is most often 2–3 cm in length. Approximately 1–2 cm from its origin, it divides into the common hepatic, splenic, and left gastric arteries. The splenic artery supplies blood to the spleen, pancreas, left half of the greater omentum, greater curvature of the stomach, and part of the fundus of the stomach. The common hepatic artery supplies the liver, gallbladder, stomach, pancreas, duodenum, and greater omentum.[1,2]

Sonographic and Doppler Characteristics. The celiac artery can be located as it arises from the anterior wall on a longitudinal image of the proximal aorta. It is best demonstrated, however, in the transverse scan plane of the aorta, as it is quite often tortuous. At its bifurcation into the common hepatic and splenic arteries, it assumes a "seagull" appearance, as these branches arise almost perpendicular to the celiac trunk (Fig. 11–12).

The splenic artery, the largest branch of the celiac, is most often tortuous. It courses along the posterosuperior margin of the pancreas and terminates within the hilum of the spleen.[1,2] It is most easily imaged along its course in the transverse plane beneath the body of the pancreas. The distal segment of the artery can be interrogated in the splenic hilum using a left lateral scan plane with a splenic window.

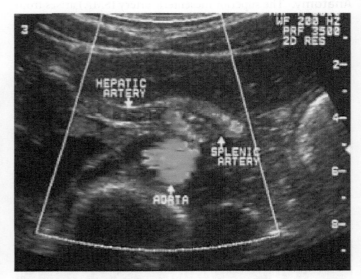

FIGURE 11-12. Transverse image of celiac artery bifurcation. Note "seagull" appearance created by position of the common hepatic and splenic arteries.

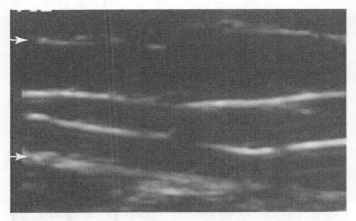

FIGURE 11-11. Real-time image of aortic dissection. Echogenic intima noted to be separated from arterial wall (arrows).

From its origin at the celiac bifurcation, the common hepatic artery courses along the superior border of the pancreatic head.[1,2] It gives rise to the gastroduodenal artery between the duodenum and the anterior surface of the head of the pancreas. It then courses superiorly and gives rise to the right gastric artery before entering the porta hepatis where it becomes the proper hepatic artery. The proper hepatic artery branches into the right and left hepatic arteries within the liver. These branches then divide into the segmental and subsegmental hepatic artery branches that course parallel to the bile ducts and portal vein branches.[1,2] The hepatic artery can be imaged from its origin to its termination within the liver. Its course and flow patterns are best delineated with color-flow imaging. The intrahepatic branches are most easily interrogated using a coronal oblique image plane.

The left gastric artery is occasionally seen longitudinally for approximately 1–2 cm but is not commonly visualized sonographically due to its small diameter and anatomic course.[6] The artery courses along the lesser curvature of the stomach, sending branches to the anterior and posterior segments of the stomach and esophagus.[1,2]

The celiac artery and its branches supply the low-resistance vascular beds of the liver and spleen. For this reason, these vessels will normally demonstrate a low-resistance waveform pattern characterized by constant forward diastolic flow (Fig. 11–13). The peak systolic velocity is less than 200 cm/s with an end-diastolic velocity less than 55 cm/s. Flow is laminar in the absence of significant disease. Postprandially, there is little to no increase in systolic or diastolic velocities, as the liver and spleen do not alter their vascular resistance in response to digestion.[5]

Superior and Inferior Mesenteric Arteries

Anatomy. The superior mesenteric artery (SMA) arises from the anterior wall of the aorta approximately 1–3 cm inferior to the celiac artery origin at about the level of the first lumbar vertebra.[1,2] In a small percentage of patients, the celiac artery and SMA may share a common trunk or the right hepatic

artery may originate from the proximal segment of the SMA, also known as a replaced hepatic artery. Just beyond its origin, the SMA arcs anteriorly and then courses inferiorly to parallel the anterior aortic wall to the level of the ileocecal valve.[1,2] From the transverse scan plane of the aorta, it can be seen that the SMA lies anterior to the left renal vein and duodenum and posterior to the pancreas. Unlike the celiac, the SMA has multiple branches that supply the pancreas, duodenum, jejunum, ileum, cecum, and the ascending and transverse colon. However, because of their small size, these vessels are not typically visualized sonographically.

The IMA originates from the left anterolateral wall of the aorta. It provides important collateral pathways when there is occlusive disease in the celiac or SMA circulation. The IMA is normally smaller in diameter than the SMA and can most often be identified from the transverse scan plane using surface anatomy as a landmark. Color-flow imaging facilitates identification of the artery's origin approximately two finger widths above the level of the umbilicus. The IMA supplies the left third of the transverse colon, the descending colon, sigmoid colon, and most of the rectum.[1,2]

Sonographic and Doppler Characteristics. The SMA can be visualized along its length from a longitudinal image plane. It will appear as a tubular structure that courses parallel to the anterior aortic wall originating just distal to the origin of the celiac artery (Fig. 11–14). It courses posterior to the splenic vein and pancreas and left of the superior mesenteric vein. From a transverse image plane, it is located superior to the left renal vein and appears disc-like with a dense echogenic ring caused by a fatty collar. From this image plane, it is noted that a portion of the body of the pancreas drapes over the SMA.

Because the SMA supplies the muscular tissues of the duodenum, jejunum, and colon, it will exhibit a high-resistance flow pattern characterized by low diastolic flow in its fasting state (Fig. 11–15). Following ingestion of a meal, vascular resistance decreases to meet the metabolic demands for additional blood flow that are associated with digestion (Fig. 11–16). To meet this demand, systolic and diastolic velocities normally increase at least twofold. Doppler spectral waveforms from

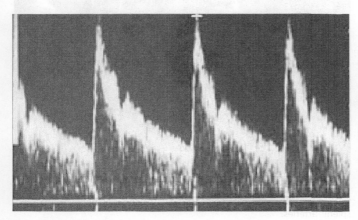

FIGURE 11–13. Classic low-resistance Doppler spectral waveform of the celiac artery.

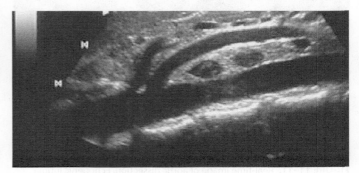

FIGURE 11–14. Real-time image of abdominal aorta demonstrating origins of the celiac and superior mesenteric arteries. Also note the adjacent lymphadenopathy.

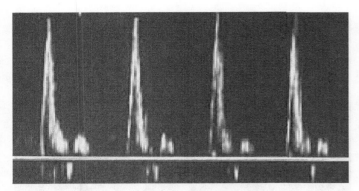

FIGURE 11–15. High-resistance spectral waveform pattern from a normal fasting superior mesenteric artery (SMA).

the IMA mimic those of the SMA in both the fasting and postprandial states.

Splanchnic Arterial Disease

Stenosis and Occlusion.
Flow-limiting disease involving the celiac artery and its branches or the SMA and IMA is most often caused by atherosclerosis and is commonly located at the vessel origins or at points of bifurcation. While the prevalence of mesenteric occlusive disease is low, women are affected more often than men, and in general, mesenteric disease is a problem of the elderly. Under normal circumstances, the visceral arteries receive 25–30% of the cardiac output and, in the fasting condition, contain one-third of the total blood volume.[6,7] When the flow demand in the gastrointestinal circulation cannot be met due to arterial stenosis or occlusion (usually in at least two of the three major splanchnic vessels), patients complain of postprandial abdominal angina, that is, pain associated with ingestion of a meal. As a result of pain associated with eating, they develop a "fear of food" syndrome and subsequent gastrointestinal impairment and significant weight loss. Even though the progression of atherosclerotic disease may be slow and insidious, the vascular compromise can lead to bowel infarction. Occasionally, patients suffer acute occlusion of the mesenteric arteries and will present with severe abdominal pain. This should be considered a

surgical emergency as delayed revascularization may result in gastrointestinal catastrophe.

Flow impairment may also be caused by compression of the splanchnic arteries. During normal respiration, the celiac artery may be intermittently compressed by the median arcuate ligament of the diaphragm. The ligament slides off the celiac artery allowing it to return to normal diameter when the patient takes a deep breath. The proximal SMA may be compressed in the mesentery or the duodenum may be "trapped" between the SMA and the aorta. This leads to SMA compression syndrome, which is characterized by an epigastric bruit, colicky abdominal pain, and occasionally malabsorption.

The visceral arterial circulation is richly collateralized with a network of vessels that connect the celiac and its branches with the branches of the superior and inferior mesenteric arteries.[2] When the celiac artery is critically stenosed or occluded, the pancreaticoduodenal arcade, a complex of small arteries surrounding the pancreas and duodenum, provides a collateral pathway. Collateral flow through branches of the IMA via the arc of Riolan or the marginal artery of Drummond, or the pancreaticoduodenal arcade may be apparent when there is occlusion of the SMA.

Sonographic and Doppler Characteristics.
Although disease may be found in any segment of the visceral arteries, atherosclerotic disease occurs most often at the vessel origins as an extension of plaque found on the aortic wall. B-mode imaging will detail the location and extent of plaque. The severity of luminal compromise may be estimated visually using color or power Doppler to define residual lumen. If stenosis is severe, a color bruit that is characterized by a mosaic color pattern and perivascular color artifact may be apparent.

Flow-limiting stenosis (>60–70% diameter reduction) of the celiac artery will demonstrate peak systolic velocities in excess of 220 cm/s and end-diastolic velocities greater than 55 cm/s.[3,5,7] A post-stenotic signal must be confirmed to differentiate elevated velocities due to focal stenosis from those associated with collateral compensatory flow. Median arcuate ligament compression of the celiac artery will result in high-velocity signals during normal respiration with return to normal velocity ranges when the patient takes a deep breath.

Peak systolic velocity in the SMA will be greater than 275 cm/s with an end-diastolic velocity exceeding 45 cm/s when the diameter of the SMA is reduced more than 70%.[3,5,7] As with the celiac artery, a post-stenotic signal must be confirmed to ensure identification of focal flow-limiting disease.

Arterial occlusion should be confirmed using spectral, color, or power Doppler optimized to show low-velocity flow.

Standard contrast arteriography with selective lateral views of the aorta provides confirmation of stenosis or occlusion of the visceral arteries and defines the presence and extent of collateral circulation prior to revascularization. In recent years, CT scanning has demonstrated a valuable role in localization of disease and display of relational anatomy.[8]

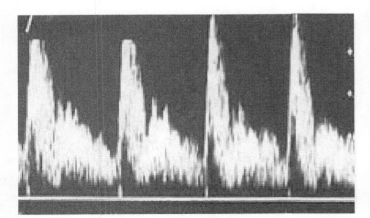

FIGURE 11–16. Low-resistance spectral waveform pattern from a postprandial SMA. Note the increase in diastolic flow.

RENAL ARTERIES

Anatomy

The renal arteries arise from the lateral, posterolateral, or anterolateral wall of the abdominal aorta at the level of the second or third lumbar vertebrae.[1,2] Most often they are single, but in approximately 35% of the population, there may be multiple renal arteries on each side.[5,6] This anomaly occurs more often on the left than on the right. The right renal artery is longer than the left and courses superiorly in its proximal segment and then courses posterior to the IVC to enter the hilum of the right kidney. The left renal artery courses through the flank posterior to the left renal vein to enter the hilum of the left kidney. The main renal artery gives rise to branches that supply blood to the adrenal gland and the ureter and then divides into anterior and posterior branches within the renal hilum. These in turn subdivide into the segmental arteries within the renal sinus and then give rise to the interlobar arteries that parallel the renal pyramids. The interlobar arteries divide into the arcuate arteries that curve around the bases of the pyramids. The arcuate arteries further subdivide into the small lobular arteries that supply the renal cortex.[1,2,5]

Sonographic and Doppler Characteristics

The proximal-to-mid segments of the renal arteries can most often be visualized from the transverse scan plane of the aorta at the level of the left renal vein (Fig. 11–17). Alternatively, the proximal segments of the arteries can be seen arising laterally from the aorta by scanning in a coronal plane through the liver so that the IVC and aorta are superimposed on each other (Fig. 11–18). The origin of the right renal artery can frequently be visualized on longitudinal images of the IVC as a small disc-shaped structure lying posterior to the IVC (Fig. 11–19). The distal-to- mid segments of the renal arteries are best seen with transverse imaging of the kidney using a subcostal or intercostal approach.[5,7] Quite often this approach will provide excellent

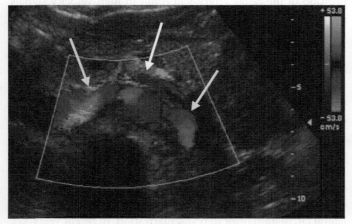

FIGURE 11–17. Transverse color-flow image of the proximal to mid segments of the renal arteries (yellow arrows) at the level of the left renal vein (white arrow).

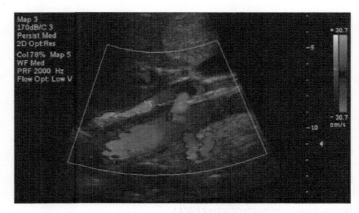

FIGURE 11–18. Longitudinal color-flow image of the inferior vena cava (IVC) and abdominal aorta demonstrating origins of renal arteries from the coronal plane.

images of the length of the renal artery from the hilum to its origin at the lateral wall of the aorta (Fig. 11–20). In an adult, kidney length is normally 11–13 cm and the width is 5–7 cm (Fig. 11–21). The anteroposterior thickness averages 2–3 cm, with the left organ being slightly larger than the right.[6]

The normal renal arterial waveform exhibits the classic features associated with flow to low-resistance end-organs; it is characterized by constant forward flow throughout diastole (Fig. 11–22). The peak systolic and end-diastolic velocities decrease proportionally from the main renal artery to the segmental arteries within the renal sinus to the arcuate arteries within the cortex of the kidney. Peak systolic velocity within the main renal artery is normally less than 120 cm/s with end-diastolic velocities averaging 30–50% of the peak systolic velocity.[5,7] A resistive index (RI) may be calculated to demonstrate evidence of impedance to arterial inflow. A normal RI in an adult is less than 0.70, while the indices are notably higher in premature infants and children younger than 4 years (0.70–1.0).[6]

Renal Arterial Disease

Stenosis and Occlusion. Atherosclerotic renal artery stenosis is the most common curable cause of renovascular hypertension. Atherosclerotic plaque occurs most frequently at the renal

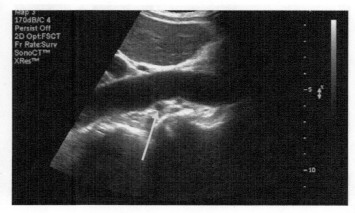

FIGURE 11–19. Real-time longitudinal image of the IVC. Note the disc-like appearance of the right renal artery posteriorly (yellow arrow).

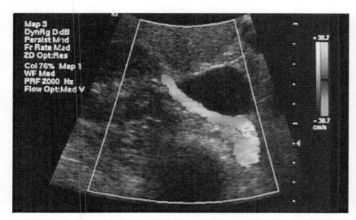

FIGURE 11–20. Color-flow image of the right renal artery as it courses from the hilum of the kidney to the aortic wall.

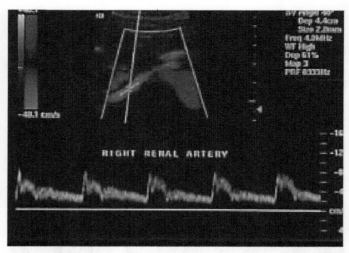

FIGURE 11–22. Color-flow image and Doppler spectral waveforms from a normal renal artery. Note the classic low-resistance waveform pattern.

artery ostium (origin) or within the proximal third of the renal artery. Ostial disease represents extension of plaque from the aortic wall. Medial fibromuscular dysplasia of the renal artery or its segmental branches is the second most common cause of renovascular hypertension.[7] This is a nonatherosclerotic disease entity that causes concentric regions of narrowing and dilation in the mid-to-distal segment of the renal artery (Fig. 11–23). In addition to atherosclerosis and fibromuscular dysplasia, causes of renal artery dysfunction include arteritis, aneurysm, congenital renal artery stenosis, congenital fibrous bands, neoplasms, vascular malformations, emboli, thrombus, trauma, fistulas, pheochromocytoma, neurofibromatosis, middle aortic syndrome, aortic coarctation, irradiation, and perirenal hematoma. Although patients with renal artery stenosis or occlusion may be asymptomatic, the majority present with systolic hypertension (>140 mm Hg), a flank bruit, congestive heart failure, or renal failure, or they are outside the normal age range for hypertension.

Medical renal disease (intrinsic parenchymal disease) should be included in the differential diagnosis for patients with hypertension. Parenchymal vascular disorders will cause elevated renovascular resistance. This may occur secondary to renal artery stenosis or be the primary etiology for elevated blood pressure.

Sonographic and Doppler Characteristics. B-mode imaging may reveal narrowed segments along the course of the renal artery, but confirmation of stenosis will be facilitated with color or power Doppler imaging (Fig. 11–24). In regions of flow-limiting disease, color Doppler will exhibit disordered flow patterns; a perivascular color artifact may be present if the stenosis is severe enough to cause a bruit. If the renal artery is occluded, no flow should be evident using spectral, color, or power Doppler optimized for slow flow. Low-amplitude, dampened spectral waveforms with tardus parvus ("late to rise") characteristics will be found within the renal parenchyma as a result of collateral flow. As renal artery stenosis progresses, renal length

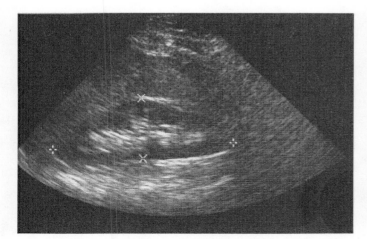

FIGURE 11–21. Gray-scale image of a kidney illustrating measurement of length and thickness.

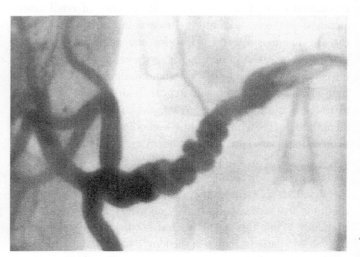

FIGURE 11–23. Arteriogram illustrating the concentric narrowing and dilation associated with renal arterial medial fibromuscular dysplasia.

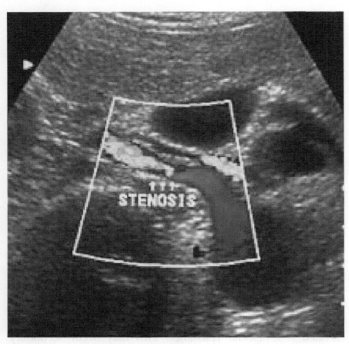

FIGURE 11–24. Color-flow image of the right renal artery demonstrating a region of disordered flow associated with stenosis.

decreases. There is commonly a difference in renal length greater than 3 cm side-to-side. Pole-to-pole length of the kidney will most often be less than 8 cm if the renal artery is occluded.[5,7]

Flow-limiting renal artery stenosis causes elevation in the peak systolic velocity. This velocity can be compared to the aortic velocity as a ratio of the angle corrected aortic peak systolic velocity recorded at the level of the celiac artery and the highest angle-corrected velocity in the main renal artery. When the renal-aortic velocity ratio (RAR) exceeds 3.5, there is evidence of flow-limiting renal artery stenosis (>60% diameter reduction). Care must be taken to ensure that the aortic peak systolic velocity is greater than 40 cm/s but less than 100 cm/s, as use of the RAR when velocity is outside these values will result in overestimation or underestimation of the severity of renal artery stenosis.[7] If the RAR cannot be used to confirm flow-limiting disease due to suspect aortic velocities, attention should be given to the peak systolic velocity in the renal artery and presence or absence of a classic post-stenotic signal. Recognition of hemodynamically significant stenosis is dependent on a renal artery peak systolic velocity greater than 180 cm/s and a post-stenotic signal. Stenosis that is hemodynamically significant (<60% diameter reducing) can be recognized when the renal artery peak systolic velocity is more than 180 cm/s, but no post-stenotic signal is present.[7]

Renal artery stenosis may also be identified using indirect methods that assess the distal renal artery and its segmental branches. While this technique has not been well validated, it has value in patients in whom the length of the renal artery cannot be adequately interrogated due to excessive abdominal gas,

body habitus, post-interventional, or traumatic causes. Using a 0-degree angle of insonation and a slow sweep speed, Doppler spectral waveforms are recorded from the distal renal artery and the segmental branches within the renal sinus. An acceleration time (time from onset of systole to the early systolic peak, which is seen on the systolic upstroke prior to peak systole) greater than 100 ms indicates more than 60% diameter-reducing renal artery stenosis. An acceleration index may also be used to identify flow-limiting renal artery disease. The index is defined as the change in distance between the onset of systolic flow and the peak systolic velocity divided by the acceleration time. An index less than 291 cm/s² is consistent with significant renal artery stenosis.[7,9]

Many types of medical renal diseases are accompanied by elevation of vascular resistance apparent in the intersegmental and arcuate arteries within the renal parenchyma. Normally, the end-diastolic velocity is at least 30–50% of the peak systolic velocity. As vascular resistance increases, diastolic flow decreases and a ratio of systolic to end-diastolic velocities within the intrarenal vessels will be greater than 0.20.[5,7]

Hydronephrosis is characterized by abnormal dilation of the renal calyces and renal pelvis caused by obstruction of the urinary tract. Sonographically, the renal sinus exhibits a hypoechoic or cystic area that may be variable dependent on the severity of the obstructive process (Fig. 11–25). The RI is commonly elevated with values greater than 0.70 in patients with obstructive hydronephrosis but may also be increased in patients with intrinsic renal parenchymal disease, perinephric or subcapsular hematoma, hypotension, and decreased heart rate.[4]

Although standard contrast arteriography remains the gold standard for confirmation of renal artery stenosis and occlusion, other imaging modalities may be used for confirmation of the sonographic examination or clinical findings. These include CT or MRI scanning, radionuclide renography, and intravenous pyelography.

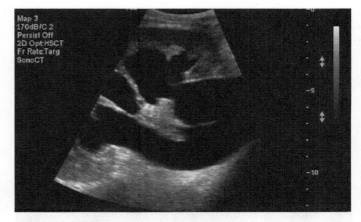

FIGURE 11–25. Real-time image of a kidney with hydronephrosis. Note the cystic appearance of the renal sinus.

INFERIOR VENA CAVA

Anatomy

The common iliac veins come together to form the IVC at approximately the level of the umbilicus or the fourth lumbar vertebra. The distal IVC ascends superiorly toward the diaphragm coursing to the right of the aorta and the spine. Although it will parallel the aorta along most of its course, it curves anteriorly in its proximal segment to enter the right atrium of the heart. The IVC receives blood from the hepatic, renal, right gonadal, right suprarenal, inferior phrenic, and lumbar veins (Fig. 11–26).[1,2] Normally, the IVC diameter is less than 2.5 cm, with slight increase in diameter above the entry level of the renal veins because of the increased volume of blood that is returned from the kidneys.[6] Diameter of the IVC is dependent on the patient's body habitus, the stage of respiration, and right atrial pressure. Anatomic anomalies may be noted, including duplication (0.2–3.0% of the population) or absence of the IVC (<0.2%) or transposition to the left side (0.2–0.5%).[1,2]

Sonographic and Spectral Doppler Characteristics

The IVC normally appears as an anechoic, tubular structure, the diameter of which varies with changes in respiration. Deep inspiration causes increased abdominal pressure and impedes venous return from the abdomen. This results in dilation of the IVC. Dilation can also occur in the presence of congestive heart failure, tricuspid regurgitation, or any condition that results in increased right atrial pressure.

Spectral Doppler demonstrates pulsatility in the proximal segment of the IVC because of the reflected right atrial pressure. Velocities are variable but remain low. The Doppler spectral

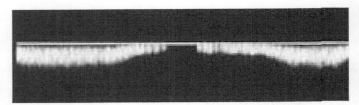

FIGURE 11–27. Doppler spectral waveforms from the infrarenal IVC. The respirophasicity is similar to that seen in the lower extremity veins.

waveform in the distal IVC demonstrates phasicity, similar to that seen in the lower extremity veins (Fig. 11–27). Color-flow imaging reveals directional variations associated with respirophasicity in the distal segment of the vein and reflected right atrial pulsations proximally.

Inferior Vena Caval Disease

Thrombosis is the most common vascular problem affecting the IVC and most often results from migration of thromboembolic material from the lower extremities or pelvic veins. IVC thrombosis is likely to occur with any condition that promotes stasis of blood flow in the abdominal veins, trauma to the vein wall, or hypercoagulability (Virchow's triad). Conditions that are associated with these features include dehydration, generalized sepsis, shock, retroperitoneal infection, pelvic inflammatory disease, caval filters or catheters, and extremity or abdominal surgery. Tumor thrombus may also be noted in association with carcinomas of the kidney, adrenal gland, pancreas, or liver. Other malignancies may involve the IVC, including ovarian and uterine neoplasms, lymphatic metastases from the prostate, pheochromocytomas, and Wilms' tumor.

While IVC thrombosis may be asymptomatic, the majority of patients will present with lower extremity edema and discomfort or symptoms characteristic of malignant conditions.

Sonographic and Doppler Characteristics. Thrombosis of the IVC causes dilation at the site of outflow obstruction. Acute thrombus will appear hypoechoic and a free-floating thrombus tail may be seen in the very acute phase (Fig. 11–28). The IVC will be noncompressible or partially compressible

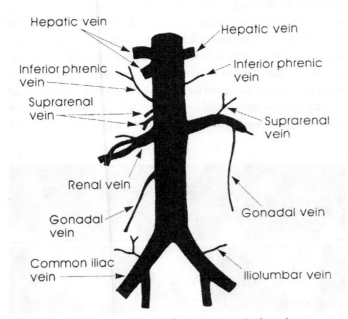

FIGURE 11–26. Diagram of the IVC illustrating its major branches.

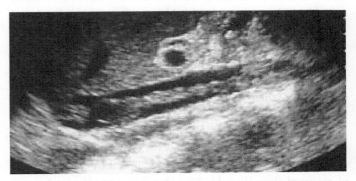

FIGURE 11–28. Real-time longitudinal image of the IVC demonstrating acute, free-floating thrombus.

with transducer pressure applied directly over the vein in the transverse imaging plane. As the thrombus ages, it will initially increase in echogenicity but then progresses through a variety of characteristics ranging from acoustic heterogeneity with anechoic regions to homogeneity. The acoustic features return to heterogeneity and the vein walls contract as the thrombus becomes chronic.

Doppler spectral waveforms demonstrate continuous, nonphasic flow patterns with partial obstruction of the caval lumen. No flow will be demonstrated by optimized spectral, color, or power Doppler when the lumen is totally obstructed. Low-amplitude, continuous waveforms may be recorded distal to the site of thrombosis if recanalization or collateralization of the thrombosed segment has occurred.

Correlative imaging is achieved with venocavography, MRI, or CT scanning.

HEPATIC AND PORTAL VEINS

Anatomy of the Hepatic Veins

The hepatic veins drain into the IVC and are the largest tributaries to the IVC. There are three major hepatic veins: the right, middle, and left. These large veins serve as boundary markers between the hepatic lobes and have multiple smaller branches throughout the liver parenchyma. The left and middle hepatic veins frequently share a common trunk at the IVC confluence, while the right hepatic vein remains independent. Occasionally, an accessory (inferior) right hepatic vein may be noted; one or more of the hepatic veins may be absent. The middle hepatic vein courses within the main interlobar fissure thus, dividing the liver into right and left lobes. The right lobe of the liver is divided into posterior and anterior segments by the right hepatic vein. The left hepatic vein divides the left lobe of the liver into medial and lateral segments.[1,2,5]

Sonographic and Spectral Doppler Characteristics.

The hepatic veins are best imaged from a subcostal approach, angling the transducer cephalad under the xiphoid process or from a right intercostal plane of view. Most often all three branches can be visualized. When only two branches are imaged from the subcostal approach, the veins mimic the head and ears of a rabbit. This is referred to as the "Playboy bunny sign" (Fig. 11–29). B-mode images normally reveal anechoic tubular structures that lack echogenic walls. While the diameter of the hepatic vein branches may appear small within the parenchyma of the liver, their diameters increase as they course toward the IVC.[6]

The Doppler spectral waveform from normal hepatic veins is pulsatile with two forward-flow cycles corresponding to the two phases of atrial filling. This is followed by a brief period of reversed flow (Fig. 11–30). This "W-shaped" waveform is dependent on variations in central venous pressure. The waveform is also influenced by respiration and compliance of the

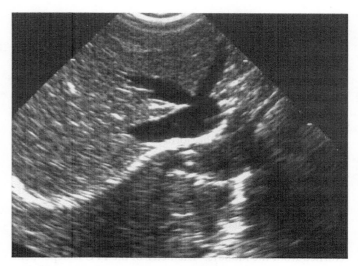

FIGURE 11–29. Real-time image of two hepatic veins at the hepatocaval confluence. The image illustrates the "Playboy Bunny" sign.

liver parenchyma. Flow direction in the hepatic veins is normally hepatofugal (away from the liver).

Anatomy of the Portal Vein

The portal vein is formed by the confluence of the splenic and superior mesenteric veins and carries nutrient-rich blood from the gastrointestinal tract, gallbladder, pancreas, and spleen to the liver where it is processed and filtered. The portal vein is responsible for carrying approximately 75–80% of the blood to the liver, while the hepatic artery supplies the remaining 20%.

Beyond the confluence of the splenic and superior mesenteric veins, the main portal vein courses to the right and cephalad to enter the porta hepatis where it bifurcates into right and left branches. The confluence of the splenic and portal veins is posterior to the neck of the pancreas. The inferior mesenteric vein drains into the splenic vein immediately to the left of this confluence. The coronary (left gastric) vein most often enters the splenic vein superiorly near the superior mesenteric/portal venous confluence and courses in a cranio-caudad plane.[10] The main portal vein lies anterior to the IVC, cephalad to the head of the pancreas, and caudal to the caudate lobe. It enters the liver along with the hepatic artery and common bile duct.[1,2,6,10] This

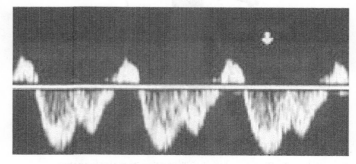

FIGURE 11–30. Classic Doppler spectral waveform pattern from normal hepatic veins.

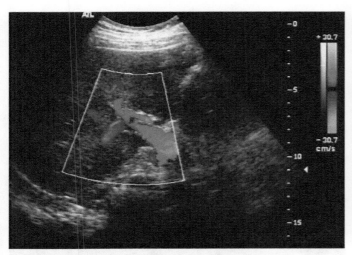

FIGURE 11–31. Color-flow image of the main portal vein from a right intercostal approach.

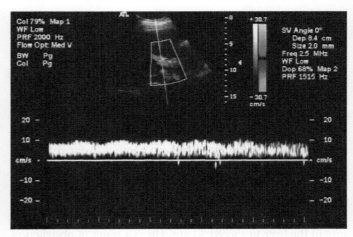

FIGURE 11–32. Color-flow image and Doppler spectral waveforms demonstrating normal hepatopetal flow direction and minimal phasicity.

portal triad travels as a unit throughout the liver parenchyma bound together by a collagenous membrane (Glisson's capsule).[6]

Within the porta hepatis, the main portal vein divides into the right and left portal vein branches. The right portal vein divides into anterior and posterior branches; the left divides into medial and lateral branches.[1,2]

Sonographic and Spectral Doppler Characteristics.

The portal vein can be followed sonographically from a transverse plane at the level of the splenic confluence and the porta hepatis. The course of the vein, its branches, and flow direction can be defined by using a right intercostal approach with the transducer angled toward the porta hepatis (Fig. 11–31). It should be noted that in contrast to the hepatic vein walls, the walls of the main portal vein and its branches are echogenic. This feature is attributed to the acoustic properties of collagen fibers found in the intimal and medial layers of the vein. While hepatic veins are boundary formers and course longitudinally toward the IVC, portal veins branch horizontally and are oriented as branches from the porta hepatis. The diameters of the left and right portal veins are greater at their origin in the region of the porta hepatis; minimal changes in diameter are noted during respiration. The diameter of the main portal vein is normally less than 13 mm in the segment just anterior to the IVC. An increase in diameter occurs during expiration, while inspiration results in decreased diameter. These changes are regulated by the volume of blood entering the visceral arterial system and the volume outflow through the systemic venous channels.

Doppler spectral waveforms from the portal veins normally demonstrate hepatopetal flow (toward the liver) with minimal phasicity and mean velocity ranging from 20 to 30 cm/s in the supine, fasting patient (Fig. 11–32). Mean velocity decreases slightly with inspiration and increases with expiration. Pulsatility of the portal veins may be apparent in patients with tricuspid insufficiency or congestive heart failure.

Hepatoportal Disease

Budd–Chiari Syndrome.
Obstruction of the outflow veins, or Budd–Chiari syndrome, results from high-grade stenosis or occlusion of some or all of the hepatic veins. Its occurrence is uncommon and is most often caused by membranous obstruction of the suprahepatic or infrahepatic portion of the IVC, but it may be related to tumor invasion or thrombosis. Budd–Chiari syndrome also occurs secondary to pregnancy, use of oral contraceptives, trauma, hypercoagulable states, polycythemia vera, radiation therapy, Behçet's syndrome, or hepatic abscesses. The hepatic veins may recanalize or they may become fibrotic. Parenchymal fibrosis, hemorrhage, and vascular congestion are associated with chronic hepatic veno-occlusive disease. While many patients may remain asymptomatic, the majority will present with right-upper-quadrant discomfort or pain, abdominal distention secondary to ascites, hepatomegaly, and superficial collateral veins. Budd–Chiari syndrome can be confirmed with CT or MRI scanning. Both modalities can demonstrate narrowing or absence of the hepatic veins. Venography may be used to confirm partial or complete obstruction of the IVC and the presence and extent of collateralization.

Portal Vein Thrombosis.
Portal vein thrombosis is most commonly associated with biliary atresia, cirrhosis, tumor, trauma, hypercoagulable states, portal hypertension, and inflammatory conditions such as pancreatitis or inflammation of the bowel. Other conditions may lead to thrombosis, including dehydration and blood disorders. Interventional procedures such as endoscopic esophageal sclerotherapy or percutaneous injection of ethanol for ablation of hepatocellular carcinoma may occasionally result in portal vein thrombosis. Periportal collaterals may form in the porta hepatis (cavernous transformation) or venous recanalization may be apparent following thrombosis of the extrahepatic portal vein. While cavernous transformation occurs in adults secondary to cirrhosis, pancreatitis, or malignancy, it is not commonly seen in patients

with liver disease but, surprisingly, is frequently encountered in patients with healthier livers.[10] It has been noted in neonates in association with omphalitis, systemic infection, abdominal inflammation, or dehydration or as a result of exchange transfusion or umbilical vein catheterization.

Portal venography is most often used to confirm the sonographic findings and to determine portal venous pressure. CT with contrast enhancement and MRI are also used to demonstrate portal vein thrombosis and cavernous transformation.

Portal Hypertension.

Normally, blood pressure within the liver is low (5–10 mm Hg) and commonly only slightly higher than that in the IVC. Portal hypertension causes the blood pressure in the liver to exceed 30 mm Hg as a result of obstruction to venous outflow.[5] In Western countries, cirrhosis is the usual cause of portal hypertension followed by hepatic vein thrombosis and portal venous occlusion. As resistance to normal portal venous flow increases, pressure within the liver increases and alternative routes for blood flow spontaneously develop. Flow in the main portal vein most often becomes hepatofugal in direction and normal portal tributaries enlarge to serve as collateral pathways.

Portal hypertension is classified into three categories: prehepatic, intrahepatic, and posthepatic. Prehepatic (presinusoidal) portal hypertension is caused by thrombosis or obstruction of the main portal vein before it enters the liver. Intrahepatic (sinusoidal) portal hypertension is the most common and is due to impedance to portal venous flow within the liver. Posthepatic (post-sinusoidal) portal hypertension occurs secondary to obstruction of the outflow veins or suprahepatic IVC.

Historically, standard contrast angiography has been used for confirmation of portal hypertension, determination of portal venous pressure, and demonstration of portosystemic collaterals. Angiography is also used to direct placement of coils or foam for embolization of varices and catheters for transjugular intrahepatic portosystemic shunts (TIPSs).

Sonographic and Doppler Characteristics of Hepatoportal Disease.

Budd–Chiari syndrome causes the liver to enlarge and may result in development of ascites. Splenomegaly is usually present and the caudate lobe may be enlarged as a result of increased outflow through the caudate veins. Sonographically, the liver parenchyma appears heterogeneous with increased echogenicity. While intraluminal echoes consistent with thrombus may be apparent in the acute stages, most commonly the hepatic veins are difficult to visualize because of reduced or absent flow. Spectral, color, and/or power Doppler optimized for very low flow should be used to demonstrate the presence of collateral pathways and to confirm patency or occlusion of the hepatic veins. Continuous, low-velocity Doppler spectral waveforms are commonly apparent proximal to stenotic segments while markedly elevated velocities are found at the site of stenosis. This pattern will be altered if the IVC is obstructed;

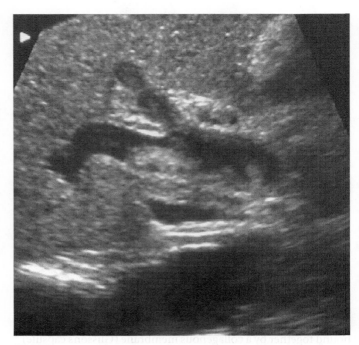

FIGURE 11–33. Real-time image demonstrating acute thrombus within the lumen of the portal vein.

low-velocity signals will be noted even in stenotic segments of the hepatic veins.

If the portal vein is acutely thrombosed, it will be dilated with acoustically homogeneous echoes within the lumen (Fig. 11–33). The thrombotic process may be segmental with sparing of one or more of the main tributaries.[5] Chronic thrombosis may cause the portal vein and its branches to be difficult to visualize because of a decrease in vein diameter and the presence of increased intraluminal echogenicity resulting from fibrosis. Total obstruction of the portal vein can be demonstrated with color or power Doppler to show the absence of flow. Thrombosis can then be confirmed with optimized spectral Doppler. Color or power Doppler will demonstrate flow around the thrombus when the vein is partially obstructed. Spectral Doppler waveforms will be nonphasic, consistent with the absence of respiratory variation as a result of increased venous pressure. If cavernous transformation has replaced the main portal vein, multiple small tubular structures will be noted in the porta hepatis (Fig. 11–34). They will appear anechoic but will demonstrate low-velocity, minimally phasic spectral waveforms characteristic of portal venous flow. When flow in the portal vein is compromised, the hepatic artery assumes responsibility for supplying the majority of oxygenated blood to the liver. As a result of flow demand, the hepatic artery may enlarge, vascular resistance in the hepatic artery decreases, and velocity may increase.

Tumor infiltration of the portal vein occurs most often in patients with hepatocellular carcinoma or liver metastases. Color Doppler will define multiple small vessels throughout the tumor-filled portal vein. While cavernous transformation of the portal vein will demonstrate venous signals in the small

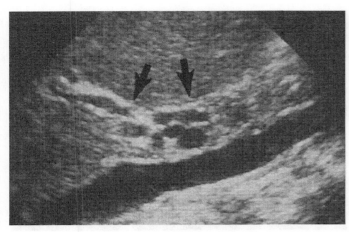

FIGURE 11-34. Real-time image of the porta hepatis demonstrating small, serpiginous venous collaterals. This finding is consistent with cavernous transformation of the portal vein.

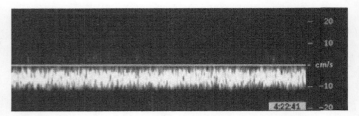

FIGURE 11-36. Doppler spectral waveform demonstrating continuous, low-velocity hepatofugal flow in the portal vein. This finding is suggestive of portal hypertension.

channels, tumor blood flow is characterized by low-resistance arterial waveforms.

Portal hypertension can be characterized by its sonographic findings. The portal vein is commonly enlarged, decompression of the liver results in changes in normal blood flow patterns and direction of flow, and collateral pathways and varices (enlarged veins) develop (Fig. 11–35). Hepatic cirrhosis results in loss of respirophasicity in the portal vein and its branches. As portal venous pressure increases, the Doppler spectral waveform may become bidirectional, demonstrating both hepatopetal and hepatofugal flow. Continuous hepatofugal portal venous flow

is consistent with portal hypertension and velocity commonly is less than 12 cm/s (Fig. 11–36). Portal vein diameter at the level of the IVC is frequently greater than 13 mm and respiratory variation in vein diameter disappears.[10] Periportal fibrosis causes increased echogenicity of the portal venous walls and the vein may become comma-shaped. The coronary vein diameter usually increases to exceed 5 mm. Additionally, the diameter of the splenic and superior mesenteric veins may increase to more than 10 mm, but most often, there is less than 20% increase in diameter of these veins from quiet respiration to deep inspiration. Varices may be noted in the splenic hilum and the region of the gallbladder.

There are other sonographic findings that characterize portal hypertension. Commonly there is fatty infiltration of the liver and portosystemic collaterals are apparent within the liver parenchyma and the splenic hilum (splenorenal and splenocaval), as well as a recanalized paraumbilical vein. Identification of the collateral pathways is facilitated with color-flow imaging which will define their presence and confirm flow direction. Splenomegaly may be present (>13 cm), while liver size decreases to less than 10 cm anteroposteriorly, less than 15 cm in length, and less than 20 cm in width.[6] Dilated, tortuous superficial veins may be obvious surrounding the umbilicus (caput medusa). These arise from a recanalized paraumbilical vein, which can be imaged in a longitudinal or transverse scan plane in the region of the falciform ligament (Fig. 11–37).[10] The

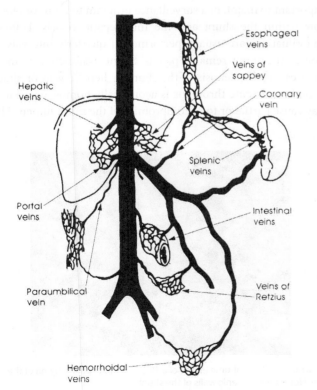

FIGURE 11-35. Diagram illustrating portosystemic collateral pathways.

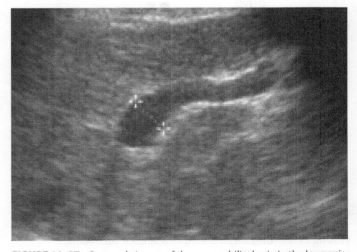

FIGURE 11-37. Gray-scale image of the paraumbilical vein in the long axis within the falciform ligament.

umbilical vein will appear as a "bull's eye" when imaged in the transverse plane.

TRANSJUGULAR INTRAHEPATIC PORTOSYSTEMIC SHUNTS

The current nonsurgical procedure of choice for reduction of venous pressure, variceal bleeding, and ascites is diversion of blood from the portal vein to the systemic venous circulation by way of an intrahepatic shunt. The shunt is created by catheter entry through the right internal jugular vein. The catheter is then advanced to the superior vena cava (SVC) and the hepatic (usually right or middle) vein. The catheter traverses the liver parenchyma and enters the main portal vein. A metallic stent is placed over the catheter and balloon dilated to create a shunt between the portal venous system and the hepatic vein (Fig. 11–38).

Sonographic and Doppler Characteristics of TIPS

Prior to placement of the TIPS, sonography has shown value in confirming patency and flow direction in the portal vein and its branches, demonstration of a recanalized paraumbilical vein or other portosystemic collaterals, varices, and location and extent of ascites. Attention is given to assessment of the internal jugular vein to ensure its patency.

Following placement of the TIPS, the shunt is evaluated to obtain baseline information on shunt velocity, direction of flow in the main portal vein and its intrahepatic branches, and the hepatic veins. Flow velocities in the main portal vein usually exceed 80 cm/s, with a waveform pattern mimicking the pulsatile flow common to the hepatic veins (Fig. 11–39). Because most of the intrahepatic flow will be toward the shunt (low resistance), hepatofugal flow direction is expected in the portal vein branches. Flow in the hepatic veins should remain hepatofugal.

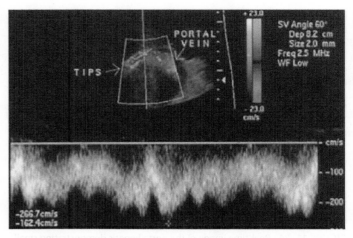

FIGURE 11–39. Color-flow image and Doppler spectral waveforms demonstrating normal flow in a TIPS.

A change in normal flow direction in the intrahepatic venous channels signifies shunt dysfunction and stenosis or occlusion of the shunt should be determined.[9]

High-resolution B-mode imaging is used to define location of the shunt within the hepatic and portal veins; the shunt should extend well into both vessels. Sonographically, the shunt will appear as an echogenic tubular structure extending along a curved path from the portal vein to the hepatic vein (Fig. 11–40). Most often, it measures 8–10 mm in diameter.

Recognition of TIPS Dysfunction

Because TIPSs are susceptible to malfunction over time, it is important to maintain a surveillance program to monitor blood flow within the shunt and the intrahepatic vessels. Follow-up evaluations are usually performed at quarterly intervals as long as the shunt remains patent. Shunt dysfunction is most often caused by stenosis of the shunt or hepatic vein or shunt thrombosis. Acute thrombus is acoustically homogeneous and may cause partial or total compromise of the shunt lumen. The

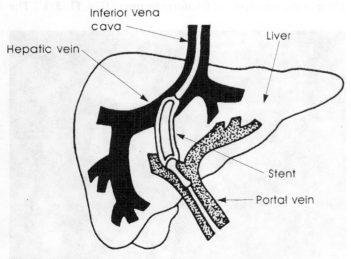

FIGURE 11–38. Diagram illustrating a transjugular intrahepatic portosystemic shunt (TIPS).

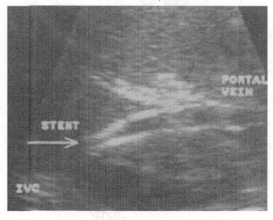

FIGURE 11–40. Real-time image of a TIPS within the parenchyma of the liver. Note the echogenic walls of the shunt.

presence and extent of the thrombus may be defined with color Doppler imaging, while total obstruction of the shunt must be confirmed with optimized spectral Doppler. The direction of flow in the main portal vein may revert to hepatofugal with decreased velocities and varices may recur.

Intimal hyperplasia is the primary factor in shunt stenosis and is caused by a buildup of collagenous material between the shunt and its endothelial surface. While it commonly occurs in the early post-shunt period, it may develop any time within the first year. Acoustically, it is homogeneous and will be noted to compromise the lumen of the shunt. The extent of compromise can be defined with color-flow imaging and the severity of stenosis determined by velocity spectral waveform parameters.

While problems may be encountered in the portal vein, body of the shunt, or the hepatic outflow vein, most often the obstruction is on the hepatic end of the conduit. B-mode imaging will confirm a reduction in the internal diameter of the shunt when compared to the baseline measurement. Magnified views will facilitate comparative measurements. Color-flow imaging will define narrow segments, regions of disordered flow, and changes in flow direction in the portal and hepatic veins. Additional signs of shunt dysfunction include recurrence of varices and portosystemic collaterals and new onset of ascites.

Changes in velocity and flow direction when compared to the baseline evaluation are key to identification of shunt dysfunction. Depending on the severity of stenosis, velocities may either increase or decrease compared to the previous examination. TIPS velocities are typically higher than those of native vessels, but an interval increase or decrease in velocity exceeding 50 cm/s has been shown to be consistent with stenosis, while actual velocities less than 60 cm/s are diagnostic of flow limitation that is clinically significant.[3,9]

RENAL VEINS

Anatomy of the Renal Veins

The renal veins return blood from the kidneys to the IVC. The intrarenal subcapsular veins converge to form the stellate veins. These veins drain into the interlobular veins, which empty into the interlobar veins. The interlobar veins form the main renal vein. The right renal vein courses superiorly to the right renal artery to the lateral wall of the IVC and is the shorter of the two renal veins. The left renal vein courses from the hilum of the left kidney to cross the aorta anteriorly and the pancreas inferiorly before entering the IVC. As it crosses the aorta, it is visualized posterior to the SMA.[1,2] The vein may be compressed in the mesentery between the aorta and SMA, resulting in the "nutcracker sign." Multiple venous branches are common.

Sonographic and Doppler Characteristics

Sonographically, the renal veins appear as anechoic tubular structures extending from the renal hila to the posterolateral

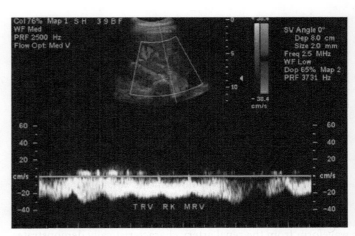

FIGURE 11–41. Color-flow image and Doppler spectral waveforms from a normal renal vein.

walls of the IVC (Fig. 11–41). The renal veins are routinely evaluated with optimized spectral and color Doppler to determine patency and flow direction. The Doppler spectral waveform pattern demonstrates low-velocity respirophasicity with flow away from the renal hilum.

Renal Venous Disorders

Renal Vein Thrombosis. Renal vein thrombosis most commonly occurs secondary to trauma or tumor. Trauma frequently causes extrinsic compression of the vein or endothelial damage, which leads to flow obstruction and thrombosis. Renal tumors often advance to the renal vein. In the neonate, thrombosis may result from infection, dehydration, hypotension, or maternal diabetes. Primary renal disorders, including membranous glomerulonephritis and nephrotic syndrome, are frequently the etiology for this condition in adults. Systemic causes must also be considered, including lupus erythematosus, amyloidosis, diabetes mellitus, and sickle cell anemia.

Renal vein thrombosis is encountered more often in the left renal vein and children are affected more often than adults. Patients may present initially with proteinuria, microscopic hematuria, and epigastric discomfort or pain. Adults may present acutely with dehydration, vascular congestion, or hypercoagulopathies. Clinical symptoms may also include pulmonary embolism.

Sonographic and Doppler Characteristics of Renal Venous Disorders. Acute renal vein thrombosis causes the kidney to increase in size while cortical echogenicity decreases. The renal sinus becomes hypoechogenic, the pyramids are prominent with poor definition and the corticomedullary junction is indistinct. Thrombosis causes the renal vein to dilate. Acute thrombus will appear acoustically homogeneous; chronicity leads to increased echogenicity. Color and power Doppler imaging may facilitate differentiation of partial from total venous obstruction by outlining the filling defect.

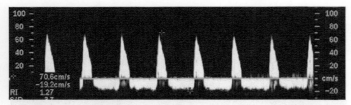

FIGURE 11–42. Doppler spectral waveforms from a renal artery with outflow to a thrombosed renal vein.

Continuous, nonphasic flow is associated with partial thrombosis, while the absence of flow due to total obstruction can be confirmed with optimized spectral, color, and power Doppler. When the renal vein is thrombosed, the Doppler spectral waveform from the renal artery characteristically demonstrates increased resistance as having a rapid systolic upstroke, rapid deceleration, and reversed, blunted diastolic flow (Fig. 11–42).

LIVER, RENAL, AND PANCREAS TRANSPLANTS

Liver Transplantation

Liver transplantation is the treatment of choice for end-stage liver disease. With current surgical techniques and immunosuppressive therapy, the expected survival rate at 1 year exceeds 85%.[9] Sonography plays a major role in the preoperative and postoperative evaluation. Children with biliary atresia may have an associated polysplenia syndrome with intestinal malrotation, bilateral symmetry of the major bronchi, and abnormal location of the portal vein to a position anterior to the duodenum. Additionally, the IVC may be interrupted. Hepatic artery anatomic variants and the presence and flow patterns associated with portacaval or mesocaval shunts must be defined. It is critical that these conditions are identified prior to transplantation.

The donor liver may be cadaveric (orthotopic) in origin or the patient may retain his or her own liver and a portion of a donor liver is transplanted (heterotopic). The vascular anatomy and anastomotic sites will differ with each type of procedure. If an orthotopic cadaver liver transplant (OLTx) is used, the recipient's liver and gallbladder are removed and a cadaveric donor liver is transplanted (Fig. 11–43). The arterial and venous anastomoses include the extrahepatic portal vein, hepatic artery, and suprahepatic and infrahepatic IVC. Biliary drainage is achieved with a Roux-en-Y cholecystojejunostomy or choledochostomy with a T-tube. With heterotopic transplantation, the vascular anastomoses are to the suprahepatic IVC, hepatic artery, and portal vein. Biliary drainage is temporary through a choledochojejunostomy.[7]

Sonographic and Doppler Characteristics of Liver Transplants.
Sonography is generally performed pre-transplantation and post-transplantation. Preoperatively, the abdomen is assessed for fluid collections and masses, hepatomegaly, splenomegaly, patency of the hepatic artery and its

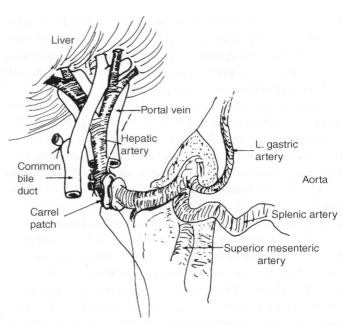

FIGURE 11–43. Diagram illustrating liver transplant procedure.

branches, portal vein and its branches, superior mesenteric vein, splenic artery and vein, and the IVC. Particular attention is given to the measurements of the liver and spleen and to detection of malignancy. The post-transplant evaluations are directed to confirmation of vessel patency and flow patterns at the anastomotic sites. Flow velocities may be slightly elevated in the early post-transplant period due to vascular accommodation, extrinsic compression due to tissue edema, and slight diameter mismatch. Even so, there is normally no evidence of remarkable velocity increase in any vessel or post-stenotic turbulence associated with flow-limiting compromise of vessel lumen. Color-flow imaging may facilitate identification of the hepatic artery and hepatic veins and confirmation of appropriate flow direction in all vessels.

Recognition of Liver Transplant Complications

Organ Rejection. Rejection of the liver transplant is a primary cause of organ dysfunction. Clinically, patients experience fever, malaise, anorexia, and hepatomegaly. Sonography is neither sensitive nor specific for the identification of hepatic transplant rejection but has value in excluding stenosis or thrombosis of the hepatic artery, portal vein, or IVC, as well as biliary complications. Laboratory tests are valuable in refining the suspected diagnosis and include elevated serum bilirubin, alkaline phosphatase, and serum transaminase. Confirmation of rejection is achieved most commonly with needle biopsy.

Hepatic Artery Thrombosis. Thrombosis of the hepatic artery post-transplant is considered a critical complication as it jeopardizes transplant viability and the possibility of re-transplantation. While it may be difficult to demonstrate intraluminal thrombus with real-time imaging, optimized spectral, color, or power

Doppler will confirm absence of flow. Standard contrast angiography has historically been chosen to validate the sonographic findings.

Hepatic Artery Stenosis. Kinking, coiling, or curling of the extrahepatic segment of the hepatic artery may occur as a result of excessive length of the anastomosed vessel. Flow-reducing stenosis can occur in any of the segmental branches of the artery within the liver parenchyma. Color-flow imaging will define regions of disordered flow and occasional evidence of perivascular color artifact characteristic of an arterial bruit associated with chaotic flow patterns. Hepatic arterial Doppler spectral waveforms exhibit peak systolic velocities in excess of 180 cm/s, with evidence of post-stenotic turbulence and a systolic acceleration time greater than 0.8 seconds (Fig. 11–44). Distal to the site of narrowing, the Doppler waveform is usually dampened with low velocity forward diastolic flow (RI <0.5).[4,7]

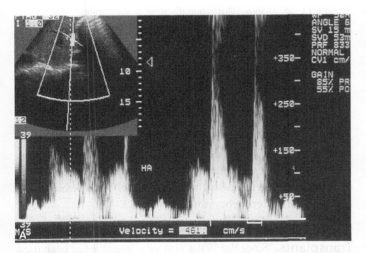

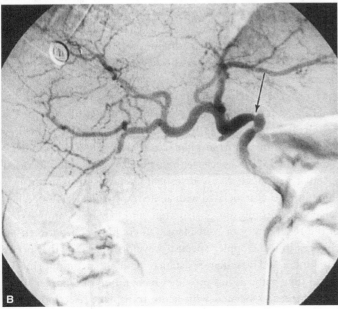

FIGURE 11–44. Arteriogram with associated Doppler spectral waveforms from a liver transplant hepatic artery stenosis.

Portal Vein Thrombosis. Post-transplant thrombosis of the portal vein is associated with early transplant failure and a high mortality rate. High-resolution B-mode imaging will demonstrate dilation of the portal vein and acoustically homogeneous intraluminal echoes. The thrombus may be partially or totally obstructive. Color or power Doppler imaging may be used effectively to highlight flow around a thrombus that is partially occluding a vein lumen or confirm absence of flow when total obstruction is suspected. Thrombosis may extend beyond the main portal vein and include the right and left branches and their tributaries. Attention should be given to identification of periportal collaterals and patency of the hepatic artery that may continue to provide flow to the liver.

Portal Vein Stenosis. Stenosis of the portal vein is an uncommon complication following liver transplantation. When present, it is most often found in the region of the portal vein anastomosis as an irregularity of the vein wall or a band-like stricture. Aneurysmal dilation and portal hypertension may be associated with chronic stenosis.

Inferior Vena Cava Thrombosis and Stenosis. Flow may be compromised in the IVC post-transplant as a result of an anastomotic stricture or extrinsic compression from tissue edema, hematomas, or fluid collections adjacent to the IVC anastomoses. Real-time imaging will demonstrate acoustically homogeneous or heterogeneous intraluminal echoes dependent on the age of the thrombus. Partial versus total obstruction can be determined with color or power Doppler and confirmed with optimized spectral Doppler interrogation. Luminal compromise may cause elevation of IVC velocities in the region of narrowing with dampening of the distal signal.

Biliary Complications. Obstruction and leaks are the most common biliary complications post-transplantation. Obstruction is considered to be present if the common bile duct diameter exceeds 6 mm. This complication is most often caused by strictures associated with surgical technical errors, infection, chronic rejection, or ischemia. Additional causes may be related to dysfunction of T-tubes or stents, redundancy of the common bile duct, biliary stones, and mucoceles of the remnant of the cystic duct. Bile leaks are identified sonographically as anechoic fluid collections in the biliary system. Bilomas may be present in the gallbladder fossa and porta hepatis. These will appear cyst-like with internal echoes and demonstrate acoustic enhancement. Most often, they are irregularly shaped.

Pseudoaneurysms. Pseudoaneurysms occur when at least two of the three layers of the arterial wall have been punctured, allowing blood to escape into the surrounding tissue. Pseudoaneurysms (false aneurysms) may occur when there is leakage of blood through an anastomotic site or from an artery that has mistakenly been punctured during the transplant procedure or post-transplantation biopsy. This is an uncommon complication and is most often associated with graft needle biopsy or

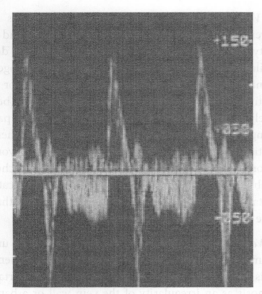

FIGURE 11–45. Characteristic "to-and-fro" Doppler spectral waveform pattern recorded in the neck of a pseudoaneurysm.

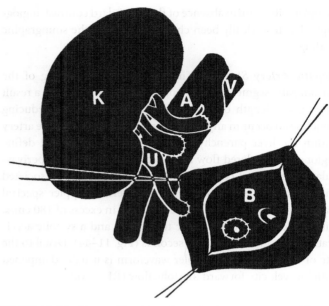

FIGURE 11–46. Diagram illustrating the surgical anastomoses used for renal transplantation. K is kidney; A is arterial; V is vernous; U is ureter; B is bladder.

infection. Recognition of pseudoaneurysms is facilitated with color-flow imaging and differentiation of pseudoaneurysm from true aneurysmal dilation is dependent on documentation of a to-and-fro Doppler spectral waveform in the tract that connects the false aneurysm to the punctured artery (Fig. 11–45).

Correlative imaging modalities for confirmation of liver transplant dysfunction are chosen based on the clinical presentation. Standard contrast arteriography is used to demonstrate patency of the primary arteries and veins and for assessment of organ perfusion. Radionuclide scintigraphy has shown value for evaluation of liver perfusion, hepatocyte function, and assessment of bile excretion. While bilomas and abscesses may be identified sonographically, hepatobiliary scintigraphy is used to confirm these lesions. CT imaging has value for confirmation of biliary necrosis; however, cholangiography is the procedure of choice for confirmation of biliary system compromise.

Renal Transplantation

Renal transplantation was first introduced in the 1950s and has become the procedure of choice for patients with end-stage renal disease. Survival rates are excellent in the current surgical era as a result of improved surgical procedures and advances in immunosuppression. Multiple causes of post-transplantation renal failure still exist, however, and many of these can be identified sonographically. Real-time imaging, coupled with spectral, color, and power Doppler, has shown value as a tool for preoperative assessment and post-transplantation surveillance of tissue and flow characteristics that are consistent with renal transplant dysfunction.

If a living-related donor kidney is used, sonography plays an important preoperative role in ensuring that the arterial and venous circulations are normal and that the recipient aorta and external iliac arteries are free of atherosclerotic debris. Following transplantation, sonographic surveillance is employed to identify increased renovascular resistance associated with acute rejection, acute tubular necrosis (ATN), transplant renal artery stenosis/occlusion, and arteriovenous (AV) communication.

In adult patients, the transplanted kidney is most often placed superficially in the right lower abdomen. The donor renal artery is anastomosed to the right external or internal iliac artery, while the transplant renal vein is anastomosed to the external iliac vein. Drainage from the ureter into the bladder is achieved via ureteroneocystostomy (Fig. 11–46).

Sonographic and Doppler Characteristics of Renal Transplants. Since the 1980s, real-time imaging has been used to identify acute renal transplant rejection. The more popular characteristics include increased renal volume, enlargement of the renal pyramids, decrease in the amount of renal sinus fat, increased cortical echogenicity, decreased echogenicity of the renal parenchyma, indistinct corticomedullary boundaries, and thickening of the renal pelvis. These criteria are neither sensitive nor specific for renal allograft rejection when correlated histologically.

Greater emphasis has been placed on assessment of the flow patterns within the transplant renal artery and vein and the parenchymal vessels because these patterns alter with increased vascular resistance. Many investigators have shown that elevation of the RI is associated with acute transplant rejection, ATN, renal vein thrombosis, obstruction, and extrinsic compression of the renal artery or transplant. Others have concentrated on changes in the Doppler spectral waveform patterns that occur with increased vascular resistance. Sequential monitoring of blood flow patterns has provided recognition of Doppler spectral patterns associated with acute transplant rejection, ATN, transplant renal artery stenosis/occlusion, renal vein thrombosis, and AV fistulas.[4,9]

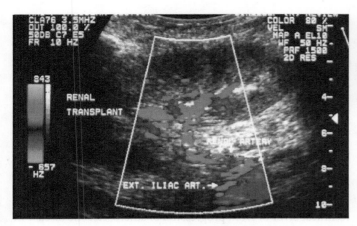

FIGURE 11–47. Color-flow image illustrating the iliac arterial and venous anastomoses and flow within the parenchyma of a renal transplant.

Sonographically, the normal renal transplant will appear as an elliptical organ lying in close proximity to the psoas muscle in the lower right iliac fossa. The ureter may be difficult to image unless it is enlarged due to obstruction. The region surrounding the transplant should be surveyed for fluid collections and care should be taken to identify hydronephrosis or inappropriate echogenicity of the renal tissues. Color-flow imaging will facilitate identification of the anastomoses of the transplant renal artery and vein to the external iliac artery and vein and confirmation of flow throughout all segments of the renal medulla and cortex (Fig. 11–47). AV fistulas and stenosis associated with kinking or intrinsic narrowing of an artery will present on the color-flow image as regions of disordered flow and mosaic coloration. Tissue infarction is best confirmed with optimized power and spectral Doppler to show absence of flow.

Doppler spectral waveforms from the normal external iliac artery demonstrate phasicity with forward flow in the segment of the artery proximal to the anastomosis of the transplant renal artery. The relatively low-resistant flow pattern is caused by the flow demand of the transplanted organ. In the segment of the external iliac artery distal to the renal artery anastomosis, the Doppler spectral waveform will be triphasic, characteristic of the high-resistance peripheral arterial system of the lower extremities (Fig. 11–48). The external iliac vein normally

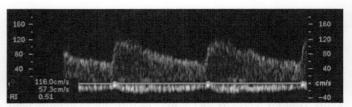

FIGURE 11–49. Normal low-resistance Doppler spectral waveforms from a renal transplant.

demonstrates respirophasicity consistent with venous flow patterns in the extremities.[3,9]

Slight flow disturbance may be apparent at the renal artery anastomosis due to slight deviation of the flow stream. High-velocity, turbulent flow patterns are not normally seen. The Doppler spectral waveform demonstrates a low-resistance pattern with constant forward flow throughout diastole. This pattern is propagated throughout the transplant renal artery and the vessels within the medulla and cortex of the organ (Fig. 11–49). The peak systolic and end-diastolic velocities decrease proportionally from the main renal artery to the arcuate vessels within the cortex. Although venous respirophasicity may decrease, continuous nonphasic flow is not normal.[3,9]

Recognition of Renal Transplant Complications

Acute Renal Transplant Rejection. Real-time imaging details an enlarged organ with a slightly irregular renal outline, indistinct corticomedullary boundaries, decreased echogenicity of the pyramids, decreased echogenicity of the renal sinus, increased cortical echogenicity, and irregular fluid-filled areas within the renal cortex.

Acute vascular rejection is characterized by proliferative endovasculitis, which causes the arterial intima to thicken. Blood flow is impeded by the arterial narrowing and vascular resistance increases (RI >0.8). The increase in resistance is characterized by a decrease in diastolic flow. This is evident in the Doppler spectral waveform pattern throughout the kidney (Fig. 11–50). As the severity of the rejection episode continues to advance, the diastolic flow component of the waveform may

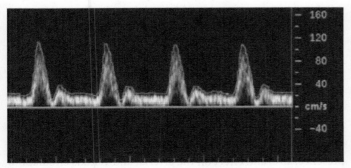

FIGURE 11–48. Doppler spectral waveforms demonstrating the flow pattern in the external iliac artery in the region of the transplant renal artery anastomosis.

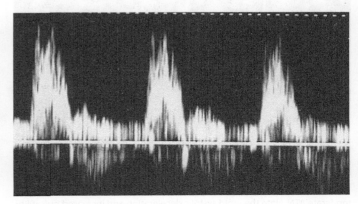

FIGURE 11–50. High-resistance Doppler spectral waveform pattern associated with acute renal transplant rejection.

deteriorate from low to zero to a reversed flow phase. In the most critical cases of rejection, diastolic flow may be altogether absent. Platelet-fibrin aggregates may form to the extent that the intersegmental and arcuate arteries of the transplant thrombose; this results in organ failure.[9]

Acute Tubular Necrosis. ATN may be difficult to identify with real-time imaging, as the tissues appear normal. Mild ATN is characterized by peritubular necrosis and medullary arterial-venous shunting. As the necrotic process becomes more severe, tubular and interstitial edemas are apparent and impedance to arterial inflow to the transplanted organ increases. Resistive indices will increase, but this quantitative method of assessment only signifies increased renovascular resistance and does not define its etiology. We have shown a continuum of Doppler spectral patterns associated with mild, moderate, and severe ATN.[5,9]

Mild ATN produces a spectral pattern that appears normal except for rapid deceleration from the systolic peak to an increased diastolic forward-flow component. This is thought to be the result of the arterial-venous medullary shunting. Moderate ATN is associated with a spectral waveform that demonstrates rapid systolic deceleration and increased pulsatility (Fig. 11–51). As the severity of the necrotic process increases, vascular resistance increases and diastolic flow decreases further. The Doppler spectral pattern for severe ATN demonstrates a reduction in the amount of diastolic flow, amplitude of the signal, and descent of the diastolic flow component. The waveform may be indistinguishable from the pattern associated with severe acute rejection.[5,9]

Transplant Renal Artery Stenosis and Occlusion. Transplant renal artery stenosis has been shown to occur in as many as 12% of cases. This is most often the result of one of two complications. The first is due to sharp angulation of the transplant renal artery at the anastomosis to the external iliac artery. The kinking may result in flow reduction in the renal artery. The second

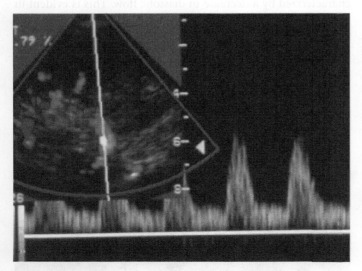

FIGURE 11–51. Doppler spectral waveform pattern associated with moderate ATN. Note the rapid systolic deceleration and increased pulsatility compared to the normal spectral pattern.

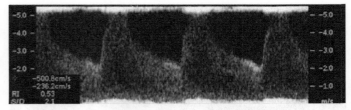

FIGURE 11–52. Flow-reducing transplant renal artery stenosis is characterized by high-velocity, turbulent signals and a renal-iliac artery ratio greater than 3.0.

type may result from anastomotic stricture as a consequence of technical error or from progression of atherosclerotic disease in the iliac artery. The second type may also be related to arterial injury during harvesting, chronic rejection, or post-transplant intimal hyperplasia. Clinically, patients present with new onset hypertension, elevated serum creatinine levels, and perhaps a bruit in the region of the transplant renal artery anastomoses.

If anastomotic kinking is present, real-time imaging will define sharp angulation at the anastomotic site; color or power Doppler can be used to confirm narrowing of the arterial lumen. Spectral Doppler waveforms from the external iliac and transplant renal artery reveal high-velocity, turbulent flow and a renal-iliac artery ratio of more than 3.0 (Fig. 11–52).[5]

Severe vascular rejection may lead to thrombosis of the transplant renal artery or the vessels within the sinus and cortex of the kidney. Infarction may be complete or segmental. Immediate surgical or lytic intervention is required to salvage the organ. High-resolution B-mode imaging details a hyperechoic organ or regions of ischemic tissue. Occlusion of the transplant renal arteries is suggested when there is no evidence of flow using optimized spectral, color, or power Doppler.

Thrombosis of the transplant renal vein is most often caused by surgical technical complications or from extrinsic compression of the vein postoperatively by hematoma, seroma, or tissue edema. Sonographically, the vein appears dilated with acoustically homogeneous intraluminal echoes. Spectral, color, or power Doppler will confirm the absence of flow in the transplant renal vein and throughout the renal parenchymal venous tree. The Doppler spectral waveform from the renal arteries is characterized by a sharp systolic upstroke followed by rapid deceleration to a reversed and blunted diastolic flow component as previously described.

Arteriovenous Fistulas. Acute renal transplant rejection has historically been confirmed with cortical needle biopsy. These procedures may result in development of AV communications within the parenchyma of the organ. These AV fistulas rarely severely compromise blood flow to the kidney and are usually self-limiting. Color-flow imaging can be used to define the presence, size, and effect on the arterial and venous circulation. Doppler spectral waveforms detail the pressure-flow gradient in the fistula as evidenced by high-velocity, turbulent flow in the feeding arteries and pulsatile, arterialized flow patterns in the draining veins.

Pseudoaneurysms. Percutaneous biopsy or anastomotic leakage may result in formation of pseudoaneurysm at the site of arterial puncture or breakthrough. The majority of pseudoaneurysms are small and self-limiting; the patient remains asymptomatic. Some, however, may be quite large and can compromise flow to the transplanted kidney or rupture. As described earlier, blood escapes from the artery into the surrounding tissue and is connected to the artery by a neck or pedicle. High-pressure flow enters the false aneurysm through the neck during systole and returns to the artery during the low-pressure diastolic phase of the cardiac cycle. This results in the classic "to-and-fro" Doppler spectral waveform that is diagnostic for flow patterns associated with pseudoaneurysms (see Fig. 11–45).

Consistent with liver transplantation, correlative imaging modalities chosen for confirmation of renal transplant dysfunction are based on the clinical presentation. MRI or radionuclide imaging is chosen to evaluate perfusion and functional status of the transplanted kidney. Standard contrast arteriography has historically been used for vascular evaluation, while CT imaging has shown value for both pre-transplantation and post-transplantation assessment.

Pancreas Transplantation

Most often, pancreatic transplantation is performed in patients with end-stage renal disease secondary to type I diabetes and to reverse the complications related to progression of disease. The pancreas is transplanted in conjunction with a renal transplant or may be transplanted alone in diabetic patients who do not have renal failure.

The first segmental pancreas transplantation was performed in 1966 and survival rates have increased in the present era as a result of improved surgical techniques and immunosuppressive regimens. Graft failure is often the consequence of acute rejection, vascular thrombosis, pancreatitis, fluid collections, infection, pseudocysts, and anastomotic leaks. The most serious complications occur in the early post-transplantation period and are commonly related to thrombosis of the splenic vein.

The pancreatic transplant is placed superficially in the pelvic area in a manner similar to that used in renal transplantation. When both organs are transplanted together, the pancreas is placed on the patient's right side and the kidney on the left side (Fig. 11–53). The celiac artery and SMA are harvested from the donor aorta on a Carrel patch and anastomosed to the recipient's external iliac artery. The tail of the pancreas is perfused by the splenic artery, which is left intact during transplantation. The donor portal vein is anastomosed to the external iliac vein; the splenic vein drains the tail of the pancreas transplant. A section of the donor's duodenum is attached to the recipient bladder to achieve exocrine drainage.[9]

Clinical features of acute pancreas transplant rejection include elevated serum amylase, glucose, and lipase levels.

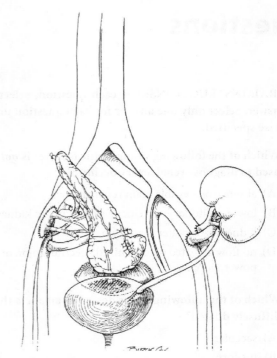

FIGURE 11–53. Diagram illustrating the surgical procedure used for transplantation of a kidney and pancreas. *(Reproduced with permission from Neumyer MM: Ultrasonographic Assessment of Renal and Pancreatic Transplants, J Vas Tech. 1995;19(5-6);321-329.)*

Recognition of Pancreas Transplant Complications

Acute Rejection. In contrast to its use as a valuable aid to detection of acute rejection in renal transplants, sonography has demonstrated little value in identification of rejection in pancreas transplants. Real-time imaging may demonstrate acoustic inhomogeneity, poor margination of the organ, dilated pancreatic duct, and relative changes in attenuation.

Thrombosis. Thrombosis is most often seen in the early postoperative period but may occur later as a consequence of rejection of the transplanted organ or infection. Venous thrombosis is most serious when it affects the splenic vein and can threaten organ viability.[9] When multiple venous segments are involved, arterial inflow is compromised and organ survival is jeopardized. Color-flow imaging is used to confirm patency of the arterial and venous anastomoses and perfusion of the transplanted organ. Most importantly, it has been the procedure of choice for confirming patency of the splenic vein throughout its tortuous course along the posterior aspect of the organ.[8]

Pancreatitis. Pancreatitis may occur as an inflammatory response to reperfusion of the organ at the time of transplantation. In most cases, this is a mild episode but, if severe, can compromise organ viability. Sonographically, in the acute phase, the pancreas is slightly enlarged with a hypoechoic, fluffy-looking texture as a result of tissue edema. Fibrosis and calcifications may be noted if the condition is long-standing.[6]

Questions

1. Which of the following sonographic features is *not* used to diagnose renal artery occlusion?

   (A) absence of a visible main renal artery

   (B) low-amplitude, low-velocity signals in the kidney

   (C) kidney size greater than 9 cm

   (D) no flow detected by optimized spectral, color, or power Doppler

2. Which of the following terms describes an aorta that is diffusely dilated?

   (A) saccular

   (B) fusiform

   (C) spindle-shaped

   (D) ectatic

3. What is the first major branch of the abdominal aorta?

   (A) lumbar artery

   (B) renal artery

   (C) celiac artery

   (D) SMA

4. Which of the following terms is used to describe concentric, spindle-shaped dilation of the abdominal aorta?

   (A) ectatic

   (B) fusiform

   (C) saccular

   (D) dissecting

5. The branches of which of the following arteries form a "seagull" appearance on a sonographic image?

   (A) IMA

   (B) renal artery

   (C) SMA

   (D) celiac artery

6. What are the branches of the celiac artery?

   (A) proper hepatic, superior mesenteric, and left gastric arteries

   (B) splenic, left gastric, and common hepatic arteries

   (C) right gastric, splenic, and inferior mesenteric arteries

   (D) left gastric, superior mesenteric, and splenic arteries

7. Abdominal pain that increases in severity with an upright position is symptomatic of which of the following conditions?

   (A) aortic dissection

   (B) pancreatitis

   (C) ruptured aortic aneurysm

   (D) acute mesenteric ischemia

8. Where are AAAs most often located?

   (A) in the juxtarenal aorta

   (B) in the suprarenal aorta

   (C) in the infrarenal aorta

   (D) at the aortic bifurcation

9. The splanchnic circulation does *not* include which of the following arteries?

   (A) renal, superior, and inferior mesenteric arteries

   (B) gastric, celiac, and superior mesenteric arteries

   (C) celiac, superior, and inferior mesenteric arteries

   (D) superior mesenteric, celiac, and gastroduodenal arteries

10. A 50–74% diameter-reducing stenosis of the abdominal aorta is characterized by which of the following findings?

    (A) a 20% increase in peak systolic velocity compared to the proximal normal arterial segment

    (B) a twofold increase in peak systolic velocity compared to the proximal normal arterial segment

    (C) a fourfold increase in peak systolic velocity compared to the proximal normal arterial segment

    (D) a 50% increase in peak systolic velocity compared to the proximal normal arterial segment

11. When an aortic stent graft is used to repair an AAA, which of the following statements about the aneurysm is true?

    (A) It is allowed to remain.

    (B) It is resected.

    (C) It is wrapped around the aortic graft.

    (D) It is ligated and bypassed.

12. Which of the following findings is *not* usually associated with aortic dissection?

    (A) pregnancy
    (B) Marfan's syndrome
    (C) hypertension
    (D) advanced age

13. Real-time images demonstrating the echogenic intima separated from the aortic wall are suggestive of which of the following diagnoses?

    (A) AAA
    (B) arterial dissection
    (C) false aneurysm
    (D) mycotic aneurysm

14. The common hepatic artery gives rise to which of the following arteries?

    (A) gastroduodenal artery and right gastric artery
    (B) coronary artery and celiac artery
    (C) proper hepatic artery and left gastric artery
    (D) gastroduodenal artery and right hepatic artery

15. The splenic artery does *not* supply blood to which of the following structures?

    (A) spleen
    (B) gallbladder
    (C) pancreas
    (D) stomach

16. Which of the following arteries is the largest branch of the celiac artery?

    (A) gastroduodenal artery
    (B) left gastric artery
    (C) hepatic artery
    (D) splenic artery

17. The left gastric artery is most often visualized in real-time

    (A) longitudinally
    (B) arising from the SMA
    (C) inferior to the celiac artery
    (D) along the greater curvature of the stomach

18. The Doppler spectral waveform from the normal celiac artery is characterized by all of the following, *except*

    (A) constant forward diastolic flow
    (B) peak systolic velocity less than 200 cm/s

    (C) end-diastolic velocity greater than 75 cm/s
    (D) rapid systolic upstroke

19. The accompanying Doppler spectral waveform is from a fasting SMA. This waveform is characteristic of

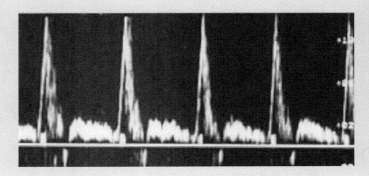

    (A) a normal SMA
    (B) more than 70% diameter-reducing SMA stenosis
    (C) a post-stenotic signal
    (D) SMA stenosis that is not hemodynamically significant

20. Anatomically, the SMA courses

    (A) anterior to the left renal vein
    (B) posterior to the duodenum
    (C) perpendicular to the aorta
    (D) anterior to the pancreas

21. Which of the following is *not* a classic symptom associated with chronic mesenteric ischemia?

    (A) post-prandial pain
    (B) "fear of food" syndrome
    (C) weight loss
    (D) acute, severe abdominal ischemia

22. The Doppler spectral waveform associated with flow-reducing SMA stenosis is *not* characterized which one of the following findings?

    (A) turbulence
    (B) an SMA-aortic ratio greater than 3.5
    (C) peak systolic velocity greater than 275 cm/s
    (D) end-diastolic velocity greater than 45 cm/s

23. A high-velocity celiac artery Doppler signal that normalizes with deep inspiration is suggestive of which of the following diagnoses?

    (A) flow-reducing celiac artery stenosis
    (B) portal hypertension
    (C) median arcuate ligament compression
    (D) mesenteric ischemia

24. A collateral pathway to compensate for occlusion of the celiac and/or SMA does *not* include which of the following?

    (A) the arc of Riolan
    (B) the pancreaticoduodenal arcade
    (C) the marginal artery of Drummond
    (D) the inferior epigastric artery

25. Which of the following imaging procedures is historically used for confirmation of visceral artery stenosis or occlusion and demonstration of the extent of collateralization?

    (A) standard contrast arteriography with selective lateral views
    (B) CT
    (C) MRI
    (D) contrast-enhanced sonography

26. The left renal vein courses

    (A) posterior to the IVC
    (B) posterior to the aorta
    (C) between the aorta and the SMA
    (D) parallel to the superior mesenteric vein

27. The arcuate arteries of the kidney

    (A) subdivide into the intersegmental arteries
    (B) curve around the bases of the pyramids
    (C) lie within the renal hilum
    (D) demonstrate a high-resistance Doppler spectral waveform

28. Renal artery flow-reducing stenosis is indicated if which of the following findings is seen?

    (A) The renal-aortic ratio is less than 3.0, and the peak systolic velocity is greater than 180 cm/s.
    (B) The peak systolic renal artery velocity is less than 180 cm/s and a post-stenotic signal is found.

(C) The end-diastolic renal artery velocity is greater than 20 cm/s, and the acceleration time is greater than 1.0.
(D) The renal-aortic ratio is greater than 3.5 and a post-stenotic signal is found.

29. The RAR can be used to diagnose renal artery stenosis if the aortic velocity is

    (A) less than 30 cm/s
    (B) between 40 and 100 cm/s
    (C) greater than 120 cm/s
    (D) between 30 and 80 cm/s

30. As renal vascular resistance increases, what happens to diastolic flow initially?

    (A) decreases
    (B) reverses
    (C) becomes quasi-steady
    (D) increases

31. The renal RI would *not* usually be increased in patients with which of the following conditions?

    (A) intrinsic renal parenchymal disease
    (B) perinephric or subcapsular hematoma
    (C) decreased heart rate
    (D) mild ATN

32. A Doppler spectral waveform demonstrating high resistance features would normally be found in which of the following arteries?

    (A) hepatic artery
    (B) IMA
    (C) renal artery
    (D) splenic artery

33. What is the second most common cause of renovascular hypertension?

    (A) ostial atherosclerotic plaque
    (B) anastomotic stenosis
    (C) fibromuscular dysplasia
    (D) renal artery aneurysm

34. Tardus parvus Doppler spectral waveforms within the renal parenchyma indicate which of the following findings?

    (A) renal artery stenosis or occlusion
    (B) medical renal disease
    (C) hydronephrosis
    (D) pyelonephritis

35. Renal artery occlusion is *not* indicated by

 (A) a kidney pole-to-pole length less than 8 cm

 (B) low-amplitude, low-velocity cortical signals

 (C) a difference in kidney length less than 2 cm

 (D) absence of color Doppler in imaged renal artery

36. An end-diastolic to systolic velocity ratio of less than 0.20 from a renal intersegmental artery indicates which of the following diagnoses?

 (A) medical renal disease

 (B) renal artery stenosis

 (C) renal artery occlusion

 (D) fibromuscular dysplasia

37. The common iliac veins come together to form the IVC at the level of the

 (A) second lumbar vertebra

 (B) fourth lumbar vertebra

 (C) ileocecal valve

 (D) inguinal ligament

38. What is the most common vascular problem affecting the IVC?

 (A) tumor extension

 (B) thrombosis

 (C) extrinsic compression

 (D) transposition

39. Carcinomas of the kidney, adrenal gland, and liver frequently involve which of the following vessels?

 (A) abdominal aorta

 (B) hepatic veins

 (C) renal arteries

 (D) IVC

40. Which of the following is *not* likely to cause IVC thrombosis?

 (A) stasis

 (B) sepsis

 (C) abdominal surgery

 (D) pregnancy

41. In a normal adult, the renal artery RI should not be greater than

 (A) 0.03

 (B) 0.35

 (C) 0.70

 (D) 1.05

42. If the IVC is partially obstructed, the Doppler spectral waveforms will be

 (A) phasic

 (B) pulsatile

 (C) continuous

 (D) absent

43. Which of the following would *not* be used for confirmation of IVC thrombosis?

 (A) venocavography

 (B) contrast angiography

 (C) MRI

 (D) computed tomographic scan

44. The liver is divided into right and left lobes by which of the following veins?

 (A) right hepatic vein

 (B) middle hepatic vein

 (C) portal vein

 (D) left hepatic vein

45. The "Playboy bunny" sign refers to the

 (A) hepatic artery

 (B) portal veins

 (C) common bile duct

 (D) hepatic veins

46. Which vessel receives drainage from the hepatic veins?

 (A) IVC

 (B) portal vein

 (C) splenic vein

 (D) superior mesenteric vein

47. The Doppler spectral waveform from the hepatic veins is normally

 (A) nonphasic

 (B) pulsatile

 (C) quasi-steady

 (D) continuous

48. Which of the following vessels supplies the majority of oxygenated blood to the liver?

 (A) aorta

 (B) hepatic artery

 (C) SMA

 (D) portal vein

49. **The portal vein is formed by the confluence of which of the following veins?**

    (A) hepatic and splenic veins

    (B) superior mesenteric and splenic veins

    (C) hepatic and superior mesenteric veins

    (D) inferior and superior mesenteric veins

50. **Where does the main portal vein lie?**

    (A) inferior to the superior mesenteric vein

    (B) inferior to the head of the pancreas

    (C) cephalad to the caudate lobe

    (D) anterior to the IVC

51. **Which three vessels form the portal triad?**

    (A) portal vein, superior mesenteric vein, splenic vein

    (B) portal vein, common bile duct, hepatic artery

    (C) portal vein, hepatic artery, SMA

    (D) portal vein, common bile duct, middle hepatic vein

52. **Which of the following is true regarding hepatic veins?**

    (A) are boundary formers and course horizontally toward the IVC

    (B) are not boundary formers and are oriented toward the porta hepatis

    (C) are not boundary formers and course longitudinally toward the porta hepatis

    (D) are boundary formers and course longitudinally toward the IVC

53. **Doppler spectral waveforms from the portal veins do *not* normally demonstrate which of the following?**

    (A) pulsatility

    (B) minimal phasicity

    (C) hepatopetal flow

    (D) velocity ranging from 20 to 30 cm/s

54. **Which of the following terms is used to describe obstruction of the hepatic veins?**

    (A) fibromuscular dysplasia

    (B) cavernous transformation

    (C) Budd–Chiari syndrome

    (D) hemangioma

55. **Which of the following statements describes hepatic veins?**

    (A) They can be compressed with a Valsalva maneuver.

    (B) They have thick, echogenic walls.

    (C) They course horizontally within the liver parenchyma.

    (D) They divide the liver into segments.

56. **In the Western countries, portal hypertension is most often caused by which of the following?**

    (A) hepatitis

    (B) sclerosing cholangitis

    (C) cirrhosis

    (D) hepatocellular carcinoma

57. **Cavernous transformation is found in association with**

    (A) hepatic vein thrombosis

    (B) portal vein thrombosis

    (C) superior mesenteric vein thrombosis

    (D) IVC thrombosis

58. **What is the normal blood pressure within the liver?**

    (A) 5–10 mm Hg

    (B) 20–30 mm Hg

    (C) 0–5 mm Hg

    (D) more than 30 mm Hg

59. **What is the most common type of portal hypertension?**

    (A) suprahepatic

    (B) extrahepatic

    (C) intrahepatic

    (D) posthepatic

60. **Which of the following signs is *not* consistent with portal hypertension?**

    (A) portal vein diameter greater than 13 mm

    (B) portal vein velocity less than 12 cm/s

    (C) respiratory variation in portal vein signals

    (D) hepatofugal portal venous flow

61. **Which of the following causes mycotic aneurysms?**

    (A) Marfan's syndrome

    (B) trauma

    (C) penetrating injuries

    (D) infection

62. **The paraumbilical vein is a branch of which of the following veins?**

    (A) coronary vein

    (B) left gastric vein

    (C) left portal vein

    (D) middle hepatic vein

63. Which of the following veins assumes a "bull's eye" appearance in the transverse image plane in the region of the falciform ligament and after exiting the liver may form the caput medusa in the region of the umbilicus in patients with portal hypertension?

    (A) paraumbilical vein

    (B) coronary vein

    (C) left hepatic vein

    (D) right gastric vein

64. A TIPS is placed in the liver to shunt blood from which of the following veins?

    (A) right hepatic artery to left hepatic vein

    (B) left portal vein to right hepatic artery

    (C) main portal vein to right hepatic vein

    (D) right portal vein to left hepatic vein

65. The color-flow image and Doppler spectral waveforms below are suggestive of which of the following findings?

    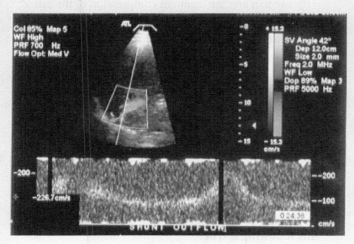

    (A) TIPS stenosis

    (B) obstruction in the hepatic outflow vein

    (C) IVC thrombosis

    (D) portal vein thrombosis

66. Following placement of a functioning TIPS, flow in the hepatic veins should be

    (A) hepatopetal

    (B) phasic

    (C) hepatofugal

    (D) continuous

67. The B-mode image below demonstrates

    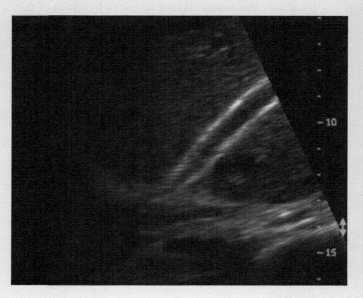

    (A) a TIPS within the liver

    (B) hepatocellular carcinoma

    (C) hemangioma

    (D) stenosis of the right hepatic vein

68. Following placement of a TIPS, velocity within the shunt is 180 cm/s, flow in the portal vein is 110 cm/s, flow in the main portal vein is hepatopetal, flow in the left portal and hepatic veins is hepatofugal. What are these findings most consistent with?

    (A) occlusion of the TIPS

    (B) TIPS stenosis

    (C) normally functioning TIPS

    (D) hepatic outflow obstruction

69. Following placement of a TIPS, velocity within the shunt is 55 cm/s, flow in the portal vein is 58 cm/s, flow in the main portal vein is hepatopetal, flow in the left portal and hepatic veins is hepatopetal. What are these findings most consistent with?

    (A) occlusion of the TIPS

    (B) TIPS stenosis

    (C) normally functioning TIPS

    (D) hepatic outflow obstruction

70. The Doppler spectral waveform pattern that suggests renal vein thrombosis is characterized by which of the following findings?

    (A) rapid systolic upstroke, rapid deceleration, and low diastolic flow

    (B) delayed systolic upstroke, rapid deceleration, and high diastolic flow

    (C) rapid systolic upstroke, rapid deceleration, and reversed, blunted diastolic flow

    (D) delayed systolic upstroke, rapid deceleration, and high, blunted diastolic flow

71. Which of the following symptoms is *not* associated with renal vein thrombosis?

    (A) hematuria

    (B) pulmonary embolism

    (C) epigastric pain

    (D) fever

72. The Doppler spectral waveforms shown below illustrate

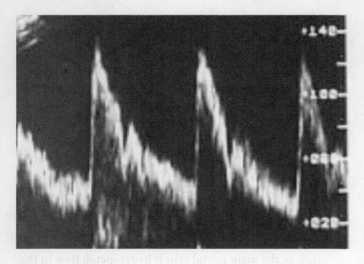

    (A) flow-reducing celiac artery stenosis

    (B) flow-reducing renal artery stenosis

    (C) normal flow in the celiac artery

    (D) normal flow in the renal artery

73. The Doppler spectral waveforms shown below are diagnostic of

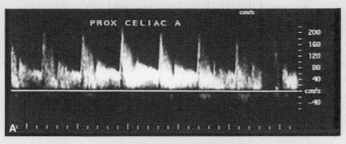

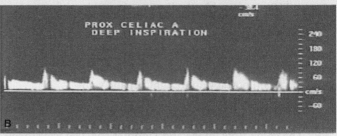

    (A) atherosclerotic stenosis of the celiac artery

    (B) median arcuate ligament compression of the celiac artery

    (C) postprandial celiac artery flow

    (D) collateral compensatory flow in the celiac artery

74. If the urethra is obstructed, which of the following is true?

    (A) Hydronephrosis will not occur.

    (B) Hydronephrosis will be unilateral.

    (C) Hydronephrosis will be bilateral.

    (D) Renal calculi are the cause.

75. Acute renal vein thrombosis is suggested if which of the following is true?

    (A) The renal sinus becomes hyperechogenic.

    (B) The corticomedullary junction is indistinct.

    (C) The Doppler spectral waveform demonstrates pulsatility.

    (D) The kidney is smaller than normal.

76. The kidney exhibits a hypoechoic, cystic-appearing area within the echogenic renal sinus. What is this finding most consistent with?

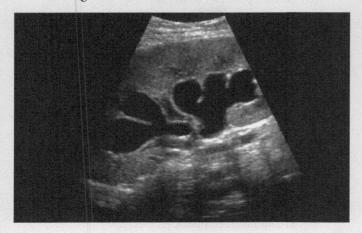

(A) renal calculus

(B) hydronephrosis

(C) renal infarction

(D) renal artery occlusion

77. With obstructive hydronephrosis, the RI is

(A) less than 0.50

(B) more than 1.2

(C) more than 3.5

(D) more than 0.70

78. Which of the following terms is used to describe a cadaveric liver transplant?

(A) orthotopic

(B) heterogeneous

(C) heterotopic

(D) homogeneous

79. The arterial and venous anastomoses for a cadaveric liver transplant include the

(A) extrahepatic portal vein, hepatic artery, right hepatic vein, suprahepatic and infrahepatic IVC

(B) the left portal vein, hepatic artery, right hepatic vein, and IVC

(C) extrahepatic portal vein, hepatic artery, suprahepatic and infrahepatic IVC

(D) right portal vein, splenic vein, suprahepatic and infrahepatic IVC

80. Which of the following is *not* a valued tool for confirmation of liver transplant rejection?

(A) sonography

(B) standard contrast arteriography

(C) radionuclide scintigraphy

(D) CT

81. Which of the following is considered a critical complication following liver transplantation?

(A) hepatic artery stenosis

(B) hepatic vein thrombosis

(C) IVC stenosis

(D) hepatic artery thrombosis

82. Post-liver transplantation, the hepatic artery Doppler spectral waveforms demonstrate a peak systolic velocity greater than 180 cm/s, systolic acceleration time greater than 0.8 s, and RI less than 0.5. What are these findings most consistent with?

(A) normal hepatic artery

(B) hepatic artery stenosis

(C) hepatic artery thrombosis

(D) portal vein obstruction

83. Pseudoaneurysms are associated with

(A) an intimal tear

(B) low-resistance Doppler spectral waveforms

(C) to-and-fro flow patterns

(D) a post-stenotic signal

84. The diameter of the portal vein is measured as it crosses anterior to the IVC in a patient lying supine. The diameter should not exceed

(A) 5 mm

(B) 10 mm

(C) 13 mm

(D) 15 mm

85. The gastroduodenal artery is a branch of which of the following arteries?

(A) celiac artery

(B) hepatic artery

(C) splenic artery

(D) gastric artery

86. Which of the following is not a significant cause of renal transplant failure?

(A) acute rejection

(B) ATN

(C) renal artery stenosis

(D) fibromuscular dysplasia

87. In adults, the transplant renal artery is most often anastomosed to which of the following arteries?

    (A) aorta

    (B) common iliac artery

    (C) external iliac artery

    (D) hepatic artery

88. Real-time imaging characteristics of renal transplant rejection include

    (A) decreased renal volume, decreased cortical echogenicity, thickening of the renal pelvis

    (B) decreased renal volume, increased cortical echogenicity, thickening of the renal pelvis

    (C) decreased renal sinus fat, increased cortical echogenicity, thickening of the renal pelvis

    (D) increased renal volume, increased cortical echogenicity, thickening of the renal pelvis

89. The Doppler spectral waveform pattern associated with acute renal transplant rejection demonstrates

    (A) rapid systolic upstroke, rapid deceleration, low or absent diastolic flow

    (B) rapid systolic upstroke, delayed deceleration, forward diastolic flow

    (C) delayed systolic upstroke, rapid deceleration, low or absent diastolic flow

    (D) delayed systolic upstroke, delayed deceleration, forward diastolic flow

90. Moderate ATN is associated with a Doppler spectral pattern demonstrating

    (A) rapid systolic upstroke, rapid deceleration, absent diastolic flow

    (B) rapid systolic upstroke, rapid deceleration, increased pulsatility

    (C) delayed systolic upstroke, delayed deceleration, low or absent diastolic flow

    (D) delayed systolic upstroke, delayed deceleration, acceleration index greater than 3.78

91. Flow-reducing transplant renal artery stenosis is suggested by

    (A) a RAR greater than 3.5

    (B) a peak systolic renal artery velocity greater than 180 cm/s

    (C) a renal-iliac velocity ratio greater than 3.0

    (D) an end-diastolic to peak systolic velocity ratio greater than 0.2

92. Which of the following does *not* apply to the right renal artery?

    (A) courses posterior to the IVC

    (B) arises from the aortic wall at the level of the first or second lumbar vertebrae

    (C) demonstrates a spectral waveform with constant forward diastolic flow

    (D) gives rise to branches that supply the adrenal, pancreas and ureter

93. Doppler spectral waveforms from a renal transplant arteriovenous fistula are characterized by

    (A) low velocity, low-amplitude arterial signals, and pulsatile venous flow

    (B) high-velocity, turbulent arterial signals, and low amplitude, continuous venous flow

    (C) high-velocity, turbulent arterial signals, and pulsatile venous flow

    (D) low-velocity, low-amplitude arterial signals, and continuous venous flow

94. What is the most serious complication of pancreas transplantation?

    (A) SMA stenosis

    (B) hepatic artery thrombosis

    (C) splenic vein thrombosis

    (D) celiac artery stenosis

95. Normally, portal venous flow is

    (A) pulsatile

    (B) hepatopetal

    (C) hepatofugal

    (D) bidirectional

96. Severe portal hypertension may be accompanied by all of the following, *except*

    (A) a patent paraumbilical vein

    (B) a patent coronary vein

    (C) increased portal venous flow volume

    (D) a caput medusa

97. TIPSs are used to

    (A) treat recurrent gastrointestinal bleeding and refractory ascites

    (B) treat hepatocellular carcinoma

    (C) shunt blood from the splenic vein to the renal vein

    (D) shunt blood from the jugular vein to the IVC

98. **Renal artery occlusion is suggested by all of the following,** *except*

   (A) absence of flow in the renal artery using optimized power Doppler imaging

   (B) low-amplitude, low-velocity Doppler spectral waveforms throughout the renal parenchyma

   (C) a side-to-side difference in renal length of 1.5 cm

   (D) a kidney length less than 8 cm

99. **The renal artery acceleration index is defined as**

   (A) the time interval from the onset of systole to the early systolic peak

   (B) the time interval from the onset of systole to peak systole divided by Doppler frequency

   (C) the change in distance between the onset of systolic flow and the early systolic peak

   (D) the change in distance between the onset of systolic flow and the peak systolic velocity divided by the acceleration time

100. **The term "flow-reducing stenosis" signifies arterial narrowing of**

   (A) 20–30%

   (B) 30–40%

   (C) 50–60%

   (D) 100%

101. **The postprandial Doppler spectral waveform from the normal SMA will exhibit**

   (A) rapid systolic upstroke, rapid deceleration, reversed diastolic flow

   (B) rapid systolic upstroke, rapid deceleration, forward diastolic flow

   (C) rapid systolic upstroke, delayed deceleration, low diastolic flow

   (D) rapid systolic upstroke, blunt systolic peak, delayed run-off

102. **The best image of the celiac, common hepatic, and splenic arteries is obtained from the**

   (A) transverse plane at the level of the left renal vein

   (B) sagittal plane to the right of midline

   (C) transverse plane at the level of the SMA

   (D) sagittal plane at the level of the SMV

103. **A perivascular color artifact is noted in the region of a transplant renal artery anastomosis. What is this most likely associated with?**

   (A) a bruit

   (B) an arteriovenous fistula

   (C) transplant renal artery occlusion

   (D) a pseudoaneurysm

104. **A "to-and-fro" Doppler spectral waveform is associated with**

   (A) saccular aneurysm

   (B) dissecting aneurysm

   (C) pseudoaneurysm

   (D) fusiform aneurysm

105. **Acute occlusion of a renal artery would likely result in**

   (A) low-amplitude, low-velocity Doppler waveforms throughout the kidney

   (B) increased flow in the contralateral renal artery

   (C) Doppler waveforms with absent diastolic flow in the cortical vessels

   (D) no evidence of collateral flow

106. **An AAA greater than 6 cm in anteroposterior diameter should be**

   (A) followed with sonograms at 6-month intervals

   (B) followed with CT scan at yearly intervals

   (C) treated emergently to prevent risk of rupture

   (D) treated with ultrasound probe compression

107. **What is the second most common cause of renovascular hypertension?**

   (A) fibromuscular dysplasia

   (B) atherosclerotic renal artery stenosis

   (C) renal artery occlusion

   (D) chronic renal failure

108. **The longitudinal image of the aorta seen below illustrates**

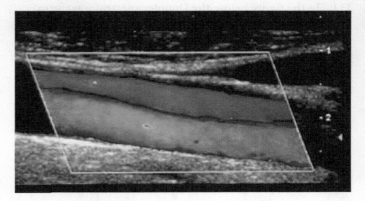

   (A) saccular aneurysm

   (B) fusiform aneurysm

   (C) mycotic aneurysm

   (D) aortic dissection

109. The transverse image of the aorta seen below illustrates

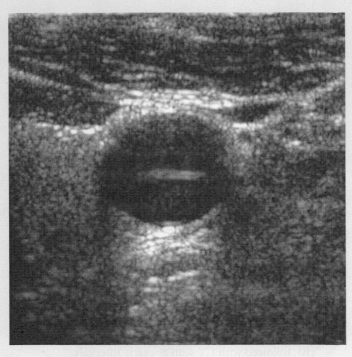

(A) saccular aneurysm
(B) fusiform aneurysm
(C) mycotic aneurysm
(D) aortic dissection

110. Which artery is *not* routinely evaluated during a mesenteric duplex study?

(A) superior mesenteric
(B) splenic
(C) left gastric
(D) celiac

111. In the figure below, the Doppler spectral waveform from the SMA indicates

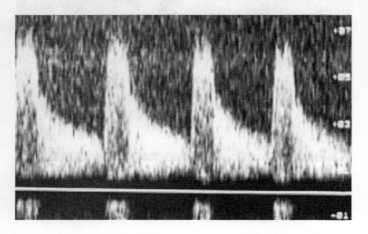

(A) collateralization
(B) fasting state
(C) postprandial state
(D) flow-limiting stenosis

112. A rapid decrease in velocity and turbulent flow distal to arterial stenosis is the result of

(A) a pressure-flow gradient
(B) narrowing of the diameter of the vessel
(C) an increase in kinetic energy at the distal end of the stenosis
(D) tandem lesions

113. What is the best image plane to use for visualization of the left renal vein?

(A) transverse
(B) coronal
(C) oblique
(D) longitudinal

114. The color-flow image seen below illustrates

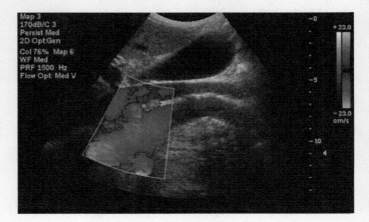

(A) normal renal artery
(B) multiple renal arteries
(C) renal artery occlusion
(D) retroaortic left renal vein

115. The transducer is placed in the right intercostal space directed toward the porta hepatis. The color bar indicates flow toward the transducer is red and flow away is blue. Using this scan plane and color setting, flow in the normal portal vein will be

(A) blue
(B) red
(C) bidirectional
(D) absent

116. Power Doppler imaging demonstrates all of the following, *except*

(A) power spectrum

(B) perfusion

(C) intensity

(D) direction

117. Distal to an 80% stenosis in the proximal renal artery, the Doppler spectral waveform will exhibit

(A) rapid systolic upstroke

(B) early systolic peak

(C) tardus parvus morphology

(D) absence of diastolic flow

118. Heterotopic partial transplantation is

(A) frequently used with pancreas transplantation

(B) frequently used for patients with renal failure

(C) the most common type of liver transplantation

(D) used with cadaveric livers

119. The abdominal aorta is considered aneurysmal if its diameter exceeds

(A) 1 cm

(B) 2 cm

(C) 3 cm

(D) 1 times the diameter of the proximal normal segment

120. Which vessel is *not* interrogated during routine evaluation of a renal transplant?

(A) external iliac artery

(B) external iliac vein

(C) intersegmental artery

(D) IVC

121. Which vessel is not routinely interrogated during evaluation of a pancreas transplant?

(A) hepatic artery

(B) splenic vein

(C) SMA

(D) portal vein

122. Clinically, patients with portal hypertension may have

(A) bleeding from gastroesophageal varices

(B) ascites

(C) hepatomegaly

(D) all of the above

123. Increased velocity due to stenosis can be differentiated from collateral compensatory flow by noting that

(A) the post-stenotic signal is present with a flow-reducing stenosis but not with collateral flow

(B) the high velocity will be seen throughout the visualized length of the artery in both cases

(C) A but not B

(D) both A and B

124. Which of the following is a complication associated with aortic stent grafts that may require lifelong follow-up?

(A) risk of kinking

(B) crossed limbs

(C) endoleaks

(D) stenosis

125. Which of the following is *not* associated with aortic endoleaks?

(A) flow within the residual aneurysm sac

(B) increased risk for rupture

(C) graft and endoleaks waveforms differ

(D) turbulent chaotic flow pattern

126. The right renal artery can be imaged from

(A) transverse approach at the level of the left renal vein

(B) longitudinal image of the IVC from a right paramedian scan plane

(C) transverse view of the kidney through an intercostal approach

(D) all of the above

127. The left portal vein divides into

(A) the paraumbilical and coronary veins

(B) medial and lateral branches

(C) left gastric and coronary veins

(D) anterior and posterior branches

128. The coronary vein enters which of the following veins near the confluence of the superior mesenteric and portal veins?

(A) inferior mesenteric

(B) renal

(C) portal

(D) left gastric

129. The Doppler spectral waveform from the normal portal vein is

    (A) pulsatile
    (B) minimally phasic
    (C) continuous and nonphasic
    (D) high resistant

130. In patients with portal hypertension, it is common to find spontaneous venous shunting between the

    (A) IVC and hepatic artery
    (B) coronary vein and the paraumbilical vein
    (C) splenic vein and renal vein
    (D) superior mesenteric vein and portal vein

131. Velocity parameters diagnostic of flow-reducing SMA stenosis are

    (A) peak systolic velocity less than 250 cm/s; end-diastolic velocity less than 45 cm/s
    (B) peak systolic velocity greater than 275 cm/s; end-diastolic velocity greater than 55 cm/s
    (C) peak systolic velocity less than 250 cm/s; end-diastolic velocity less than 45 cm/s and a post-stenotic signal
    (D) peak systolic velocity greater than 275 cm/s; end-diastolic velocity greater than 45 cm/s and a post-stenotic signal

132. The caput medusa associated with portal hypertension is identified

    (A) in the region of the portal confluence
    (B) as periportal collaterals in the porta hepatis
    (C) as superficial collaterals surrounding the umbilicus
    (D) as varices in the splenic hilum

133. Which of the following arteries is *not* part of the renal arterial system?

    (A) segmental arteries
    (B) arcuate arteries
    (C) cruciate arteries
    (D) interlobar arteries

134. The adult kidney is normally

    (A) 8–10 cm in length, 2–4 cm in width, and 4–5 cm in anteroposterior thickness
    (B) 10–14 cm in length, 3–5 cm in width, and 2–3 cm in anteroposterior thickness
    (C) 12–15 cm in length, 2–4 cm in width, and 4–5 cm in anteroposterior thickness
    (D) 11–13 cm in length, 5–7 cm in width, and 2–3 cm in anteroposterior thickness

135. The peak systolic velocity in the adult aorta is normally

    (A) 30–70 cm/s
    (B) 40–100 cm/s
    (C) 70–140 cm/s
    (D) 140–160 cm/s

136. Elevated RI in a renal transplant can be associated with

    (A) acute rejection
    (B) ATN
    (C) increased transducer pressure over the transplant
    (D) all of the above

137. The Doppler spectral waveform from the suprarenal aorta may be

    (A) triphasic
    (B) biphasic
    (C) A but not B
    (D) both A and B

138. The Doppler spectral waveform pattern for severe ATN is indistinguishable from the pattern associated with severe acute rejection. Both patterns demonstrate

    (A) rapid systolic upstroke, rapid deceleration, constant forward diastolic flow
    (B) rapid systolic upstroke, rapid deceleration, low diastolic flow
    (C) delayed systolic upstroke, rapid deceleration, constant forward diastolic flow
    (D) delayed systolic upstroke, delayed deceleration, low diastolic flow

139. Which type of aneurysm forms an "outpouching" from the aortic wall?

    (A) mycotic aneurysm
    (B) pseudoaneurysm
    (C) saccular aneurysm
    (D) fusiform aneurysm

140. An epigastric bruit that is present during normal respiration but disappears with deep inspiration is most likely due to

    (A) median arcuate ligament compression of the celiac artery
    (B) atherosclerotic aortic stenosis
    (C) SMA Nutcracker syndrome
    (D) renal artery stenosis

141. The RAR should *not* be used when the aortic peak systolic velocity is

(A) 50–60 cm/s

(B) 90 cm/s

(C) less than 30 cm/s

(D) 100 cm/s

142. The inferior mesenteric vein drains into the splenic vein

(A) to the left of the confluence of the portal and splenic veins

(B) to the right of the confluence of the portal and splenic veins

(C) inferior to the confluence of the portal and splenic veins

(D) superior to the confluence of the portal and splenic veins

143. Which vessel is not usually visualized sonographically?

(A) IMA

(B) cystic vein

(C) paraumbilical vein

(D) inferior right hepatic vein

144. Pulsatility of the portal venous Doppler waveform indicates

(A) right heart failure

(B) tricuspid regurgitation

(C) portal hypertension

(D) all of the above

145. When measured in the cranio-caudad plane, the spleen is considered to be enlarged when its length exceeds

(A) 8 cm

(B) 10 cm

(C) 13 cm

(D) 15 cm

146. In patients with portal hypertension, the most common portosystemic collateral is the

(A) paraumbilical vein

(B) coronary vein

(C) splenic vein

(D) cystic vein

147. The coronary vein is considered to be enlarged when its diameter exceeds

(A) 2 mm

(B) 4 mm

(C) 6 mm

(D) 8 mm

148. The normal flow direction in the coronary vein is

(A) toward the splenic and portal vein

(B) away from the splenic and portal vein

(C) hepatofugal

(D) toward the IVC

149. The portal vein travels throughout the liver with the

(A) middle hepatic vein and left hepatic artery

(B) hepatic vein and common bile duct

(C) paraumbilical vein and hepatic artery

(D) hepatic artery and common bile duct

150. To obtain the correct dimensions of an AAA, it is important to scan following

(A) the axis of the spine

(B) the axis of the aorta

(C) the axis of the IVC

(D) all of the above

Figure 11-54. This color Doppler image was taken 5 days post-liver transplant.

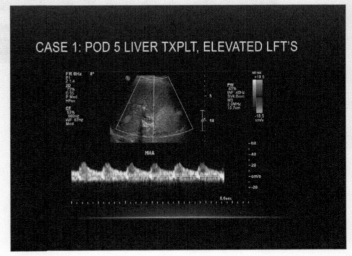

FIGURE 11-54.

151. The following statement is true.

(A) There is a "tardus-parvus" waveform.

(B) The velocities are too low.

(C) The waveform is normal.

(D) The spectral Doppler is not of the main hepatic artery.

152. Concerning the above image, the most likely diagnosis is

    (A) hepatic artery thrombosis

    (B) hepatic artery stenosis

    (C) liver transplant rejection

    (D) normal

Figure 11-55. This is a color Doppler sonogram of a transplanted liver whose surgery was 70 days ago.

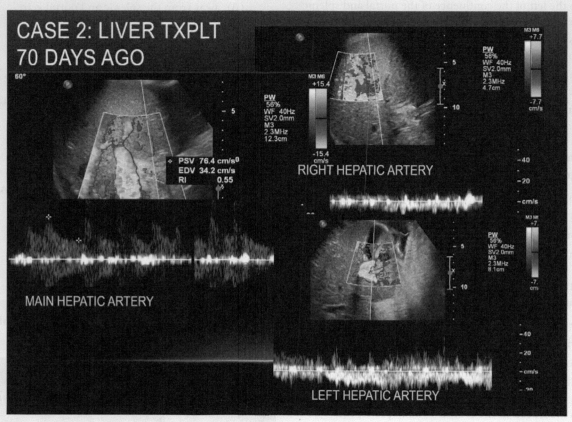

FIGURE 11-55.

153. The abnormal finding is

    (A) possible hepatic artery thrombosis

    (B) normal flow in right hepatic artery

    (C) normal flow in left hepatic artery

    (D) normal flow in main hepatic artery

154. The most likely diagnosis is

    (A) thrombosis of the main hepatic artery

    (B) thrombosis of the right hepatic artery

    (C) thrombosis of the left hepatic artery

    (D) normal

Figure 11-56. Gray scale (left) and color Doppler sonography (right) of transplanted liver prior to liver biopsy.

Figure 11-57. A & B. Gray scale (A) and color Doppler (B) images of a liver transplant.

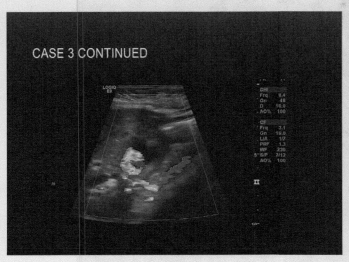

FIGURE 11-56.

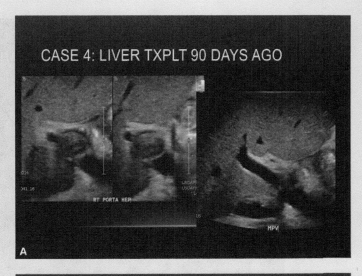

155. The abnormal finding is

    (A) hepatic artery pseudoaneurysm

    (B) normal flow in the inferior vena cava

    (C) flow within the gallbladder fossa

    (D) flow within the hepatic cyst

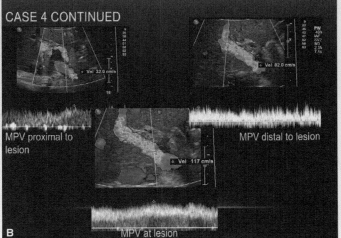

FIGURE 11-57

156. The abnormal finding is

    (A) a significant gradient across the portal vein anastomosis

    (B) abnormal hepatic artery velocities

    (C) a thrombus within the main portal vein

    (D) rejection

157. The most likely diagnosis is

    (A) stenosis of the portal vein at anastomosis

    (B) rejection

    (C) hepatic artery thrombosis

    (D) pseudoaneurysm

Figure 11-58. Color and spectral Doppler sonogram of the main renal artery.

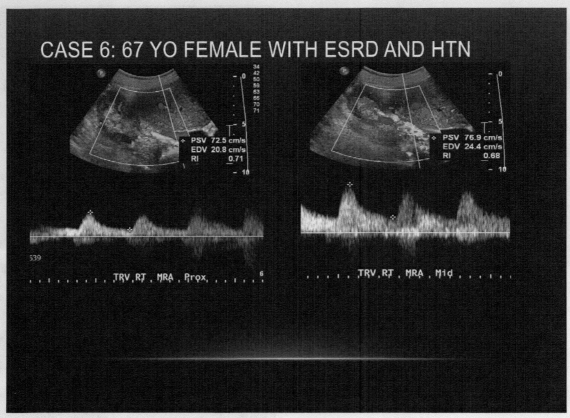

FIGURE 11-58.

158. **The abnormal finding is**

(A) "tardus parvus" waveform

(B) low velocities

(C) high velocities

(D) absent flow

159. **The most likely diagnosis is**

(A) renal artery stenosis

(B) rejection

(C) renal artery thrombosis

(D) renal vein thrombosis

Figure 11-59. A & B. Gray scale (A) and color Doppler (B) of
the kidneys.

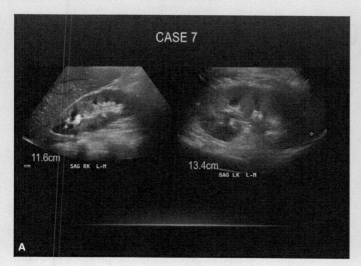

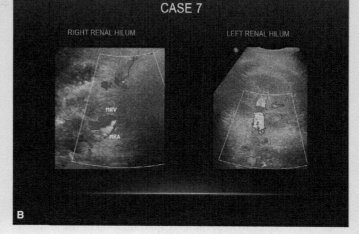

FIGURE 11-59

160. The abnormal finding is

(A) unilateral renal enlargement due to tumor

(B) shrunken atrophic kidney

(C) hydronephrosis

(D) rejection

161. The abnormal finding on color Doppler sonography is

(A) lack of renal vein flow on left

(B) lack of renal vein flow on right

(C) artifacts due to motion

(D) no flow within the kidneys

Answers and Explanations

1. **(C)** Renal size decreases as the compromise to blood flow increases. The kidney size is generally less than 9 cm when the renal artery is occluded.

2. **(D)** A vessel that is diffusely dilated is considered "ectatic." Saccular, fusiform, and spindle-shaped are terms used to describe the shape of aneurysms.

3. **(C)** The first major branch of the abdominal aorta is the celiac artery, which originates from the anterior wall of the aorta just inferior to the diaphragm. One to two centimeters distal to the origin of the celiac artery, the SMA arises from the anterior aortic wall. These vessels may share a common trunk.

4. **(B)** A concentric, spindle-shaped dilation of the abdominal aorta is termed "fusiform" and is used to describe aneurysms. A saccular aneurysm is created by an outpouching from the aortic wall. Dissecting is a term used to describe a tear in the intimal lining of an artery allowing blood to course between the intima and the media. Ectasia refers to a vessel that is diffusely dilated.

5. **(D)** The branches of the celiac artery (common hepatic and splenic) form a "seagull" appearance in the transverse imaging plane. They arise almost perpendicular to the celiac trunk at its bifurcation.

6. **(B)** The three branches of the celiac artery are the common hepatic, splenic, and left gastric.

7. **(C)** Patients with a ruptured aortic aneurysm usually present with abdominal or back pain that worsens in the upright or erect position.

8. **(C)** Aortic aneurysms are most often located below the renal arteries and in the common iliac arteries.

9. **(A)** The splanchnic circulation supplies blood flow to the gastrointestinal system and is composed of the celiac artery, the superior and inferior mesenteric arteries, and their branches. The renal arteries are part of the urogenital system.

10. **(B)** A doubling of velocity across segments of a vessel of similar diameter is consistent with more than 50% reduction in diameter; a fourfold increase in velocity signifies a narrowing more than 75%.

11. **(A)** The aortic stent graft (endograft) is inserted percutaneously over a catheter advanced into the aorta from the femoral artery. The endograft excludes the aneurysm which remains. With surgical repair, the aneurysm is most often treated with graft replacement of the aorta.

12. **(C)** Hypertension is not a common cause of aortic dissection although it results in increased pressure on the arterial wall. Because the medial layer of the arterial wall weakens with age, this is the most predisposing condition for aortic dissection.

13. **(B)** Arterial dissection is characterized by a tear in the intima of the arterial wall. This allows blood to course between the intima and media, creating a true and false lumen. The intimal flap can be seen on real-time images as an echogenic, pulsating structure within the lumen of the artery.

14. **(A)** The common hepatic artery divides into the gastroduodenal artery in the hepatoduodenal ligament and the right gastric artery at the liver hilum.

15. **(B)** Gallbladder. The splenic artery supplies blood to the spleen, pancreas, left half of the greater omentum, greater curvature of the stomach, and part of the fundus of the stomach. The common hepatic artery supplies the gallbladder.

16. **(D)** The splenic artery is the largest branch of the celiac artery.

17. **(A)** Approximately 1–2 cm of the left gastric artery may be seen longitudinally. This artery is not routinely examined during evaluation of the mesenteric arterial circulation.

18. **(C)** The normal celiac artery Doppler spectral waveform exhibits the characteristics of blood flow to low-resistance end-organs. It has rapid systolic upstroke, rapid deceleration, and constant forward diastolic flow. The peak systolic velocity is normally less than 200 cm/s and the end-diastolic velocity is less than 55 cm/s.

19. **(A)** The waveform demonstrates low diastolic flow and the absence of turbulence. These are features of a normal vessel supplying blood to a high-resistance end-organ. Flow-reducing SMA stenosis would cause the peak systolic and end-diastolic velocities to increase to more than 275 cm/s and 45 cm/s, respectively. A post-stenotic signal would be evident immediately distal to the stenosis as a consequence of the pressure-flow gradient that develops with significant vessel narrowing.

20. **(A)** The SMA originates from the anterior wall of the aorta 1–2 cm below the celiac artery and behind the pancreas. It courses anterior to the left renal vein and parallels the aorta as it moves caudally.

21. **(D)** Acute, severe abdominal ischemia is associated with sudden occlusion of one or more of the mesenteric arteries. Chronic mesenteric ischemia has an insidious onset as a consequence of progression of atherosclerotic disease. Clinically, patients present with a triad of symptoms: postprandial pain, "fear of food" syndrome, and weight loss.

22. **(B)** The diagnostic criteria for flow-reducing SMA stenosis are peak systolic velocity greater than 275 cm/s, end-diastolic velocity greater than 45 cm/s, and a classic turbulent post-stenotic signal.

23. **(C)** The median arcuate ligament of the diaphragm can compress the celiac artery origin during respiration. Compression occurs during normal respiration but is relieved with deep inspiration and breath holding because of relaxation of the diaphragmatic crus. While portal hypertension may cause increased hepatic artery velocity, this would not vary with respiration and is uncommonly transmitted to the celiac artery. Flow-reducing celiac artery stenosis, and mesenteric ischemia due to significant disease in one or more mesenteric arteries, would cause velocity elevation in the celiac artery. The velocities would not vary with respiratory maneuvers.

24. **(D)** The inferior epigastric artery is a collateral pathway for occlusive disease involving the aorto-iliac system. Occlusion of the proximal mesenteric arteries is compensated through collaterals that commonly arise from the IMA and its branches or through the pancreaticoduodenal arcade.

25. **(A)** Standard contrast arteriography with selective lateral views has historically been used to confirm the sonographic findings and to define collateral pathways prior to revascularization. In recent years, CT scans have been used to localize disease and display relational anatomy.

26. **(C)** The left renal vein courses from the hilum of the left kidney, crosses the aorta anteriorly between the aorta and SMA, and moves inferior to the pancreas before entering the IVC.

27. **(B)** Arcuate arteries arise from the interlobar arteries. They curve around the base of the pyramids where they give rise to the lobular arteries that supply the cortex of the kidney. Their flow pattern is normally low resistance like that of the main renal artery and its larger branches.

28. **(D)** Flow-reducing renal artery stenosis is indicated if the renal-aortic ratio is greater than 3.5, the peak systolic renal artery velocity is greater than 180 cm/s, and there is a post-stenotic signal.

29. **(B)** If the RAR is used to determine severity of renal artery stenosis, care must be taken to assure that the aortic velocity is between 40 and 100 cm/s. Use of velocities outside those values in the calculation can result in over or underestimation of the severity of disease. Example: renal artery velocity = 150 cm/s and the aortic velocity = 30 cm/s. The renal-aortic ratio = 5.0, suggesting significant renal artery stenosis. Similarly, if the renal artery velocity = 320 cm/s and the aortic velocity = 120 cm/s, the renal-aortic ratio will be 3.0 and flow-limiting renal artery stenosis would not be indicated.

30. **(A)** This inverse relationship is caused by the impedance to arterial inflow that results from intrinsic disease. Such conditions are generally associated with endovasculitis and interstitial edema. In cases of marked renovascular resistance, the diastolic flow component of the Doppler spectral waveform may approach zero or reverse.

31. **(D)** The Doppler spectral waveform associated with mild ATN may be indistinguishable from the signal recorded in a normal kidney. Most often, there is increased diastolic flow as a result of arterial-venous shunting. This is evident in a normal RI. As AT progresses in severity, renovascular resistance increases and the RI is elevated.

32. **(B)** The fasting, normal IMA demonstrates a high-resistance waveform pattern typical of arteries feeding resting, muscular tissues (fasting SMA, peripheral arteries). The features of such waveforms are rapid systolic upstroke, rapid deceleration, and low diastolic flow. There may be a brief period of early diastolic flow reversal. The hepatic, renal, and splenic arteries supply high flow demand organs and their waveform is characterized by constant forward diastolic flow.

33. **(C)** The most common curable cause of renal-related hypertension is atherosclerotic renal artery stenosis. The second most common cause is due to medial fibromuscular dysplasia. This is a nonatherosclerotic disease entity that commonly affects the mid-to-distal segment of the renal artery in young, hypertensive women.

34. **(A)** The term "tardus parvus" refers to the delayed systolic upstroke and run-off evident in the dampened Doppler spectral waveforms recorded distal to flow-limiting stenosis or arterial occlusion. Medical renal disease, hydronephrosis, and pyelonephritis cause increased renovascular resistance. The resultant waveform would demonstrate low diastolic flow.

35. **(C)** When kidney size differs by more than 3.0 cm, occlusion of the renal artery on the side with the smaller kidney should be suspected. A small kidney with absent Doppler signals in the renal artery and dampened signals within the renal parenchyma from collateral vessels is consistent with renal artery occlusion.

36. **(A)** A diastolic to systolic velocity ratio less than 0.20 is consistent with renal parenchymal disease (medical renal disease). Renal artery stenosis, occlusion, and fibromuscular dysplasia do not result in elevated vascular resistance in the kidney unless there is associated medical renal disease.

37. **(B)** The right and left common iliac veins come together to form the IVC at the level of the fourth or fifth lumbar vertebrae.

38. **(B)** The pathologic condition that most often affects the IVC is thrombosis. Primary tumors of the IVC are uncommon but tumor extension or compression of the IVC may occur.

39. **(D)** Carcinomas of the kidney, adrenal gland, and liver often extend into the IVC via paracaval lymph nodes.

40. **(D)** Pregnancy can result in extrinsic compression of the IVC but prolonged, severe stasis is uncommon and caval thrombosis is an infrequent complication of pregnancy. Stasis due to prolonged inactivity, including surgery, can lead to venous thrombosis. Conditions that lead to dehydration, such as sepsis, promote development of thrombosis.

41. **(C)** A RI less than 0.70 is considered normal for an adult.

42. **(C)** Continuous, nonphasic Doppler spectral waveforms will be recorded when the lumen of the IVC is partially compromised.

43. **(B)** Contrast arteriography would not be a procedure of choice for confirmation of inferior vena caval thrombosis. Arteriography will enhance definition of the lumen of arteries, but it is limited in its ability to define filling defect or absence of flow in the outflow circulation.

44. **(B)** The right hepatic vein divides the right lobe of the liver into anterior and posterior segments. The middle hepatic vein divides the liver into right and left lobes. The left hepatic vein separates the medial and lateral segments of the left lobe of the liver. The portal vein enters the liver through the porta hepatis.

45. **(D)** The "Playboy Bunny" sign refers to the real-time image of at least two of the three major hepatic veins obtained with oblique, cephalic angulation of the transducer from a right paramedian approach under the xiphoid process.

46. **(A)** The three major hepatic veins drain into the IVC. The portal vein is formed by the confluence of the splenic and superior mesenteric veins and carries oxygenated blood into the liver.

47. **(B)** The spectral waveform from the normal hepatic veins demonstrates somewhat chaotic, pulsatile flow. There are two cycles of forward flow toward the heart as a result of reflections of right atrial and ventricular diastole. These are followed by a third cycle which is brief and reversed, accompanying atrial systole.

48. **(D)** The portal vein carries more than 50% of the oxygen required by the liver. While its responsibility for blood supply to the liver may increase when the portal venous flow is compromised, the hepatic artery most often supplies only 30% of the blood flow. The aorta and SMA do not provide flow directly to the liver.

49. **(B)** The portal vein is formed by the confluence of the superior mesenteric and splenic veins.

50. **(D)** The portal vein lies anterior to the IVC, cephalad to the head of the pancreas, and caudal to the caudate lobe.

51. **(B)** The portal triad is composed of the portal vein, hepatic artery, and the common bile duct.

52. **(D)** Hepatic veins are boundary formers which divide the segments of the liver. They course longitudinally toward

the IVC, increasing in diameter as they approach the hepato-caval confluence. Portal veins course horizontally toward their origin at the porta hepatis.

53. **(A)** Portal venous flow exhibits low velocity, minimally phasic variation as a result of respiration-related changes in thoracic pressure. Flow direction is normally hepatopetal (toward the liver). Pulsatility is common to the hepatic venous circulation.

54. **(C)** Occlusion of one or more of the hepatic veins is termed Budd–Chiari syndrome. Cavernous transformation may follow portal vein thrombosis and appears as periportal collaterals in the porta hepatis. Hemangioma is a benign tumor of the liver. Fibromuscular dysplasia is a nonatherosclerotic disease entity that causes concentric narrowing and dilation of arteries. This condition is observed in renal and carotid arteries.

55. **(D)** Hepatic veins divide the liver into segments, coursing longitudinally toward the vena cava. For this reason, they are considered "boundary formers." Unlike the portal veins which have echogenic walls due to the collagen within their boundaries, the hepatic vein walls lack echogenicity. The veins usually are not compressed during a Valsalva maneuver, which increases abdominal pressure.

56. **(C)** In Western nations, portal hypertension is most often caused by cirrhosis. Cirrhosis may be caused by hepatitis, but is not the direct cause of portal hypertension. Hepatocellular carcinoma and sclerosing cholangitis may be found in association with portal hypertension but are not the primary causes of this condition.

57. **(B)** Portal vein thrombosis may be followed by development of serpiginous periportal collaterals within the hepatic hilum. This is referred to as cavernous transformation.

58. **(A)** Normal blood pressure within the liver is 5–10 mm Hg. Portal hypertension is present when the pressure gradient from the portal vein to the hepatic veins or IVC exceeds 10 mm Hg.

59. **(C)** The most common type of portal hypertension is intrahepatic due to sinusoidal obstruction resulting from cirrhosis.

60. **(C)** Portal hypertension causes the portal vein velocity to decrease due to increased resistance to flow and the flow pattern becomes continuous as respiratory variation disappears as a result of increased hepatic pressure. The portal vein enlarges to more than 13 mm in diameter and with severe disease, the flow direction in the portal vein reverses to decompress the liver.

61. **(D)** Mycotic aneurysms are arterial dilations that are infected. Marfan's syndrome is associated with stretching and weakening of the aortic wall which may lead to development of an aneurysm. Injuries that cause penetration of the arterial wall may result in pseudoaneurysms.

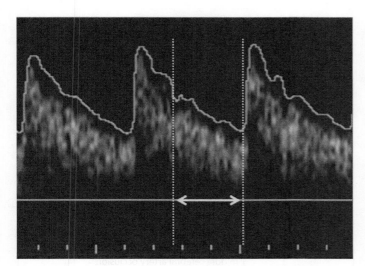

FIGURE 12–3. Spectral waveform from the internal carotid artery (ICA). The diastolic flow component of the cardiac cycle is outlined by the dotted yellow lines. Note that there is continuous forward flow (flow above the baseline) throughout the cardiac cycle.

PHYSIOLOGY AND HEMODYNAMICS

Peripheral resistance of a vascular bed is one factor that determines the amount of blood flow to a region of the body. The resistance is primarily controlled by the vasoconstriction and vasodilatation of the arterioles within that vascular bed. Vasodilatation decreases the peripheral resistance allowing blood to move in that direction. Vasoconstriction increases the resistance, and blood tends to move in the direction of lower resistance. The resistance within a given system is reflected in the diastolic component of the Doppler spectral waveform.

The brain is a very low-resistance vascular bed that allows for continuous blood supply throughout the cardiac cycle so that continuous forward flow is expected throughout diastole in all vessels that directly provide blood to the brain (Fig. 12–3).[10] These include the ICA and vertebral arteries, which in general will yield very similar Doppler spectral waveforms. The ECA, however, perfuses the areas of the face and smaller structures of the head and generally will yield very little flow in diastole.

Accordingly, there is a distinct difference in the Doppler waveforms that represent these vessels. It is extremely important for the examiner to recognize this difference so as to allow proper identification of the bifurcation vessels. Since the CCA is common to the ICA and ECA, it yields characteristics belonging to both vessels (Fig. 12–4).

SIGNS AND SYMPTOMS

Physical Examination

Physical examination of the extracranial carotid circulation includes palpation of common carotid, internal carotid, and temporal artery pulses. Acquisition of the bilateral brachial artery blood pressures can be performed routinely or per a prescribed algorithm and can be useful in the evaluation of patients with suspected vertebrobasilar symptoms as mentioned earlier. Auscultation of the carotid arteries is also part of the physical examination. Patients with evidence of cerebrovascular disease may in fact be asymptomatic. An asymptomatic stenosis is defined as any pre-occlusive lesion in the common carotid, carotid bifurcation, or ICA in a patient with no ipsilateral monocular or cerebral hemispheric symptoms.

Cervical or carotid bruit is often the only indication for screening in patients with suspected hemodynamically significant carotid artery disease. Information about the incidence of carotid bruit in asymptomatic patients is available from the Framingham study. This found that 3.5% of men and women had carotid bruits at 44–54 years. This increased to 7.0% at 65–79 years.[31]

Auscultation is performed by placing a stethoscope over the carotid artery. The patient is asked to take a deep breath and hold while the examiner listens for bruits (Fig. 12–5). A bruit is the result of vibration in the tissue that is transmitted to the surface of the skin. Bruits in the neck can be the result of the turbulent blood flow that is seen distal to a hemodynamically significant stenosis. They can also be heard in patients with loops, coils, kinks, and tortuosity of the ICA, or they can be cardiac in origin. Not all patients with these findings, however, will

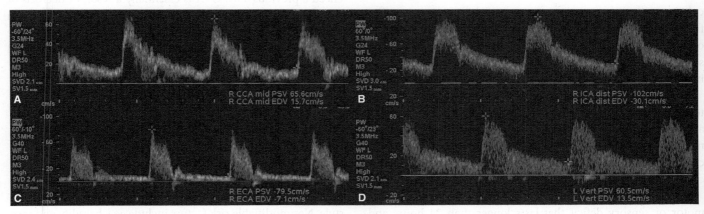

FIGURE 12–4. Ultrasound images with corresponding Doppler spectral waveforms from the common carotid (**A**), internal carotid (**B**), external carotid (**C**), and vertebral (**D**) arteries.

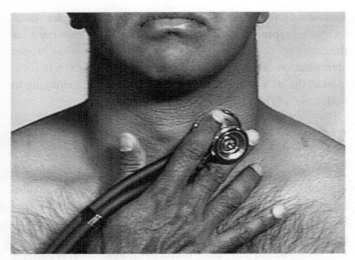

FIGURE 12–5. A stethoscope is placed over the cervical carotid artery and the examiner listens while the patient takes a deep breath.

present with a carotid bruit. Other causes may include external compression from thoracic outlet syndrome, arteriovenous malformations, and tumors.[32,33]

Auscultation for carotid artery bruit during routine examination has a low specificity that requires the support of ultrasound investigation. Due to the relatively low prevalence of carotid artery disease in the community, a national screening program is not cost-effective. However, patients in whom a bruit is heard should have further investigations in order to prevent the sequelae of carotid artery disease.[34,35]

Acute neurological deficits are differentiated as transient ischemic attacks (TIA) or strokes, based on whether the deficit resolves within, or persist longer than 24 hours. A TIA is any neurological dysfunction that lasts for less than twenty-four hours and completely resolves. Transient symptoms, however, are often a precursor to more serious complications. The neurological dysfunction may be described by the patient as some variation of a motor or sensory deficit (Table 12–2). A TIA typically lasts for just a few minutes or even seconds and is a result of deprivation of blood supply to a focal area of the brain. This may be caused by emboli or severe stenosis in the carotid circulation, either intracranial or extracranial. Patients may suffer from repeated symptoms that are similar in nature but get worse or occur with increased frequency. This is referred to as crescendo TIA and is important to identify, as this may be a sign of impending stroke and requires urgent/emergent intervention.

Other temporary symptoms involve the vertebrobasilar system (posterior circulation). Symptoms include vertigo, syncope, ataxia, drop attacks, and any other symptom that is bilateral in nature. Although these types of symptoms are indications for cerebrovascular evaluation, they typically are not caused by carotid disease, as there are many other differential diagnoses.[36]

CVA, commonly referred to as stroke, is defined as any motor or sensory deficit that lasts longer than 24 hours and does not completely resolve. Due to both the physical and

TABLE 12–2 • Common Signs and Symptoms of Cerebrovascular Disease (Transient Ischemic Attacks and Strokes)	
Signs or Symptoms	**Definition**
Amaurosis fugax	Transient blindness, either partial or complete often "shade coming down over one eye"; caused by embolism to the ophthalmic artery or one of its branches
Hemiparesis/ hemiplegia	Unilateral paralysis either partial or complete
Hemianopia	Blindness in one-half of the field of vision; can be bilateral or unilateral and may be from middle cerebral artery occlusion
Dysarthria	Difficulty with speech secondary to impaired muscles used for speech
Dysphasia	Difficulty with the coordination of speech or failure to arrange words in context
Dysphagia	Difficulty with swallowing
Ataxia	Unsteady gait
Diplopia	Double vision
Vertigo	Loss of equilibrium sometimes described as the room spinning

chemical changes that occur in the brain with stroke, damage can continue to occur for several days. This is called a stroke-in-evolution. Sometimes, a patient may experience a stroke which lasts more than 24 hours and settles within a week. This is called a reversible ischemic neurologic deficit (RIND). A stroke in which there is no further ischemia or loss of functional activity is a completed stroke. 75% of patients with stroke have experienced a previous TIA. CVA is essentially a result of necrosis or death of brain tissue. Major CVA can be debilitating resulting in permanent paralysis and potentially death. In addition, it is quite possible for patients to have had a stroke and never have suffered any symptoms. Most of these are found incidentally on a CT scan of the head that is usually performed for some other reason.

MECHANISMS OF DISEASE

Epidemiology and Risk Factors for Stroke

Some stroke risk factors are hereditary, while others are a function of natural processes. Still others result from a person's lifestyle. Nonmodifiable risk factors include age, heredity and race, gender, and prior stroke, TIA or heart attack.[11]

Advancing age is a risk factor for stroke. The chance of having a stroke approximately doubles for each decade of life after age 55. While stroke is common among the elderly, many people under 65 also suffer from strokes.

Heredity (family history) and race play an important role. It is well known that stroke risk is greater if a parent, grandparent, sister, or brother has had a stroke. African Americans have a much higher risk of death from a stroke than Caucasians do. This is partly because African Americans have higher risks of high blood pressure, diabetes, and obesity.

Stroke is the fifth leading cause of death in the United States, kills about 140,000 Americans each year (approximately 1 out of every 20 deaths) and is more common in men than in women.[80] In most age groups, more men than women will have a stroke in a given year. However, more than half of total stroke deaths occur in women. At all ages, more women than men die of stroke. Use of birth control pills and pregnancy pose special stroke risks for women.

Someone in the United States has a stroke every 40 seconds and every 4 minutes, someone dies of stroke. Every year, more than 795,000 people in the United States have a stroke. Approximately 610,000 of these are first or new strokes. About 185,000 strokes (nearly 25%) are in people who have had a previous stroke. Most strokes (85–90%) are ischemic strokes, in which blood flow to the brain is blocked. Stroke costs the United States an estimated $34 billion each year.[2] This total includes the cost of health care services, medicines to treat stroke, and missed days of work. Stroke is a leading cause of serious long-term disability and reduces mobility in more than half of stroke survivors age 65 and over.[81] The risk of stroke for someone who has already had one is many times that of a person who has not. Episodes of TIA are "warning signs" that produce stroke-like symptoms but no permanent damage. This will be discussed further in the text. TIAs are strong predictors of stroke and a person who has had one or more TIAs is almost 10 times more likely to have a stroke than someone of the same age and sex who has not. Recognizing and treating TIAs can reduce the risk of a major stroke.

The modifiable risk factors for stroke include hypertension, diabetes, cigarette smoking, hyperlipidemia, carotid artery stenosis, atrial fibrillation, excessive alcohol consumption, and physical inactivity (Table 12–3).[12]

The most important controllable risk factor is hypertension, which increases the risk of stroke two- to fourfold.[13] This higher risk is seen in both systolic and diastolic hypertension as well as in isolated systolic hypertension in the elderly. Blood pressure control significantly reduces the risk of stroke; it has been shown to prevent 30 strokes for every 1000 patients treated. Many people believe the effective treatment of high blood pressure is a key reason for the accelerated decline in the death rates for stroke. According to the current recommendation of the Stroke Council of the American Heart Association (AHA), blood pressure should be maintained at less than 140/90 mm Hg (lower for diabetics).[11]

TABLE 12–3 • Risk Factors: Modifiable and Non-Modifiable

- Advanced age
- Atrial fibrillation
- Carotid artery stenosis
- Cigarette smoking
- Diabetes
- Excessive alcohol consumption
- Family history of stroke
- Heart disorders
- History of transient ischemic attacks
- Hypercholesterolemia
- Hyperlipidemia
- Hypertension
- Obesity
- Physical inactivity
- Use of oral contraceptives

Diabetes mellitus is an independent risk factor for stroke. Diabetes increases stroke risk 1.8- to 6-fold. Many people with diabetes are also obese and have high blood pressure and high blood cholesterol, which increases their risk even more. While diabetes is treatable, the presence of the disease still increases the risk of stroke.

In recent years, studies have shown cigarette smoking to be an important risk factor for stroke. Approximately 27% of men and 22% of women in the United States smoke cigarettes. Smokers have a relative risk of stroke in the range of 1.8, and the estimated population attributable risk of stroke due to smoking is 18%. The nicotine and carbon monoxide in cigarette smoke damage the cardiovascular system in many ways. The use of oral contraceptives combined with cigarette smoking greatly increases stroke risk. Fortunately, this increased risk disappears within 5 years of smoking cessation.[11,12]

Hyperlipidemia is a risk factor for a stroke. Lipid disorders have been shown to increase the risk of stroke by 1.8- to 2.6-fold. Most of the information regarding the effect of lowering cholesterol on stroke risk comes from secondary analyses of trials on the prevention of coronary disease, but it is prudent to use these guidelines when evaluating patients for stroke risk. Tighter control of hyperlipidemia is indicated for patients who have a history of stroke or cardiovascular disease.[12]

Carotid artery disease (also called carotid artery stenosis) or other artery disease results in an increased risk for stroke since the carotid arteries supply blood to the brain. A carotid artery narrowed by fatty deposits from atherosclerosis may become blocked by a blood clot. Peripheral artery disease can result in the narrowing of blood vessels carrying blood to leg and arm muscles. People with peripheral artery disease have a higher risk of carotid artery disease, which raises their risk of stroke.

Atrial fibrillation is a heart rhythm disorder that raises the risk for stroke. The heart's upper chambers do not beat effectively, which can lead to pooling of blood causing clot formation. If a clot breaks off, enters the bloodstream and lodges in an artery leading to or in the brain, a stroke can result. People with coronary artery disease or heart failure have a higher risk of stroke than those with hearts that function normally. Dilated cardiomyopathy (an enlarged heart), heart valve disease, and some types of congenital heart defects also raise the risk of stroke.

Sickle cell disease is a genetic disorder that mainly affects African American and Hispanic children. "Sickled" red blood cells are less able to carry oxygen to the body's tissues and organs. These cells also tend to stick to blood vessel walls, which can block arteries to the brain and cause a stroke. Stroke is the second leading killer of people under 20 who suffer from sickle-cell anemia.[14]

Physical inactivity and obesity can increase risk of high blood pressure, high blood cholesterol, diabetes, heart disease, and stroke.

Atherosclerosis

Atherosclerosis is a chronic systemic disease that affects the arterial system and occurs within the arterial wall, typically within or beneath the intima. It is a chronic inflammatory response in the walls of arteries, in large part due to the accumulation of macrophage white blood cells and promoted by low density (especially small particle) lipoproteins (plasma proteins that carry cholesterol and triglycerides) without adequate removal of fats and cholesterol from the macrophages by functional high-density lipoproteins (HDL). It is commonly referred to as a "hardening" of the arteries.

Plaque formation may begin as simple layers of lipids called fatty streaks that are deposited in the wall. Over time, plaques on the walls may progress to a more fibrous component that includes the accumulation of lipids, collagen, and fibrin that is soft and gelatinous in texture appearing as a hypoechoic structure along the arterial wall. Eventually, the plaque may proliferate further into the lumen causing narrowing, also known as stenosis. The walls may harden secondary to a more calcium and collagen component. Unstable plaques or plaques that have areas that are weak, compared to more firm or well-integrated plaque within the wall, potentially can be a source of embolic debris.[15,16]

The atheromatous plaque is divided into three distinct components:

1. The atheroma, which is the nodular accumulation of a soft, flaky, yellowish material at the center of large plaques, composed of macrophages nearest the lumen of the artery

2. Underlying areas of cholesterol crystals

3. Calcification at the outer base of older/more advanced lesions.

Atherosclerosis is commonly seen at origins and bifurcations of vessels. Since flow divides and changes its laminar characteristics, a shearing force is created at the flow divider which over time is responsible for the wear of the intima.[15] For this reason, the carotid bifurcation is a prime location for carotid artery disease.

Atherosclerosis typically begins in early adolescence, and is usually found in most major arteries, yet is asymptomatic and not detected by most diagnostic methods during life. Autopsies of healthy young men that died during the Korean and Vietnam Wars showed evidence of the disease.[17,18] It most commonly becomes seriously symptomatic when interfering with the coronary circulation supplying the heart or cerebral circulation supplying the brain, and is considered the most important underlying cause of strokes, heart attacks, various heart diseases including congestive heart failure, and most cardiovascular diseases, in general. Atheroma in arm, or, more often, leg arteries, that results in decreased blood flow, is called peripheral artery occlusive disease (PAOD).

According to United States data for the year 2004, for about 65% of men and 47% of women, the first symptom of atherosclerotic cardiovascular disease is heart attack or sudden cardiac death (death within one hour of onset of the symptom). Most artery flow disrupting events occur at locations with less than 50% residual lumen.

Embolus

An embolus can be a solid, liquid, or a gas that travels through the bloodstream. Embolic strokes are usually caused by a blood clot that forms elsewhere in the body or plaque debris and travels through the bloodstream to the brain. Embolic strokes often result from heart disease or heart surgery and occur rapidly and without any warning signs. About 15–50% of embolic strokes occur in people with atrial fibrillation, the rest are attributable to a variety of causes, including (1) left ventricular dysfunction secondary to acute myocardial infarction or severe congestive heart failure, (2) paradoxical emboli secondary to a patent foramen ovale, and (3) atheroemboli. These latter vessel-to-vessel emboli often arise from atherosclerotic lesions in the aortic arch, carotid arteries, and vertebral arteries. In paradoxical embolism, a deep vein thrombosis embolizes through an atrial or ventricular septal defect in the heart then into the brain.[19] This phenomenon may manifest itself as symptoms of TIA or even CVA more commonly known as a stroke. By identifying these lesions with duplex ultrasound, the risks associated with significant atherosclerotic disease can be prevented with appropriate treatment.

Subclavian Steal

Subclavian steal refers to a phenomenon of flow reversal in the ipsilateral vertebral artery to supply the distal subclavian artery in the presence of a proximal subclavian or innominate artery

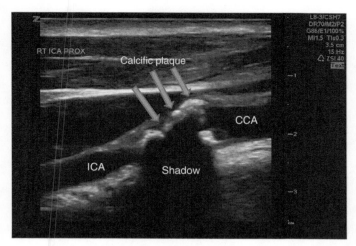

FIGURE 12–6. This diagram depicts the anatomy and physiology of a subclavian steal. Flow in the right vertebral artery is antegrade (toward the brain) to the basilar. Flow then reverses in the contralateral vertebral to perfuse the left subclavian artery in the presence of a hemodynamically significant stenosis in the left subclavian artery proximal to the left vertebral artery origin.

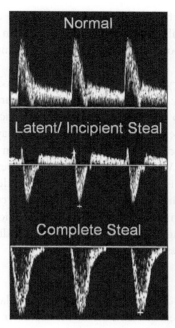

FIGURE 12–7. Doppler waveforms of the vertebral artery in various degrees of subclavian artery stenosis. Top is a normal waveform. Middle is an alternating flow waveform, and bottom demonstrates complete reversal of flow.

obstruction (Fig. 12–6). This phenomenon demonstrates the hemodynamic effects of severe stenosis and the compensatory nature of the circulatory system. In most cases, subclavian steal is asymptomatic (ie, subclavian steal phenomenon), does not warrant invasive evaluation or treatment, and represents an appropriate physiological response to proximal arterial disease. True subclavian steal syndrome cannot occur without retrograde blood flow in a vertebral artery associated with proximal ipsilateral subclavian artery stenosis or occlusion. The syndrome implies the presence of significant symptoms due to arterial insufficiency in the brain (ie, vertebrobasilar insufficiency) or upper extremity, which is supplied by the subclavian artery. It is more common on the left since the left subclavian is an isolated artery and does not communicate with the carotid artery. Therefore, the anatomy of the innominate artery is protective. Patients with this condition can experience vertebrobasilar symptoms in response to exercise of the ipsilateral arm. Arm/hand ischemia is rare in these patients, although a significant difference in blood pressure often exists between the two arms. A decreased radial artery pulse, combined with symptoms of vertebrobasilar insufficiency exacerbated by arm exercise is pathognomonic. The diagnosis is confirmed angiographically by late films demonstrating filling of the distal subclavian by retrograde vertebral blood flow or by duplex ultrasound detection of reversed flow in the vertebral artery.[20] A vertebral artery Doppler signal can also yield an alternating (toward and away) flow pattern (Fig. 12–7). This alternating pattern can transition to complete flow reversal with exercise of the ipsilateral upper extremity or after reactive hyperemia testing and can be demonstrated by observation of the vertebral artery Doppler signal after exercise or release of a blood pressure cuff that has been inflated to a suprasystolic blood pressure for approximately 3 minutes. A standard transcranial Doppler (TCD) evaluation

with particular attention to the blood flow direction and the velocities in the vertebral arteries and the basilar artery can also be useful. Blood flow is normally away from the transducer (suboccipital approach) in the vertebrobasilar system. If flow is toward the transducer at rest or with provocative maneuvers, there is evidence of a steal.[21]

Dissection and Kinking

Dissection and kinking of the carotid artery are nonatherosclerotic conditions that can affect the cerebral circulation. Dissection is usually the result of trauma that causes a sudden tear in the intimal lining of the vessel. The intima then separates from the media and adventitia (Fig. 12–8). This separation creates a

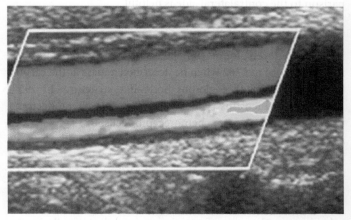

FIGURE 12–8. This is an ultrasound image of a common carotid artery (CCA) dissection with two patent flow lumens.

"false" lumen wherein blood may pulsate. The dissection may extend proximally or distally and may remain asymptomatic or may thrombose and cause neurological symptoms when it is flow limiting.

There is very little research about the hemodynamic variation induced by carotid kinking in the literature and whether this can lead to cerebral ischemia remains unclear. Although uncommon, the significantly kinked ICA may be clinically significant and cause cerebral ischemia, even in the absence of atherosclerosis. When this is suspected it is imperative to evaluate the vessel distal to the kink to assess for decreased blood flow velocities and waveform changes that are commonly seen in patients with flow-reducing lesions. Additionally look for other supporting evidence such as decreased diastolic flow in the proximal vessels.

Aneurysm

An aneurysm is defined as a permanent focal dilation of an arterial segment greater than 50% of the diameter of the normal adjacent vessel. Aneurysms of the extracranial carotid artery are rare (Fig. 12–9); several decades ago, such aneurysms were often attributed to syphilitic arteritis and peritonsillar abscesses. Currently, the most common causes are trauma, cystic medial necrosis, fibromuscular dysplasia (FMD), and atherosclerosis.[22] Neurologic manifestations are varied and include (1) cranial nerve involvement, which may produce dysarthria (hypoglossal nerve), hoarseness (vagus nerve), dysphagia (glossopharyngeal nerve), or tinnitus and facial tics (facial nerve); (2) compression of the cervical sympathetic chain and Horner's syndrome; and (3) ischemic syncopal attacks, resulting from embolism or interference with blood flow. Commonly, patients with an extracranial carotid aneurysm present to their physician with a cervical or parapharyngeal mass. Sometimes, an unsuspecting physician will perform a needle biopsy, which is followed by significant bleeding, hematoma formation, or a stroke.[23] An aneurysm of the carotid artery must not be misdiagnosed as a large carotid bulb. Keep in mind that the carotid bulb presents in various sizes and locations (Fig. 12–10), in addition, a comparison to the contralateral side is helpful.

Carotid Body Tumors

Haller introduced glomus tumors of the head and neck into the medical record in 1762 when he described a mass at the carotid bifurcation that had a glomus body–like structure. In 1950, Mulligan renamed this type of neoplasm as a chemodectoma to reflect its origins from chemoreceptor cells. In 1974, Glenner and Grimley renamed the tumor paraganglioma on the basis of its anatomic and physiologic characteristics. They also created a classification method based on the location, innervation, and microscopic appearance of the tumors.

Carotid body tumors, also called chemodectomas, are vascular tumors that arise from the paraganglionic cells in the outer layer of the carotid artery at the level of the bifurcation

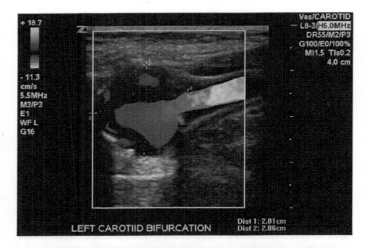

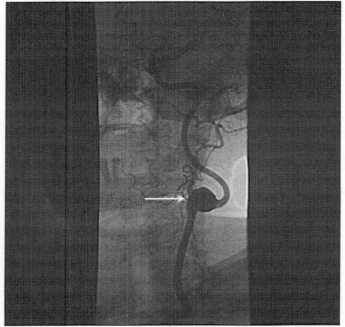

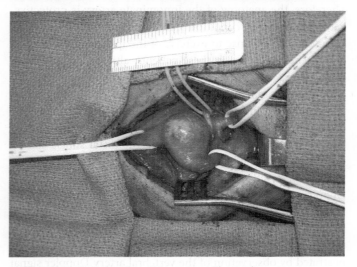

FIGURE 12–9. Patient with an ICA aneurysm. The top figure is a sagittal ultrasound image of an ICA aneurysm. The middle image is the confirmatory arteriogram, and the bottom image shows the intraoperative finding.

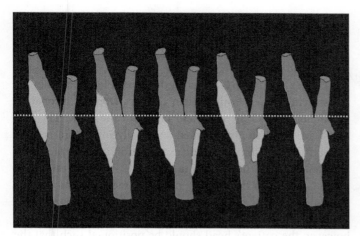

FIGURE 12–10. This cartoon illustrates the variable location of the carotid "bulb" outlined in aqua blue. Note that although the level of the bifurcation (dotted white line) is unchanged, the bulb may encompass any or all parts of the bifurcation, internal or external carotid arteries. Therefore, the level at which the CCA divides into the internal and external carotid arteries should be referred to as the carotid bifurcation and not the carotid "bulb."

(Fig. 12–11). This disease, which may be hereditary, is more common in South America than in North America. Tumors can become sizeable before causing symptoms, such as a painless, pulsating mass in the upper neck, and, eventually can cause difficulty swallowing. Ten percent of these tumors are bilateral. Although these can be noted on duplex ultrasonography,[24,25] they are definitively diagnosed using computed tomography (CT) or magnetic resonance imaging (MRI) scans, and sometimes angiography.[26] These tumors are generally benign; only about 5–10% are malignant. Treatment includes surgery and occasionally radiation therapy.[27]

Fibromuscular Dysplasia

The normal artery wall consists of three layers: the tunica intima, the tunica media, and the tunica adventitia. The tunica intima consists of the endothelium, connective tissue, and a basal layer of elastic tissue called internal elastic lamina. The tunica media is characterized by the presence of concentric layers of vascular smooth muscle cells and elastin-rich extracellular matrix. The tunica adventitia is the outer layer of the vascular wall, and it consists of fibroblasts, collagen, mast cells, nerve endings, and vasa vasorum.

Fibromuscular Dysplasia (FMD) is a nonatherosclerotic disease that usually affects the media of the arterial wall due to abnormal cellular development that causes stenosis of the renal arteries, carotid arteries, and less commonly, other arteries of the abdomen and extremities. This disease can cause hypertension, strokes, and arterial aneurysms and dissections.

FMD is often diagnosed incidentally in the absence of any signs or symptoms during an imaging study. Angiography with contrast will show a characteristic "string of beads" morphology in a vessel affected by FMD (Fig. 12–12). This pattern is caused by multiple arterial dilations separated by concentric stenosis. FMD tends to occur in females between 14 and 50 years of age. However, it has been found in children under the age of 14, both male and female. Up to 75% of all patients with FMD will have disease in the renal arteries.[28] The second most common artery affected is the carotid artery. More than one artery may have evidence of FMD in 28% of people with this disease.[29] If evidence of disease is noted in one vascular bed, all relevant arteries must be checked.

In the carotid system, it predominantly occurs in the mid segment of the ICA, is bilateral in approximately 65% of the cases, and is usually found in females. Color Doppler imaging may reveal a disturbed, nonlaminar flow pattern adjacent to the

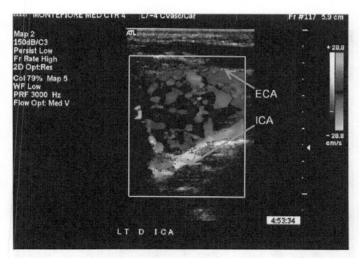

FIGURE 12–11. Color-flow duplex image of a carotid body tumor. Note the typical splaying of the bifurcation vessels secondary to the location of the tumor between the ICA and ECA, which are indicated by the green arrows. Hypervascularity is evident by the color Doppler.

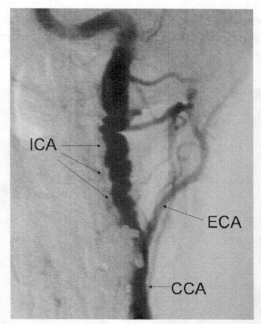

FIGURE 12–12. Angiographic presentation of fibromuscular dysplasia. Notice the classic "string of beads" appearance in the distal segment of the extracranial ICA. (ECA: external carotid artery; CCA: common carotid artery.)

arterial wall, with absence of atherosclerotic plaque in the proximal and distal segments of the ICA.[21,24,25]

Neointimal Hyperplasia

Neointimal hyperplasia accounts for most re-stenoses occurring within the first 2 years following vascular interventions. Development of the neointimal hyperplastic lesion involves the migration of smooth muscle cells from the media to the neointima, their proliferation, and their matrix secretion and deposition. Thus, mechanisms of smooth muscle cell migration are key to the formation of neointima, early re-stenosis, vessel occlusion, and ultimate failure of vascular interventions. This is often a factor in patients who experience restenosis after carotid endarterectomy (CEA).[30]

TESTING FOR CEREBROVASCULAR DISEASE

Duplex Ultrasound Technique[37,38]

The examination is explained and a history (including risk factors and symptoms) is obtained from the patient. Brachial artery pressures are recorded bilaterally (<20 mm Hg difference is within normal limits) and the presence of cervical bruits if present are documented.

Suggested instrument setups for carotid duplex imaging are as follows: (1) use a high frequency (5–10 MHz) linear array transducer; (2) image orientation: brain (distal) to the left of the monitor, heart (proximal) to the right; (3) color assignment: although color is based on the direction of blood flow (toward or away) in relation to the transducer, red is usually assigned to arteries and blue to venous blood flow; (4) the color scale (pulse repetition frequency [PRF]) should be adjusted throughout the examination to evaluate the changing velocity patterns; (5) the wall filter is set low; (6) the color "*box*" width affects frame rates (number of image frames per second) so the color display should be kept as small as possible; and (7) the color gain should be adjusted throughout the examination as the signal strength changes.

Duplex evaluation is primarily done in the long axis since the assessment of the carotid system requires Doppler insonation throughout the CCA, ICA, and origin of the ECA. The vertebral arteries also are included, especially in the presence of vertebrobasilar symptoms. The examination is performed with the patient in the supine position (Fig. 12–13). Anything that restricts access to the entirety of the extracranial carotid system from the base of the neck to the angle of the mandible is removed (Fig. 12–14). Pillows may be used to support the neck, however, the patient's head should be positioned such that the chin is pointed up and the head slightly turned away from the side being examined.

The examination begins with a transverse sweep of the carotid system examining the vessels of interest from the origin of the CCA to its bifurcation where the origins of the internal and external carotid artery are identified. This allows for a preview of all the vessels and surrounding structures (Fig. 12–15). Any abnormalities including extracarotid pathology such as thyroid masses are noted. The sonographic appearance and size of these structures is included in the final report. Location of plaque, plaque characteristics, and location of the bifurcation is assessed as well.

Sagittal to the long axis of the vessel, follow the course of the CCA from its origin (or as proximal as can be obtained) to the bifurcation. The origin of the right CCA can almost always be imaged since its origin is from the innominate artery (Fig. 12–16). In contrast, because access is limited secondary to depth and adjacent bony and muscular structures, the left CCA origin may be very difficult to visualize. Imaging with a sector transducer is an alternative and should be used when a significant stenosis is suspected at the origin of the left CCA. Using color-flow Doppler

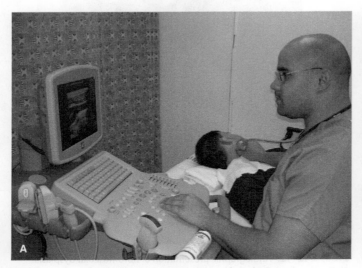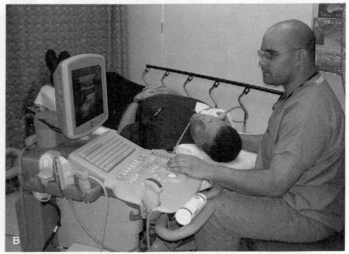

FIGURE 12–13. The examination is performed in the supine position while the examiner is either (**A**) at the head of the patient or (**B**) standing or sitting beside the patient.

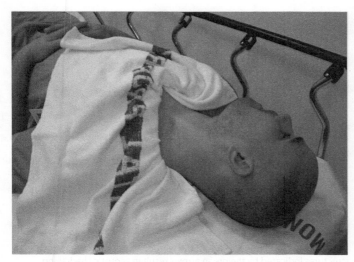

FIGURE 12–14. All restrictive garments such as turtleneck shirts and jewelry are removed to allow easy access to the neck, and the patient's head is turned slightly away from the side that is examined.

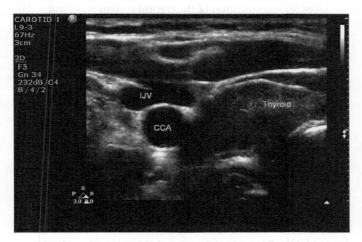

FIGURE 12–15. Transverse ultrasound image of the CCA and surrounding structures.

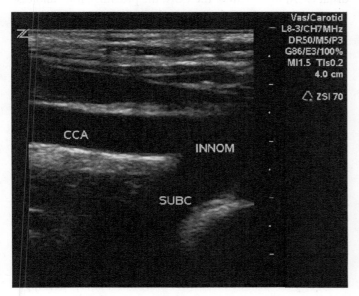

FIGURE 12–16. Ultrasound image of the right CCA off the innominate.

TABLE 12–4 • Differentiating the ICA from the ECA*

Characteristics	ICA	ECA
Extracranial branches	None	Yes (eight in number)
Doppler waveform	ICA yields a low-resistance waveform with continuous forward flow throughout the cardiac cycle and will always have more diastolic flow than the ECA in normal conditions	ECA yields a high-resistance waveform with less diastolic flow than internal; sometimes a reversed flow component in early diastole
Size and location at bifurcation	Larger and located posterior and lateral to the ECA	

*Tapping on the superficial temporal artery causes oscillations in the ECA waveform (although this is thought to be a very weak parameter). As oscillation is sometimes noted in both the ICA and the ECA.

imaging as a guide, interrogate the length of the CCA with pulsed Doppler, noting peak systolic and end-diastolic velocities. The CCA bifurcation is a common place for atherosclerotic plaque and is also the site of what is commonly referred to as the carotid bulb, although the location of the bulb itself may be variable (Fig. 12–10). This area should be assessed from multiple views. At this point the ICA and ECA are followed individually, and it is important to distinguish the ICA from the ECA. Although the spectral waveform pattern is the primary determinant, other parameters are useful (Table 12–4).

Follow the course of the ICA from its origin at the CCA bifurcation as far distal as possible. Using color-flow Doppler as a guide, interrogate the length of the vessel with pulsed Doppler and measure the peak systolic and end-diastolic velocities. Imaging from a posterolateral or lateral approach usually provides the best image. Where significant plaque is visualized multiple views and Doppler assessment is imperative to ensure the data obtained is accurate and reproducible. Typically, atherosclerotic disease occurs within the first few centimeters of the ICA, and elevated velocities at this segment in the presence of disease will be categorized based primarily on the spectral Doppler velocities. The distal ICA may be difficult to image secondary to depth and tortuosity. The clinical implication of tortuosity has yet to be proven as a significant finding, however, it should be noted that normal flow disturbances occur and elevated velocities may be recorded as a result of rapid changes in Doppler angles between the insonation beam and the acute changes in geometry of the blood vessel (Fig. 12–17).[39] Consideration is therefore recommended before interpreting high velocities as indicative of hemodynamically significant disease.

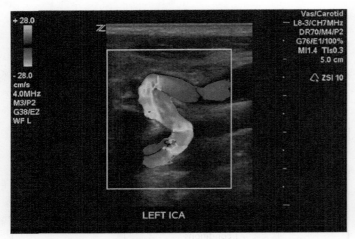

FIGURE 12–17. Color duplex image of a tortuous ICA. Notice the changes in the color-flow pattern that indicate rapid changes in the Doppler angle and not necessarily elevated velocities associated with stenosis.

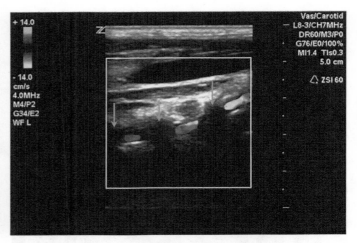

FIGURE 12–19. Long-axis view of the vertebral artery. Note that the bony structures indicated by the green arrows result in acoustic shadowing.

Look for other visual evidence of disease on the B-mode image and for the presence of post-stenotic turbulence.

A Doppler waveform is obtained at the origin of the ECA. This is done to document patency and to help distinguish this vessel from the ICA (Fig. 12–18).

The vertebral artery lies deeper than the CCA and can be located by angling the transducer slightly laterally from a longitudinal view of the mid/proximal CCA. To reliably identify the vertebral artery, it should be followed distally, and periodic shadowing should be visualized from the transverse processes of the vertebrae (Fig. 12–19). The vertebral artery is accompanied by the vertebral vein, and proper identification of the artery is made by evaluation of the Doppler signal. Once the vertebral artery has been identified, it should be followed as far proximally as possible. The use of color Doppler will greatly assist in locating the vertebral artery, its origin, and evaluating the direction of blood flow.

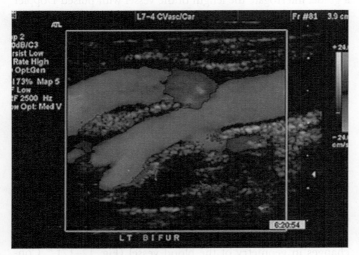

FIGURE 12–18. Color duplex illustrating branches of the external carotid artery (ECA). This is helpful for identification of the internal carotid artery versus the ECA.

Doppler interrogation of the carotid system is performed in the longitudinal plane using a 45–60-degree angle between the ultrasound beam and the vessel walls, and the angle cursor parallel to the vessel wall (placement of the Doppler sample volume parallel to the color jet has not undergone extensive validation criteria). Using a relatively constant Doppler angle permits comparison of repeated studies in the same individual over time. Insonation angles greater than 60 degrees should never be used for data acquisition and analysis as significant measurement error is introduced in even small changes in the Doppler angle of insonation. The Doppler sample volume is moved slowly through the artery searching for the highest velocity. The color Doppler display will help to guide the proper placement of the sample volume and is useful in locating sites of disease as evidenced by the presence of aliasing of the color-flow image.

Doppler signals are recorded from the proximal, mid, and distal CCA; the origin of the ECA; the proximal, mid, and distal ICA; the origin of the vertebral artery; and the subclavian artery bilaterally. In a normal vessel, the Doppler sample volume placement should be at the center of the lumen. The pulsed Doppler sample volume placement width is set at 1–2 mm to detect discrete changes in blood flow and minimize artifactual spectral broadening inherent in current transducer technology. When a stenosis is identified, a thorough interrogation of the stenotic area is performed. In the presence of disease, color-flow Doppler imaging should be used as a guide to aid in the optimal placement of the pulsed Doppler sample volume where the highest velocity may be obtained. Be sure to profile the lesion by moving the sample volume back and forth through the lesion to elicit the highest velocity within the stenosis. A Doppler waveform is obtained at the site of stenosis, where the highest velocity is suspected (Figs. 12–20 and 12–21), and a second Doppler waveform is obtained distal to the lesion for documentation of post-stenotic turbulence that almost always accompanies a hemodynamically significant stenosis. It is important to

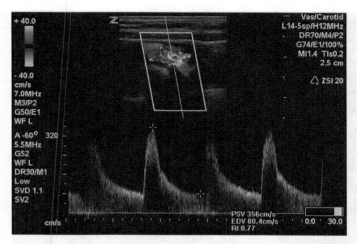

FIGURE 12–20. Internal carotid artery stenosis evident by the significant elevation of the velocity.

evaluate all Doppler signals bilaterally to correctly perform a carotid duplex imaging examination.

The location of any plaque, as well as its surface characteristics (smooth versus irregular) and echogenicity (homogeneous, heterogeneous, or calcified), visualized during the examination should be described (Fig. 12–22).

Interpretation and Diagnostic Criteria

The accurate interpretation of a carotid duplex imaging examination depends upon the quality and the completeness of the evaluation. Often the patient's body habitus will affect the quality of the image and the sonographer's ability to search the entire carotid system with Doppler. The sonographer must be

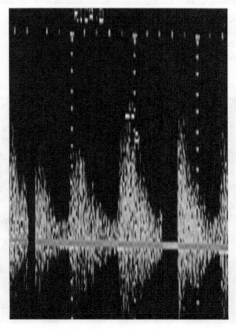

FIGURE 12–21. Spectral Doppler waveform that demonstrates post-stenotic turbulence as evident by flow above and below the baseline; spectral broadening; and irregular picket-fence configuration of the envelope of the spectral waveform throughout the cardiac cycle.

prepared to switch transducers when necessary to complete the carotid examination and have a complete understanding of the equipment controls to optimize the duplex imaging system. In addition to the peak systolic velocity (PSV), end diastolic velocity, direction of blood flow, the shape of the Doppler spectral waveform should be compared at the same level bilaterally. Abnormal waveform shape (increased or decreased pulsatility) may be an indicator of more proximal (innominate, subclavian) or distal (intracranial) disease (Fig. 12–23). The PSV is the most frequently used measurement to gauge the severity of the stenosis but the end-diastolic velocity, spectral configuration, and the carotid index (or peak internal carotid artery velocity to common carotid artery velocity ratio) provide additional information. It is important to understand that all of the criteria that have been published, unless otherwise noted, are used to categorize stenosis at the origin of the ICA only.

To determine the degree of stenosis present, a complete Doppler evaluation of the artery is necessary. There should be an elevated velocity through the narrowed segment and post-stenotic disturbances distal to the stenosis. The highest velocity obtained from a stenosis is used to classify the degree of narrowing. Doppler signals obtained distal to the area of post-stenotic flow disturbance may be normal or diminished, and the upstroke of the distal Doppler spectral waveform may be slowed.

Impact of the North American Symptomatic Carotid Endarterectomy Trial (NASCET)[40]

The results from NASCET demonstrated that in experienced surgical hands CEA is safe and effective in the near term and remarkably effective in the longer term in preventing recurrence of ipsilateral carotid ischemia and, in particular, in preventing disabling ipsilateral stroke and recommended CEA for high-grade carotid stenosis (70–99%). Prior to this, University of Washington criteria was traditionally and widely used to categorize disease at the origin of the ICA (Table 12–5). However, because CEA trials like NASCET,[40] the Asymptomatic Carotid Atherosclerosis Study (ACAS),[41] and the European Carotid Surgery Trial (ECST)[42] used specific thresholds for surgical treatment, updated and validated ultrasound criteria for ICA stenosis more than 70% and more than 60% were needed to estimate disease and classify patients. Investigators have found that an ICA/CCA peak systolic velocity (PSV) ratio is useful in grading ICA stenosis more than 70%[43] and more than 60% (Table 12–6).[44] The ratios are calculated using the highest PSV from the origin of the ICA divided by the highest PSV from the CCA (approximately 2–3 cm proximal to the bifurcation).

In the presence of a contralateral ICA occlusion, the velocity from the ipsilateral ICA may be elevated. This may lead to over estimating the extent of ipsilateral ICA disease.[45,46] To avoid overestimation of the ICA stenosis, new velocity criteria have been suggested. A PSV of more than 140 cm/s is used for a stenosis greater than 50% diameter reduction and an end-diastolic

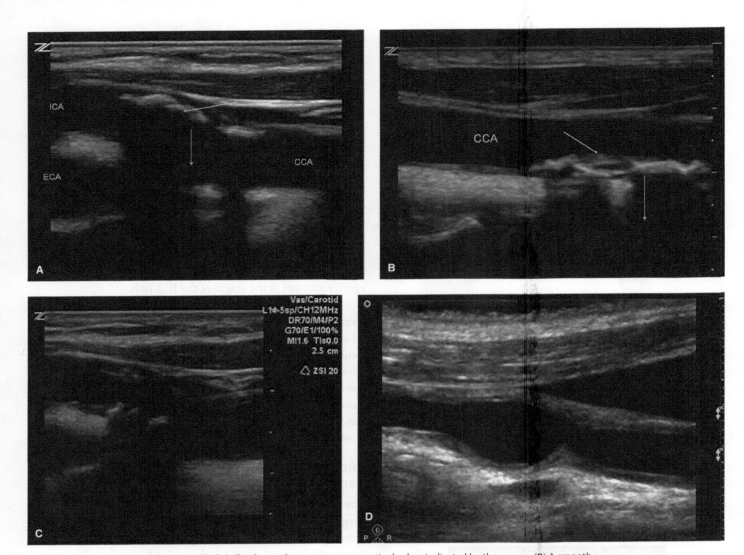

FIGURE 12–22. (**A**) Calcific plaque that creates an acoustic shadow indicated by the arrows. (**B**) A smooth plaque that is heterogeneous in texture with a calcific component that causes an acoustic shadow indicated by the dotted arrow. (**C**) A plaque with an irregular border and heterogeneous in texture. (**D**) A smooth and predominantly homogeneous plaque. (CCA: common carotid artery; ECA: external carotid artery; ICA: internal carotid artery.)

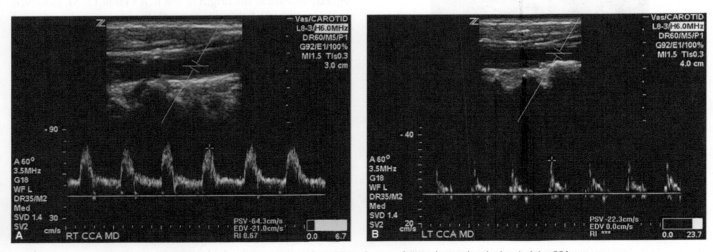

FIGURE 12–23. This is a comparison of the spectral Doppler waveforms obtained at the level of the CCA bilaterally in a patient with a left ICA occlusion. (**A**) Normal spectral Doppler waveform of the right CCA. (**B**) On the contralateral side, a high-resistance spectral Doppler waveform with no diastolic flow suggestive of the distal ICA occlusion on the ipsilateral side.

TABLE 12–5 • Strandness Criteria for Grading ICA Stenosis		
Diameter Reduction	Peak Systolic Velocity	End-Diastolic Velocity
<50%	<125 cm/s	
50–79%	≥125 cm/s	
80–99%		>140 cm/s
Occlusion	no signal	no signal

velocity of more than 155 cm/s for a stenosis greater than 80% diameter reduction of the lumen.[46]

Anatomic features, such as a high carotid bifurcation (<1.5 cm from the angle of the mandible), excessive distal extent of plaque (>2.0 cm above the carotid bifurcation), or a small distal ICA diameter (≤0.5 cm), or a redundant or kinked ICA can complicate CEA. In the past, arteriography was the only preoperative study capable of imaging these features. Accordingly, in the presence of ICA stenosis, other important information to include in the evaluation and interpretation of a carotid duplex imaging examination is (1) the location of the bifurcation relevant to the angle of the mandible (or some other external landmark), (2) the distal extent of the plaque beyond the ICA origin, (3) patency and diameter of the distal ICA, (4) the presence of tortuosity or kinking of the vessels, and (5) plaque characteristics (ie, smooth versus irregular surface, and calcifications). This information is particularly relevant in patients undergoing CEA based on the duplex scan findings alone.[47]

The Carotid "Bulb"

The ICA origin an important anatomical site as it is here where carotid artery disease is most likely to develop. The origin of the ICA is sometimes slightly dilated hence the term the carotid bulb. Flow at this bulbous segment will often be helical and somewhat disturbed and is often referred to as flow separation. It is important to note that the anatomic distribution of the carotid bulb can vary and may encompass the most distal segment of the CCA as well and/or any combination of the internal and external carotid arteries. In some patients, the carotid bulb

TABLE 12–6 • NASCET and ACAS Criteria for Grading ICA Stenosis	
Diameter Reduction	ICA/CCA PSV Ratio
70–99%	>4[40]
60–99%	>3.2[41]

is absent. Often ultrasound reports describe carotid plaque as being located within the bulb or bifurcation. These terms are used interchangeably; however, they can refer to two distinct regions. Defining plaque as being present within the carotid bulb is ambiguous since this usually applies to more than one vessel. It is more appropriate to define plaque by using terms such as proximal, mid or distal. Carotid bifurcation refers to a specific anatomic region and would be acceptable as defining the location of disease. Given carotid bulb variability, the term "carotid bulb" should be removed from common use within carotid duplex interpretations.[82]

Diagnosis of Internal Carotid Artery Occlusion

Atherosclerosis is by far the most common cause of occlusion of the extracranial carotid arteries; however, FMD and dissection are additional causes. Most occlusions occur in the ICA.[48] ICA occlusion is not amenable to surgical intervention, and a false-positive diagnosis will preclude the potential for treatment in this patient population. It is, therefore, important for patient management to differentiate between high-grade stenosis versus occlusion of the ICA. Differentiation of these two clinical entities was a major concern in ultrasound in the era before color-flow Doppler. However, with the advent of and technological advances in the 2D image and in color and power Doppler imaging, ICA occlusion can now very accurately be distinguished from high-grade stenosis.[48–50]

In the presence of a suspected ICA occlusion, the artery should be evaluated with spectral Doppler, color Doppler, and power Doppler to rule out the presence of trickle flow. Power Doppler is sometimes referred to as color power angio (CPA or amplitude Doppler). Power Doppler provides information commensurate with the amplitude of the Doppler shift but not on the shift itself. It is advantageous in that it is very sensitive in small vessel and low flow/low velocity states but is hampered by excessive movement (eg, vessel pulsatility, labored breathing, coughing, and swallowing) sometimes resulting in nondiagnostic images. Secondary ultrasound characteristics of a ICA occlusion are echogenic material filling the lumen, lack of arterial pulsations, reversed color blood flow near the origin of the occlusion, and increased resistance with loss of diastolic blood flow in the ipsilateral CCA (proximal to the occlusion) (Figs. 12–23B and 24).

It is important to employ several technical strategies[51]: (1) the ultrasound instrument must be adjusted to allow for the detection of very low flow velocities. The operator must take care to assure the appropriate PRF, this is referred to as the scale on some instruments. The wall filter must be adjusted so that it does not exclude low-frequency signals; (2) make sure to obtain the best possible image of the vessel in question and inspect the lumen for any evidence (2D or Doppler) of active blood flow. This may require multiple angle views and approaches so that both the 2D and Doppler analysis have been optimized; (3) interrogate all visualized segments of the ICA with spectral Doppler.

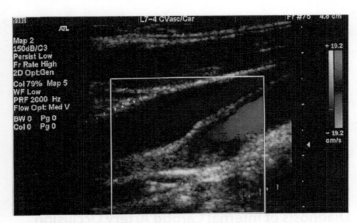

FIGURE 12–24. Color duplex image of a carotid artery occlusion.

If flow is detected, be careful to assure the correct flow direction so as to not mistake an adjacent vein for a patent ICA; (4) use both the saggital and transverse planes to evaluate the suspected occlusion for any potential flow channels; (5) if possible, image the very distal ICA. In the presence of a suspected occlusion, the presence of antegrade flow distally is likely to mean that a patent lumen proximally has been overlooked.

Pitfalls in the diagnosis of ICA occlusion include calcific plaques (Fig. 12–25). These will cause acoustic shadowing that limit or prevent visualization of the vessel of interest. Other pitfalls include high bifurcations and deep vessels that can limit the investigation, and a pulsatile jugular vein that can be mistaken for a patent ICA.

CCA occlusion/stenosis occurs much less often than ICA occlusion and it can be accompanied by stroke or other neurologic events or it can be asymptomatic. Often these patients present after radiation therapy to the neck region. Atherosclerosis is a less likely cause.

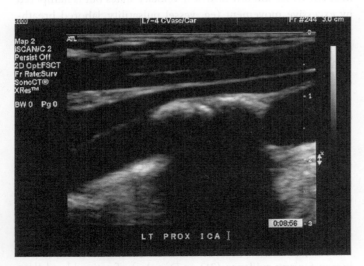

FIGURE 12–25. Color duplex image of a calcific plaque that in many cases limits and sometimes prohibits adequate visualization of the carotid bifurcation. These plaques must be imaged from multiple approaches to achieve an adequate evaluation.

Plaque Characterization

While the Doppler-derived velocity remains the primary and most reliable method for determining the degree of stenosis and for evaluation ICA disease, the role of plaque characterization as part of the duplex carotid examination is becoming more important as the significance and relationship of vulnerable and/or unstable plaque relative to stroke become better understood.

A normal carotid artery has smooth vessel walls and no visible plaque extending into the vessel lumen. The intima media layer is easily seen as a thin line on the innermost part of the wall uniformly throughout the vessel. The lumen of the vessel is anechoic although it is not uncommon for echoes to be present within the lumen of the carotid artery in both planes as a function of the reverberation artifact of the wall of the internal jugular vein. As it is a relatively straight and superficial vessel, most abnormalities of the carotid artery are detectable on B-mode imaging. These include plaque formation, intraluminal defects such as dissections and thrombus, and iatrogenic injuries (pseudoaneurysms and arteriovenous fistulas). Atherosclerotic plaque initially presents as an increase in the thickness of the intima and media layers of the artery wall and subsequently by echogenic material that encroaches on the arterial lumen.

B-mode imaging can provide detailed information on both the surface features and internal composition of atherosclerotic plaque. Plaque is evaluated most accurately with gray scale, without the use of conventional color or power Doppler imaging and should be evaluated in both the transverse and sagittal projections. Plaque can occur along any segments of the extracranial carotid system however most commonly forms at the carotid artery bifurcation and will often involve the distal CCA and origins of the internal and external carotid artery.

Plaque extent and severity is defined as the location and the approximate length of the plaque and to the plaque thickness and degree of luminal narrowing. Plaque severity is more difficult to define using ultrasound because plaque can vary in thickness from one location to another. Transverse (short-axis) images provide the best evaluation of carotid plaque thickness as they most accurately reveal the maximum thickness of the plaque and degree of luminal narrowing. Plaque extent and severity are reported using generic terms, such as minimal, moderate, and severe.

The surface of the plaque can be described as smooth or irregular. Use of the term ulcerated is generally discouraged. Ulceration is the loss of the vascular endothelium and although some irregular plaques may be ulcerated, this is not a finding that is reliably predicted by ultrasound. Homogeneous plaque is uniform in appearance and is often of relatively low echogenicity. In general low echogenicity correlates with a high lipid content and the presence of fibro-fatty tissue. A smooth appearing fibrous cap may also be present. Heterogeneous or mixed echogenicity plaque may be comprised of fatty material in areas of calcium that tend to cause brighter echoes and sometimes acoustic shadowing. Acoustic shadowing occurs when calcium attenuates the transmission of ultrasound and creates a shadow deep to the calcified area.

Assessment of luminal narrowing/stenosis must always be performed in conjunction with the waveform and velocity information acquired by the pulsed Doppler as plaque severity can be grossly over or underestimated by the sonographic evaluation alone.

Transcranial Doppler and Imaging[83,84]

Originally introduced by Rune Aaslid in 1982 and applied to patients with vasospasm secondary to subarachnoid hemorrhage (SAH) transcranial Doppler (TCD) and transcranial duplex imaging (TCDI) provide information in patients in a variety of clinical settings [52] TCD, and more recently, transcranial color Doppler and power imaging, give detailed information about the flow velocity in brain arteries and veins (Fig. 12–26). This hemodynamic information is routinely used in diagnosis of cerebrovascular disease. TCD can be used to monitor for emboli in patients with or at risk for TIA or stroke and is especially useful for monitoring during carotid or cardiac procedures and following coil or stent deployment for intracranial aneurysms. Additionally, it is used to assess for intracranial stenosis, in vasospasm from a SAH, for detection of cardiac shunts (patients with a patent foramen ovale), in the assessment of brain death and in evaluating children with sickle cell disease. and other problems, this relatively quick and inexpensive test is growing in popularity in the United States.[53,54] It is often used in conjunction with other tests such as MRI, MRA, carotid duplex ultrasound (CDU), and CT scans.

One fact to keep in mind when utilizing TCD is that the value obtained for a particular artery is the velocity of blood flowing through the vessel, and unless the diameter of that vessel is established by some other means, it is not possible to determine the actual blood flow. Thus, TCD is primarily a technique for measuring relative changes in flow. The utility of the technique is now well established for a number of different disease processes.[54-64]

Two methods of recording may be used for this procedure. The first uses the B-mode image in combination with the Doppler information. Once the desired blood vessel is found, blood flow velocities may be measured with a pulsed Doppler, which records velocities over time. This is referred to as transcranial duplex imaging (TCDI) and is performed using the duplex scanner. The second method of recording uses only the Doppler probe function, relying instead on the training and experience of the clinician in finding the correct vessels. This is referred to subsequently as TCD.

The operator must be aware that the Doppler spectral waveforms obtained during a TCDI examination are based on hemodynamics, and that the waveforms obtained do not provide anatomic information. TCDI is an advancement of intracranial ultrasound techniques since it combines the hemodynamic information with anatomic landmarks, enabling the accurate identification of the intracranial arteries. Increases in intracranial arterial velocity may be due but not limited to: increased volume flow without a lumen diameter change, a decrease in lumen diameter (stenosis) without a change in volume flow, or by a combination of an increase in volume flow and a decrease in lumen diameter.

The accurate interpretation of a patient's TCDI examination may be difficult without knowledge of the location and the extent of atherosclerotic disease present in the extracranial vasculature.

The TCD technique was introduced as a method to detect cerebral arterial vasospasm following SAH. During the past 20 years, the list of clinical applications for TCD has grown (Table 12–7), and the addition of new areas of research will

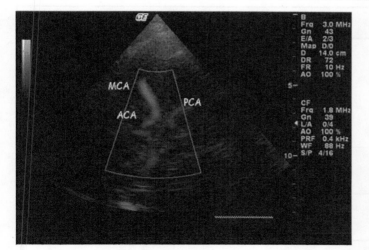

FIGURE 12–26. Power Doppler image of a portion of the circle of Willis.

TABLE 12–7 • Transcranial Doppler Applications
1. Diagnosis of intracranial vascular disease
2. Monitoring vasospasm in subarachnoid hemorrhage
3. Screening of children with sickle cell disease
4. Assessment of intracranial collateral pathways
5. Evaluation of the hemodynamic effects of extracranial occlusive disease on intracranial blood flow
6. Intraoperative monitoring
7. Detection of cerebral emboli
8. Monitoring evolution of cerebral circulatory arrest
9. Documentation of subclavian steal
10. Evaluation of the vertebrobasilar system
11. Detection of feeders of arteriovenous malformations
12. Monitoring anticoagulation regimens or thrombolytic therapy
13. Monitoring during neuroradiologic interventions
14. Testing of functional reserve
15. Monitoring after head trauma

permit better understanding of intracranial cerebrovascular hemodynamics.

Examination Protocols and Techniques

TCDI.[65-67] The quality of the intracranial image is dependent upon proper adjustment of many instrument controls. Increasing the power setting and the color gain to the appropriate levels during a TCDI study are probably the most important instrument control adjustments. Adjusting the focal zone in the range of 6–8 cm will improve the image and color resolution. Maintaining a small image sector width and color box width will keep the highest possible frame rates. Checking for the appropriate color PRF, sensitivity, and persistence settings is also very important to obtain good quality color Doppler intracranial images.

The color display is important because it assists in the proper placement of the Doppler sample volume. The interpretation of the TCDI examination is made from the Doppler spectral waveform information. Therefore, Doppler signals are obtained from various depths along the artery's path (Table 12–8). The color Doppler display helps guide the operator, as the Doppler sample volume is "swept" through the intracranial arteries to obtain the Doppler spectral waveforms. At each depth setting, it is important to adjust the position of the sample volume on the color display and angle the transducer to optimize the Doppler signal.

Conventional color orientation for TCDI examinations is set for shades of red indicating blood flow toward the transducer and shades of blue indicating blood flow away from the transducer. By keeping this color assignment constant, intracranial blood flow direction in the arteries can be readily recognized. The appearance of intracranial arterial blood flow is dependent upon many instrument controls that can affect its presentation.

Therefore, estimations of arterial size are not accurate from the color Doppler display.

The Doppler evaluation of the intracranial arteries is performed with a low frequency (2–3 MHz) phased-array imaging transducer. A large sample volume is used to obtain a good signal-to-noise ratio. With TCDI, a smaller gate (ie, 5–10 mm) can be placed on a specific arterial segment that is readily identified from a color-flow image. Intracranial arterial velocities acquired with TCDI are acquired assuming a zero-degree angle.

Additionally, with the use of TCDI, many investigators are reporting results using peak systolic and end-diastolic velocities instead of the traditionally accepted mean velocities (time average peak velocities). Each institution will have to decide which velocity value to report, and adjust the diagnostic criteria accordingly.

TCD is a "blind" technique that encompasses many of the concepts described above but employs a Doppler probe only without the image component to analyze the intracranial vasculature.[66,67] Using various windows (Fig. 12–27) and depths, mean velocities are acquired, and a diagnosis can be rendered (Table 12–8).

Intima-Media Thickness

Large observational studies and atherosclerosis regression trials of lipid-modifying pharmacotherapy have established that intima-media thickness (IMT) of the carotid and femoral arteries, as measured noninvasively by B-mode ultrasound, is a valid surrogate marker for the progression of atherosclerotic disease.[68] IMT is a measurement that can be obtained at the level of the carotid bifurcation (Fig. 12–28). Although automated software is required to ensure accurate and reproducible data to assess a patient's risks for such events, we can comment on the

TABLE 12–8 • Mean Velocities Using Various Doppler US Approaches

Window	Artery	Depth (mm)	Mean Velocity (cm/s)
Transtemporal	Middle cerebral	30–67	62 ± 12
	Anterior cerebral	60–80	50 ± 11
	Terminal internal carotid	60–67	39 ± 9
	Posterior cerebral	55–80	39 ± 10
	Posterior communicating		
	Anterior communicating		
Transorbital	Ophthalmic	40–60	21 ± 5
	Internal carotid (siphon)	60–80	47 ± 10
Suboccipital	Vertebral	40–85	38 ± 10
	Basilar	>80	41 ± 10
Submandibular	Distal internal carotid	35–70	37 ± 9

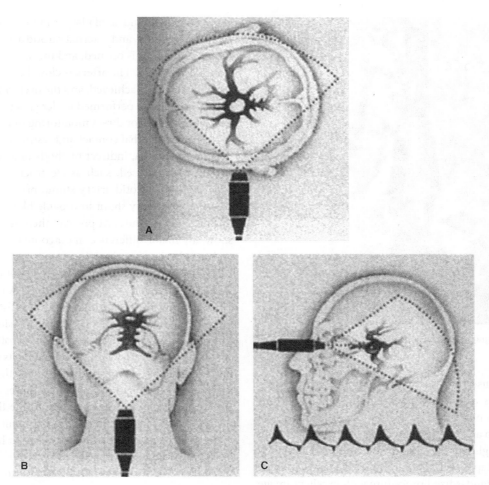

FIGURE 12–27. Transcranial Doppler is accomplished using the following approaches: (**A**) transtemporal, (**B**) suboccipital, (**C**) transorbital.

integrity of the vessel wall and look for variations of wall thickness along its length. Measuring the IMT is simply a screening tool and is mentioned here as an attempt to increase its awareness and utilization.[69]

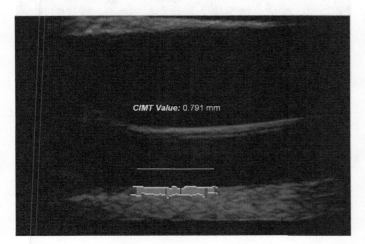

FIGURE 12–28. Carotid intima-media thickness (CIMT) measurement using proprietary software (Prowin).

Other Diagnostic Imaging Modalities[85]

Other tests commonly used in the diagnosis and management of patients with known or suspected cerebrovascular diseases include contrast cerebral angiography (CA), magnetic resonance angiography (MRA), and CT.

Angiography or more specifically carotid arteriography is a catheter-based technique that may include assessment of the aortic arch as well as selected injections of individual subclavian and carotid arteries with anteroposterior, lateral, and oblique views to evaluate the intracranial and extracranial vessels (Fig. 12–29).[20,71] It is the gold standard for the preoperative assessment of patients considered for carotid interventions, although the reported complications of stroke and death range between 0.2% and 0.7%. Noninvasive modalities such as duplex ultrasound, TCD, and MRA combined duplex ultrasound are attractive because they avoid the contrast and catheter-related complication associated with arteriography. In many institutions, duplex ultrasound has emerged as the sole preoperative imaging study prior to carotid and other arterial and venous interventions.[46,70]

CT of the head is useful in identifying silent infarcts, determining the timing of surgery, evaluating the risk of surgery, and

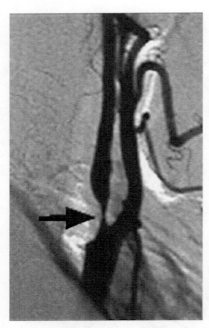

FIGURE 12–29. Angiographic diagnosis of an internal carotid artery stenosis.

ruling out other causes of disease or symptoms. CT provides radiographic images of the body from many angles. A computer combines the pictures into two- and three-dimensional images. This test can also be performed with the administration of contrast dye to highlight the cerebrovasculature.[19] Computed tomography angiography (CTA) of carotid arteries and vertebrobasilar system is a standardized procedure with excellent image quality, but radiation exposure remains a matter of concern.

MRA is increasingly being used as a noninvasive method for analyzing the carotid bifurcation. Many studies comparing duplex, MRA, CTA, and angiography have now been performed. While initial reports on MRA suggest it to be accurate for identifying carotid occlusion, MRA appears less reliable than duplex ultrasound for categorizing stenosis in areas of moderate to severe narrowing where flow is turbulent and it tends to overestimate disease. MRA remains an adjunct to CTA, duplex ultrasound, or angiography.[72-75]

Treatment

The management options for patients with carotid artery stenosis include the following on their own or in combination: (1) conservative management (risk factor modification), (2) CEA, (3) balloon angioplasty and stenting (CAS), or (4) transcarotid artery revascularization (TCAR).[13]

The standard surgical procedure is CEA, while the newer minimally invasive endovascular intervention is called carotid artery angioplasty with stenting. Common indications for these procedures are transient ischemic attacks (TIAs) or cerebrovascular accidents (CVAs, strokes), although CEA can also be performed in asymptomatic patients with carotid stenosis. CAS and TCAR are typically reserved for more high-risk patients.[13]

CEA is the removal of plaque on the inside of an artery. The internal, common, and external carotid arteries are clamped, the lumen of the ICA is opened, and the atheromatous plaque substance is removed. The artery is closed usually with the use of a patch, hemostasis achieved, and the overlying layers closed. The procedure may be performed under general or local anesthesia. The latter allows for direct monitoring of neurological status by intraoperative verbal contact and testing of grip strength. With general anesthesia, indirect methods of assessing cerebral perfusion must be used, such as electroencephalography (EEG), TCD analysis, carotid artery stump pressure monitoring, and/or use of a temporary shunt to provide blood supply to the brain during the procedure. At present, there is no good evidence to show any major difference in outcome between local and general anesthesia.

Angioplasty and stenting of the carotid artery are undergoing investigation as alternatives to CEA (Fig. 12–30). CAS is a less invasive procedure that can be performed via a percutaneous approach or through a small incision for intra-arterial access. A catheter is advanced into the carotid artery to the area of stenosis. This catheter has a balloon at its tip, which may vary in size. Once the balloon is advanced over the lesion, the balloon is inflated. Inflation of the balloon compresses the plaque in the artery and makes a larger opening inside the artery to restore the lumen for improved blood flow. A stent (a tiny, expandable metal coil) is often deployed at the site to help keep the artery from narrowing or closing again (recoil).

Because of the potential for emboli to the brain that may cause stroke, embolic prevention devices (EPD) are being used during CAS. One type of EPD has a filter-like basket attached to a catheter that is positioned in the artery so as to "catch" any clots or small debris that may break loose from the plaque during the procedure. This technique may help reduce the incidence of stroke during CAS.[76]

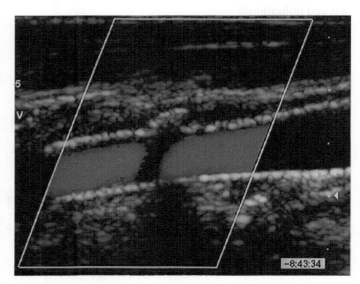

FIGURE 12–30. Ultrasound image of a carotid stent. Notice the plaque that has been pushed against the wall as a result of balloon angioplasty.

Yet another hybrid technique used in adjust to angioplasty and stenting of the carotid artery is TCAR. A small incision is made in the neck to expose the CCA. A soft, flexible sheath is placed directly into the carotid artery and connected to a system that reverses the flow of blood away from the brain to protect again any clots, small debris, or fragments of plaque that may break loose during the procedure. The blood is filtered and return through another sheath placed in the femoral vein. This system allows for angioplasty and stenting to be performed while blood flow is reversed.[86]

Intraoperative Carotid Duplex Imaging

The assessment of the CEA site by duplex imaging for technical adequacy has been shown to be an effective method to improve the results of the operation. Intraoperative duplex imaging identifies disturbed blood flow and anatomic abnormalities such as residual plaque, thrombus, and platelet aggregation. The detection of peak systolic velocities more than 150 cm/s with the presence of an anatomic defect warrants correction because of its potential to progress. Investigators have reported that the use of intraoperative carotid duplex imaging has had a favorable impact on the stroke rate and incidence of restenosis of the carotid artery. However, it is recommended that each institution should establish its own diagnostic criteria whether for use in the operating room or for diagnosis of atherosclerotic lesions.[77–79]

References

1. Stephens RB, Stillwell DL. *Arteries and Veins of the Human Brain*. Springfield, IL: Charles C Thomas; 1969.

2. McVay CB. *Anson and McVay Surgical Anatomy*. 6th ed. Philadelphia: WB Saunders; 1984.

3. Clemente CD (ed). *Gray's Anatomy of the Human Body*. 30th American ed. Philadelphia: Lea and Febiger; 1985.

4. Meyer JS (ed). *Modern Concepts of Cerebrovascular Disease*. New York: Spectrum Books; 1975.

5. Fields WS, Breutman ME, Weibel J. *Collateral Circulation to the Brain*. Baltimore: Williams and Wilkins; 1965.

6. Strandness DE Jr. *Collateral Circulation in Clinical Surgery*. Philadelphia: WB Saunders; 1969.

7. Bendick PJ, Glover JL. Vertebrobasilar insufficiency: evaluation by quantitative duplex flow measurements. *J Vasc Surg*. 1987;5:594-600.

8. Bendick PJ, Glover JL. Hemodynamic evaluation of vertebral arteries by duplex ultrasound. *Surg Clin North Am*. 1990;70:235-244.

9. Bendick PJ. Duplex examination. In: Berguer R, Caplna LR (eds). *Vertebrobasilar Arterial Disease*. St. Louis: Quality Medical Publishers; 1992, pp. 93-103.

10. Strandness DE Jr. Extracranial artery disease. In: Strandness DE Jr, ed. *Duplex Scanning in Vascular Disorders*. 2nd ed. New York: Raven Press; 1993, pp. 113-157.

11. Hallett JW, Brewster DC, Darling RC. *Handbook of Patient Care in Vascular Surgery*. 3rd. ed. Boston: Little, Brown & Co.; 1995.

12. Goldstein LB, Adams R, Becker K, et al. Primary prevention of ischemic stroke: a statement for healthcare professionals from the Stroke Council of the American Heart Association. *Circulation*. 2001;103:163-182.

13. Fazel P, Johnson K. Current role of medical treatment and invasive management in carotid atherosclerotic disease. *Proc (Bayl Univ Med Cent)* 2008;21(2):133-138.

14. National Institute of Neurological Disorders and Stroke (NINDS) (1999). Stroke: Hope Through Research.

15. Maton A, Hopkins J, McLaughlin CW, et al. *Human Biology and Health*. Englewood Cliffs, NJ: Prentice Hall; 1993.

16. Patterson RF. Basic science in vascular disease. *J Vasc Technol*. 2002;26(1).

17. Tuzcu EM, Kapadia SR, Tutar E, et al. High prevalence of coronary atherosclerosis in asymptomatic teenagers and young adults: evidence from intravascular ultrasound. *Circulation*. 2001; 103(22):2705–2710.

18. Fishbein MC, Schoenfield LJ. Heart Attack Photo Illustration Essay. Available at: MedicineNet.com.

19. Feigin VL. Stroke epidemiology in the developing world. *Lancet* 2005;365(9478):2160–2161.

20. Panetta TF. Cerebrovascular disease. In: Sales CM, Goldsmith J, Veith FJ, eds. *Handbook of Vascular Surgery*. St. Louis, MO: Quality Medical Publishing; 1994.

21. Katz ML. Extracranial/intracranial cerebrovascular evaluation. In: Hagen-Ansert SL, ed. *Textbook of Diagnostic Ultrasonography*. 5th ed. St. Louis, MO: Mosby; 2001.

22. Smullens SW. Surgically treatable lesions of the extracranial circulation, including the vertebral artery. *Radiol Clin N Am*. 1986;23:453-460.

23. Ito M, Nitta T, Sato K, Ishii S. Cervical carotid aneurysm presenting as transient ischemic and recurrent laryngeal nerve palsy. *Surg Neurol*. 1986;25:346-350.

24. Gritzmann N, Herold C, Haller J, et al. Duplex sonography of tumors of the carotid body. *Cardiovasc Intervent Radiol*. 1987;10(5):280-284.

25. Jansen JC, Baatenburg de Jong RJ, Schipper J, et al. Color Doppler imaging of paragangliomas in the neck. *J Clin Ultrasound*. 1997 Nov-Dec;25(9):481-485.

26. Alkadhi H, Schuknecht B, Stoeckli SJ, Valavanis A. Evaluation of topography and vascularization of cervical paragangliomas by magnetic resonance imaging and color duplex sonography. *Neuroradiology*. 2002 Jan;44(1):83-90.

27. Antonitsis P, Saratzis N, Velissaris I, et al. Management of cervical paragangliomas: review of a 15-year experience. *Langenbecks Arch Surg*. 2006 Aug;391(4):396-402. Epub 2006 May 6.

28. Fenves AZ, Ram CV. Fibromuscular dysplasia of the renal arteries. *Curr Hypertens Rep*. 1999 Dec;1(6):546-549.

29. Lüscher TF, Keller HM, Imhof HG, et al. Fibromuscular hyperplasia: extension of the disease and therapeutic outcome. Results of the University Hospital Zurich Cooperative Study on Fibromuscular Hyperplasia. *Nephron*. 1986;44 Suppl 1:109-114.

30. Samson RH, Yungst Z, Showalter DP. Homocysteine, a risk factor for carotid atherosclerosis, is not a risk factor for early recurrent carotid stenosis following carotid endarterectomy. *Vasc Endovascular Surg*. 2004 Jul-Aug;38(4):345-348.

31. Gillett M, Davis WA, Jackson D, et al. Prospective evaluation of carotid bruit as a predictor of first stroke in type 2 diabetes: the Fremantle Diabetes Study. *Stroke*. 2003 Sep;34(9):2145-2151. Epub 2003 Aug 7.

32. Murie JA, Sheldon CD, Quin RO. Carotid artery bruit: association with internal carotid stenosis and intraluminal turbulence; *Br J Surg*. 1984 Jan;71(1):50-52.

33. LaBan MM, Meerschaert JR, Johnstone K. Carotid bruits: their significance in the cervical radicular syndrome; *Arch Phys Med Rehabil*. 1977 Nov;58(11):491-494.

34. Magyar MT, Nam EM, Csiba L, et al. Carotid artery auscultation—anachronism or useful screening procedure? *Neurol Res*. 2002 Oct;24(7):705-758.

35. Hill AB. Should patients be screened for asymptomatic carotid artery stenosis? *Can J Surg*. 1998 Jun;41(3):208-213.

36. Soteriades ES, Evans JC, Larson MG, et al. Incidence and prognosis of syncope. *N Engl J Med*. 2002 Sep 19;347(12):878-885.

37. Labropoulos N, Erzurum V, Sheehan MK, Baker W. Cerebral vascular color flow scanning technique and applications. In: Mansour MA, Labropoulos N, eds. *Vascular Diagnosis*. Philadelphia PA: Elsevier Saunders; 2005. Chapter 9.

38. SVU Vascular Technology Professional Performance Guideline. Extracranial Cerebrovascular Duplex Ultrasound Evaluation. Available at http://www.svunet.org.

39. Hoskins SH, Scissons RP. Hemodynamically significant carotid disease in duplex ultrasound patients with carotid artery tortuosity. *J Vasc Technol*. 2007;31(1):11-15.

40. North American Symptomatic Carotid Endarterectomy Trial Collaborators. Beneficial effect of carotid endarterectomy in symptomatic patients with high grade carotid stenosis. *N Engl J Med*. 1991;325:445-453.

41. Executive Committee Asymptomatic Carotid Atherosclerosis Study. Endarterectomy for asymptomatic carotid artery stenosis. *JAMA*. 1995;273:1421.

42. Randomized trial of endarterectomy for recently symptomatic carotid stenosis: final results of the MRC European Carotid Surgery Trial (ECST). *Lancet*. 1998;351:1379-1387.

43. Moneta GH, Edwards JM, Chitwood RW, et al. Correlation of North America Symptomatic Carotid Endarterectomy Trial (NASCET) angiographic definition of 70-99% internal carotid artery stenosis with duplex scanning. *J Vasc Surg*. 1995;17:152-159.

44. Moneta GH, Edwards JM, Papanicolaou G, et al. Screening for asymptomatic carotid internal carotid artery stenosis: duplex criteria for discriminating 60-99% stenosis. *J Vasc Surg*. 1995;21:989-994.

45. Fujitani Rm, Mills JL, Wang LM, Taylor SM. The effect of unilateral internal carotid artery occlusion upon contralateral duplex study: criteria for accurate interpretation. *J Vasc Surg*. 1992;16:459-468.

46. Spadone DP, Barkmeier LD, Hodgson KJ, et al. Contralateral internal carotid artery stenosis or occlusion: pitfall of correct ipsilateral classification—a study performed with color-flow imaging. *J Vasc Surg*. 1990;11:642-649.

47. Wain RA, Lyon RT, Veith FJ, et al. Accuracy of duplex ultrasound in evaluating carotid artery anatomy before endarterectomy. *J Vasc Surg*. 1998 Feb;27(2):235-242; discussion 242-244.

48. Chang YJ, Lin SK, Ryu SJ, et al. Common carotid artery occlusion: evaluation with duplex sonography. *Am L Neuroradiol*. 1995;16:1099-1105.

49. Mattos MA, Hodgson K, Ramsey DE, et al. Identifying total carotid occlusion with colour flow duplex scanning. *Eur J Vasc Surg*. 1992;6:204-210.

50. Lee DH, Gao FQ, Rankin RN, et al. Duplex and color Doppler flow sonography of occlusion and near occlusion of the carotid artery. *Am J Neuroradiol*. 1996;17:1267-1274.

51. Zwiebel WJ, Pellerito JS. Carotid occlusion, unusual carotid pathology and tricky carotid cases. In: Zwiebel WJ; Pellerito JS, eds. *Introduction to Vascular Ultrasonography*. Chapter 10. Philadelphia, PA: Elsevier Saunders; 2005.

52. Aaslid R, Markwalder TM, Nornes H. Noninvasive transcranial Doppler ultrasound recording of flow velocity in basal cerebral arteries. *J Neurosurg*. 1982 Dec;57(6):769-774.

53. Sloan MA, Alexandrov AV, Tegeler CH, et al. Therapeutics and Technology Assessment Subcommittee of the American Academy of Neurology. Assessment: transcranial Doppler ultrasonography: report of the Therapeutics and Technology Assessment Subcommittee of the American Academy of Neurology. *Neurology*. 2004 May 11;62(9):1468-1481.

54. Newell D, Aaslid R. *Transcranial Doppler*. New York: Raven Press; 1992.

55. Babikian VL, Feldmann E, Wechsler LR, et al. Transcranial Doppler ultrasonography: year 2000 update. *J Neuroimaging*. 2000 Apr;10(2):101-115. Review.

56. Adams RJ, McKie VC, Hsu L, et al. Prevention of a first stroke by transfusions in children with sickle cell anemia and abnormal results on transcranial Doppler ultrasonography. *N Engl J Med*. 1998;339:5-11.

57. Alexandrov AV, Bladin CF, Norris JW. Intracranial blood flow velocities in acute ischemic stroke. *Stroke*. 1994;25:1378-1383.

58. Alexandrov AV, Demchuck AM, Wein TH, Grotta JC. The accuracy and yield of transcranial Doppler in acute cerebral ischemia. *Stroke*. 1999;30:238.

59 Wilterdink JL, Feldmann E, Furie KL, et al. Transcranial Doppler ultrasound battery reliably identifies severe internal carotid artery stenosis. *Stroke*. 1997;28:133-136.

60. Razumovsky AY, Gillard JH, Bryan RN, Hanley DF, Oppenheimer SM. TCD, MRA and MRI in acute cerebral ischemia. *Acata Neurol Scand*. 1999;99:65-76.

61. Di Tullio M, Sacco RL, Venketasubramanian N, et al. Comparison of diagnostic techniques for the detection of patent foramen ovale in stroke patients. *Stroke*. 1993;24:1020-1024.

62. Petty GW, Mohr JP, Pedley TA, et al. The role of transcranial Doppler in confirming brain death: sensitivity, specificity, and suggestions for performance and interpretation. *Neurology*. 1990;40:300-303.

63. Ducrocq X, Hassler W, Moritake K, et al. Consensus opinion on diagnosis of cerebral circulatory arrest using Doppler-sonography: Task Force Group on cerebral death of the Neurosonology Research Group of the World Federation of Neurology. *J Neurol Sci*. 1998;159:145-150.

64. Ringelstein EB. CO_2-reactivity: dependence from collateral circulation and significance in symptomatic and asymptomatic patients. In: Caplan LR, Shifrin EG, Nicolaides, Moore WS, eds. *Cerebrovascular Ischemia: Investigation and Management*. London: Med-Orion; 1996, pp. 149-154.

65. Spencer MP. Transcranial Doppler monitoring and causes of stroke from carotid endarterectomy. *Stroke*. 1997;28:685-691.

66. Katz ML, Alexandrov AV. *A Practical Guide to Transcranial Doppler Examinations*. Littleton, CO: Summer Publishing Company; 2003.

67. Katz ML. Intracranial cerebrovascular evaluation. In: *Textbook of Diagnostic Ultrasonography*. St. Louis, MO: Mosby; 2001.

68. Bots ML, Hoes AW, Koudstaal PJ, et al. Common carotid intima-media thickness and risk of stroke and myocardial infarction: the Rotterdam Study. *Circulation*. 1997;96:1432-1437.

69. Bortel L. What does intima–media thickness tell us? *J Hypertens*. 2005;23:37-39.

70. Hingorani A, Ascher E, Marks N. Preprocedural imaging: new options to reduce need for contrast angiography. *Semin Vasc Surg*. 2007 Mar;20(1):15-28.

71. Redmond PL, Kilcoyne RF, et al. Principles of angiography. In: Rutherford RB, ed. *Vascular Surgery*. 3rd ed. Philadelphia: WB Saunders; 1989, pp. 143-157.

72. Khaw KT. Does carotid duplex imaging render angiography redundant before carotid endarterectomy. *Br J Radiol*. 1997;70:235-238.

73. Alvarez-Linera J, Benito-León J, Escribano J, et al. Prospective evaluation of carotid artery stenosis: elliptic centric contrast-enhanced MR angiography and spiral CT angiography compared with digital subtraction angiography. *AJNR Am J Neuroradiol*. 2003 May;24(5):1012-1019.

74. Hirai T, Korogi Y, Ono K, et al. Prospective evaluation of suspected stenoocclusive disease of the intracranial artery: combined MR angiography and CT angiography compared with digital subtraction angiography. *AJNR Am J Neuroradiol*. 2002 Jan;23(1):93-101.

75. Saloner D. Preoperative evaluation of carotid artery stenosis: comparison of contrast-enhanced MR angiography and duplex ultrasonography with digital subtraction angiography. *AJNR Am J Neuroradiol*. 2003 Jun-Jul;24(6):1034-1035.

76. Yadav JS, Wholey MH, Kuntz RE, et al. Protected carotid-artery stenting versus endarterectomy in high-risk patients. *N Engl J Med*. 2004;351:1493-501.

77. Bandyk DF, Mills JL, Gahtan V, Esses GE. Intraoperative duplex scanning of arterial reconstructions: fate of repaired and unrepaired defects. *J Vasc Surg*. 1994;20:426-433.

78. Baker WH, Koustas AG, Burke K, et al. Intraoperative duplex scanning and late carotid artery stenosis. *J Vasc Surg*. 1994;19:829-833.

79. Kuntz KM, Polak JF, Whittemore AD, et al. Duplex ultrasound criteria for the identification of carotid stenosis should be laboratory specific. *Stroke*. 1997;28:597-602.

80. Vital Signs: Recent trends in stroke death rates—United States, 2000-2015. *MMWR*. 2017;66.

81. Benjamin EJ, Blaha MJ, Chiuve SE, et al. on behalf of the American Heart Association Statistics Committee and Stroke Statistics Subcommittee. Heart disease and stroke statistics—2017 update: a report from the American Heart Association. *Circulation*. 2017; 135:e229-e445.

82. Thornton JB, Kupinski AM, et al. Anatomic distribution of the carotid bulb as determined by duplex ultrasound. *J Vasc Ultrasound*. 2007;31(2):87–91. Available at: https://doi.org/10.1177/154431671503900105.

83. Alexandrov AV, Sloan MA, Wong LKS. Practice Standards for transcranial Doppler Ultrasound Part I—test performance. *J Neuroimaging*. 2006;17:11-18.

84. Alexandrov AV, Sloan MA, Tegeler CH, et al. Practice Standards for transcranial Doppler Ultrasound Part II—clinical indications and expected outcomes. *J Neuroimaging*. 2012;22:215-224.

85. Furie KL. Evaluation of carotid artery stenosis. https://www.uptodate.com/contents/evaluation-of-carotid-artery-stenosis.

86. TCAR. A safe, less invasive option to treat carotid disease. https://silkroadmed.com/the-tcar-procedure/

Questions

GENERAL INSTRUCTIONS: For each question, select the best answer. Select only one answer for each question unless otherwise specified.

1. **What is the annual rank of stroke in the United States as a cause of death?**

    (A) 1st with 800,000 deaths each year

    (B) 2nd with 600,500 deaths each year

    (C) 3rd with 500,000 deaths each year

    (D) 5th with 140,000 deaths each year

2. **Common imaging diagnostic modalities are used to directly image the internal carotid artery include all, *except***

    (A) carotid duplex ultrasound (CDU)

    (B) computerized tomography angiography (CTA)

    (C) magnetic resonance imaging (MRI) diffusion imaging

    (D) Positron emission tomography (PET)

3. **Which of the following best defines stroke?**

    (A) a sudden increase of blood flow to the brain causing syncope

    (B) a sudden increase in blood flow to the brain causing eye damage

    (C) any motor or sensory deficit that lasts greater than 24 hours

    (D) any motor or sensory deficit that lasts less than 24 hours

Match the following terms with the correct definition.

4. Transient ischemic attack (TIA) _____

5. Stroke in evolution (SIE) _____

6. Reversible ischemic neurologic deficit (RIND) _____

7. Completed stroke _____

8. Crescendo TIA _____

    (A) neurologic symptoms that last longer than 24 hours, but completely resolve

    (B) this is caused by either lack of blood supply or effect of blood outside of normal vessels

    (C) ischemic neurologic symptoms that last less than 24 hours and completely resolve

    (D) stroke in which there is no further ischemia or loss of functional activity.

    (E) repeated ischemic neurologic symptoms that last less than 24 hours and completely resolve

9. **Modifiable risk factors for stroke include all, *except***

    (A) hypertension

    (B) renal artery stenosis

    (C) smoking

    (D) hyperlipidemia

10. **TIA/stroke symptoms referable to ICA stenosis include all of the following, *except***

    (A) paralysis on the side contralateral to the stenosis

    (B) decreased level of consciousness

    (C) amaurosis fugax

    (D) ataxia

11. Which of the following is a neurologic symptom related to atherosclerotic disease in the posterior circulation (vertebrobasilar disease)?

    (A) amaurosis fugax
    (B) contralateral extremity weakness
    (C) orthostatic hypotension
    (D) vertigo

12. Brachial artery pressure difference of _____ is within normal limits.

    (A) less than 20 mm Hg
    (B) between 20 and 25 mm Hg
    (C) between 25 and 30 mm Hg
    (D) more than 30 mm Hg

13. Color Doppler ultrasound reliably provides all of the following, *except*

    (A) real-time imaging
    (B) Doppler waveform analysis
    (C) ophthalmic artery pressure
    (D) color depiction of the flow characteristics

14. The optimal transducer for carotid duplex imaging is

    (A) 2.5–5 MHz linear array
    (B) 5–10 MHz curved array
    (C) 5–10 MHz linear array
    (D) 7.5–10 MHz curved array

15. Doppler interrogation in the extracranial carotid system is performed using which of the following angles?

    (A) 60–70-degree angle to the artery
    (B) 0-degree angle to the artery
    (C) 45–60-degree angle to the artery
    (D) 20–35-degree angle to the artery

16. Which of the following is the most frequently utilized measurement for estimation of percentage diameter ICA stenosis?

    (A) end-diastolic velocity
    (B) peak diastolic velocity divided by end-diastolic velocity
    (C) peak systolic velocity
    (D) mean systolic velocity

17. Which of the following is a pulsed Doppler artifact generated by a wide sample (>2 mm) volume?

    (A) spectral broadening
    (B) turbulence
    (C) aliasing
    (D) mirror image

18. Which of the following is an advantage of power Doppler?

    (A) extremely sensitive to high flow state of intracranial arteries
    (B) more sensitive to frequency shift information
    (C) beneficial in defining occluded vessels
    (D) is dependent on beam angle and free from aliasing artifact

Match the following three layers of an artery wall with the correct definition.

19. Media _____   (A) elastic inner layer

20. Adventitia _____   (B) layer of muscle and elastic tissue

21. Intima _____   (C) outer loose filmy layer

22. Which of the following terms best describes mixed echogenicity plaque?

    (A) homogeneous
    (B) calcified with acoustic shadowing
    (C) ulcerated with irregular margins or craters
    (D) heterogeneous

23. The left carotid artery arises from which of the following?

    (A) vertebral artery
    (B) aortic arch
    (C) internal thoracic
    (D) innominate artery

24. Which vessel often reverses flow to supply the distal subclavian artery in the presence of a proximal subclavian or innominate artery obstruction?

    (A) vertebral
    (B) internal thoracic
    (C) thyrocervical and costocervical trunk
    (D) dorsal scapular

Match the following to Fig. 12–31.

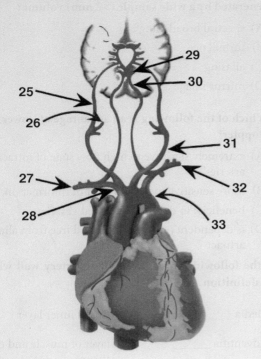

FIGURE 12–31.

25. _____   (A) basilar artery

26. _____   (B) right external carotid artery

27. _____   (C) left subclavian artery

28. _____   (D) right common carotid artery

29. _____   (E) left vertebral artery

30. _____   (F) right subclavian artery

31. _____   (G) left common carotid artery

32. _____   (H) aortic arch

33. _____   (I) brachiocephalic trunk

                     (J) right internal carotid artery

34. **This important anatomical site is where carotid artery disease is most likely to develop:**

(A) internal carotid artery

(B) vertebral artery

(C) common carotid artery

(D) external carotid artery

Match the following arteries with the correct spectral analysis description.

35. internal carotid artery _____

(A) exhibits a complicated turbulent flow pattern

36. external carotid artery _____

(B) demonstrates a rapid increase in velocity during systole with a clear window and a continuous antegrade flow during diastole

37. common carotid artery _____

(C) combination of the pattern of internal and external carotid arteries

38. carotid bulb _____

(D) demonstrates a brisk systolic upstroke, sharp peak, abrupt downstroke

Match the following extracranial waveforms with the proper normal waveform.

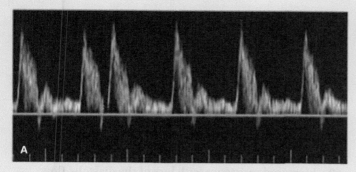

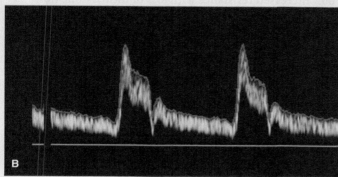

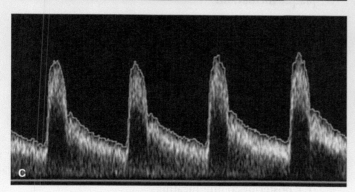

39. external carotid artery _____

40. internal carotid artery _____

41. common carotid artery _____

42. Which of the following is the "gold standard" for carotid imaging?

   (A) carotid duplex ultrasound

   (B) computed tomography angiography

   (C) magnetic resonance arteriography

   (D) contrast arteriography

Place the following steps in the proper order per the examination protocol described in the study guide.

43. _____   (A) Using color-flow Doppler as a guide, interrogate the length of the vessel with pulsed Doppler and measure the peak systolic and end-diastolic velocities.

44. _____   (B) Sagittal to the long axis of the vessel, follow the course of the CCA from its origin (or as proximal as can be obtained) to the bifurcation.

45. _____   (C) Brachial artery pressures are recorded bilaterally.

46. _____   (D) a transverse sweep of the carotid system

47. _____   (E) The examination is explained and a history (including risk factors and symptoms) is obtained from the patient.

Match the following gray-scale image to the normal extracranial carotid arteries.

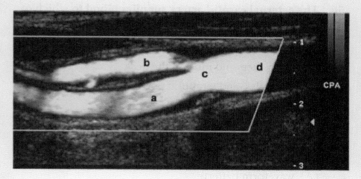

48. _____ external carotid artery.   A

49. _____ internal carotid artery   B

50. _____ common carotid artery.   C

51. _____ carotid bulb.   D

52. Which of the following terms is used to describe expected flow in the bulbous segment of the carotid artery?

   (A) laminar

   (B) turbulent

   (C) helical

   (D) parabolic

53. Disturbed flow at the carotid bulb is often referred to as

   (A) plug flow

   (B) flow separation

   (C) reversed flow

   (D) alternating flow

54. The first branch of the internal carotid artery is the

   (A) superior thyroid

   (B) occipital

   (C) ophthalmic

   (D) superficial temporal

55. The internal carotid artery supplies blood to which of the following structures?

   (A) cerebral hemispheres of the brain only

   (B) external occipital protuberance

   (C) posterior portion of the brain and face

   (D) ophthalmic artery, anterior portion of the brain, and the circle of Willis

56. The external carotid artery supplies blood to which of the following structures?

   (A) cerebellum

   (B) scalp, face, and most of the neck

   (C) face, eyes, and temporal portion of the brain

   (D) anterior part of the brain

57. Which is the primary determinant for distinguishing the ICA from the ECA?

   (A) waveform pattern

   (B) Absence of branches

   (C) temporal tapping

   (D) velocity

58. Which common carotid artery arises directly from the aortic arch?

   (A) the right common carotid artery

   (B) the left common carotid artery

   (C) the right subclavian artery

   (D) the left innominate artery

59. The spectral Doppler flow pattern beyond a hemodynamically significant stenosis will almost always exhibit

   (A) plug flow

   (B) post-stenotic dilatation

   (C) post-stenotic turbulence

   (D) helical flow

60. Increased resistance with loss of the diastolic flow component in the common carotid artery may indicate which of the following?

   (A) occlusive disease proximal to the sample site

   (B) occlusive disease distal to the sample site

   (C) occlusive disease at the sample site

   (D) sample volume site placed too close to the arterial wall

61. What is the most common site for atherosclerotic plaque formation?

   (A) distal internal carotid artery

   (B) distal common carotid artery

   (C) carotid bifurcation

   (D) vertebral artery origin

62. Which branch of the internal carotid artery is seen extracranially?

   (A) Ophthalmic

   (B) cavernous

   (C) posterior communicating

   (D) none of the above

Identify the following plaque morphology with the appropriate image.

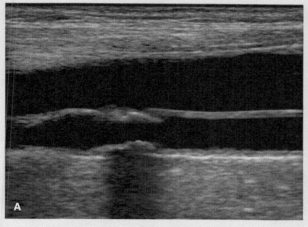

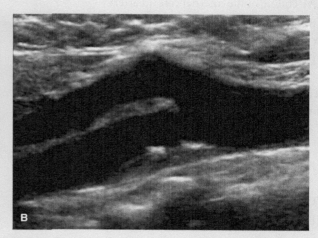

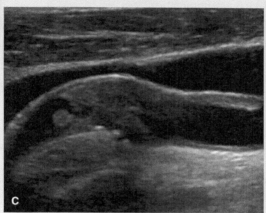

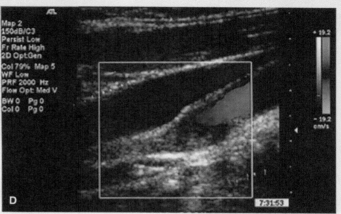

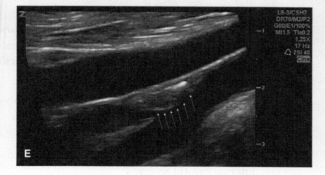

63. Homogenous _____

64. Heteregenous _____

65. Irregular surface_____

66. Calcified _____

67. ICA occlusion _____

68. **Which of the following best describes carotid body tumors?**

(A) They almost always appear bilaterally.

(B) They are best evaluated using duplex ultrasound.

(C) They appear at the carotid bifurcation.

(D) They are almost always malignant.

69. **Which of the following carotid artery findings can be associated with symptoms of cerebral ischemia?**

    (A) coiling of the internal carotid artery

    (B) kinking of the internal carotid artery

    (C) tortuosity of the internal carotid artery

    (D) looping of the internal carotid artery

70. **The North American Symptomatic Carotid Endarterectomy Trial (NASCET) recommends**

    (A) carotid endarterectomy for lesions less than 50% diameter reducing

    (B) treating all patients with aspirin therapy and perform carotid Doppler exam once a year

    (C) medical treatment for high-grade ICA stenosis

    (D) carotid endarterectomy for high grade ICA stenosis

Match the following vessels to Fig. 12–32.

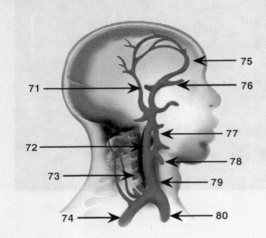

FIGURE 12–32.

71. _____

72. _____

73. _____

74. _____

75. _____

76. _____

77. _____

78. _____

79. _____

80. _____

(A) superficial temporal artery

(B) supraorbital artery

(C) subclavian artery

(D) internal carotid artery

(E) ophthalmic artery

(F) common carotid artery

(G) external carotid artery

(H) superior thyroid artery

(I) brachiocephalic trunk

(J) vertebral artery

81. **Which of the following is *not* a branch of the subclavian?**

    (A) vertebral

    (B) internal thoracic

    (C) thyrocervical trunk

    (D) hypophyseal

82. **The extracranial posterior circulation is composed of which of the following?**

    (A) paired vertebral arteries in the back of the neck

    (B) basilar artery

    (C) brachiocephalic

    (D) posterior cerebral arteries

83. **In most cases subclavian steal**

    (A) is asymptomatic

    (B) warrants invasive evaluation or treatment

    (C) does not represent an appropriate physiological response to proximal arterial disease

    (D) causes blurred vision bilaterally

84. **True subclavian steal syndrome** _____

    (A) is associated with a blood pressure difference of less than or equal to 10–20 mm Hg between the two arms

    (B) is not associated with proximal ipsilateral subclavian artery stenosis or occlusion

    (C) cannot occur without retrograde blood flow in a vertebral artery

    (D) does not include reversal of vertebral artery flow

85. **Which of the following are normal characteristics of the vertebral artery spectral waveform?**

    (A) high-resistance or multiphasic flow similar to external carotid artery

    (B) monophasic flow, dampened flow

    (C) low-resistance waveform pattern similar to the internal carotid artery

    (D) multiphasic flow seen in peripheral vessels

86. **The vertebral artery is best visualized by**

    (A) positioning the transducer medial to the jugular

    (B) using the transverse approach just lateral to the common carotid artery

    (C) imaging in a longitudinal plane at the level of the common carotid with the transducer angled laterally until the vertebral is seen

    (D) identifying the carotid bifurcation and angling medially

Match the following arteries in Fig. 12–33.

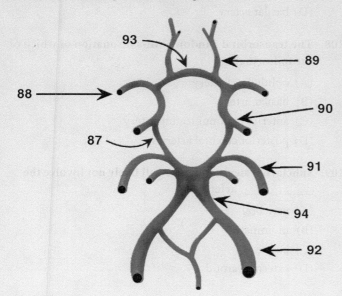

FIGURE 12–33.

87. _____   (A) anterior cerebral artery

88. _____   (B) posterior communicating artery

89. _____   (C) anterior communicating artery

90. _____   (D) middle cerebral artery

91. _____   (E) basilar artery

92. _____   (F) internal carotid artery

93. _____   (G) vertebral artery

94. _____   (H) posterior cerebral artery

95. **Which of the following transducer characteristics is required for performing a transcranial Doppler examination?**

(A) high-frequency continuous-wave transducer

(B) high-frequency linear array

(C) low-frequency (2 MHz) phased-array imaging transducer

(D) high frequency hockey stick configuration

96. **Which of the following vessels is imaged from the suboccipital window examine?**

(A) vertebral arteries

(B) anterior communicating arteries

(C) anterior cerebral arteries

(D) distal internal carotid arteries

97. **Which of the following best describes transcranial Doppler?**

(A) invasive technique that measures and visualizes the major intracranial vessels

(B) displays intracerebral hemorrhages

(C) used to measure the velocity of blood flow in the intracranial brain vessels

(D) performed to exclude significant external carotid artery stenosis

98. **Which of the following arteries is the largest branch of the internal carotid artery?**

(A) ophthalmic artery

(B) middle cerebral artery

(C) anterior cerebral artery

(D) superior hypophyseal artery

99. **The middle cerebral artery does not supply blood to which of the following lobes of the brain?**

(A) occipital lobe

(B) frontal lobe

(C) temporal lobe

(D) cerebellum

100. **The ophthalmic artery communicates via an extensive collateral pathway with which of the following arteries?**

(A) anterior communicating artery

(B) anterior cerebral artery

(C) middle cerebral artery

(D) external carotid artery

101. **The anterior cerebral artery and its branches do not supply blood to which of the following structures?**

(A) frontal and parietal lobes

(B) brain stem

(C) septum pellucidum

(D) corpus callosum

102. The vertebral arteries unite to form which of the following arteries?

    (A) posterior communicating artery
    (B) posterior cerebral artery
    (C) basilar artery
    (D) subclavian artery

103. The brainstem is supplied by which of the following arteries?

    (A) middle cerebral artery
    (B) posterior communicating artery
    (C) basilar artery
    (D) external carotid artery

104. The basilar artery gives rise to which one of the following?

    (A) anterior inferior cerebellar artery
    (B) posterior communicating artery
    (C) superior cerebellar artery
    (D) posterior cerebral arteries

105. The transtemporal window allows insonation of all, *except* the

    (A) middle cerebral artery (M1–M2 segments)
    (B) basilar artery
    (C) posterior cerebral artery
    (D) anterior cerebral artery

106. The Suboccipital window allows insonation of which of the following?

    (A) carotid siphon
    (B) vertebral and basilar arteries
    (C) anterior communicating artery
    (D) distal internal carotid artery

107. The Submandibular window allows insonation of which of the following?

    (A) ophthalmic artery
    (B) carotid siphon

    (C) distal internal carotid artery
    (D) basilar artery

108. The transorbital window allows insonation of which of the following?

    (A) ophthalmic artery
    (B) basilar artery
    (C) anterior communicating artery
    (D) posterior cerebral arteries

109. Subclavian steal syndrome will likely not involve the _____ artery.

    (A) vertebral
    (B) inominate
    (C) basilar
    (D) external carotid

110. Intracranial vessel stenosis will likely exhibit which of the following characteristics?

    (A) focal increase in the mean blood flow velocity distal to the stenosis
    (B) focal increase in the mean blood flow velocity at the site of the vessel stenosis
    (C) turbulent flow proximal to the stenosis
    (D) aneurysmal dilatation

111. Which of the following intracranial vessels is the most often occluded in stroke?

    (A) basilar artery
    (B) anterior cerebral artery
    (C) ophthalmic artery
    (D) middle cerebral artery

112. Transcranial color Doppler in all these clinical settings, *except*_____.

    (A) brain death
    (B) concussion syndrome
    (C) arteriovenous malformations
    (D) detecting cardiac shunts

Answers and Explanations

1. **(D)** Stroke is the 5th leading cause of death in the United States, kills about 140,000 Americans each year (approximately 1 out of every 20 deaths) and is more common in men than in women. (Reference 80.)

2. **(D)** Four diagnostic modalities are used to directly image the internal carotid artery: cerebral angiography (CA), carotid duplex ultrasound (CDU), magnetic resonance angiography (MRA), computed tomographic angiography (CTA).

3. **(C)** Any sensory or motor deficit lasting more than 24 hours.

4. **(C)** Transient ischemic attack is an acute neurologic symptom that lasts less than 24 hours and completely resolves.

5. **(E)** Stroke in evolution is ischemic symptoms that actively worsen during a period of observation.

6. **(A)** Reversible ischemic neurologic deficit is a neurologic symptom that lasts longer than 24 hours and completely resolves.

7. **(D)** Completed stroke is a stable neurologic deficit that had sudden onset and persists longer than 3 weeks.

8. **(E)** Repeated TIA symptoms that are similar in nature but get worse or occur with increased frequency.

9. **(B)** The modifiable risk factors for stroke include hypertension, diabetes, cigarette smoking, hyperlipidemia, carotid artery stenosis, atrial fibrillation, excessive alcohol consumption, and physical inactivity.

10. **(D)** Ataxia, also called dystaxia, is a symptom of vertebrobasilar insufficiency, not internal carotid artery symptoms.

11. **(D)** Vertigo is a neurologic symptom of vertebrobasilar disease.

12. **(A)** Brachial artery pressures are recorded bilaterally. Pressure can vary from right to left however a less than 20 mm Hg difference is within normal limits.

12. **(A)** Brachial artery pressures are recorded bilaterally. Pressure can vary from right to left however a less than 20 mm Hg difference is within normal limits.

13. **(C)** Duplex ultrasound does not measure pressure.

14. **(C)** A 5–10 MHz linear array is the optimal transducer for high-resolution gray-scale imaging of the carotid arteries.

15. **(C)** 45–60-degree angle to the artery gives the best Doppler information.

16. **(C)** Peak systolic velocity is the most utilized of the Doppler criteria for estimation of percentage diameter reduction.

17. **(A)** Spectral broadening is an artifact that occurs with pulsed Doppler.

18. **(C)** Power Doppler is beneficial in defining occluded vessels and it is not dependent on frequency shift.

19. **(B)** The arterial layer of muscle and elastic tissue is the media.

20. **(C)** The outer loose filmy layer of the artery wall is the adventitia.

21. **(A)** The elastic inner layer of the artery wall is the intima.

22. **(D)** Mixed echogenicity plaque is described as heterogeneous.

23. **(B)** Except for the origin of the common carotid arteries, the right and left carotid artery circulation are identical. The right carotid artery circulation begins at the level of the right clavicle where the brachiocephalic trunk divides and becomes the right common carotid artery (CCA) and right subclavian artery. The left common carotid artery and the left subclavian artery both originate directly from the aortic arch.

24. **(A)** Subclavian Steal Syndrome refers to the reversal of flow in the ipsilateral vertebral artery to supply the distal subclavian artery in the presence of a proximal subclavian or innominate artery obstruction.

25. **(J)** Right internal carotid artery.

26. **(B)** Right external carotid artery.

27. **(F)** Right subclavian artery.

28. **(I)** Brachiocephalic trunk.

29. **(A)** Basilar artery.

30. **(E)** Left vertebral artery.

31. **(G)** Left common carotid artery.

32. **(C)** Left subclavian artery.

33. **(H)** Aortic arch.

34. **(A)** Internal carotid artery.

35. **(B)** The internal carotid artery demonstrates a rapid increase in velocity during systole with a clear window and continuous antegrade flow during diastole.

36. **(D)** The external carotid artery has a brisk systolic upstroke, sharp peak, and abrupt downstroke because it supplies a high-resistance system.

37. **(C)** The common carotid artery combines the pattern of the internal and the external carotid artery.

38. **(A)** The Carotid "bulb" exhibits a complicated turbulent flow pattern.

39. (B) External carotid artery.

40. (C) Common carotid artery.

41. (A) Internal carotid artery.

42. (D) Contrast arteriography is the gold standard for the preoperative assessment of patients considered for carotid interventions.

The following steps are the recommended order per the examination protocol described in the study guide:

43. (E) The examination is explained and a history (including risk factors and symptoms) is obtained from the patient.

44. (C) Brachial artery pressures are recorded bilaterally.

45. (D) a transverse sweep of the carotid system is performed.

46. (B) Sagittal to the long axis of the vessel, follow the course of the CCA from its origin (or as proximal as can be obtained) to the bifurcation.

47. (A) Using color flow Doppler as a guide, interrogate the length of the vessel with pulsed Doppler and measure the peak systolic and end diastolic velocities.

48. (B) External carotid artery.

49. (A) Internal carotid artery.

50. (D) Common carotid artery.

51. (C) Carotid bifurcation.

52. (C) Flow at the bulbous segment of the carotid artery will often be helical and somewhat disturbed.

53. (B) Flow at the bulbous segment will often be helical and somewhat disturbed and is often referred to as flow separation.

54. (C) The ophthalmic artery is the first major branch of the internal carotid artery.

55. (D) The primary role of the ICA is to perfuse the ophthalmic artery, anterior portion of the brain, and the circle of Willis.

56. (B) The external carotid artery supplies blood to the face, scalp, and neck which primarily feed the thyroid, tongue, tonsils, and ears.

57. (A) The spectral waveform pattern is the primary determinant although other parameters are useful.

58. (B) The left common carotid artery.

59. (C) The Doppler flow waveform obtained distal to a hemodynamically significant lesion will reveal post-stenotic turbulence.

60. (B) Increased resistance in the common carotid artery can indicate stenotic or occlusive disease distal to the sample site. Total occlusion of the internal carotid artery can cause a decrease in diastolic flow in the common carotid artery because of increased resistance to flow.

61. (C) The carotid bifurcation is the most common site for atherosclerotic plaque formation.

62. (D) None of the above. There are no branches of the ICA outside of the skull (extracranial).

Identification of plaque morphology:

63. (E)

64. (B)

65. (C)

66. (A)

67. (D) Occlusion of the internal carotid artery.

68. (C) Carotid body tumors are vascular tumors that arise from the paraganglionic cells in the outer layer of the carotid artery at the level of the bifurcation.

69. (B) Kinking of the internal carotid artery can be associated with the symptom of ischemia.

70. (D) The results from NASCET demonstrated that in experienced surgical hands carotid endarterectomy (CEA) is safe and effective in the near term and remarkably effective in the longer term in preventing recurrence of ipsilateral carotid ischemia and, in particular, in preventing disabling ipsilateral stroke and recommended CEA for high-grade carotid stenosis (70–99%).

71. (A) The superficial temporal artery.

72. (D) The internal carotid artery.

73. (J) The vertebral artery.

74. (C) The subclavian artery.

75. (B) The supraorbital artery.

76. (E) The ophthalmic artery.

77. (G) The external carotid artery.

78. (H) The superior thyroid artery.

79. (F) The common carotid artery.

80. (I) The brachiocephalic trunk.

81. (D) The hypophyseal is not a branch of the subclavian.

82. (A) The extracranial posterior circulation is composed of paired vertebral arteries in the back of the neck.

83. (A) In most cases, subclavian steal is asymptomatic does not warrant invasive evaluation or treatment and represents an appropriate physiological response to proximal arterial disease. Subclavian steal *syndrome* implies the presence of significant symptoms due to arterial insufficiency in the brain or upper extremity, which is supplied by the subclavian artery.

84. **(C)** True subclavian steal syndrome cannot occur without retrograde blood flow in a vertebral artery associated with proximal ipsilateral subclavian artery stenosis or occlusion.

85. **(C)** The normal vertebral artery spectral analysis will depict low-resistance waveform pattern similar to the internal carotid artery.

86. **(C)** The vertebral artery can be visualized by the longitudinal plane at the level of the common carotid with the transducer angled laterally until the vertebral is seen passing through the transverse processes.

87. **(B)** The posterior communicating artery.

88. **(D)** The middle cerebral artery.

89. **(A)** The anterior cerebral artery.

90. **(F)** The internal carotid artery.

91. **(H)** The posterior cerebral artery.

92. **(G)** The vertebral artery.

93. **(C)** The anterior communicating artery.

94. **(E)** The basilar artery.

95. **(C)** The transcranial Doppler examination requires a low frequency (2 MHz) transducer .

96. **(A)** The suboccipital window examines vertebral arteries and basilar artery.

97. **(C)** The transcranial Doppler is described as a noninvasive technique to measure the velocity of blood flow in the major intracranial brain vessels by using pulsed-waved Doppler.

98. **(B)** The middle cerebral artery is the largest branch of the cerebral internal carotid artery.

99. **(D)** The middle cerebral artery supplies blood to the frontal lobe, the temporal lobe, and the parietal lobe.

100. **(D)** The ophthalmic artery forms extensive anastomoses with the external carotid artery.

101. **(B)** The anterior cerebral artery and its branches supply the frontal and parietal lobes, the corpus callosum, the septum pellucidum, the basil ganglia, and the anterior limb of the internal capsule.

102. **(C)** The vertebral arteries unite with the basilar artery.

103. **(C)** The basilar artery supplies the various parts of the brainstem.

104. **(D)** The basilar artery then terminates at the circle of Willis where the right and left posterior cerebral arteries originate.

105. **(B)** The basilar artery.

106. **(B)** The vertebral and basilar arteries.

107. **(C)** The distal internal carotid artery.

108. **(A)** The ophthalmic artery.

109. **(D)** Subclavian steal syndrome can be detected in intracranial vessels of the intracranial vertebral arteries and basilar artery.

110. **(B)** Intracranial vessel stenosis will exhibit characteristics of focal increase in the mean blood flow velocity at the site of the stenosis and color-flow Doppler will show multiple color patterns.

111. **(D)** The middle cerebral artery is the most common intracranial vessel to occlude and is seen with acute stroke.

112. **(B)** Detecting cardiac shunts.

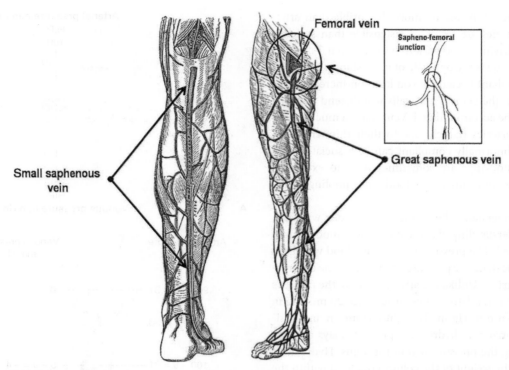

FIGURE 13-11. Small saphenous vein and tributaries. Great saphenous vein and branches. *(Reproduced with permission from Goss CM: Anatomy of the Human Body. Philadelphia, PA: Lea & Febiger; 1973.)*

perforator veins in each lower extremity. Using microinjection techniques, van Limborgh found approximately 60 perforator veins in the thigh, 8 in the popliteal fossa, 55 in the leg, and 28 in the foot.

The lower extremity perforators consist of four main groups: foot, medial calf, lateral calf, and thigh perforators. The most important perforators are the direct medial calf perforators, which cross the superficial posterior compartment. Historically, some veins had eponymous names such as Dodd's perforator at the inferior one-third of the thigh, Boyd's perforator at the knee level, Cockett's perforators at the inferior two-thirds of the leg (usually there are three: superior, medium, and inferior Cockett's perforators). However, according to the International Federation of Associations of Anatomists (IFAA) and the Federative International Committee on Anatomical Terminology (FICAT), the lower extremity perforators are grouped according to their topography and descriptive terms designating location are now used to name them.[91] These perforating veins allow blood in the superficial veins to remain at manageable levels. Perforator veins penetrate the fascia, hence, the name perforating. In the thigh, there is a constant perforating vein in the distal thigh (Hunterian perforator) that connects the femoral vein to the GSV, however more numerous and more important are the perforating veins in the calf.

When functioning properly, valves in the perforating or communicating veins direct the flow from the superficial veins toward the deep system only (Fig. 13–12).

NORMAL VENOUS HEMODYNAMICS[9,10]

Arteries and veins possess relative percentage of distensibility, elasticity, and compliance. Distensibility is defined as the ability of a blood vessel wall to expand and contract passively with

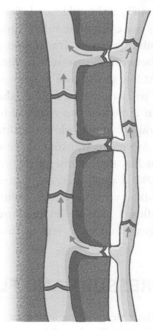

FIGURE 13-12. Venous flow pattern. Superficial to deep veins via the perforators.

changes in pressure. Veins are 8x more distensible than arteries. Pulmonary arteries are 6x more distensible than systemic arteries. Pressure driving blood back to heart is about 7 mm Hg. Compliance of a vessel is the opposite of its elastance. The veins are said to be compliant because if you keep on increasing the volume of blood in the veins, their walls will distend allowing for more blood to be accommodated. Veins have a much higher compliance than arteries (largely due to their thinner walls). Veins which are abnormally compliant can be associated with edema. Pressure stockings are sometimes used to externally reduce compliance, and thus keep blood from pooling in the legs.

In order to understand the changes that occur with disease, a general understanding of normal venous hemodynamics needs to be achieved. The pressure within any blood vessel is a result of, in part, the dynamic pressure produced by the contraction of the left ventricle. Unlike the arterial system, the pressure in the venous system is relatively low, around 15–20 mm Hg in the venules and 0–6 mm Hg in the right atrium. In any position other than horizontal, hydrostatic pressure plays a major role in determining the pressure within the veins. Hydrostatic pressure is due to the weight of the column of blood within the vessel. Hydrostatic pressure is equal to the density of the blood multiplied by the acceleration due to gravity multiplied by the height of the column of blood. In the human body, the level of the right atrium is used as the reference point by which to measure hydrostatic pressure. When supine, the arteries and veins are all approximately the same height as the heart. Therefore, the hydrostatic pressure is negligible and the pressure will approximate the dynamic pressure. The pressure within the veins at the level of the ankle is about 15 mm Hg. When standing, an individual who is approximately 6 feet tall will add a hydrostatic pressure of 102 mm Hg at the ankle level (Fig. 13–13).

Because veins are collapsible tubes, their shape is determined by transmural pressure. Transmural pressure is equal to the difference between the pressure within the vein and the tissue pressure. At low transmural pressures (when a person is supine), a vein will assume a dumbbell shape. As the pressure within a vein increases, the vein will become elliptical. At high transmural pressures (while standing), the vein will become circular. As venous transmural pressure is increased from 0 to 15 mm Hg, the volume of the vein may increase by more than 250%. A small increase in pressure is required to change an elliptical vein into a high-volume circular vein; however, a significant increase in pressure is required to stretch the venous wall once the vein has assumed a circular configuration.[8-10]

VENOUS PRESSURE AND FLOW

The first characteristic we associate with arterial flow is pulsatility; however, the direct influence of the pulsating heart on the venous system is minimal. Most veins do not yield pulsatile flow,

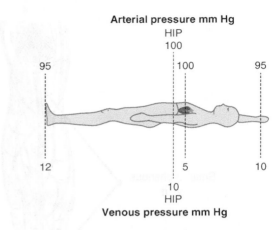

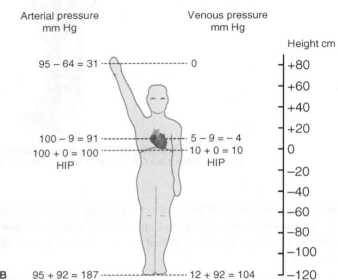

FIGURE 13–13. Graph showing changes in venous pressure caused by changes in body position. *(Reproduced with permission from Strandness DE. Sumner DS. Hemodynamics for Surgeons. New York, NY: Grune & Stratton; 1975.)*

but there are two full and one partial exceptions to that rule. Because of the proximity to the heart, the internal jugular vein and subclavian vein are normally pulsatile. The axillary vein may or may not be pulsatile depending on the individual. Pulsatility in the axillary vein is not considered abnormal but rather an individual variation. Nonpulsatility is normal in all but the great veins. The characteristic of flow typical of veins is called phasicity. Augmentation can also be performed. Augmentation of flow is elicited by squeezing the leg, typically the calf or distal thigh, at a level below the area of insonation. If the subsequent increased venous flow is transmitted to the level of evaluation, it suggests that no occlusive thrombus exists between the level of compression and insonation.

The term phasicity in reference to the venous system refers to the ebb and flow that occurs in normal veins in response to respiration. All deep veins normally exhibit phasicity, even those that are somewhat pulsatile. Respiration has this ebb-and-flow influence because unlike the strong-walled arteries, veins are collapsible.

The two phases of respiration are inspiration (breathing in) and expiration (breathing out). The way in which the blood moves in phase with respiration differs according to the part of the body affected and the position in which the body is placed.

When a body is standing upright, breathing produces pressure gradients that influence the movement of venous blood. As the lungs fill with air during inspiration, the thoracic cavity expands. When the thorax expands, the diaphragm drops, and consequently the abdominal cavity becomes smaller. The veins located within the chest and abdomen are affected by these changes in pressure. As the thoracic cavity gets larger, pressure within it decreases and pressure within the right atrium and the thoracic portion of the vena cava is also reduced. At the same time, the abdominal cavity is getting smaller, raising the pressure within the abdomen and the abdominal veins.

Fluids move from areas of high pressure to areas of low pressure. During inspiration, the result is collapse of the IVC and decreased or no flow from the lower extremities. With expiration, the process reverses itself; the intra-abdominal pressure decreases and the intrathoracic pressure increases, resulting in increasing venous blood flow to the heart from the lower extremities and in general decreased flow from the upper extremities.[8,9] Flow is normally phasic and spontaneous in veins of the lower extremity above the knee. Due to the low volume of flow in veins below the knee, spontaneous flow may not be present.

Venous Return from the Upper Extremities

Respiration affects venous return from the upper extremities, but to a lesser extent than it affects the lower body. Again, phasicity in the upper extremity veins also can vary according to circumstances. In the brachial vein for instance, inspiration may produce either a reduced or an increased sound. If the lowered or negative intrathoracic pressure causes more blood to move from the brachial vein to the subclavian vein, flow from the brachial vein will increase. Sometimes, however, expansion of the lungs on inspiration will physically compress the subclavian vein. When this happens, less venous blood will move from the chest into the arms and the sound on the brachial vein will diminish. From a clinical standpoint, this is important in that phasic changes should be detectable in all deep veins in relation to breathing.

Venous Return from the Lower Extremities

In the presence of a deep venous thrombosis, venous pressure is increased due to an increase in venous resistance. The change in venous resistance will depend on the location of the obstructed venous segment, the length of the obstruction, and the number of veins involved. Oscillations in the venous flow from the leg may be reduced or absent and flow may become continuous.

Edema is a consistent sign of increased venous pressure. The Starling equilibrium equation describes the movement of fluid across the capillary. Forces that act to move fluid out of the capillary are the intracapillary pressure and the interstitial osmotic pressure. Forces that favor the reabsorption of fluid from the interstitium are the interstitial pressure and the capillary osmotic pressure. Normally, the forces are balanced so that there is little overall fluid loss out of the vascular space into the interstitial space. While standing, the increased capillary pressure is no longer balanced by the reabsorptive forces and fluid loss from the vascular system occurs. Edema formation is limited by the action of the muscle of the calf muscle pump. Contraction of the calf muscles acts to empty the veins and decrease venous pressure. In the presence of venous thrombosis, venous pressure is increased. This increased venous pressure will be transmitted back through the vascular system to the capillary level resulting in increased capillary pressure which will lead to edema formation. Use of compression stockings will decrease interstitial pressure, which will favor increased fluid reabsorption. This decreases edema formation. Elevating the legs will reduce the intracapillary pressure by reducing the hydrostatic pressure, which will also limit edema formation.[8]

VENOUS DYNAMICS WITH EXERCISE

The calf muscle pump aids in the return of blood from the legs against the force of gravity. The muscles act as the power source. The intramuscular sinusoids (especially the gastrocnemius and soleus) and the deep and superficial veins all play a part in this mechanism. The valves are necessary to ensure efficient action of the muscle pump. Closure of the valves in the deep veins decreases the length of the column of blood, which aids in reducing venous pressure. At rest, blood pools in the leg and it is only propelled passively by the dynamic pressure gradient created by the contraction of the left ventricle. Contraction of the calf muscles can generate pressures more than 200 mm Hg. This compresses the veins forcing blood upward in both the deep and superficial veins. The valves are closed in the perforating veins and in the veins in the distal calf to prevent reflux of blood. Upon relaxation, since these veins in the calf are empty, blood is drawn into this area from the superficial veins via perforators. More distal veins also help fill the calf veins upon relaxation.[8,10]

VENOUS RESISTANCE

When distended, the cross-sectional area of the vein is about three to four times that of the corresponding arteries. It is not surprising then that the extrapulmonary veins contain about two-thirds of the blood in the body. Nevertheless, it is somewhat surprising that despite their large diameter, veins offer about the same resistance to flow as arteries. This is explained by the collapsible nature of the vein walls. Veins are seldom completely full. In the partially empty state, they assume a flattened or elliptical cross section, which offers a great deal more resistance to blood flow than a circular cross section. The ability to go from an elliptical to a circular cross section is distinctly advantageous. It permits the veins to accommodate a great increase in blood flow without an increase in the pressure gradient from the periphery to the heart. In other words, as the rate of flow increases, the vein becomes more circular, lessening resistance.

DEEP VEIN THROMBOSIS: MECHANISMS OF DISEASE AND PATHOLOGY

Etiology, Pathology, and Pathophysiology of Deep Vein Thrombosis[11]

Venous obstruction is almost always the result of venous thrombosis. Less frequently, extrinsic compression may lead to total obstruction, such as on the subclavian vein, sometimes due to a thoracic outlet issue, although this is rare. This is sometimes referred to as effort thrombosis or Paget–Schroetter syndrome (Fig. 13–14).[12,13] Compression can also occur in the area of the left common iliac vein (May Thurner syndrome[14,15]). Deep vein thrombosis (DVT) in the lower limbs is a relatively common condition and is particularly important because of the risk of pulmonary embolism (PE). This is the primary clinical concern when DVT is suspected. In the past, it was thought that deep venous thrombosis inevitably caused chronic edema, hyperpigmentation, and other changes of chronic venous insufficiency. This often occurs in the first 1–2 years after the DVT. Some evidence of symptoms and signs is present in 50% of cases after DVT, but it is only severe in 10–20% of cases. Now, it is well known that approximately one-third of thrombi will lyse quickly. In vein segments that experience total lysis within 3–5 days, valvular function is often maintained.[16] Because of the risk for pulmonary embolization, urgent diagnosis is made by imaging techniques and treatment is by immediate anticoagulation. Acute anticoagulation is achieved with heparin and chronic anticoagulation with warfarin. Thrombolytic therapy may be used in special clinical situations.[17–23]

Deep vein thrombi can vary from a few millimeters in length to long tubular masses that fill the main veins. They can form in veins greater than 1 or 2 mm in diameter and generally in large- or medium-sized vessels. Thrombi begin as microscopic nidi, and then grow by an additive process and become visible. Small thrombi are commonly found in valve pockets throughout various deep veins of the leg and thigh and in saccules of the soleal veins. Clinicians consider the soleal veins to be critical in the origination of DVT and PE.[92,93] It is from these that the long tubular structures grow. Initially, there is propagation in the direction of the venous stream by deposition of successive layers of thrombus coagulum from the blood, the primary microscopic nidus thus becomes visible. Additional further layers, both longitudinally and circumferentially, increase the length and diameter of the thrombus. Such thrombi at first are attached to the vein only at their points of origin and float almost freely in the blood system (Fig. 13–15). If further propagation occurs, venous obstruction may result and this often leads to retrograde thrombosis back to the next patent vessel.[24,25] After a DVT episode, there is an acute inflammatory response in the vein wall and in the thrombus itself, leading to a dynamic process in which the thrombus regresses due to recanalization. The process of recanalization of the veins of the lower limbs after an episode of acute deep venous thrombosis is part of the natural evolution of the remodeling of the venous thrombus in patients on anticoagulation with heparin and vitamin K inhibitors. Recanalization is defined as the return of blood flow to a venous segment that had previously been occluded. This process may take days to weeks, may not be complete and often results in valve incompetence.[94,95] Additionally, for these reasons "aging of thrombus"

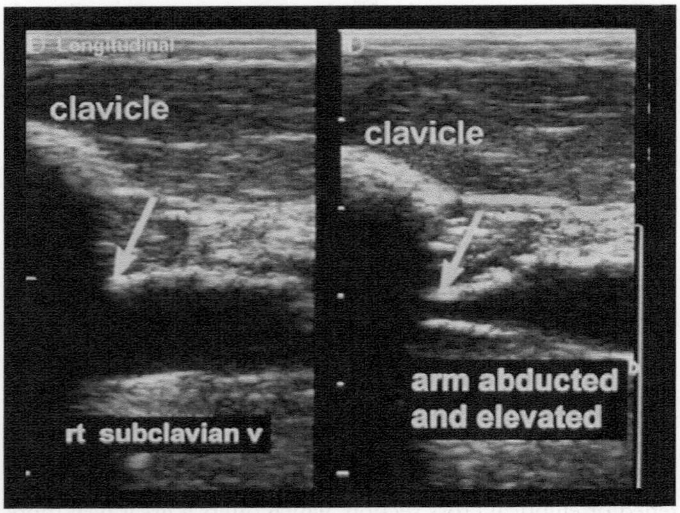

FIGURE 13–14. Sonograms demonstrating normal subclavian vein on the left image and compression with abduction of upper extremity on right image.

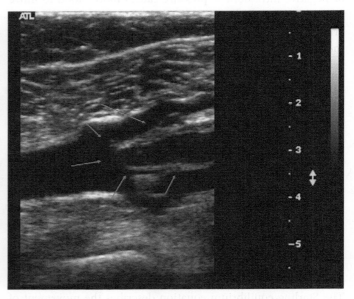

FIGURE 13–15. Sonogram with red arrows demonstrating thrombus within the lumen of a vein.

is often difficult or impossible to distinguish by ultrasound. For this reason, the term indeterminate (equivocal) age is preferred over subacute DVT when the ultrasound features are of neither acute DVT or chronic post-thrombotic change (although subacute DVT can be used in the follow-up of a known acute DVT). The term chronic post-thrombotic change is preferred over chronic or residual DVT to prevent overtreatment with anticoagulation.[96]

Pathophysiology of Calf Vein Thrombosis. Despite observations that most thrombi begin in the calf and that proximal thrombi are often an extension of calf vein thrombosis, limited data suggest that there are pathophysiological differences between proximal and isolated calf vein thrombosis. Patients with isolated calf vein thrombosis have fewer risk factors and a lower incidence of malignancy. Among 499 patients with an acute DVT, those with calf vein thrombosis had a median of one risk factor in comparison to two risk factors in those with proximal thrombosis.[16] Consistent with these observations, patients with isolated vein thrombosis appear to be less hypercoagulable. Such data suggest the isolated calf vein thrombi are not simply early thrombi that have yet to propagate but rather reflect a more limited prothrombotic state.

Incidence of Deep Vein Thrombosis[26,27]

Clinically recognized acute DVT has been estimated to have an incidence of up to 250,000–300,000 new cases per year in the United States. A number of studies have focused specifically on the epidemiology of venous thromboembolism (VTE). In these studies, involving predominantly Caucasian populations, the incidence of first-time symptomatic VTE directly standardized for age and sex to the U.S. population ranged from 71 to 117 cases per 100,000 population.[27–32]

Based on potential differences in the incidence of acute and chronic complications, these episodes are commonly defined as involving the proximal lower extremity veins, extending from the popliteal to the iliac vein confluence or isolated to the calf veins. Isolated calf vein thrombosis may involve the peroneal, posterior tibial or anterior tibial veins, the gastrocnemius veins, or the soleal veins. Although lower extremity DVT is thought to usually originate in the calf veins, most *symptomatic* thromboses involve the proximal veins. The incidence of isolated calf vein thrombosis has varied among series but has rarely been insignificant. As many as one-third of thrombi detected by duplex ultrasonography are isolated to the calf veins.[16]

Risk Factors

Patient's with one or more elements of Virchow's triad (Table 13–1) are susceptible to thrombosis.[33–35] Most cases arise during the course of another illness and a connection with confinement to bed and advancing age has been known for a long time. Post-trauma, orthopedic, gynecologic, obstetric, and surgical patients are at risk, but many medical patients such as those with heart attacks, congestive heart failure, acute strokes, and

TABLE 13–1 • Virchow's Triad

Virchow's triad can be summarized as follows:
- Venous stasis
  - More time for clotting
  - Small clots not washed away
  - Increased blood viscosity
- Vessel wall damage
  - Accidental trauma
  - Surgical trauma
- Blood coagulability increase
  - Increase in tissue factor
  - Presence of activated factors
  - Decrease in coagulation inhibitors (antithrombin III [ATIII])

paraplegia are as well. Additionally, DVT occurs as a primary state in healthy ambulatory men and women without apparent cause, and it is now recognized as a hazard in patients taking therapeutic estrogen and in women taking oral contraceptives. Other recognized predisposing factors are obesity and previous thrombosis (Table 13–2).

Isolated iliac vein thrombosis is thought to be rare. However, it is well known that pregnancy and pelvic abnormality such as cancer, trauma, and recent surgery can also predispose to iliac vein thrombosis.[36] The true incidence of isolated pelvic DVT in these patients, however, is not known, as duplex diagnosis of iliac thrombosis is often difficult and its accuracy, compared to the diagnosis of lower extremity DVT, is yet to be established.

While axillary-subclavian venous thrombosis represents a small fraction of all cases of DVT, in fact it is an important clinical entity. In the past, it was thought to be benign and self-limiting, and conservative measures were advocated. More recently, it has been recognized that considerable morbidity may occur, and aggressive management is dominant in today's practice.[37] Similarly, in the past, spontaneous axillary-subclavian venous thrombosis, referred to as effort thrombosis, was associated with a variety of physical activities. Now because of the increasing use of central venous catheters and pacemaker wires, a more frequent cause is traumatic and iatrogenic with an increasing incidence of upper extremity DVT being reported. Some patients with upper extremity venous thrombosis will have abnormal clotting factors (Fig. 13–16).

Central lines are widely used for anything from rapid fluid resuscitation, to drug administration, to parenteral nutrition, and for administering hemodialysis. Types of catheters vary and the choice and selection of the catheter depends largely on the nature and duration of intended treatment. They can include tunneled and nontunneled catheters, implanted ports, dialysis catheters, and peripherally inserted central catheters (PICC line). The subclavian (most common), internal jugular and the femoral vein are three common sites used for central line

TABLE 13–2 • Risk Factors for Venous Thromboembolism

	Risk Factors for Venous Thromboembolism			
Stasis/Endothelial Injury	Thrombotic Disorders	Medical Conditions	Drugs	Other
Indwelling vein devices	Activated Protein C resistance	Malignancy (solid tumor and myeloproliferative disorders)	Oral contraceptive use	Advancing age
Surgery (especially pelvic or orthopedic)	Factor V Leiden	Pregnancy	Hormone replacement therapy	
Major trauma, fractures	Prothrombin gene mutation G20210A	Myocardial infarction	Chemotherapy (including tamoxifen)	
Prolonged travel	Hyperhomocysteinemia	Congestive heart failure		
Paralysis (including anesthesia >30 minutes)	Anticardiolipin antibodies	Stroke		
Varicose veins	Lupus anticoagulant	Obesity		
History of DVT	Elevated factor VIII level	Inflammatory bowel disease		
Prolonged bed rest	Protein C deficiency Protein S deficiency Dysfibrogenemia Dysplasminogenemia	Nephrotic syndrome History of DVT Heparin induced thrombocytopenia Paroxysmal nocturnal hemoglobinuria		

insertion. In most scenarios, establishing central venous access with ultrasound guidance is considered the standard of care.[97]

There are several complications associated with central line use, regardless of the site of insertion. Complications that occur during or closely following a central line insertion are

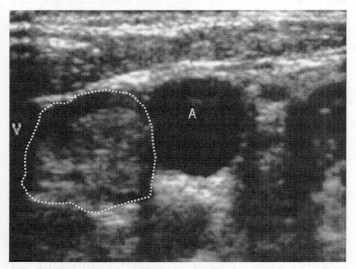

FIGURE 13–16. Transverse sonogram of deep vein thrombosis (DVT) in the upper extremity.

categorized into cardiac, vascular, pulmonary, and catheter placement complications.[98]

The immediate vascular complications seen during a central line insertion are arterial injury, venous injury, bleeding, and hematoma formation. Ultrasound guidance has been shown to greatly reduce the risk of vascular complications.[99] Arterial injury tends to occur most commonly in cases of femoral vein central lines and least commonly in subclavian vein central lines. Past research has demonstrated that ultrasound guidance can decrease the incidence of complications at all central line access sites.

Delayed onset complications include deep venous thrombosis. Patients often experience symptoms of ipsilateral extremity erythema, edema, and paresthesia. The thrombosis can extend to the central venous system causing superior vena cava syndrome (SVCS) in some patients. The incidence of SVC syndrome in patients is one in every 1000. Subclavian central lines have the lowest rate of thrombosis and femoral vein central lines have the highest rate of thrombosis. Cancer patients have amongst the highest risk of thrombosis at 41% cases.[100] A long-standing central line can lead to the development of venous stenosis (often a cause of hemodialysis access failure). The risk of venous stenosis has a prevalence of 41% and is often asymptomatic. Symptomatic patients can be treated with stenting of the stenosis site. PICC line insertion can cause vascular complications like AV fistula formation and superficial vein thrombophlebitis.

Symptoms and Physical Findings

Difficulty in diagnosing DVT is based on the presence of nonspecific symptoms in many patients. The clinical presentation of DVT can be totally asymptomatic or may progress to flagrant phlegmasia cerulea dolens and venous gangrene. The clinical diagnosis based on a physical examination is known to be notoriously inaccurate. Homans' sign (calf pain with passive dorsiflexion of the foot) is also a poor predictor for the presence of DVT. This has led to the investigation and use of pretest probability algorithms. Wells et al. suggested an algorithm based on the determination of pretest probability and compression ultrasound screening.[38] When thrombi develop in the deep venous system of the lower extremity, the findings may include acute inflammation, pain, and/or swelling, or it may be an entirely bland pathologic process. While the thrombus can produce a venous occlusion, such blockage may be partial or so well compensated that the distal limb swelling does not occur. Therefore, definitive diagnosis remains elusive except by imaging techniques.

The findings of DVT will vary with the location of the thrombus as well as whether it occurs in isolated fashion or in multiple venous segments. It is the proximal iliofemoral veins that present the greatest risk for fatal PE and often produce the most dramatic manifestations (Fig. 13–17). There can be massive swelling, pain, and tenderness of the lower extremity as is seen in phlegmasia cerulean dolens, a severe form of iliofemoral thrombus that causes significant obstruction to venous outflow. This is characterized by cyanosis, which rarely progresses to gangrene. Phlegmasia alba dolens is another form characterized by arterial spasm and a pale cool leg with diminished pulses. Thrombi in the distal or calf veins present the least risk for pulmonary embolus.[39]

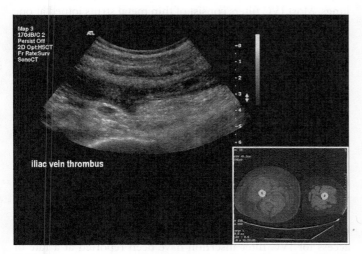

FIGURE 13–17. Sonogram of an iliac vein thrombus. In lower right edge of the image is a corresponding CT scan with increased size of the right leg in this patient with phlegmasia.

Superficial Thrombophlebitis. The terminology describing this entity is appropriate because it truly describes an inflammatory process. It is commonly believed that thrombosis of the deep and superficial venous system represents the same process. However, there does not appear to be any evidence to support that theory.

Contributing Factors. The most common cause of superficial thrombophlebitis is intravenous infusions that inflict a chemical injury on the vein wall that leads to inflammation and then inevitably thrombosis of the involved vein or veins. In the lower limbs, superficial thrombophlebitis most commonly occurs in varicose veins. This commonly follows a traumatic event that may or may not be severe. The development of migratory superficial phlebitis may be the first sign of an underlying malignancy (Trousseau's sign)[40] and has also been associated with Buerger's disease (thromboangiitis obliterans).[41]

Risk Factors and Clinical Manifestations. Varicose veins in the lower extremity and intravenous therapy in the upper extremity predispose a patient to phlebitis. The clinical presentation of superficial thrombophlebitis consists of severe pain, redness, inflammation, swelling, and pyrexia (fever). This is evident simply on physical examination of the involved area, and because the process leads to the development of thrombosis, a palpable cord is often seen.

Differential Diagnosis. The most common entities that can be confused with superficial thrombophlebitis are lymphangitis and cellulitis. In most case, the differential diagnosis is not too difficult, particularly if the examiner realizes that cellulitis and lymphangitis do not typically lead to thrombosis of the superficial veins.

Diagnostic Approach. Phlebitis in a superficial vein is readily diagnosed clinically. Physical diagnosis of superficial thrombophlebitis can be made by detecting an erythematous streaking in the distribution of the superficial veins. Tenderness is present and the extent of thrombus is identified by a palpable cord. Because superficial thrombophlebitis leads to thrombosis of the involved veins, continuous-wave Doppler is the ideal method for establishing the diagnosis. The finding of a patent vein in the area of inflammation rules out phlebitis. Although the diagnosis can be made by physical examination, accurate estimation of the proximal extent of the disease process or deep venous involvement is based on objective testing in the vascular laboratory. If there is any concern over the extent of the thrombosis, particularly whether it involves the deep venous system, it is important to use duplex scanning to depict both the thrombus and its proximal extent.

Clinical Implications. Although the initial diagnosis can be made clinically, it is now known that approximately 20% of patients with superficial vein thrombosis will have an associated occult DVT. Further, in approximately one-third of those who present with only superficial phlebitis initially, the thrombus will eventually extend into the deep venous system via the SFJ or perforating vein. Phlebitis of the long saphenous vein above the knee is particularly susceptible to progression to DVT. Therefore, it is prudent to perform a duplex examination for DVT and in selective cases, a follow-up examination in patients with suspected or proven ascending superficial phlebitis.

Evaluation of the lower extremity venous system for DVT has revealed thrombosis of the GSV in approximately 1% of limbs. Thus, examination of the SFJ should be part of the examination of the lower extremity venous system when DVT is suspected.

Upper Extremity Findings. Symptomatic patients with axillary-subclavian venous thrombosis often present with a swollen forearm, upper arm, and shoulder. A visible pattern of venous distention may be present across the anterior aspect of the shoulder and chest wall. There may be venous distention of the antecubital veins as well as those in the hand. If a tender palpable cord is present in the neck and/or axilla, this is due to a superficial thrombophlebitis accompanying the DVT. A bluish or cyanotic discoloration is commonly present in the hand and fingers and an aching pain in the forearm, exacerbated by exercise is also a common complaint.

PULMONARY EMBOLISM

Pulmonary embolism (PE) is a common medical condition that can contribute substantially to individual patient morbidity and mortality as well as global health care costs. There are an estimated 600,000 cases of PE each year in the United States, with an in-hospital case-fatality rate attributable to PE of approximately 2%.[42,43] These statistics clearly underestimate the extent of the problem, as this does not include patients with DVT, many more patients with PE die *with* PE (even if not *from* PE), and the mortality with these conditions continues to increase after hospital discharge. In fact, mortality rates from 3 months to 3 years after hospital discharge frequently range from 15% to 30%.[43–45] For patients with hemodynamic compromise, the mortality with PE is substantially higher, in the range of 20–30%, while still in the hospital.[42] Mortality rates are higher in men than women and in African American individuals compared with Caucasian individuals, yet mortality rates overall are declining temporally.[46–49]

Ninety percent of PEs arise from DVT of the lower extremities and pelvis; the rest originate from the upper extremities, heart, or pulmonary arteries. While in most patients with established PE, diagnosis of DVT may be confirmed by noninvasive testing or venography, and only about 30% will present with clinical manifestations of venous thrombosis. In the appropriate clinical setting, suspicion usually is aroused by the sudden onset of chest pain, dyspnea, and hemoptysis and by low PO_2.[50–53] Findings, however, have almost no predictive value. Tachycardia, tachypnea, and low PCO_2 are perhaps more indicative of PE.[54,55]

TREATMENT

The treatment of acute DVT is directed at preventing its primary complications, recurrent VTE, and the post-thrombotic syndrome. Without appropriate treatment, 20–50% of patients with proximal thrombosis will sustain a PE. The data with respect to calf vein thrombosis is less sound, although the incidence of PE is thought to be significantly less than for proximal DVT.[50–53]

The embolic potential of isolated calf vein thrombosis continues to be debated; however, approximately 20% of such thrombi will propagate to a more proximal level at which point the risk for pulmonary embolus is increased. Although the incidence of post-thrombotic sequelae may be less than after proximal thrombosis, between one-fourth and one-half of patients will have mild-to-moderate symptoms 1–3 years later. Isolated calf vein thrombosis should, therefore, not be regarded as trivial and cannot be ignored.

Current consensus recommendations in patients without contraindications include antithrombotic treatment, including unfractionated heparin, warfarin, low-molecular-weight heparin, and thrombolytic agents presently to treat venous thromboembolic disease. However, improved anticoagulants are being developed. Gradient elastic stockings, filters, stents, and thrombectomies can also be used in the therapeutic armamentarium, when appropriate. Thrombolytic therapy is suggested for patients with massive iliofemoral DVT at risk of limb gangrene. Venous thrombectomy is suggested in related patients with massive iliofemoral DVT at risk of gangrene. These modalities are often employed in patients with massive, severely symptomatic phlegmasia cerulea or alba dolens.

Inferior Vena Cava Interruption.

Inferior Vena Cava (IVC) filters help reduce the risk of PE. IVC filters are typically deployed just distal to the renal veins to by trap large clots and prevent them from reaching the heart and lungs. Most IVC filters consist of thin metal struts joined at one end to form a cone shape. They are used in patients who do not respond to or cannot be given conventional medical therapy such as blood thinners or with a contraindication for, or complication of, anticoagulant therapy as well as recurrent or progression of DVT despite adequate anticoagulation. The IVC filter can be placed through a small incision in a vein in your groin or neck. Until recently, IVC filters were available only as permanently implanted devices. Newer filters, called optionally retrievable filters, may be left in place permanently or have the option to be removed later. This removal may be performed when the risk of pulmonary embolus has passed.

Complications. Procedure complications from vascular access for IVC filter insertion have been reported at a rate of 4–11%. Arteriovenous fistula (AVF) is a rare complication of IVC filters thought to arise from trauma to adjacent arteries during the procedure. The reported incidence rate based upon review of published case series up to 2004 was 0.02%. Patency of the IVC proximal and distal to the filter can be evaluated with duplex ultrasound. Echogenic material in and around the filter represents thrombus that has been captured. Rarely, an IVC filter strut can perforate the IVC causing hematoma, however, this is better evaluated by CT scan.

Filter complications include the following:

1. *Filter Tilt.* Presence of IVC filter tilt is defined as greater than 15 degrees' angulation of the filter from the long axis of the vena cava and is seen in all filters except for the Bird's Nest filter. Tilt was found to be the most commonly cited cause for failure to retrieve filters. There is no increased risk of thrombosis with filter tilt of less than 15 degrees.

2. *Filter Migration.* Significant filter migration is defined as a 2 cm or greater superior or inferior movement from the initial placement location. Filter migration can be due to a variety of causes. A filter being undersized for the vena cava may lead to migration. The original Greenfield filter was associated with significant migration which prompted a design change in 1991 in which filter hooks were modified to prevent this complication. With contemporary filters, migration rates are much lower with all filters having less than 1% incidence of migration except the G2 filter which has a 4.5% incidence of

migration. Migration of the filter into the cardiopulmonary system requires immediate intervention as this can have fatal consequences. An endovascular approach is preferred, however open surgery may be required in few cases.

3. *Incomplete Opening of the Filter.* Incomplete opening of the filter can be due to a defect in the filter, operator error, or an unidentified thrombus in the IVC leading to an abnormal and asymmetric configuration of the filter following deployment.

Finally, serial noninvasive follow-up to exclude proximal propagation is a reasonable alternative in patients with contra-indications to anticoagulation.[17]

Lower Extremity Venous Duplex Ultrasound

Full diagnostic capabilities for the ultrasound evaluation and diagnosis of DVT include Doppler spectral analysis, color-flow Doppler imaging transducer compression, and high-resolution B-mode imaging. Normal ultrasound findings include unidirectional flow, compressibility of the vein, and a lumen free of internal echoes. In order to demonstrate the compressibility of a normal vein, minimal external compression is needed with the transducer in the transverse position (Fig. 13–18). Unidirectional flow is best demonstrated with color-flow Doppler imaging. Doppler spectral analysis is beneficial in evaluating venous

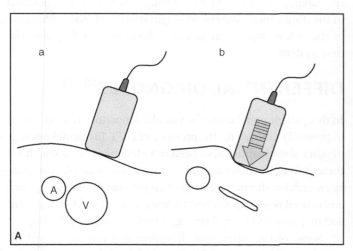

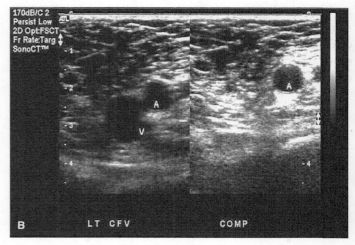

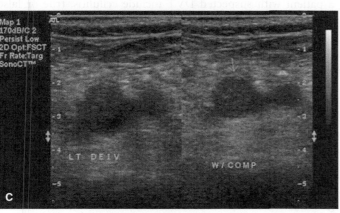

FIGURE 13–18. (A) Schematic illustrating external compression with the transducer in the transverse position, (*a*) noncompression (*b*) compression. (B) Sonogram demonstrating the effect of noncompression and compression a normal vein. (C) Sonogram demonstrating the effect of compression on a vein with thrombus.

flow, which normally changes during the respiratory cycle as described earlier.

For the average person, a 5 MHz linear transducer is the scan head of choice. Often, transducers are changed during an examination depending on the depth of the vessel and the patient's body habitus. For larger patients, a lower frequency transducer of 2.5 MHz or 3.75 MHz can be used with the trade-off of slightly reduced resolution.

Examination Protocol. The following protocol has been described in detail in the Society for Vascular Ultrasound's Vascular Technology Professional Performance Guideline.[56] The routine protocol calls for careful examination of the common femoral vein, GSV, deep femoral vein origin, femoral vein in the thigh, popliteal vein, and the calf veins, including the posterior tibial and peroneal veins.

The examination is performed with the patient in the supine position and the examination table in slight reverse Trendelenburg with the leg externally rotated (Fig. 13–19). This is the position of choice for viewing the common femoral vein, femoral vein in the thigh, deep femoral vein, GSV, popliteal vein, and the anterior and distal posterior tibial veins. The patient may be turned prone or lateral to view the popliteal vein, peroneal and proximal posterior tibial veins, and small saphenous and soleal veins.

When indicated, and if possible, the iliac veins are also evaluated. The anterior tibial veins are not routinely evaluated, as in the absence of symptoms in their distribution, their involvement in the thrombotic process is rare. The sonographer should carefully study all vessels using a combination of long- and short-axis images. Special care must be taken not to miss duplicated vessels. This is especially true of the femoral vein in the

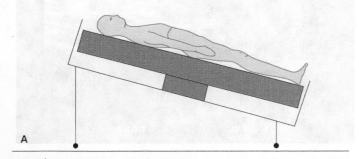

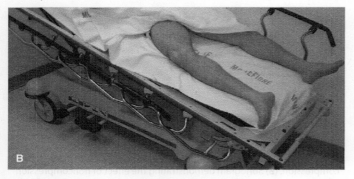

FIGURE 13–19. **(A)** Examination table in reverse Trendelenburg position. **(B)** Patient lying down in a reverse Trendelenburg position.

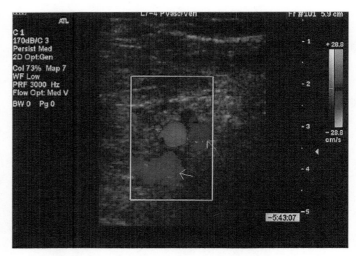

FIGURE 13–20. Duplex image of a duplicated popliteal vein.

thigh and the popliteal vein below the knee (Fig. 13–20). Several reports have demonstrated that multiple femoral veins were present in 177 (46%) of 381 venograms, a much higher rate than the generally accepted frequency of duplication of 20–25%.[57,58]

Images with and without compression and using the color flow to detect directional flow are all useful. Doppler spectral analysis helps in assessing phasicity and augmentation responses and is particularly helpful as a secondary means of evaluating the patency of the iliac veins. Although the GSV is not included in the deep venous system, its origin is often visualized because of the risk of saphenous thrombophlebitis extending into the deep system.[56-59]

DIFFERENTIAL DIAGNOSES[60-71]

In this patient population, the vascular laboratory is accustomed to primarily evaluate for the presence of DVT. Incidental findings of other abnormalities have been reported; however, a search for these entities is neither routine nor standard protocol. A systematic search for alternative causes of the patient's signs or symptoms and official reporting of these findings is beneficial to the patient and may avoid additional testing or prolonged hospitalization.

Some of the differential diagnoses that may be present in a patient with suspected DVT include cellulitis, true or false aneurysms, arterial venous fistulas, and feeder sources for hematomas. In addition, the surrounding tissues may contain masses such as cysts and hematomas and enlarged lymph nodes may also be present.

Incidental Pathology

Cellulitis is rarely associated with DVT.[60] In these cases, the vascular laboratory may be asked to exclude DVT or evaluate for the presence of abscess formation. Soft-tissue thickening and edema are a common finding in these patients. Abscess typically presents as a discrete fluid collection with variable echogenicity. There may be neovascularity of the wall.[61]

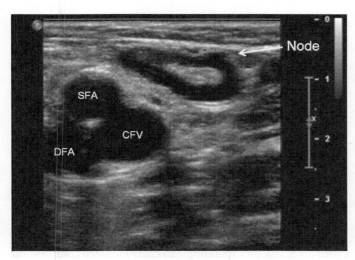

FIGURE 13–21. Sonogram of a inguinal node near the femoral vessels.

In the case of conspicuous swelling of the extremity, lymphedema can be suspected when markedly enlarged lymph nodes are visualized in the groin with normal venous hemodynamics. The inguinal nodes lie in the groin near the femoral vessels and appear enclosed in a dense fibrous capsule (Fig. 13–21). Lymphadenopathy is an enlargement of lymph nodes, which can be the result of an inflammatory or a neoplastic process. Swelling and localized tenderness can occur secondary to lymphatic obstruction or extrinsic venous compression. It may be possible to distinguish a benign enlarged lymph node from a malignant lymph node by shape and vascular patterns. A benign node generally will maintain an ovoid shape with bright echoes reflecting the hilum and surrounding hypoechogenic regions for the remainder of the node. Vascularity is seen entering in the hilar region. With malignancy, the node may become more spherical with loss of the echogenic hilum and more irregular vascularity.

A bursa is a sac of fluid. Dilated bursae communicating with the knee form cysts in the area of the popliteal fossa. These popliteal cysts commonly cause pain, swelling, and tenderness and if large enough, compression of adjacent vascular structures. Popliteal cysts are avascular, which may be helpful in the diagnosis of a structure in this region. They are found in patients with osteoarthritis, rheumatoid arthritis, and injury to the knee. Dilated bursae that lie between the gastrocnemius muscle and the semimembranous tendons, posterior and medial to the knee joint are known as Baker's cysts. Baker's cysts have an oval and often septated appearance that is mostly hypoechoic in character and are typically located posteromedial to the popliteal vessel in the popliteal space. Ruptured cysts can dissect downward into the muscular fascial planes of the calf muscles producing irregular borders and pointed inferior end and may yield the appearance of a thrombosed vessel. Therefore, care should be taken to demonstrate that it is distinct from the vein and artery (Fig. 13–22).

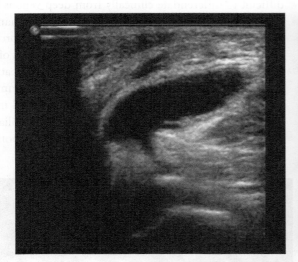

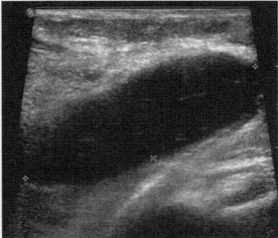

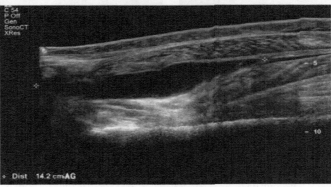

FIGURE 13–22. Sonographic images demonstrating various shapes of Baker's cyst.

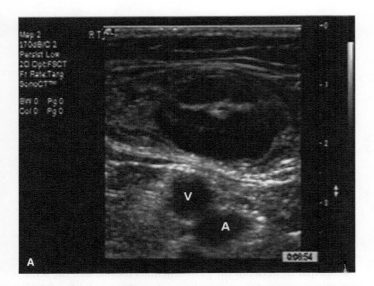

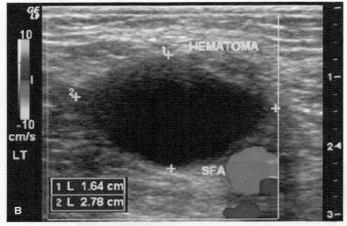

FIGURE 13–23. (**A** and **B**) Sonographic variations of hematomas.

Following trauma to an extremity, extravascular blood may accumulate. The resulting hematoma may appear quite similar to a Baker's cyst yet can become more echogenic with time. Characteristically, they appear as heterogeneous areas within a muscle or between muscle planes, although their appearance can be quite variable (Fig. 13–23). Differentiation between a hematoma and abscess is not possible based on ultrasound alone and usually requires aspiration for a definitive diagnosis.

Peripheral masses that develop acutely are usually accompanied by a history of previous trauma or surgical intervention. The incidence of pseudoaneurysm complication is 0.5–1.0% and the most common site is the common femoral artery. This mass is easily recognized by persistent circular swirling of blood between the site of rupture and the arterial lumen. False aneurysms are at risk for expanding, can cause localized compression of adjacent structures, and may rupture. True venous aneurysms are rare and obvious from their overtly large size. AVFs are also common following catheter insertion and can be identified by high-velocity turbulent signals within the vein, high-velocity, low-resistance flow within the communicating neck, and an easily visible color Doppler bruit. Congenital AVFs are rarely seen and are usually diagnosed early in life. These entities are discussed in detailed in Chapter 14.

On rare occasions extravascular sources such as tumors can cause extrinsic compression and swelling. These masses are difficult to differentiate clinically from deep venous thrombosis. Sonographically, hypervascularization and enhanced color fill within these structures are suggestive of this problem and warrant further investigation. This phenomenon is often noted at the iliac vein level and should be suspected in patients with abnormally continuous venous flow within the common femoral vein when there is no evidence of DVT noted in the legs. These findings should prompt examination of the iliac veins to exclude a compression syndrome versus a thrombotic process or a combination of the two (Fig. 13–24).

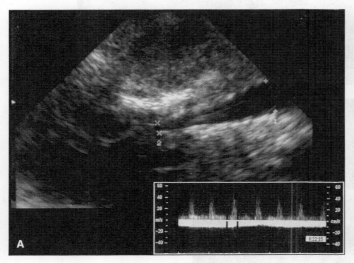

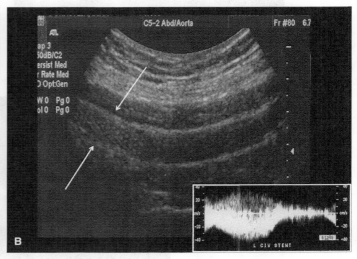

FIGURE 13–24. (**A**) Extrinsic compression of the iliac vein. Spectral Doppler on lower right of image demonstrates a continuous flow. (**B**) White arrows pointing to a stent repair in a iliac vein. Bottom right image demonstrate normal phasic flow pattern.

DIFFERENTIATION OF ACUTE VERSUS CHRONIC DEEP VEIN THROMBOSIS

Duplex ultrasound is the most common method utilized today for the diagnosis of acute DVT.[72] Three diagnostic criteria have been utilized to document the presence of *acute* DVT (Fig. 13–25).

1. Intraluminal echoes are seen. There may be soft/deformable intraluminal material with a smooth surface and/or apparently "free floating" edge or tail of thrombus (often significant for the proximal extent of clot).

2. The vein is incompressible. The vein will sometimes be significantly distended (often the diameter of the vein will be up to twice that of the accompanying artery). Increased vein size is a very specific sign of an acute process; however, not all patients with acute DVT will present with this finding.

3. There is no Doppler (color or spectral) evidence of blood flow with or without provocative maneuvers.

In most laboratories, the result of the duplex scan is the basis for clinical decisions regarding the need for anticoagulant therapy in patients suspected of DVT. The ability of duplex imaging to differentiate between acute and chronic disease is somewhat controversial but important in its use in patients with symptoms of recurrent deep venous obstruction. Generally speaking, chronic post-thrombotic changes will present as veins with normal or decreased venous diameter, damaged valves, rigid intraluminal material, irregular surface, synechiae or bands (sclerotic), calcifications (rare) that are thickened, with vein contents that are not compressible to any extent, although this is sometimes not distinguishable by duplex ultrasound. In the lower extremity, the diameter of the vein appears to be an important factor. Van Gemmeren et al.[73] compared duplex scan results to either histologic criteria or patient history and symptoms. A significant correlation was found between the age of thrombosis and the venous diameter. When thrombosis was less than 10 days old, the venous diameter was at least twice that of the diameter

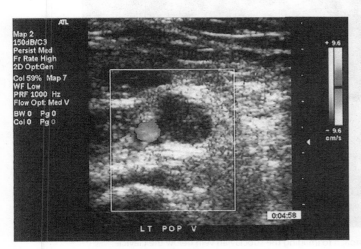

FIGURE 13–25. Color Duplex image demonstrating acute DVT.

of the accompanying artery. Two other criteria, echogenicity and margin of the vein wall, were not reliable indicators.

To increase the utility of duplex imaging in patients with recurrent disease, a baseline follow-up study should be obtained in all patients with deep venous obstruction. Gaitini et al. recommended a follow-up study 6–12 months following an acute episode.[74] An alternative approach is to obtain a baseline study at the time anticoagulant therapy is discontinued. If the patient presents with recurrent symptoms, it may be possible to interpret the results of the duplex examination without comparison to a baseline study.[75]

UPPER EXTREMITY VENOUS DUPLEX ULTRASOUND

After explaining the procedure to the patient, obtain a pertinent history and perform a physical examination of the extremities. Remove clothing so that access is not limited to the arm and neck on either side. If an indwelling catheter is in place, remove the bandages or dressings and cover the area with a sterile skin cover. The examination should be performed in a routine systematic fashion commencing at the internal jugular vein down to the brachiocephalic veins through the chest and into the arm and forearm if indicated. The asymptomatic side is always evaluated first. Comparison to the side contralateral to the involved symptomatic extremity at the same level with the patient in a similar position (supine or close to supine is best) is critical. Because the brachiocephalic, subclavian, and axillary veins are deep and protected by overlying anatomic structures and are in close proximity to the clavicle, compression ultrasound is not possible. Color and Doppler spectral flow patterns can be used to assess patency of these veins. Compression techniques can be reserved to assess the more peripheral, easily compressed deep and superficial veins in the arm.

Hemodynamics

Spontaneous flow should be present in the brachiocephalic, subclavian, and internal jugular veins. In addition, the flow signals are pulsatile due to their proximity to the right atrium. Venous flow does not reduce as dramatically during expiration in the upper extremity (particularly medial to the clavicle) and phasicity normally seen in lower extremity veins may not be appreciated. Augmentation from compression maneuvers is reduced when compared to the lower extremity veins due to the smaller venous volume of the upper extremities.

Protocol[57,76–79]

Begin the scan with the patient in the supine position and the arm at the patient's side. Using a 5 or 7 MHz linear-array transducer, the internal jugular vein is identified in the mid-neck in the transverse plane. This vessel should be examined from the level of the mandible to its confluence with the subclavian vein while compressing the vessel intermittently to assess it for the presence of intraluminal thrombus. Anatomic structures may

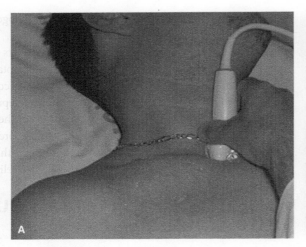
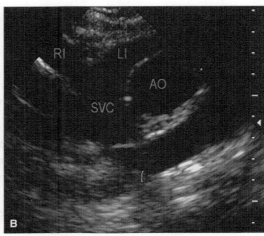

FIGURE 13-26. **(A)** Transducer position at the suprasternal notch. **(B)** Sonogram of the superior vena cava (SVC) using the suprasternal notch approach.

prevent compressibility of the very proximal internal jugular vein. Spectral waveforms are obtained in the long axis carefully noting the direction and pattern of the venous flow as the internal and external jugular veins serve as major collateral pathways to shunt flow to the contralateral side in the presence of brachiocephalic vein occlusion. Venous flow is frequently pulsatile due to the proximity of this vein to the heart.

Using color Doppler, scan in a medial direction along the cephalad border of the clavicle and follow the subclavian vein into the brachiocephalic vein. This part of the scan is performed using a small footprint transducer with a 5 MHz imaging frequency. The right brachiocephalic vein is oriented vertically and the left assumes a more horizontal plane. Color flow should outline the flow channel even when the vessel walls are poorly seen. In some patients, the brachiocephalic vein may be followed to the superior vena cava, although most often only a small section of this vein may be visualized (Fig. 13–26).

The subclavian vein is then located inferior to the clavicle and followed to the outer border of the first rib where it becomes the axillary vein (Fig. 13–27). Compression maneuvers can be

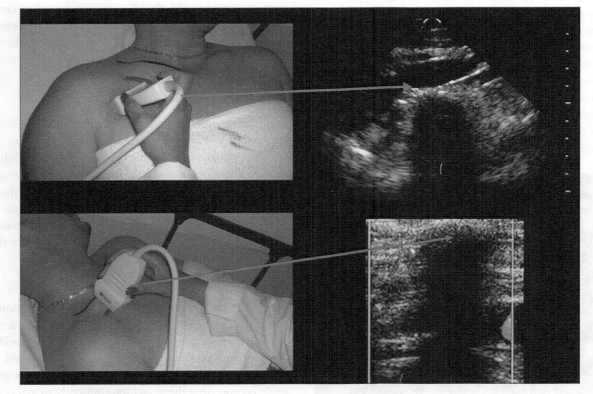

FIGURE 13-27. Demonstrate transverse and sagittal approach to imaging the subclavian vein below the clavicle (left) with corresponding sonograms (right).

attempted; however, most often color and spectral Doppler will need to be used as these vessels may be resistant to compression despite the absence of clot. If the subclavian or axillary vein is not clearly seen, abduct the arm 90 degrees from the torso and bend the arm in a pledge position to free the vessels from compression from surrounding structures. In the transverse and then longitudinal view, observe the vessel looking for the presence of internal echoes that may represent thrombus. Wall motion should also be observed as often as the vein walls will coapt in response to breathing.

The axillary vein can be followed through the deltopectoral groove into the arm where it becomes the brachial vein. The brachial veins are adjacent to the brachial artery and may be difficult to see because of their small size. They are best imaged in the transverse plane and should be compressed in a manner similar to that of the lower extremity veins to their termination at the elbow.

The cephalic vein is imaged at its confluence with the axillary vein. This vessel is best imaged using a high-frequency (7–10 MHz) transducer and is evaluated for patency using the compression technique. It is often very small and too superficial to image unless it is thrombosed. An occlusive tourniquet can be placed proximally on the upper arm to dilate this vein and make it easier to see. If signs or symptoms of cephalic vein thrombosis are present, the symptomatic segments of the vein should be imaged. The basilic and the brachial veins are continuous with the axillary vein in the upper arm, allowing these vessels to be seen in the same scan plane. The basilic vein is more posterior and is closer to the skin; however, once it has penetrated the fascia, it will be as deep as the brachial veins.

The forearm veins may be evaluated if the patient is symptomatic in this region. These veins are small and often difficult and tedious to visualize and evaluate. They are best identified by using the color-flow scan to find the adjacent artery and then using augmentation techniques to confirm the presence of flow.

Photoplethysmography (PPG) techniques assess reflux and differentiate between superficial and deep vein incompetency. These techniques provide indirect information about location and extent of venous insufficiency. These methods are less time consuming than the color-flow Doppler for screening the bilateral lower extremities and can be of great value when there are a large number of patients. PPG involves the use of a photoelectric cell placed above the medial malleolus. This photocell actually has an infrared light emitting diode and a photodetector that is attached to an amplifier and a strip chart recorder in the direct current (DC) mode. The patient is placed in a sitting position with the legs hanging in a dependent, non–weight-bearing position. Either the patient dorsiflexes the foot to contract the calf muscles or the calf is squeezed to empty the veins. The leg is allowed to relax and the refilling time of the veins is recorded. The normal venous refilling time is 20 seconds or greater.

Less than 20 seconds indicates venous incompetency (Fig. 13–28).[80] Venous incompetency can be confined to the superficial veins or involve the deep veins. It is important to discriminate which systems are involved since the superficial veins can be surgically corrected but the deep veins cannot be surgically corrected. If the initial examination is positive for incompetency, the test is repeated with a tourniquet placed above the knee to occlude the superficial veins. If the test with the tourniquet is positive it indicates the deep system is also incompetent.

Air plethysmography (APG)[81,82] is a technique that allows the measurement of limb volume changes with different maneuvers. The device consists of a cuff that is placed around the leg, a calibrated pressure transducer, and an analog chart recorder that provides a visual display. Parameters derived from performing various APG measurements with positional changes include the venous filling index, which quantitates venous reflux, the ejection fraction, which correlates with calf muscle pump function, and the residual volume fraction, which correlates with ambulatory calf venous pressure. Venous occlusion techniques allow the measurement of arterial flow into the limb and the venous outflow fraction, which can be used to evaluate venous obstruction. Differentiation of pathology in the deep venous system from that in the superficial venous system is possible. APG has been validated in the evaluation of venous insufficiency in the legs and has a place in the evaluation of symptomatic patients suspected of having deep venous thrombosis. The ability of the device to quantitate absolute arterial flow to the lower extremity makes it useful in evaluating operative results and following disease progression.

Venography (phlebography)[83,84] is defined as radiography of the veins after injection of contrast medium. It is now used infrequently because ultrasound studies are a less invasive way to get the needed diagnostic information. There are two types of venography: *ascending* and *descending* depending on the injection site. Ascending venography will be injected into a peripheral vein and the contrast material carried centripetal by the venous flow. Descending venography will be injected into a proximal vein in the leg and the contrast media carried distally by induced retrograde venous flow. Although not ideal and now rarely used, descending venography offers the ability to assess valve competence.

The normal venogram of the lower extremity demonstrates the deep and superficial system, as well as the external and common iliac veins. In some instances, special maneuvers (compression or muscular contraction) may be required to delineate the venous structures fully. The veins are quite variable among different individuals but are usually shown as deep venous trunks that are well defined and easily recognized. The valves are best seen after muscular contraction. The perforators will be defined between the deep venous trunks and the superficial veins. When venous thrombus or clot obstructs or occludes a vein it creates a filling defect on the venogram such that contrast is not seen where expected.

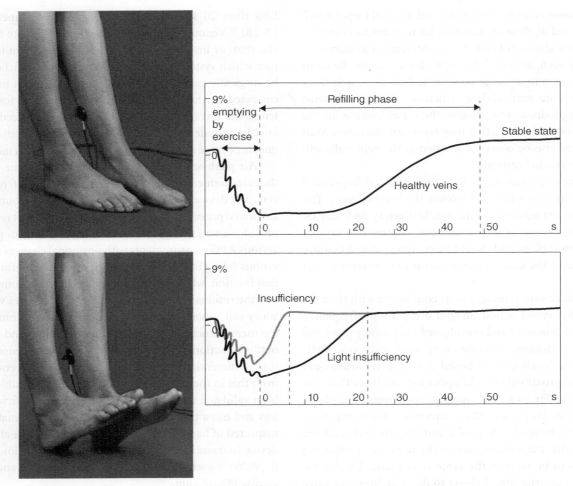

FIGURE 13–28. Images of photoplethysmography (PPG). Left upper photo demonstrate the feet in a resting position and the lower left photo demonstrate the feet in a dorsiflexion position in order to empty the calf. On the top upper right is a normal response to calf exercise. On the bottom right is an abnormal response to venous valvular incompetency.

CHRONIC VENOUS DISEASE

Venous insufficiency can be conveniently divided into primary venous insufficiency (varicose veins, telangiectasias) and chronic venous insufficiency (skin changes, secondary venous dysfunction).[85] About 10–30% of the US population has some variant of venous disease.[86] The American Venous Forum has developed the CEAP classification to help define the different degrees of venous insufficiency by different categories: C (clinical state), E (etiology), A (anatomy), P (pathophysiology).

The major components of pathophysiology in venous insufficiency are obstruction and vascular incompetence. These components may lead to venous hypertension, which is presently thought to be responsible for significant signs and symptoms in this disease class.

Signs and Symptoms

Varicose veins are dilated veins within subcutaneous tissue, which can be divided into primary (normal deep system) and secondary (abnormal deep symptoms). Factors that increase the

risk of developing varicose veins include advancing age, gender (women are more likely to develop the condition), pregnancy (during pregnancy, the volume of blood in your body increases and there is increased production of the hormone progesterone), family history, obesity, stationary standing or sitting for long periods of time, and a history of DVT.

Symptoms that may be associated with varicose veins include heaviness, itching, tiredness, burning, and cramps. Chronic venous insufficiency may be manifested by varicose veins alone or by hyperpigmentation, edema, ulceration, and lipodermatosclerosis (Fig. 13–29).[85]

History and physical examination as above can identify the diagnosis of venous insufficiency but in general cannot identify the presence, location, or extent of vascular incompetency or obstruction. Duplex scanning has become the single most important noninvasive adjunctive tool in answering these questions and, thus, provides the appropriate medical or surgical approach in this clinical setting. This modality is noninvasive, provides anatomic and physiologic information, is reproducible, and can be performed at low cost. Utilizing combinations

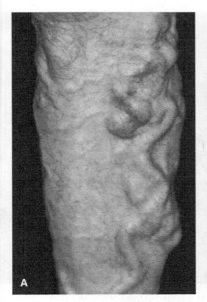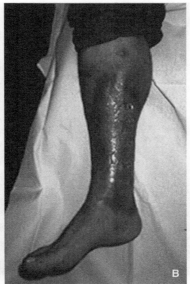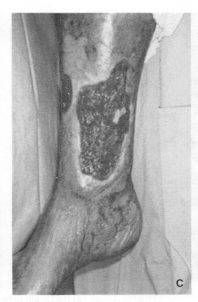

FIGURE 13–29. Images of various manifestations of chronic venous insufficiency. (**A**) large varicose veins. (**B**) Hyperpigmentation. (**C**) Venous ulcerations.

of B-mode (gray-scale) and color Doppler imaging and Doppler spectral waveform analysis vessels can be defined, presence and extent of venous obstruction can be determined, and differentiation of antegrade and retrograde blood flow can be assessed.

Vein Reflux Testing Protocols

With the advent of endovenous options for the treatment of patients with manifestations of CVI, duplex ultrasound has emerged as the gold standard test in this setting. The goal of duplex ultrasonographic imaging in patients with venous insufficiency is to map venous anatomy, identify anatomic variants, and find the sources of venous insufficiency. Duplex ultrasound is the most efficient and accurate tool for evaluation of venous insufficiency, since it is noninvasive, nonionizing, reproducible, and gives dynamic information. Duplex ultrasound is indicated for evaluation of patients with suspected venous insufficiency who are contemplating therapy and for monitoring response after therapy.

The exam may be completed in two parts.[87,88] Equipment requirements include a probe capable of gray-scale imaging at 7.5–10 MHz and pulsed-wave Doppler imaging. The examination of venous incompetence should ideally be performed with the interventionalists performing the interventional procedures, as this facilitates optimal patient and treatment selection. First, a supine protocol can be utilized using a standard DVT protocol. Comprehensive deep venous evaluation must be performed for detection of DVT and reflux. Chronic DVT findings may be subtle and manifest as webs, focal wall thickening, or calcification. Persistent or repeated venous obstructions can contribute to venous hypertension. In the second part of the exam, the proximal great saphenous can be evaluated with Valsalva in reversed Trendelenburg position, but the remainder of the exam should be completed with the patient in the standing position with the weight on the leg that is not being examined to ensure maximum venous distention. The patient will need to be able to support their weight on the opposite leg to participate in maneuvers that elicit reflux.

Slight limb flexion and outward rotation provides optimal visualization of the GSV. The entire length of the GSV is first examined using axial gray-scale technique, noting the maximal vein diameter (normally <4 mm). Any varicose tributaries are then identified and followed distally. Next, the SFJ is assessed for reflux. Color or power Doppler imaging are used in combination with rapid compression and release of distal venous segments to identify sites of reflux. Since color Doppler imaging often underestimates the degree of venous reflux, pulsed-wave Doppler imaging is preferred while performing compression and release.

For assessment of the SSV, the knee is slightly flexed and the muscles of the thigh are relaxed. Using axial gray-scale technique, the SSV is serially examined from the distal calf moving proximally to its termination at the sapheno-popliteal junction (SPJ), although the termination may vary. Again, note the maximal diameter, and assess for venous competence of the SPJ. A thigh extension of the SSV is also assessed for reflux if present. Perforating veins in the thigh and the leg are then examined in transverse and oblique planes to identify the longitudinal axis of perforator. The vessels below the knee can also be evaluated with the patient seated on a high stretcher and the legs dangling (Fig. 13–30).

The normal diameter of the GSV and SSV in upright position is 4 and 3 mm, respectively. Sudden caliber change of the vessels is an important marker of refluxing flow within that segment, as incompetent veins are dilated and tortuous.

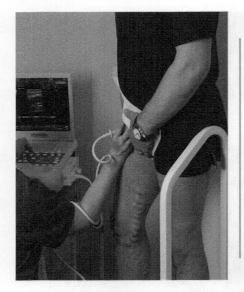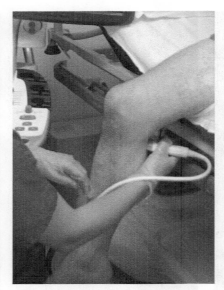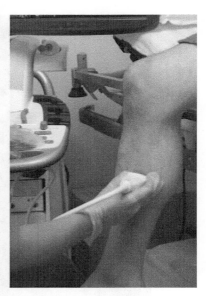

FIGURE 13–30. In the far left panel the patient is standing and the sonographer is seated in front of him allowing for easy access to the superficial veins of interest from the level of the saphena-femoral junction to the ankle. The patient can be turned to evaluate the popliteal, small saphenous, and intersaphenous veins as needed. In the middle and right, the patient is seated for comfort. In this position the technologist can evaluate the vessels below the knee located in the leg medially and posteriorly as well as the vessels near the medial malleolus.

The diameter often changes abruptly at the level of the incompetent valves in the superficial system or at the level of perforating veins communicating with an incompetent deep venous segment. There are several common tributaries in the thigh region that can contribute to GSV reflux, including anterolateral and the posterior-medial tributaries in the thigh region. Pudendal veins can also contribute to GSV reflux in pregnant women.

While reflux can be evaluated using both color and pulsed-wave Doppler, pulsed-wave Doppler is more accurate. A short duration of reflux seen by color Doppler after release of distal compression is likely physiologic and represents a small amount of retrograde flow before complete closure of valves. A competent valve will yield little to no reflux with provocative maneuvers. Reflux is generally defined as greater than 0.5 seconds of flow reversal. This may further be classified into mild, moderate, and severe, according to reflux duration (Fig. 13–31).[89]

There are numerous norms reported in the literature, with some investigators reporting a limit of 1 second for the deep venous system and 0.3 seconds for perforators, and others define 0.5 seconds for perforating veins as well.[101] Hemodynamically significant refluxing perforators are usually located central to incompetent venous channels. Perforating veins with diameters greater than 3.5 mm can also be taken as a sign of significant reflux.

Duplex Ultrasound after Treatment

Duplex ultrasound is essential for monitoring of post-procedural results, complications, and recurrence after endovenous ablation. Early post-procedure duplex ultrasound ensures satisfactory closure of ablated segments and to identify thrombotic complications (Fig. 13–32). Evaluation 1–2 weeks after endovenous ablation of a treated segment will reveal smaller noncompressible veins with wall thickening and/or no flow. After several weeks, the venous wall undergoes fibrosis and become difficult to identify after several months.

Endovenous heat-induced thrombosis (EHIT) refers to deep venous thrombosis after venous ablation. There are four categories, defined largely by the extent of thrombus. EHIT 1 describes thrombus up to but not inside the deep venous junction. EHIT 2 describes thrombosis of the femoral or popliteal vein occluding less than 50% of the cross-sectional diameter. EHIT 3 refers to greater than 50% occlusion of the cross-sectional diameter. EHIT 4 is complete occlusion.[42] A rare complication after thermal ablation is formation of an AVF.[43] AVFs can lead to partial patency of ablated segments with pulsatile flow on duplex ultrasound. AVFs between the proximal SSV and the sural artery or between the superficial external epigastric artery and proximal GSV have been described.

In some patients, it may be necessary to extend the examination proximally or to primarily evaluate the pelvic and visceral vein systems.

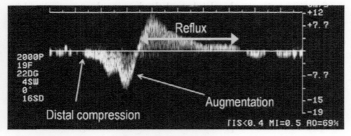

FIGURE 13–31. Doppler image demonstrating venous reflux.

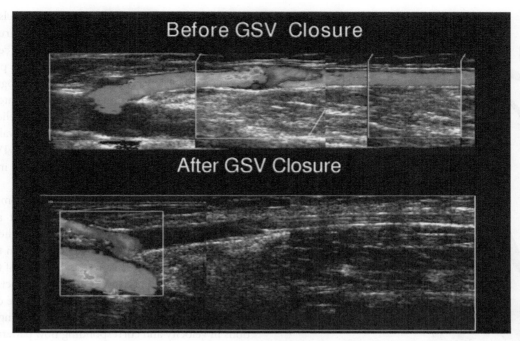

FIGURE 13–32. On the top panel is a duplex ultrasound image that shows preprocedure patency of a refluxing great saphenous vein (GSV). In the lower panel is an image post radiofrequency ablation that reveals an occluded GSV to the level of the superficial epigastric vein but not involving the deep venous system.

Duplex imaging of the ovarian veins permits identification and localization of vein valve incompetence. Imaging of the renal vein and iliac veins permits identification and localization of compression or other abnormalities.

Indications, Signs, and Symptoms

These include pelvic pain, labial varicosities, lower extremity varicose veins, varicocele, unilateral leg swelling (in the absence of DVT), pain during or after intercourse, dull ache, and pressure and/or heaviness in lower abdomen after sitting or standing all day. In males, the typical presentation for left renal vein compression is sharp unpredictable abdominal pain, difficulty with and/or painful urination with episodic hematuria and varicocele, especially on the left.

Patient Peparation

For this examination, it is recommended that the patient should fast overnight to minimize bowel gas; a bowel prep is not usually required. As with any pelvic/abdominal exam, the patient should not chew gum or smoke the morning of the exam as this may increase swallowing of air. The patient needs to drink 24 fluid oz 30 minutes prior to exam to achieve a full bladder for examination.

Patient Communication and Positioning (For This and All Vascular Lab Examinations)

After acknowledging and introducing yourself to the patient, explain the nature of the exam and how long it will take and then answer any questions the patient may have. A patient interview, history, and physical examination is performed to elucidate the patient's symptoms and obtain the patient's medical history

(with special attention regarding parity, ie, how many children they have given birth to) as ovarian vein reflux is more common in women having three or more births. Inquire about surgical history (gynecologic surgeries or prior venous surgeries), current uterine or ovarian problems (ie, fibroids/cysts), current medications (ie, medroxyprogesterone), and the results of other gynecological imaging. A visual inspection of the legs, pelvis, vaginal, and perineal areas for varicosities is important. Elicit any prior history of surgery on veins or arteries.

The exam begins with the patient in a supine position at a significant reverse Trendelenburg tilt. Standard color duplex ultrasound imaging equipment with curved linear transducers with a frequency of 3–5.0 MHz. Using a transabdominal approach, while the patient has a full bladder, image the uterus in long axis identifying the orientation of the uterus (anteverted or retroverted). The uterus/fundal and parauterine veins are then imaged. Document the bilateral adnexal regions for masses. The probe is then oriented transverse to image the fundus of the uterus. Use color-flow Doppler to image dilated fundal veins crossing over the myometrium (if present). Measure the diameter of the fundal veins if possible. Continue to image the uterus in transverse by scanning laterally in the parauterine space between the uterus and ovary. Use color-flow Doppler and measure the parauterine vein diameter on the left and right side. Measure the diameter of the parauterine veins in long axis.

With an empty bladder the IVC and left renal vein can be evaluated. Start with an image of the proximal IVC and demonstrate normal antegrade flow and then image the left renal vein as it courses between the aorta and SMA. Anatomy can vary, and some patients will present with a retroaortic or circumaortic left

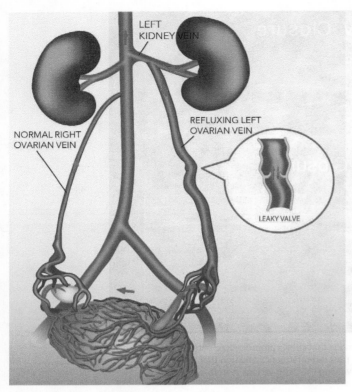

FIGURE 13–33. This is a drawing of the ovarian vein anatomy. Note the right ovarian vein empties into the inferior vena cava directly as opposed to the left which drains into the left renal vein.

renal vein. Document flow velocities and AP diameter measurements in the left renal vein at the level of the superior mesenteric artery and aorta and at sites of compression.

Left Ovarian Vein (Corresponds to the Gonadal Vein in Males) Examination

To identify this vessel, follow the left renal vein toward the kidney. The left ovarian/gonadal vein will be visualized with the probe in transverse and inferior to the left renal vein.

Visualization of the confluence of these vessels can be difficult secondary to depth and other surrounding structures. Measure the inner wall AP diameter of the proximal (central), mid, and distal (peripheral) segments and then assess patency and flow direction. Flow toward the periphery is retrograde and abnormal. If the diameter is 6 mm or greater with antegrade flow, have the patient slowly valsalva in an attempt to elicit flow reversal. The right ovarian/gonadal vein is similarly evaluated. The right ovarian vein in contrast to the left joins the IVC directly. The left ovarian/gonadal vein is more commonly involved than the right (Fig. 13–33).

The iliac veins are then evaluated for compression by surrounding structures, typically the adjacent artery. Potential compression sites can occur at the level of the proximal common iliac veins and external iliac veins (from the internal iliac artery) (Fig. 13–34). Measure the diameter of the iliac veins at both normal segments and at areas of suspected compression. Document flow patterns and velocities at the compression site and peripheral to the compression site looking for focal elevations in velocity and corresponding flow pattern changes.

Diagnostic Criteria

The findings for abnormal examination include the following:

1. Ovarian vein diameter greater than 6 mm with retrograde flow and parauterine veins that measure 4 mm or greater.

2. Left renal vein diameter reduction of 50% or more by the B-mode image or at least two- to threefold increase in velocity at the compression site.

The angle of insonation should be kept at less than 60 degrees, and a 4–7 MHz linear array transducer is commonly used to evaluate the common femoral vein, while 2–3 MHz should be used to evaluate iliac and caval vessels. B-mode will help to compare vein diameter reduction at the smallest lumen area to that of normal vein diameter. Peak vein velocity (PVV)

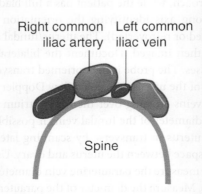

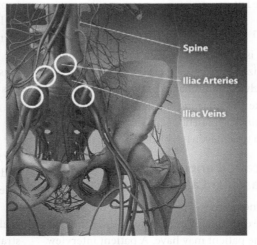

FIGURE 13–34. Common sites for iliac vein obstruction by compression. On the left panel, the left common iliac vein is compressed in the axial plane against the spine by the overlying right common iliac artery. On the right panel, the circles connote common sites of iliac vein compression from the adjacent artery.

is measured in the post-stenotic and compared to the prestenotic segment; a PVV gradient more than 2.0 is considered significant.

There is currently no gold standard diagnostic criterion in iliac vein compression syndrome. Ultrasound parameters to diagnose iliocaval stenosis include post-stenotic turbulence as indicated by the mosaic appearance (noisy signal), an abnormal Doppler signal at the area of stenosis, and sluggish and/or no spontaneous flow as well as very poor augmentation. The contralateral vasculature serves as a control if IVC thrombosis/occlusion is not present.

Historically, the presence of pathologic factors has been the main component in diagnosis; however, imaging techniques have led to a more radiologic-based diagnosis. Clinical presentations along with suggestive findings on venous duplex ultrasound are sufficient to pursue invasive venous imaging in most cases. If there is an anatomical concern that needs to be evaluated, this may best be performed using cross-sectional imaging to augment the ultrasound findings. This is usually accomplished with cross-sectional imaging (eg, CT scan with venous phase, or MR venography) as they are sensitive for estimating the location and degree of stenosis in nonthrombosed veins, identifying venous collaterals, and identifying other anatomic variations.

Catheter-based venography is warranted if there is a sufficient level of clinical suspicion for iliac vein compression in a patient with acute symptoms or if the patient has advanced clinical manifestations of chronic venous disease. Intravascular ultrasound (IVUS) is the current venous imaging standard for establishing a diagnosis of iliac vein compression as well as a valuable adjunct for treatment. When IVUS is used to make a diagnosis, venography is not necessary.

Management of venous insufficiency can be noninvasive or invasive, depending on the underlying condition of the patient. Noninvasive options include leg elevation, compression, and topical treatment.

More Invasive Options[102]

Options for the treatment of superficial venous reflux can be thermal (eg, radiofrequency or laser) and nonthermal (open surgery or liquid, foam, or glue sclerotherapy) ablation techniques, and open surgical ligation and stripping. The indications for vein ablation therapies, including endovenous laser or radiofrequency ablation, sclerotherapy, and open surgical stripping, are symptoms and signs of venous disease that persist despite a trial of medical management, and documented reflux in the target vein (ie, retrograde flow >0.5 seconds). The patient's symptoms should directly relate to the incompetent veins being treated.

Liquid, Foam, and Glue Sclerotherapy Techniques

Sclerotherapy is the most common treatment for leg veins. Sclerotherapy is a minimally invasive percutaneous technique using chemical irritants to close unwanted veins. Sclerotherapy is primarily used in the treatment of telangiectasias, reticular veins, and small varicose veins (<6 mm), which can be symptomatic, or even a source of significant distress to some patients even in the absence of symptoms. Superficial venous insufficiency of the saphenous veins or perforator veins can also be treated with sclerotherapy techniques. The most common sclerotherapy agents used in the treatment of lower extremity chronic venous disease are polidocanol, hypertonic saline, sodium tetradecyl sulfate, and glycerin. Systematic reviews of randomized trials of sclerotherapy for telangiectasias or varicose veins have found no evidence to support the use of one sclerosant over another in the short-term success of sclerotherapy.

Endovenous Ablation Techniques

These are percutaneous, minimally invasive techniques that use laser (EVLA) or radiofrequency (RFA) energy to ablate incompetent superficial veins. The axial veins are the primary target for this therapy and include the GSV, SSV, and accessory saphenous veins (ASVs).

Open Surgical Techniques

Surgical methods of vein ablation have largely been supplanted by less invasive methods but remain the standard to which minimally invasive techniques are compared. Patients with large varicose veins or complications of varicose veins are often best managed with open surgical techniques. Available techniques are chosen based upon the location, size, and extent of the patient's varicosities, and the presence or absence of venous reflux. Common procedures include the following:

- Saphenous vein inversion and removal (vein stripping)
- High saphenous ligation
- Ambulatory phlebectomy
- Transilluminated powered phlebectomy
- Conservative venous ligation (CHIVA)

References

1. Pieri A, Massimo G, Santinim M. Ultrasonographic anatomy of upper extremity veins. *J Vasc Technol.* 2002;26(3):173-180.

2. Ricci S, Georgiev M. Ultrasound anatomy of the superficial veins of the lower limb. *J Vasc Technol.* 2002;26(3):183-199.

3. Pieri A, Gatti M, Santini M, Marcelli F, Carnemolla A. Ultrasonographic anatomy of the deep veins of the lower extremity. *J Vasc Technol.* 2002;26(3):201-211.

4. Hollinshead WH. *Textbook of Anatomy.* 3rd ed. New York: Harper and Row; 1974, 75.

5. Kadir S. *Diagnostic Angiography.* Philadelphia: WB Saunders; 1986, 541.

6. DeWeese JA, Rogoff SM, Tobin CE. *Radiographic Anatomy of Major Veins of the Lower Limb.* Rochester, NY: Eastman Kodak; 1965.

7. Blackburn DR. Venous anatomy. *J Vasc Technol.* 1988;12:78-82.

8. Oliver MA. Anatomy and physiology. In: Talbot SR, Oliver MA, eds. *Techniques of Venous Imaging*. Pasadena, CA: AppletonDavies; 1992, 11-20.

9. Hemodynamics of the normal arterial and venous system. In: *Duplex Scanning in Vascular Disorders*. 3rd ed. Philadelphia, PA: Lippincott, Williams & Wilkins; 2002, 32-60.

10. Strandness DE Jr, Sumner DS. *Hemodynamics for Surgeons*. New York: Grune & Stratton; 1975, 120-160.

11. Deep venous thrombosis and the post thrombotic syndrome. In: *Duplex Scanning in Vascular Disorders*. 3rd ed. Philadelphia, PA: Lippincott, Williams & Wilkins; 2002, 169-190.

12. Urschel HC Jr, Razzuck MA. Paget-Schroetter syndrome: what is the best management? *Ann Thorac Surg*. 2000;69:1663-1668.

13. Vijaysadan V, Zimmerman AM, Pajaro RE. Paget-Schroetter syndrome in the young and Active. *J Am Board Fam Med*. 2005; 18(4):314-319.

14. May R, Thurner J. The cause of the predominantly sinistral occurrence of thrombosis of the pelvic veins. *Angiology*. 1957;8(5):419-427.

15. Fazel R, Froehlich JB, Williams DM, Saint S, Nallamothu BK. Clinical problem-solving. A sinister development—a 35-year-old woman presented to the emergency department with a 2-day history of progressive swelling and pain in her left leg, without antecedent trauma. *N Engl J Med*. 2007;357(1):53-59.

16. Meissner M, Caps M, Bergelin RO, et al. Early outcome after isolated calf vein thrombosis. *J Vasc Surg*. 1997;26:749

17. Oliver MA. Medical management of acute deep vein thrombosis. *J Vasc Technol*. 2002;26:227-229.

18. Buller HR, Agnelli G, Hull RD, et al. Antithrombotic therapy for venous thromboembolic disease: the Seventh ACCP Conference on antithrombotic and thrombolytic therapy. *Chest*. 2004;126:401S-428S.

19. Weitz JW. Orally active direct thrombin inhibitors. *Semin Vasc Med*. 2003;3:131-137.

20. Ridker PM, Goldhaber SZ, Danielson E, et al. Long-term, low intensity warfarin therapy for the prevention of recurrent venous thromboembolism. *N Engl J Med*. 2003;349:631-639.

21. Kearon C, Ginsberg GS, Kovacs MJ, et al. Comparison of low-intensity warfarin therapy with conventional intensity warfarin therapy for long term prevention of recurrent venous thromboembolism. *N Engl J Med*. 2003;349:631-639.

22. Weitz JI. New anticoagulants for treatment of venous thromboembolism. *Circulation*. 2004;110:I19-I26.

23. Thromboembolic Risk Factors (THRIFT) Consensus Group. Risk of and prophylaxis for venous thromboembolism in hospital patients. *BJM*. 1991;305:567-574.

24. Kim SH, Bartholomew JR. Venous thromboembolism. Disease management project. Cleveland, OH: Cleveland Clinic; 2010.

25. Turpie AGG, Chin BSP, Lip GYH. Clinical review. ABC of antithrombotic therapy. Venous thromboembolism: pathophysiology, clinical features, and prevention. *BMJ*. 2002;325:887-890.

26. White RH. The Epidemiology of venous thromboembolism. *Circulation*. 2003;107:1-4.

27. Anderson FA Jr, Wheeler HB, Goldberg RJ, et al. A population-based perspective of the hospital incidence and case-fatality rates of deep vein thrombosis and pulmonary embolism. The Worcester DVT Study. *Arch Intern Med*. 1991;151:933-938.

28. Silverstein MD, Heit JA, Mohr DN, et al. Trends in the incidence of deep vein thrombosis and pulmonary embolism: a 25-year population-based study. *Arch Intern Med*. 1998;158:585-593.

29. Bounameaux H, Hicklin L, Desmarais S. Seasonal variation in deep vein thrombosis. *BMJ*. 1996;312:284-285.

30. Coon WW. Epidemiology of venous thromboembolism. *Ann Surg*. 1977;186:149-164.

31. Gillum RF. Pulmonary embolism and thrombophlebitis in the United States, 1970–1985. *Am Heart J*. 1987;114:1262-1264.

32. Kierkegaard A. Incidence and diagnosis of deep vein thrombosis associated with pregnancy. *Acta Obstet Gynecol Scand*. 1983;62:239-243.

33. Dickson BC. Venous thrombosis: on the history of Virchow's triad. *UTMJ*. 2004;81:166-171.

34. Owen CA. *A History of Blood Coagulation*. Rochester: Mayo Foundation for Medical Education and Research; 2001, 169-180.

35. Rosendaal F. Venous thrombosis: a multicausal disease. *Lancet*. 1999;353(9159):1167-1173.

36. Meissner M, Caps M, Bergelin R, Manzo R, Strandness DE Jr. Early outcome after isolated calf vein thrombosis. *J Vasc Surg*. 1997;26(5):749-756.

37. Hingorani A, Ascher E, Lorenson E, et al. Upper extremity deep venous thrombosis and its impact on morbidity and mortality rates in a hospital-based population. *J Vasc Surg*. 1997 Nov;26(5):853-860.

38. Wells PS, Anderson DR, Bormanis J, et al. Value of assessment of pretest probability of deep-vein thrombosis in clinical management. *Lancet*. 1997;350:1795-1798.

39. Patel AV. Diseases of the venous and lymphatic systems. In: Sales CM, Goldsmith J, Veith FJ, eds. *Handbook of Vascular Surgery*. St. Louis, MO: Quality Medical Publishing, Inc; 1994.

40. Del Conde I, Bharwani LD, Dietzen DJ, Pendurthi U, Thiagarajan P, López JA. Microvesicle-associated tissue factor and Trousseau's syndrome. *J Thromb Haemost*. 2007;5:70-74.

41. Olin JW. Thromboangiitis obliterans (Buerger's disease). *N Engl J Med*. 2000;343:864-849.

42. Saeger W, Genzkow M. Venous thromboses and pulmonary embolisms in post-mortem series: probable causes by correlations of clinical data and basic diseases. *Pathol Res Pract*. 1994;190: 394-399.

43. Kniffin WD Jr, Baron JA, Barrett J, et al. The epidemiology of diagnosed pulmonary embolism and deep venous thrombosis in the elderly. *Arch Intern Med*. 1994;154:861-866.

44. Cushman M, Tsai A, Heckbert SR, et al. Incidence rates, case fatality, and recurrence rates of deep vein thrombosis and pulmonary embolus: the Longitudinal Investigation of Thromboembolism Etiology (LITE). *Thromb Haemost*. 2001;86(suppl 1):OC2349.

45. Hansson PO, Welin L, Tibblin G, et al. Deep vein thrombosis and pulmonary embolism in the general population. "The Study of Men Born in 1913." *Arch Intern Med*. 1997;157:1665-1670.

46. Nordstrom M, Lindblad B, Bergqvist D, et al. A prospective study of the incidence of deep-vein thrombosis within a defined urban population. *J Intern Med*. 1992;232:155-160.

47. White RH, Zhou H, Kim J, et al. A population-based study of the effectiveness of inferior vena cava filter use among patients with venous thromboembolism. *Arch Intern Med*. 2000;160: 2033-2041.

48. White RH, Zhou H, Romano PS. Incidence of idiopathic deep venous thrombosis and secondary thromboembolism among ethnic groups in California. *Ann Intern Med*. 1998;128:737-740.

49. Murin S, Romano PS, White RH. Comparison of outcomes after hospitalization for deep venous thrombosis or pulmonary embolism. *Thromb Haemost*. 2002;88:407-414.

50. Fedullo PF, Tapson VF. Clinical practice. The evaluation of suspected pulmonary embolism. *N Engl J Med*. 2003;349:1247-1256.

51. Carson JL, Kelley MA, Duff A, et al. The clinical course of pulmonary embolism. *N Engl J Med*. 1992;326:1240-1245.

52. Goldhaber SZ. Pulmonary embolism. *N Engl J Med*. 1998;339:93-104.

53. Horlander KT, Mannino DM, Leeper KV. Pulmonary embolism mortality in the United States, 1979–1998: an analysis using multiple-cause mortality data. *Arch Intern Med*. 2003;163:1711-1717.

54. Turkstra F, Kuijer PMM, van Beek EJR, et al. Diagnostic utility of ultrasonography of leg veins in patients suspected of having pulmonary embolism. *Ann Intern Med*. 1997;12:775-781.

55. Wells PS, Anderson DR, Rodger M, et al. Derivation of a simple clinical model to categorize patients probability of pulmonary embolism: increasing the models utility with the SimpliRED D-dimer. *Thromb Haemost*. 2000;83:416-420.

56. Vascular Technology Professional Performance Guidelines. Lower Extremity Venous Duplex Evaluation. Available at: http://www.svtnet.org.

57. Nix L, Troillet R. The use of color in venous duplex examination. *J Vasc Technol*. 1991;15:123-128.

58. Zwiebel W. Technique for extremity venous ultrasound examination. In: *Introduction to Vascular Ultrasonography*. 5th ed. Philadelphia, PA: Elsevier Saunders; 2005.

59. Labropoulos N, Tassiopoulos AK. Vascular diagnosis of venous thrombosis. In: *Vascular Diagnosis*. 1st ed. Philadelphia: Elsevier Inc; 2005.

60. Glover JL, Bendick PJ. Appropriate indications for venous duplex ultrasonographic examinations. *Surgery*. 1996 Oct;120(4):725-730.

61. Polak JP. *Peripheral Vascular Sonography*. 2nd ed. Philadelphia: Lippincott, Williams & Wilkins; 2004, 204-209.

62. Gocke J. Lower extremity venous ultrasonography. In: Mohler ER, Gerard-Herman M, Jaff MR, eds. *Essentials of Vascular Laboratory Diagnosis*. Danvers, MA: Blackwell Futura; 2005, 199.

63. Zweibel WT. Nonvascular pathology encountered during venous sonography. In: Zweibel WT, Pellerito JS, eds. *Introduction of Vascular Technology*. Philadelphia, PA: Elsevier Saunders; 2005, 501-512.

64. Daigle RJ. *Techniques in Noninvasive Vascular Diagnosis*. Littleton, CO: Summer Publishing; 2002, 89-91.

65. Bluth EI. Leg swelling with pain or edema. In: Bluth EI et al, eds. *Ultrasonography in Vascular Diseases*. New York, NY: Thieme; 2001.

66. Labropoulos N, Tassiopoulos AK. Vascular diagnosis of venous thrombosis. In: Mansour MA, Labropoulos N, eds. *Vascular Diagnosis*. Chapter 41. Philadelphia, PA: Elsevier Saunders; 2005, 435-437.

67. Hodge M et al. Incidental finding during venous duplex examination: solitary fibrous tumor or arteriovenous malform in the left lower extremity. *J Vasc Ultrasound*. 2007;31(1):41-44.

68. Mansour MA. Vascular diagnosis of abdominal and peripheral aneurysms. In: Mansour MA, Labropoulos N, eds. *Vascular Diagnosis*. Chapter 35. Philadelphia, PA: Elsevier Saunders; 2005.

69. Kim-Gavino CS, Vade A, Lim-Dunham J. Unusual appearance of a popliteal venous aneurysm in a 16 year old patient. *J Ultrasound Med*. 2006;25:1615-1618.

70. Arger PH, Lyoob SD, eds. *The Complete Guide to Vascular Ultrasound*. Philadelphia, PA: Lippincott, Williams & Wilkins; 2004, 26.

71. Shaw M et al. Case study: cystic adventitial disease of the popliteal artery. *J Vasc Ultrasound*. 2007;31(1):45-48.

72. Gaitini D. Current approaches and controversial issues in the diagnosis of deep vein thrombosis via duplex Doppler ultrasound. *J Clin Ultrasound*. 2006 Jul-Aug;34(6):289-297.

73. van Gemmeren D, Fobbe F, Ruhnke-Trautmann M, et al. Diagnosis of deep leg vein thrombosis with color-coded duplex sonography and sonographic determination of the duration of the thrombosis. *Z Kardiol*. 1991 Aug;80(8):523-528.

74. Gaitini D, Kaftori JK, Pery M, Markel A. Late changes in veins after deep venous thrombosis: ultrasonographic findings. *Rofo*. 1990 Jul;153(1):68-72.

75. Cavezzi A, Labropoulos N, Partsch H, et al.; UIP. Duplex ultrasound investigation of the veins in chronic venous disease of the lower limbs—UIP consensus document. Part II. Anatomy. *Vasa*. 2007 Feb;36(1):62-71.

76. Nack T, Needleman L. Comparison of duplex sonography and contrast venography for evaluation of upper extremity venous disease. *J Vasc Technol*. 1992;16(2):69-73.

77. Falk RL, Smith DF. Thrombosis of upper extremity thoracic inlet veins: diagnosis with duplex Doppler sonography. *Am J Roentgenol*. 1987;149:677-682.

78. Froehlich JB, Zide RS, Persson AV. Diagnosis of upper extremity deep vein thrombosis using a color Doppler imaging system. *J Vasc Technol*. 1991;15(5):251-253.

79. Knudson GJ et al. Color Doppler sonographic imaging in the assessment of upper extremity deep vein thrombosis. *Am J Roentgenol*. 1990;154:399-403.

80. Gerlock AJ, Giyanani VL, Krebs CA. *Applications of Noninvasive Vascular Techniques*. Philadelphia: WB Saunders; 1988.

81. Asbeutah AM, Riha AZ, Cameron JD, McGrath BP. Quantitative assessment of chronic venous insufficiency using duplex ultrasound and air plethysmography. *J Vasc Ultrasound*. 2006;30(1):23-30.

82. Katz MR, Comerota AJ, Kerr R. Air plethysmography (APG®): a new technique to evaluate patients with chronic venous insufficiency. Dept of Surgery, Temple University Hospital, Philadelphia, PA. *J Vasc Technol*. 1991;15(1):23-17.

83. Kim D, Orron DE, Porter DH. Venographic anatomy, technique and interpretation. In: Kim D, Orron DE, eds. *Peripheral Vascular Imaging and Intervention*. St. Louis: Mosby-Year Book; 1996, 269-349.

84. Abrams HI. *Angiography*. 2nd ed. Vol. II. Boston: Little Brown; 1971, 1251-1271.

85. Bergan JJ et al. Chronic venous insufficiency. In: Merli GJ, Weitz HH, Carasasi AC, eds. *Peripheral Vascular Disorders*. Philadelphia, PA: Saunders; 2004, 123-129.

86. Arcelus TI, Caprini TA. Nonoperative treatment of chronic venous insufficiency. *J Vasc Technol*. 2002;26:231-238.

87. Manzo R. Duplex evaluation of chronic disease. In: Strandness DE, ed. *Duplex Scanning in Vascular Diseases.* Philadelphia, PA: Lippincott; 2002.

88. Neumyer MM. Ultrasound diagnosis of venous insufficiency. In: Zwiebel WT, Pellerito JS, eds. *Introduction of Vascular Technology.* Chapter 26. Philadelphia, PA: Elsevier Saunders; 2005.

89. Thrush A, Hartshorne T. *Peripheral Vascular Ultrasound.* London: Churchill Livingstone; 1999.

90. Belcaro G, Nicolaides AN, Veller M. *Venous Disorders.* London: Saunders; 1995.

91. Georgiev M. Regarding "Nomenclature of the veins of the lower limbs: an international interdisciplinary consensus statement. *J Vasc Surg.* 2004;39(5):1144; author reply 1144.

92. Kageyama N, Ro A, Tanifuji T, et al. Significance of the soleal vein and its drainage veins in cases of massive pulmonary thromboembolism. *Ann Vasc Dis.* 2008;1:35-39.

93. Ohgi S, Ohgi N. Relationship between specific distributions of isolated soleal vein thrombosis and risk factors. *Ann Vasc Dis.* 2014;7(3):246-255.

94. Killewich LA, Macko RF, Cox K, et al. Regression of proximal deep venous thrombosis is associated with fibrinolytic enhancement. *J Vasc Surg.* 1997;26(5):861-868.

95. Labropoulos N, Bhatti AF, Amaral S, et al. Neovascularization in acute venous thrombosis. *J Vasc Surg.* 2005;42(3):515-518. PMID: 16171599.

96. Needleman L, Cronan JJ, Lilly MP, et al. Ultrasound for lower extremity deep venous thrombosis. *Circulation.* 2018;137(14): 1505-1515.

97. Bannon MP, Heller SF, Rivera M. Anatomic considerations for central venous cannulation. *Risk Manag Healthc Policy.* 2011;4:27-39.

98. Kornbau C, Lee KC, Hughes GD, Firstenberg MS. Central line complications. *Int J Crit Illn Inj Sci.* 2015;5:170-178.

99. Vascular Access 2006 Work Group. Clinical practice guidelines for vascular access. *Am J Kidney Dis.* 2006;48:176-247.

100. Kusminsky RE. Complications of central venous catheterization. *J Am Coll Surg.* 2007;204:681-696.

101. Labropoulos N, Tiongson J, Pryor L, et al. Definition of venous reflux in lower-extremity veins. *J Vasc Surg.* 2003;38:793-798.

102. Gloviczki P, Comerota AJ, Dalsing MC, et al. The care of patients with varicose veins and associated chronic venous diseases: clinical practice guidelines of the Society for Vascular Surgery and the American Venous Forum. *J Vasc Surg.* 2011;53:2S.

Questions

1. Veins of the legs are provided with valves to
   (A) prevent DVT
   (B) ensure blood flow toward the heart
   (C) prevent pulmonary embolus
   (D) perfuse the distal extremity

2. What is the longest vein in the body?
   (A) cephalic vein
   (B) femoral vein
   (C) GSV
   (D) IVC

3. The popliteal vein passes through what structure to become the femoral vein?
   (A) profunda hiatus
   (B) adductor canal
   (C) Scarpa's triangle
   (D) flexor hallucis longus

4. Which of the following veins is *not* part of the superficial venous system?
   (A) GSV
   (B) femoral vein
   (C) small saphenous vein
   (D) basilic vein

5. Which of the following parameters is *not* typically exhibited by normal veins of the lower extremity above the knee?
   (A) spontaneous flow
   (B) phasic flow
   (C) pulsatile flow
   (D) compressibility

6. What percentage of blood in the body can be found within the venous system?
   (A) 50–60%
   (B) 60–65%
   (C) 70–80%
   (D) 80–90%

7. All of the following are true of veins, *except*
   (A) Veins have thicker walls than arteries.
   (B) Veins are more distensible than arteries.
   (C) Veins are collapsible.
   (D) Veins can be divided into deep and superficial systems.

8. Which of the following complications is the primary clinical concern in DVT?
   (A) claudication
   (B) PE
   (C) valve competency
   (D) loss of extremity

9. Duplex scanning of the deep venous system of the lower extremities is usually performed with the patient in which of the following positions?
   (A) supine position with the leg straight
   (B) supine position with the leg externally rotated
   (C) supine position with the leg internally rotated
   (D) prone position with the leg internally rotated

10. The outermost layer of the vein wall is called the tunica
    (A) media
    (B) intima
    (C) adventitia
    (D) endothelium

11. A spontaneous venous signal may not be heard in which one of the following vessels?
    (A) external iliac vein
    (B) posterior tibial vein
    (C) deep femoral vein
    (D) common femoral vein

12. Which of the following terms best describes a normal venous signal in the lower extremity?
    (A) continuous
    (B) phasic
    (C) pulsatile
    (D) oscillating

13. Extensive iliofemoral thrombosis producing a leg swelling, severe pain, and cyanotic mottled skin is commonly referred to as

    (A) Raynaud's phenomenon

    (B) claudication

    (C) Byrum trace syndrome

    (D) phlegmasia cerulea dolens

14. DVT often destroys the venous valves sometimes resulting in post-phlebitic syndrome, which can lead to all of the following, *except*

    (A) thin vessel walls

    (B) chronic induration

    (C) stasis dermatitis

    (D) ulcers

15. During inspiration, as the intra-abdominal pressure increases

    (A) blood flows smoothly throughout the body

    (B) blood flow from the lower extremities decreases

    (C) blood flow from the lower extremities increases

    (D) there is no significant effect on the venous flow patterns

16. Which of the following *cannot* be used to evaluate chronic venous insufficiency?

    (A) photoplethysmography

    (B) air plethysmography

    (C) duplex ultrasound

    (D) PET scan

17. Which of the following is *not* a component of "Virchow's triad"?

    (A) injury to the vessel wall

    (B) hypercoagulability

    (C) hypercholosterlemia

    (D) stasis

18. Which vessels' distal landmark is the area between the medial malleolus and the Achilles tendon near the skin surface?

    (A) anterior tibial veins

    (B) posterior tibial veins

    (C) small saphenous vein

    (D) GSV

19. Which layer of the vein wall are the venous valves attached to?

    (A) tunica adventitia

    (B) tunica intima

    (C) tunica media

    (D) tunica lateral

20. For IVC filters all the following are true, *except*

    (A) they are suggested for patients with a contraindication for anticoagulation therapy

    (B) can be performed via a femoral vein access

    (C) always meant to be permanently placed

    (D) used for failure of anticoagulation

21. This vessel joins the axillary vein to form the subclavian vein

    (A) costocoracoid vein

    (B) basilic vein

    (C) cubital vein

    (D) cephalic vein

22. The gastrocnemius veins drain the blood from the gastrocnemius muscle and empty into which of the following vessels?

    (A) posterior tibial vein

    (B) anterior tibial veins

    (C) popliteal vein

    (D) peroneal vein

23. The venous pressure normally measures about 15–20 mm Hg in the venules. What does it normally measure in the right atrium?

    (A) 15–20 mm Hg

    (B) 100 mm Hg

    (C) 0–6 mm Hg

    (D) 50 mm Hg

24. Which of the following is *least* likely to compromise blood flow on the basis of compression?

    (A) Baker's cyst

    (B) lymph nodes

    (C) venous reflux

    (D) hematomas

25. **Which of the following is *not* a normal characteristic of veins?**

(A) phasicity

(B) compressibility

(C) augmentation

(D) continuous flow without respiratory variation

26. **There are no valves present in which of the following veins?**

(A) brachicephalic veins

(B) axillary vein

(C) external jugular vein

(D) internal jugular vein

27. **The superficial veins of the lower extremities can be demonstrated sonographically**

(A) within the subcutaneous tissue

(B) within the connective tissue sheath

(C) just below the subcutaneous fat

(D) just above the deep fascia

28. **DVT of the upper extremity has become more frequent because of which of the following?**

(A) Increased number of patients having radiation therapy and complications

(B) Increased incidence of trauma patients with complications

(C) Increased incidence of thoracic outlet syndrome

(D) Increased use of central venous catheters

29. **Which of the following describes the normal route of venous flow in the lower extremity?**

(A) superficial veins to perforator veins to the deep veins

(B) deep veins to the perforator veins to the superficial veins

(C) deep veins to superficial veins to perforator veins

(D) superficial veins to the deep veins to perforator veins

30. **Which of the following veins is a continuation of the dorsalis pedis vein?**

(A) popliteal vein

(B) anterior tibial vein

(C) small saphenous vein

(D) peroneal vein

31. **Which one of the following is most likely to lead to hemodialysis access failure?**

(A) a large outflow vein

(B) perigraft collection

(C) outflow vein stenosis

(D) the "steal syndrome"

32. **What is sclerotherapy?**

(A) surgical removal of the superficial veins

(B) use of support stockings and appropriate exercise

(C) injection of superficial veins with agent to induce thrombosis

(D) injection of deep and superficial veins with agent to induce thrombosis

33. **Which of the following is *not* a cause of chronic venous insufficiency?**

(A) varicose veins

(B) surgery

(C) post-thrombotic syndrome

(D) chronic recurrent thrombosis

34. **Which one of the following is *not* used to augment flow in veins?**

(A) distal compression of the vein

(B) coughing

(C) Valsalva maneuver

(D) compression of the vein with the transducer probe

35. **Venography shows a clot in the venous system as**

(A) an echogenic mass within the vein

(B) a filling defect within the vein

(C) a heterogeneous mass within the vein

(D) a dilated vein with a spongy appearing mass in the lumen

36. **Acute thrombus is soft and may be compressed to a certain extent. Chronic thrombus**

(A) is not compressible to any extent

(B) may be easily compressed to a certain extent

(C) will easily compress completely

(D) with some difficulty (pressure) will compress completely

37. **Chronic venous insufficiency may be characterized by all of the following, *except***

    (A) ischemic rest pain with blue toe syndrome

    (B) varicose veins

    (C) chronic swelling of the leg

    (D) cutaneous hyperpigmentation

38. **Which of the following is *not* believed to be a contributing factor to primary varicose veins?**

    (A) pregnancy

    (B) atherosclerotic changes

    (C) history of DVT

    (D) family history

39. **Contrast venography is**

    (A) a less invasive technique to diagnose venous problems

    (B) the primary modality for evaluating valves function in the lower extremity

    (C) no longer routinely used to evaluate leg veins

    (D) a noninvasive imaging technique

40. **Which vein(s) arise(s) from and drain the plantar venous arch and superficial venous network of the foot?**

    (A) anterior tibial veins

    (B) posterior tibial veins

    (C) GSV

    (D) small saphenous vein

41. **Which vein receives both the superficial and deep venous systems of the upper extremity?**

    (A) innominate vein

    (B) cephalic vein

    (C) brachial vein

    (D) subclavian vein

42. **The communicating veins or "perforators" are located throughout the leg; in most legs, there are**

    (A) more than 50 of these veins

    (B) more than 1000 of these veins

    (C) more than 100 of these veins

    (D) more than 500 of these veins

43. **After an episode of DVT recanalization can begin**

    (A) Only after 3 months

    (B) 1–2 years after the onset of DVT

    (C) days to weeks after the onset of DVT

    (D) only if the patient is treated with bed rest and comporession

44. **Which of the following is *not* among the most significant risk factor for DVT?**

    (A) obesity

    (B) the use of oral contraception

    (C) diabetes

    (D) pregnancy

45. **Deep vein thrombus can originate anywhere in the venous system, but studies have shown the single most common site to be which of the following?**

    (A) soleal sinusoids

    (B) posterior tibial vein

    (C) iliofemoral veins

    (D) SFJ

46. **What type of venography offers the ability of assessing valvular functions?**

    (A) posterior venography

    (B) descending venography

    (C) ascending venography

    (D) visceral venography

47. **In what anatomic region is/are the venous valves found?**

    (A) tunica intima

    (B) tunica media

    (C) tunica adventitia

    (D) both A and C

48. **The left ovarian vein drains into the**

    (A) right ovarian vein

    (B) left internal iliac vein

    (C) IVC

    (D) left renal vein

49. **A valve is competent if**

    (A) It simultaneously opens and closes.

    (B) It allows both forward and reverse venous flow.

    (C) It will not allow little to no reversal of venous blood flow.

    (D) It stays open continuously allowing continuous venous flow.

Questions 50 through 58: Match the structures in Fig. 13–35 with the terms in Column B.

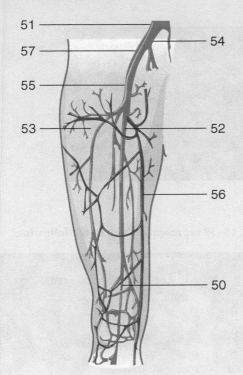

FIGURE 13–35.

COLUMN A

50. _____

51. _____

52. _____

53. _____

54. _____

55. _____

56. _____

57. _____

COLUMN B

(A) popliteal vein

(B) GSV

(C) femoral vein

(D) distal IVC

(E) common iliac vein

(F) deep femoral vein (profunda)

(G) external iliac vein

(H) common femoral vein

Questions 58 through 64: Match the structures in Fig. 13–36 with the terms in Column B.

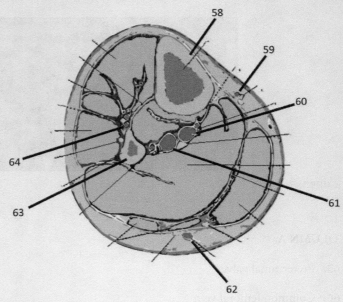

FIGURE 13–36.

COLUMN A

58. _____

59. _____

60. _____

61. _____

62. _____

63. _____

64. _____

COLUMN B

(A) GSV

(B) Posterior tibial vein

(C) Anterior tibial vein

(D) Fibula

(E) Peroneal vein

(F) Small saphenous vein

(G) Tibia

14

Vascular Sonography— Peripheral Arterial

George L. Berdejo, Fernando Amador, and William D. Suggs

Study Guide

PULMONARY CIRCULATION AND SYSTEMIC CIRCULATION

The cardiovascular system has two major pathways: the systemic circulation and pulmonary circulation. Pulmonary circulation moves blood between the heart and lungs. It transports deoxygenated blood to the lungs to absorb oxygen and release carbon dioxide. The oxygenated blood then flows back to the heart. Systemic circulation moves blood between the heart and the rest of the body.

ANATOMY OF THE ARTERIAL SYSTEMIC CIRCULATION

The circulatory system is a closed system of tubes that carry oxygenated blood away from the heart to the tissues of the body and then return deoxygenated blood to the heart. The system consists of arteries (large elastic tubes) dividing into medium size muscular arteries and into smaller arteries that branch into arterioles that branch into microscopic vessels termed capillaries. Vasa vasorum are small vessels that nourish the media and the adventitia. The systemic circulation includes all the arteries and arterioles that carry oxygenated blood from the left ventricle to the systemic capillaries plus the veins and venules that carry deoxygenated blood returning to the right atrium after flowing through the organs and tissue. Subdivisions of the systemic circulation are the coronary, cerebral, and the hepatic portal circulation.[1]

The composition of large- and medium-size arteries includes:

- *Intima (tunica interna)*: The intima is the innermost layer and is a monolayer of flattened endothelial cells and a thin underlying matrix of collagen and elastic fibers.

- *Media (tunica media)*: The media is a thick middle layer of varying amounts of smooth muscle, collagen, and elastic fibers. It has an outer border of external elastic membrane separating it from the adventitia.

- *Adventitia (tunica externa)*: The adventitia is the outermost layer of an artery composed of collagen and elastin, which provides the strength of the arterial wall (Fig. 14–1).[2]

The composition of the arteries provides two important functional properties: elasticity and contractility. The ventricles of the heart contract and eject blood from the heart, and the large arteries expand and accommodate the increased blood flow. The ventricles relax, and the elastic recoil of the arteries forces the blood onward. As the sympathetic stimulation is increased, the smooth muscle of the artery contracts and narrows the vessel lumen, which is termed *vasoconstriction*. Conversely, as the sympathetic stimulation decreases, the smooth muscle relaxes and the vessel dilates, this is termed *vasodilatation*.[2]

All systemic arteries arise from the heart, branch from the aorta, and are termed according to their location. The aorta is divided into the ascending aorta, aortic arch, the descending aorta, thoracic aorta, and abdominal aorta. The lower abdominal aorta bifurcates into the common iliac arteries to supply the pelvis and lower extremities. The arteries of the pelvis include: the common iliac arteries, internal iliac (hypogastric) arteries and external iliac arteries.[3]

THE AORTA

The systemic circulation begins with the left side of the heart.[4–6] As blood passes through the mitral valve during diastole, the left ventricle expands to allow blood to accumulate. During the systolic contraction of the left ventricle, blood will pass through

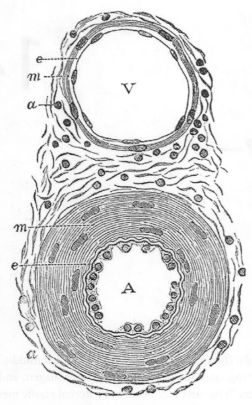

FIGURE 14–1. Transverse section of a small artery (A) and vein (V) of a child. The intima, media, and adventitia are represented by the lowercase letters *e*, *m*, and *a* respectively. *(Reproduced with permission from Wikipedia Commons https://en.wikipedia.org/wiki/Tunica_media)*

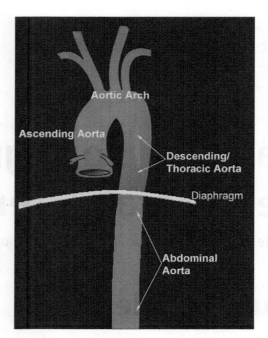

FIGURE 14–2. Cartoon displaying the four segments of the aorta.

The celiac artery and the superior and inferior mesenteric arteries are unpaired, while the renals are paired. The celiac artery is a short trunk, about 1.25 cm in length, which arises from the front of the aorta, just below the aortic hiatus of the diaphragm, and passing nearly horizontally forward, divides into three large branches, the left gastric, common hepatic,

the aortic valve and into the aortic arch. The aorta is the longest artery in the body. The aorta is divided into four main segments (Fig. 14–2):

1. Ascending aorta or aortic trunk
2. Aortic arch
3. Descending or more commonly known as the thoracic aorta
4. Abdominal aorta

The great vessels include the aortic arch and its three major branches that include the following (Fig. 14–3):

1. Innominate artery or brachiocephalic trunk
2. Left common carotid artery (CCA)
3. Left subclavian artery

The abdominal aorta begins at the aortic hiatus of the diaphragm, in front of the lower border of the body of the last thoracic vertebra, and, descending in front of the vertebral column, ends on the body of the fourth lumbar vertebra, commonly a little to the left of the middle line by dividing into the two common iliac arteries. It diminishes rapidly in size, in consequence of the many large branches that it gives off. The major branches of the abdominal aorta are the celiac, superior mesenteric, renal, lumbar, and inferior mesenteric arteries.

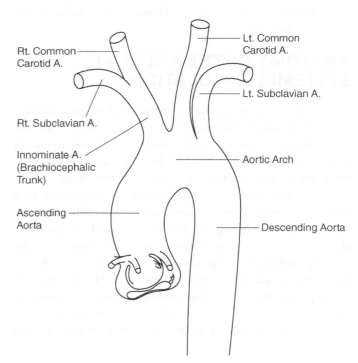

FIGURE 14–3. The aortic arch vessels include the innominate artery, which divides and gives off the right common carotid and right subclavian arteries. The next major vessel is the left common carotid and the last major arch vessel is the left subclavian artery.

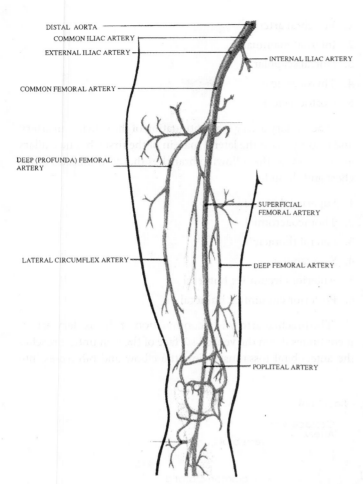

FIGURE 14–4. Anatomy of the arterial circulation from the distal abdominal aorta to the popliteal artery below the knee.

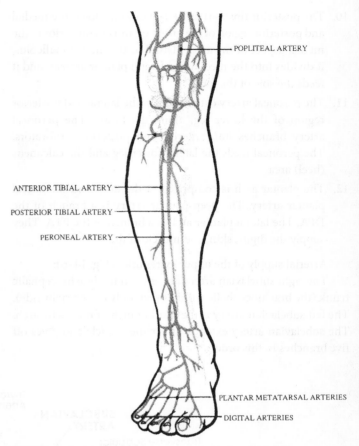

FIGURE 14–5. Anatomy of the major arteries below the knee.

and splenic; it occasionally gives off one of the inferior phrenic arteries. The renals emerge immediately distal to the level of the superior mesenteric artery to perfuse the right and left kidney.

Arterial supply of the pelvis and lower extremities (Figs. 14–4 and 14–5):

1. The abdominal aorta supplies blood to much of the abdominal cavity and ends at the fourth lumbar vertebra (L4) where it bifurcates to form the right and left common iliac arteries. The common iliac arteries divide into the internal and external iliac arteries.

2. The internal iliac arteries supply the pelvic wall, perineum, pelvic organs, and some areas of the gluteal and thigh.

3. The external iliac arteries. The two main branches are the inferior epigastric artery and deep circumflex iliac artery.

4. The common femoral artery (CFA) is a continuation of the external iliac artery. It is the segment of the femoral artery between the inferior margin of the inguinal ligament and the branching point of the deep femoral artery. It divides into the superficial and deep femoral arteries.

5. The deep femoral artery serves as important collateral when there is significant disease in the superficial femoral artery (SFA).

6. The SFA is a continuation of the CFA. It courses the length of the thigh passing through the adductor canal or Hunter's canal at the distal third of the thigh, where it becomes the above the knee popliteal artery (Pop A). The most common location of arterial lesions of the leg is the distal SFA.

7. The Pop A is a continuation of the SFA. The Pop A divides into the anterior tibial artery and tibioperoneal trunk. There are multiple branches around the knee area genicular branches, muscular branches and sural arteries.

8. The anterior tibial artery is a branch of the Pop A and carries blood to the anterior compartment of the leg and dorsal surface of the foot. The artery typically passes anterior to the popliteus muscle prior to passing between the tibia and fibula through an oval opening at the superior aspect of the interosseus membrane. It runs along the along the anterolateral aspect of the leg. The anterior tibial artery becomes the dorsalis pedis artery (DPA) at the foot.

9. The tibioperoneal trunk is the second branch of the distal Pop A. The tibioperoneal trunk branches into the posterior tibial and peroneal arteries.

10. The posterior tibial artery (PTA) extends down the medial and posterior region of the lower leg and lies posterior to the medial aspect of the ankle. Distal to the medial malleolus, it divides into the medial and lateral plantar arteries and it feeds the sole of the foot.

11. The peroneal artery extends down the lateral and posterior region of the lower leg, along the fibula. The peroneal artery branches into anterior and posterior perforators. The peroneal feeds the lateral lower leg and the calcaneus (heel) area.

12. The plantar arch is comprised of the deep and the lateral plantar artery. The deep plantar artery is a branch of the DPA. The lateral plantar arch is a branch of the PTA. They supply the digits, skin, and muscle of the foot.

Arterial supply of the upper extremities (Fig. 14–6):

The right subclavian artery arises from the brachiocephalic trunk (the brachiocephalic trunk is seen only on the right side). The left subclavian artery is the third branch of the aortic arch. The subclavian artery extends under the clavicle and gives off five branches in this order:

1. Vertebral artery
2. Internal mammary
3. Dorsal scapular
4. Thyrocervical
5. Costocervical

The axillary artery is a continuation of the subclavian artery, and its origin is at the lateral margin of the first rib. The axillary artery gives off the following branches that feed muscles of the chest and shoulder.

1. Superior thoracic
2. Thoracoacromial
3. Lateral thoracic
4. Subscapular
5. Anterior circumflex humeral
6. Posterior circumflex humeral

The brachial artery is a continuation of the axillary artery. It continues down the ventral surface of the arm until it reaches the antecubital fossa just below the elbow and bifurcates into

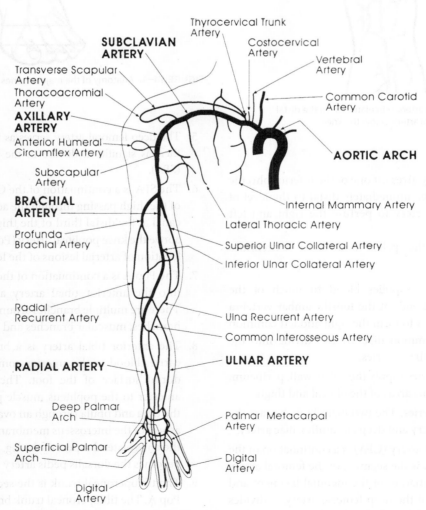

FIGURE 14–6. Arterial anatomy of the upper extremities. Major vessels are in bold print.

the radial and ulnar artery. The ulnar and radial arteries are the main arteries of the forearm.

The radial artery courses along the lateral side of the forearm to the wrist and at the hand it forms the deep palmar arch. The ulnar artery courses along the medial side of the forearm to the wrist and at the hand forms the superficial palmar arch. In the hand the volar and digital arteries supply muscle and skin of the hand and digits.

PHYSIOLOGY AND HEMODYNAMICS

The physiology of circulation is termed *hemodynamics*. Blood flows as a result of the difference in energy or pressure. The arterial system represents the high energy/pressure, and the veins represent the low energy/pressure. Energy/pressure levels decrease from the arterial to venous ends because of the lost energy as a result of blood viscosity and its inertia. There are layers and particles inherent in the vessels that create resistance and cause a loss of energy. The energy is restored by the pumping action of the heart to maintain the arterial energy/pressure difference required for the blood flow. Blood flow through the arterial system is termed *laminar flow* and is defined as blood movement in concentric layers with the highest velocity in the center of the vessel creating a parabolic flow profile[7] (Fig. 14–7). This form of flow is idealized but is nevertheless a fairly good approximation of the flow in medium- and small-sized blood vessels throughout the human circulatory system. Theoretically, the distribution of velocities in a perfectly straight, nonbranching vessel with nonpulsatile flow should be parabolic in cross section, with peak velocities at the center of the lumen. In real vessels, however, the flow profile is usually more blunted because of elasticity and pulsatility effects, even though the general laminar pattern may be maintained. When the flow profile becomes flattened in this form with a nearly uniform distribution of velocities across the lumen, the term *plug flow* (often seen in the aorta) is sometimes applied. This type of flow can be present in both normal and abnormal flow states. Plug flow can be seen in larger vessels such as the aorta or CCA. It is also present at the entrance of a vessel. In an abnormal state such as stenosis, plug flow describes the portion of blood cells that are traveling at the same velocity through the narrowed region.

$$Q = \frac{(P_1 - P_2)\, \pi r^4}{8L\eta}$$

Q = Flow
P_1 = Proximal Pressure
P_2 = Distal Pressure
π = Pi, a constant
r = Radius
L = Length
η = Viscosity

FIGURE 14–8. Poiseuille's equation.

There are several laws that govern blood flow and influence the results of the Doppler evaluation of the arterial system.

Jean Poiseuille was the first to determine the relationship between pressure, viscosity, and flow. His work described steady flow states but can be roughly applied to the pulsatile flow found in the arterial system. *Poiseuille's law* states that in a cylindric tube model, the mean linear velocity of laminar flow is directly proportional to the energy difference between the ends of the tube and the square of the radius. It is inversely proportional to the length of the tube and viscosity of the fluid. Volume flow is proportional to the fourth power of the vessel radius[7,8] (Fig.14–8). Small changes in the radius result in large changes in flow. Poiseuille's law is written as follows:

$$\Delta P = Q8L\eta/\pi r^4 \text{ or } \Delta P = V8L\eta/r^2$$

ΔP is the pressure difference, Q is the volume flow, L is the length of the tube (or vessel), η is viscosity, and r is the radius of the tube (or vessel). In the second equation, V stands for average flow velocity. When narrowing in a blood vessel causes a measurable pressure drop, it is considered hemodynamically significant. It can be seen from this equation that a pressure drop will occur with a decrease in the size of the tube (or vessel). Pressure drops across a given hemodynamically significant stenosis will increase with increasing flow and velocity and a corresponding drop in flow volume.

The factors affecting the development of turbulence are expressed by the Reynolds number (Fig. 14–9) that is included

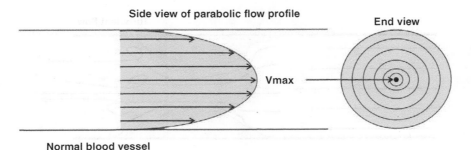

Side view of parabolic flow profile

End view

Vmax

Normal blood vessel

FIGURE 14–7. Laminar flow, sometimes known as streamline flow, occurs when a fluid flows in parallel layers, with no disruption between the layers. Note the fastest moving flow is in the center of the vessel resulting in a parabolic flow profile.

$$Re = \frac{v \times r}{\frac{n}{p}}$$

Re = Reynolds Number
v = Velocity of Blood (cm/sec)
r = Radius (cm)
n = Viscosity (poises)
p = Density

FIGURE 14–9. The equation for Reynolds number.

in the basic principles of fluid dynamics. The development of turbulence depends mainly on the size of the vessel and the velocity of flow. Laminar flow is stable, and the streamline tends to remain intact, whereas turbulent flow has broken discontinuous streamlines that produce eddy currents (circular, backward movements of the fluid) and vortices (radial rotation of the fluid within a body of fluid) (Fig. 14–10). The stability of a fluid can be reasonably predicted by the Reynolds number. Laminar flow tends to be disturbed if the Reynolds number exceeds 2000.[7,8]

Bernoulli's equation plays a central role in the quantitative applications of Doppler. The equation makes the assumption that the total energy along a streamline is constant. The energy simply changes from one form to another as the conditions of the streamline changes.

Bernoulli's equation states that the moving fluid shifts energy from one form to another, depending on the conditions. The total energy remains constant. If the flow is vertical, the hydrostatic pressure makes contribution.[8,9]

Bernoulli's Principle

$$P_1 + \rho gh_1 + 1/2\rho v_1^2 = P_2 + \rho gh_2 + 1/2\rho v_2^2 + heat$$

where   P = pressure
ρgh = hydrostatic pressure
1/2pv² = kinetic energy

The sum of velocity and kinetic energy of a fluid flowing through a tube is constant.

The volume of blood flow through tissue in a given period of time (milliliters per minute) is termed the *blood flow*. The velocity of blood flow (centimeters per second) is inversely related to the cross-sectional area of the blood vessel such that:

$$V = Q/A$$

where V is velocity, Q is flow, and A is the area of the vessel. Therefore, the blood flows slowest where the cross-sectional area is greatest. Blood pressure (BP) is the pressure exerted by blood on the wall of a blood vessel. BP is created by the contraction of the ventricles. In the aorta of a resting young adult, BP rises to approximately 120 mm Hg during systole (contraction) and drops to approximately 70–80 mm Hg during diastole (relaxation). If the carbon monoxide rises, the BP rises. If the total volume of blood in the system decreases, the BP decreases. As blood flows into small arteries, the resistance increases, and the pressure within the arteries begins to fall. The expansion and contraction of arteries after each systole of the left ventricle creates a pressure wave termed the pulse, which is transmitted down the aorta into the peripheral arteries. Normally, the pulse rate is the same as the heart rate. Resting pulse is between 70 and 80 beats/min. *Tachycardia* is the term for a rapid resting heart or pulse rate (over 100/min), and *brachycardia* is the term for a slow resting heart or pulse rate (under 60/min). If pulses are missed, it is irregular.[9] BP is usually measured in the left brachial artery using a sphygmomanometer.

In cases of arterial stenosis, specific characteristics are seen. Flow is generally disturbed in and around the stenosis. Proximal to the stenosis, blood forms a velocity gradient across the vessel lumen as it moves. The flow velocity increases upon entering the stenosis because of the decreased cross-sectional area. Blood flow and pressures are not significantly affected until at least 50% diameter reduction is seen. (equivalent of a 75% reduction in the cross-sectional area). At the orifice of the stenosis, there is usually flow separation that produces a stagnant region around the narrowing. In the narrowest point within the stenosis, the maximum high-velocity jet flows into the larger opening beyond the stenosis and creates flow reversals, eddy currents, and vortices. Inside the stenosis, the flow may be increased but the flow profile may remain stable (laminar). It maintains its streamlines and organization. Moving distally to the larger opening, there is an unstable flow pattern (poststenotic turbulence). This turbulent

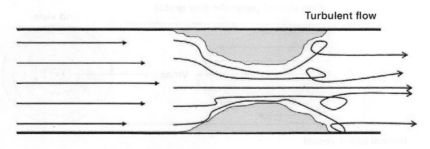

Turbulent flow

Abnormal blood vessel

FIGURE 14–10. The hemodynamics of stenosis. Exit effects beyond the stenosis result in swirling and eddying of the blood flow (turbulence).

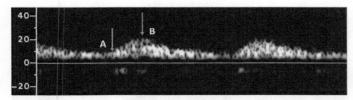

FIGURE 14–11. Tardus parvus figure. The tardus parvus waveform is a sonographic sign frequently observed in spectral Doppler of arteries distal to a stenosis or reconstituted arteries distal to an occlusion. Note the delay in rise time from the onset of systole (**A**) to the peak of systole (**B**).

flow is a chaotic form of fluid transport in which velocity components randomly fluctuate. Turbulence takes place when blood velocities exceed a critical threshold or when vascular morphology creates conditions that disrupt the laminar flow state. In the vascular system, it is not uncommon to see disturbed (nonlaminar) flow in the aorta and in the region of bifurcations. Turbulence is seen distal to areas of stenosis, although in very high grade stenosis (>90–99% diameter reducing), turbulence may not be present. In these cases, a tardus parvus (*late and weak*) pattern of flow may be seen (Fig. 14–11). This phenomenon can be seen distal to site of severe stenosis or occlusion and is due to reduced magnitude of blood flow through the narrowed vessel. Tardus refers to the late-arriving systolic peak (increased acceleration time [AT]), and parvus the decreased peak velocity. As the flow continues down the vessel, the energy present in the flow turbulence dissipates and stability returns to the flowing blood. It is important to profile all stenoses by scanning from the normal vessel through the stenosis to identify the highest velocity within the jet and past the stenosis to document the poststenotic turbulence that should be present in all stenotic lesions.

Mechanisms of Disease

Risk Factors.[10,11] There are several risk factors that contribute to the development of atherosclerosis, some which can be controlled, and some that cannot. Risk factors include:

- Documented atheroma in any artery
- Diabetes
- Dyslipidemia (cholesterol and triglyceride level disturbances)
- Higher fibrinogen blood concentrations
- Homocysteine in the upper half of the normal range, and especially elevated levels
- Aging and male gender (women have more problems after menopause, but hormone replacement therapy worsens rather than improves the risk)
- Tobacco smoking, even just once a day. This is probably the most important risk factor for peripheral vascular disease (PVD). Smoking accelerates the atherosclerotic process and causes vasospasm.
- First-degree relatives with heart disease or a stroke at a relatively young age
- High BP
- Obesity (especially central obesity, ie, fat at waist level, especially intra-abdominal (around the intestines)
- Being physically less active, especially aerobic exercise
- Several internal chemical markers indicating ongoing inflammation may also relate to relative risk

These risk factors, judging from clinical trials, operate synergistically to promote earlier and more severe disease yet still miss many who become disabled from the consequences of atherosclerosis.

Most humans develop atherosclerosis. Usually only "high-risk" patients are advised to change dietary choices, exercise, lose weight, take cholesterol-lowering mediation, and lower blood sugar levels.

Atherosclerosis

Most arterial disease is due to atherosclerosis. Atherosclerosis is a chronic systemic disease that affects the arterial system and occurs within the arterial wall, typically within or beneath the intima. There are various characteristics of the disease, among them location. Atherosclerosis is commonly seen at origins and bifurcations of vessels. Since flow divides and changes its laminar characteristics, a shearing force is created at the flow divider, and over time, this is responsible for the wear of the intima.[12]

It is a chronic inflammatory response in the walls of arteries, in large part due to the accumulation of macrophage white blood cells and promoted by low-density (LDL; especially small particle) lipoproteins (plasma proteins that carry cholesterol and triglycerides) without adequate removal of fats and cholesterol from the macrophages by functional high-density lipoproteins (HDL). It is commonly referred to as a "hardening" of the arteries.

Plaque formation may begin as simple layers of lipids called fatty streaks that are deposited in the wall. Over time plaques on the walls may progress to a more fibrous component that includes the accumulation of lipids, collagen, and fibrin that is soft and gelatinous in texture appearing as a hypoechoic structure along the arterial wall. Over time the plaque may proliferate further into the lumen causing narrowing, also known as stenosis. The walls may harden secondary to a more calcium and collagen component. Unstable plaques or plaques that have areas that are weak, compared to more firm or well integrated plaque within the wall, potentially can be a source of embolic debris.[12]

It is caused by the formation of multiple plaques within the arteries.[11,12] The atheromatous plaque is divided into three distinct components:

1. The atheroma that is the nodular accumulation of a soft, flaky, yellowish material at the center of large plaques, composed of macrophages nearest the lumen of the artery
2. Underlying areas of cholesterol crystals
3. Calcification at the outer base of older/more advanced lesions.

Atherosclerosis typically begins in early adolescence and is usually found in most major arteries, yet is asymptomatic and not detected by most diagnostic methods during life. Autopsies of healthy young men that died during the Korean and Vietnam Wars showed evidence of the disease.[13,14] It most commonly becomes seriously symptomatic when interfering with the coronary circulation supplying the heart or cerebral circulation supplying the brain, and is considered the most important underlying cause of strokes, heart attacks, various heart diseases including congestive heart failure (CHF), and most cardiovascular diseases, in general. Atheroma in arm, or, more often, leg arteries that results in decreased blood flow, is called peripheral artery occlusive disease (PAOD). Advanced disease states can lead to severe ischemia from significantly decreased blood flow to an extremity with resultant damage to or dysfunction of tissue.

According to US data for 2004, for about 65% of men and 47% of women, the first symptom of atherosclerotic cardiovascular disease is heart attack or sudden cardiac death (death within 1 hour of onset of the symptom). Most artery flow disrupting events occur at locations with less than 50% residual lumen.

Embolism is defined as an obstruction in a vessel from a foreign substance (blood clot). Most arterial embolisms are of cardiac origin and often seen in patients with atrial fibrillation, after a myocardial infarction, ventricular aneurysm, bacterial endocarditis, mechanical heart valves, atrial myxoma, and paradoxical emboli. Other sources of embolism are aneurysms or atherosclerotic plaques. Common locations of cardio-emboli are the aortic bifurcation, iliacs, femoral bifurcation, and Pop A.

Aneurysms are a permanent localized dilation of an artery with an increase in diameter of at least 50% compared to an adjacent segment. The dilation involves all three layers of the artery. Common places to find aneurysm are the infrarenal aorta and femoral and popliteal arteries. A fusiform aneurysm is a circumferential dilation of an artery. A saccular aneurysm is outer bulge of a discrete part of the artery.

Abdominal aortic aneurysms (AAA) are primarily found in the infrarenal aorta. If the diameter of the aorta is >3 cm or twice the size of the adjacent segment, it can be considered aneurysmal (Fig. 14–12). The risk factors for developing an aortic aneurysm are age (>65 years), gender (male > female), hypertension, family history, smokers, and the presence of chronic obstructive pulmonary disease. The larger the aneurysm, the greater the risk of rupture. AAAs >5 cm in diameter have a 25% rupture rate in 5 years. In addition to rupture, other complications of AAA are occlusion, embolization that may cause blue-toe syndrome, compression of adjacent periabdominal structures, infection, and aortocaval fistula.[15]

Iatrogenic pseudoaneurysm and arteriovenous fistula (AVF) are commonly seen in the groin as complications postcardiac catheterization. A pseudoaneurysm (also known as false aneurysm) is a collection of blood contained by surrounding tissue that communicates with an adjacent artery via an extravascular neck or

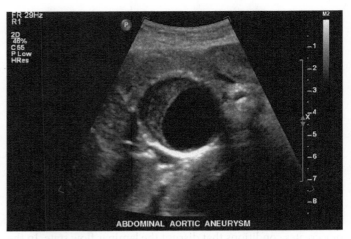

FIGURE 14–12. Transverse ultrasound image of an abdominal aortic aneurysm with laminated thrombus seen on the lateral wall to the left (patient's right).

tract (iatrogenic). It is often the result of injury to the artery, either traumatic or iatrogenic (Fig. 14–13). Pseudoaneurysms can also occur in other arteries throughout the body as a result of infection, rupture of an aneurysm, surgery, or trauma. An AVF is a communication between an artery and an adjacent vein.

The most common place to see a pseudoaneurysm is in the groin. Pseudoaneurysms are simply diagnosed and treated using ultrasound techniques. Pseudoaneurysms generally appear as round sacs in close proximity to, and often with, a connecting "neck" from an adjacent donor vessel. The internal appearance of the sac can be variable, depending on the amount and age of thrombus present within the sac. Partial rupture of the pseudoaneurysm may lead to a complex (multilobed) configuration, with multiple interconnected sacs. Ultrasound with Doppler plays a crucial role in the diagnosis of these iatrogenic injuries and is the quickest and best modality for assessment of suspected peripheral pseudoaneurysms.

Spectral Doppler documentation of a to-and-fro flow pattern within the communicating neck is essential to making the diagnosis (this depends on the diameter and length of the neck). The "to" represents the blood entering the pseudoaneurysm sac during systole, while the "fro" represents blood flowing away from the pseudoaneurysm sac during diastole. The high-velocity flow within the neck may also create an adjacent soft tissue color bruit characterized by perivascular speckling of color Doppler signals. A characteristic "yin-yang" sign may be seen on color flow within the cavity of the pseudoaneurysm (this is due to the swirling pattern of blood flow within the pseudoaneurysm sac) (Figs. 14–14A–C) Rarely, an AVF may occur in association with a pseudoaneurysm. Usually, the pseudoaneurysm is initially created at the arterial puncture, and then a second channel is created by the needle passing through the pseudoaneurysm and the adjacent vein, resulting in an AVF.

Historically, duplex-guided manual compression had routinely been used to correct these lesions; however, in

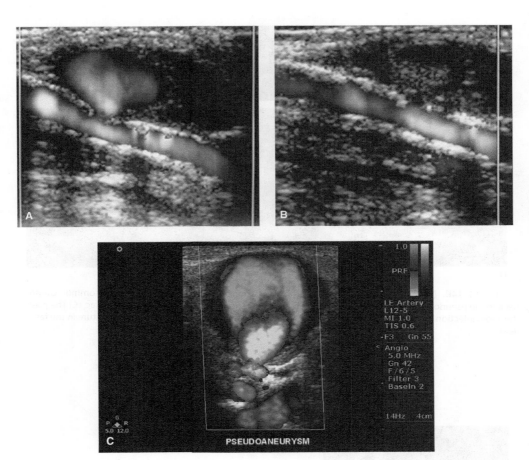

FIGURE 14–13. (**A**) A brachial artery pseudoaneurysm (PSA). Although there is flow within the sac, thrombus, seen to the right of the image, has started to form within the sac. (**B**) A postcompression scan. The PSA sac is now completely filled with thrombus after 10 minutes of duplex-guided manual compression. (**C**) A femoral artery PSA with very little thrombus formation.

recent years, ultrasound-guided thrombin injection has been employed.[16] Depending on the anatomy of the AVF, these may also be treated using duplex guided manual compression.[17]

A mycotic aneurysm is caused by an infectious process that involves the arterial wall. They often occur in multiple sites and are usually seen as a complication of bacterial endocarditis. In children, ultrasound or magnetic resonance imaging (MRI) may be used to identify and monitor treatment of the aneurysm because of the noninvasive nature and lack of radiation. The mycotic aneurysm exhibits the same ultrasound characteristics as the aneurysm.

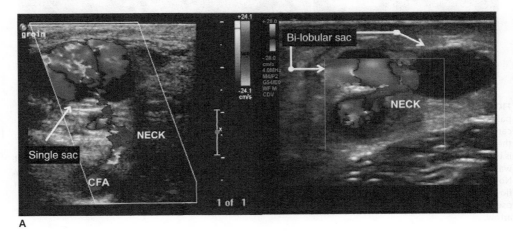

FIGURE 14–14A. Pseudoaneurysms (PA) generally appear as round sacs in close proximity to, and often with a visible connecting "neck", from an adjacent donor vessel. In image on left is a single lobe pseudoaneurysm with a relatively long neck. On the right, is a bilobe brachial artery pseudoaneurysm. Note in the image on the right, the lobe on the right is nearly completely thrombosed. Both images show the classic "yin-yang sign within the cavity of the pseudoaneurysm sac.

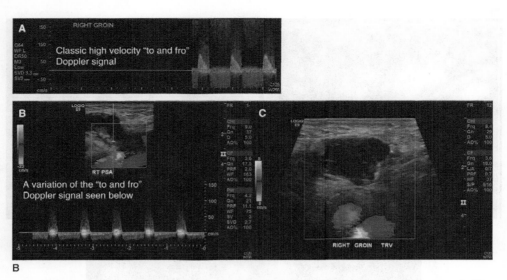

FIGURE 14–14B. (**A**) An example of a signature "to and fro" Doppler signal obtained from the communicating neck to the pseudoaneurysm sac. (**B**) A variation of the to-and-from signal and flow within the sac. (**C**) The post-thrombin injection image that shows complete thrombosis of the sac with the adjacent vasculature in the far field.

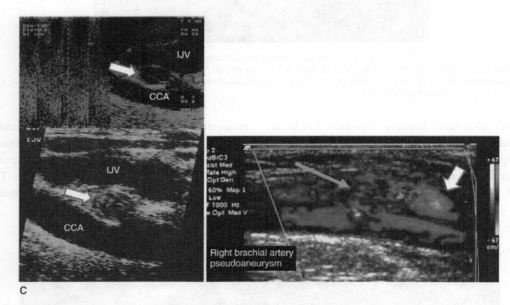

FIGURE 14–14C. In the upper and lower images on the left is a patient who presented with a loud bruit and palpable thrill over the right neck after attempted cannulation of the internal jugular vein that resulted in a carotid artery to internal jugular vein fistula with an intervening pseudoaneurysm. In this case, the flow within the neck is not to and fro but is very high velocity and low resistance (seen in the upper left image) as the flow is entering the low resistance venous system. This patient underwent duplex-guided manual compression. Clot was formed in the pseudoaneurysm sac (connoted by the white arrows) and the AVF was excluded successfully. Note the thrombus in the PA sac post compression. On the right is a color flow image that demonstrates a color flow bruit caused by vibration of tissue from the high-velocity jet within the neck to the relatively superficial pseudoaneurysm sac (in this image obscured by the color flow bruit). The PA sac is connoted by the white arrow.

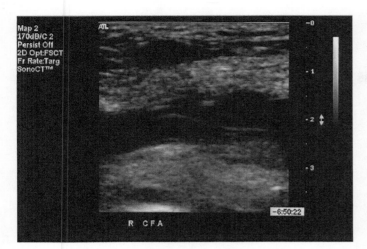

FIGURE 14–15. Ultrasound image of a common femoral artery with dissection (linear echo) that extends proximally (to the left of the image) into the external iliac artery.

Dissection is a nonatherosclerotic condition that is usually a result of trauma that causes a sudden tear in the intimal lining of the vessel (Fig. 14–15). The intima then separates from the media and adventitia. This separation creates a "false" lumen wherein blood may pulsate. Since there is no place for pulsatile flow in the false lumen, it may extend proximally or distally or may thrombose. The thrombosis may cause hemodynamic changes in the true lumen and cause neurologic symptoms when the dissection involves the carotid arteries.[15]

Nonatherosclerotic Lesions[18]

Arteritis is a disease that is characterized by inflammation of the blood vessels. This inflammatory response may lead to occlusion or narrowing of arterial lumen.

Takayasu's arteritis is a type of vasculitis or arteritis that affects large vessels as well as the aorta and its main branches (brachiocephalic, common carotid, and subclavian arteries). It is most common in young Asian women. Cardiovascular symptoms may include hypertension, diminished peripheral pulses, and aortic regurgitation.

Bechet's syndrome is a multisystem vasculitis that affects the arteries and veins. It presents with ulcer of the genital and mouth and other skin lesions. Recurrent superficial and deep vein thrombosis is common and may include cerebral venous thrombosis.

Polyarterisis nodosa is a vasculitis that involves the medium and small muscular arteries. It may lead to aneurysmal formation, renal dysfunction, CHF, and new onset of hypertension.

Kawasaki's disease is a vasculitis that may affect large, medium, and small arteries, but it is more frequent in the coronary arteries. It predominately affects boys. It presents with an unexplained fever, rash, erythema of the palms/soles, and oral mucous changes (strawberry tongue and fissure lips).

Thromboangiitis obliterans (Buerger's disease) is a segmental inflammatory disease that affects the small- and medium-sized arteries, veins, and nerve in the upper and lower extremities. It is a highly cellular inflammatory thrombus within the blood vessel, but it spares the vessel walls. It primarily occurs in young male (<40 years) heavy smokers. It begins with ischemia of the distal arteries and veins of the extremities. The patient may present with rest pain, ischemic ulcers, and or thrombophlebitis.

Raynaud's disease and Raynaud's syndrome. Raynaud's disease is characterized by episodic vasospasm on exposure to cold or with emotional stress. The classic presentation is blanching of the digits (white), the pallor is replaced by cyanosis (blue) due to an ischemic response, and finally the digits turn red during hyperemic phase although these changes may not necessarily occur in series (Fig. 14–16). For most people, it is not a serious health problem, but for some, the reduced blood flow can cause damage.

Raynaud's is classified as primary (not associated with any other disease) and secondary (associated with underlying disease, connective tissue disorder, arterial occlusive disease, trauma, neurologic disorders, drugs, and toxins). The most common site of occurrence is the fingers. Other sites are the toes, nose, and ears. The risk factors associated with the disorder are female sex, family history, and exposure to cold weather. The patient with primary Raynaud's (Raynaud's disease) presents with symptoms bilaterally (symmetric attacks) involving both hands precipitated by exposure to cold or emotional stress, normal digit pressures. Secondary Raynaud's (Raynaud's syndrome or phenomenon) presents with abnormal digit pressure, asymmetric in patients with embolization and trauma, and bilateral or symmetric symptoms in patients with systemic disorder.

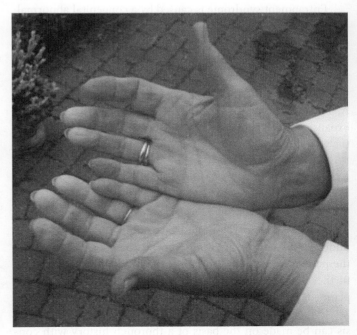

FIGURE 14–16. The hands of a patient with Raynaud's phenomenon. Note the different color changes in this patient demonstrating the various stages of the color change.

Thoracic outlet syndrome (TOS) refers to symptoms that are produced by obstruction/compression of the vascular or neurologic bundle serving the arm as it passes from the thoracocervical region to the axilla. The subclavian vessels and the lower trunk of the brachial plexus pass through three triangular channels, which make up the thoracic outlet. Neurogenic is the most common, and venous and arterial are most rare. Neck and upper extremity trauma is the most common factor in neurogenic TOS. Other cases are associated with congenital and acquired anatomic variations. Most of the patients are female and present with pain, paresthesias and weakness typically involving the hand. Compression of the subclavian vein at the thoracic outlet may occur and cause effort thrombosis (Paget-Schroetter syndrome) of the subclavian vein. The diagnosis of TOS can be challenging. Despite common presentations with pain in the neck and upper extremity, there are a host of presenting patterns that can vary within and between the subdivisions of neurogenic, venous, and arterial TOS. Depending on the subdivision of TOS suspected, diagnostic investigations are currently of varying importance, necessitating high dependence on good history taking and clinical examination. Adson's sign is the loss of the radial pulse in the arm by rotating the head to the ipsilateral side with the neck extended following deep inspiration (Adson's maneuver). It is sometimes used as a sign of TOS. Adson's sign is no longer used as a positive diagnosis of TOS since many people without TOS will show a positive Adson's and there is minimal evidence of interexaminer reliability. The mainstays of tests in arterial TOS are duplex ultrasound, arteriography, hemodynamic testing (eg, finger plethysmography) at rest, and, with provocative maneuvers, CT angiography and MR angiography.

Entrapment syndrome is caused by a congenital abnormality between the Pop A and the medial head of the gastrocnemius muscle. It is most commonly consider in young athletic male patients who present with calf pain when exercising. The symptoms are usually unilateral.

Cystic adventitial disease most commonly affects the Pop A. The cyst arises from the media or subadventitial layer with expansion into the adventitia causing stenosis or occlusion of the vessel. It is most common in young male (40 years).

HISTORY AND PHYSICAL EXAMINATION[15,18]

The value of a history and physical examination should not be underestimated in establishing a correct diagnosis. This part of the patient evaluation also builds the foundation upon which further diagnostic tests and therapeutic interventions may be planned.

In the vast majority of cases, an accurate anatomic diagnosis can be made on the basis of a thorough history with confirmation by a directed physical examination. The availability and wide array of sophisticated diagnostic tests available at the present time may facilitate the tendency for all practitioners to rely on the results of these tests and not on the physical examination. It is important for all practitioners to maintain their history taking and physical examination skills, and it is only through the frequent performance of these tasks that this can be achieved. Although much of the following discussion does not fall under the purview of the sonographer/vascular technologist, the more knowledgeable and skilled one is in patient assessment, the more likely he or she is to obtain meaningful test results. Finally, an accurate history and physical exam serve as a "control" for all vascular diagnostic ultrasound or physiologic tests that are by nature, operator dependent.

History

The first priority in the evaluation of the patient is to adequately assess the patient's chief complaint and history of present illness, that is, the reason the patient is seeking medical attention and all the events relating to this complaint. When acquiring a patient history, the examiner must pay close attention to patient demographics such as age (atherosclerosis often present after age 40) and sex (some diseases are more common in males than females).

Patients may present complaining of pain, numbness or weakness, swelling, discoloration, ulceration, or other symptoms. Whatever the chief complaint, all the aspects and characteristics of the presenting complaint should be elucidated. This includes location and radiation, that is, where the symptom occurs and whether it radiates to another part of the body. The quality and quantity (severity) of the symptom must be assessed; that is, it is it burning, dull, sharp, aching, etc. The temporal pattern is critical, that is, when did the symptoms first begin, how long have they been present for, are they constant or intermittent, is it experienced frequently or infrequently, are the symptoms improving, worsening, or remaining static. Mitigating factors that relieve or aggravate the symptom should be evaluated. Finally, symptoms in the abstract are not the critical issue, but rather, the impact on the patient's lifestyle must be evaluated. For example, for some patients two to three block claudication might be only a minor nuisance while for others it might be severely disabling.

A complete history also must include the patient's past medical history, past surgical history, medications, and allergies. Specific inquiries relating to risk factors for vascular disease should be made. These include the presence of diabetes, hypertension, elevated cholesterol, cigarette smoking, and markers of atherosclerotic problems such as myocardial infarction, previously documented coronary artery disease, angina, chest pain, transient ischemic attacks, and/or stroke. Any history of deep vein thrombosis or phlebitis should be obtained as well as a history of clotting problems and blood transfusions. The presence of renal dysfunction should be evaluated since many patients may ultimately come to angiography and also since patients who are on dialysis generally having extensive vascular calcification. Surgical history is also of importance with special attention to previous vascular and/or cardiac procedures. This will obviously impact the availability of vein for use as a conduit as well as provide the basis for the surgical or interventional treatment planning. Medications are, of course, of importance as these may contribute to or mask certain symptoms. A social history including the patient's living arrangements, occupation, and support systems may also be of critical importance especially if aggressive treatment is warranted to treat the symptoms. A brief family history may be relevant especially relating to a history of coagulopathy or excessive bleeding.

Signs and Symptoms. Pain is the most common chief complaint regardless of whether the occlusive disease is acute or chronic. Pain may present as either intermittent claudication or pain at rest.

Acute arterial occlusion is a sudden and complete blockage of a main arterial supply to the extremity. The most common etiology of an acute occlusion may be embolic or thrombotic (bypass graft or native artery). Most emboli originate in the heart (atrial fibrillation, recent myocardial infarct). Thrombosis of a diseased artery or a bypass graft is common. Another cause for acute occlusion is vascular trauma. The initial presentation is characterized by the presence of the six Ps (Table 14–1). Patients with embolic events tend to have a history of cardiac disease with no significant underlying peripheral arterial disease. Symptoms are of rapid onset. The patient with an acute thrombosis is likely to have had a previous vascular procedure either endovascular or open. In this group of patients, onset may be more gradual secondary to the development of collaterals from the chronic disease.

Chronic arterial disease often presents as intermittent claudication. This word is derived from the Latin, claudico, meaning to limp, and is pain that is brought on by exercise and relieved with rest. It is often described as a cramping sensation or a feeling of tiredness or heaviness. It is reproduced by the same level of exercise and is relieved within 2–5 minutes of rest.

The pathophysiology of claudication is that of muscle ischemia caused by diminished oxygen delivery. An occlusion or stenosis of the arteries supplying a particular muscle group will limit flow; therefore the increased metabolic demands during exercise cannot be met.[12] Most patients with calf claudication have stenosis or occlusion of the SFA. Bilateral thigh or buttock

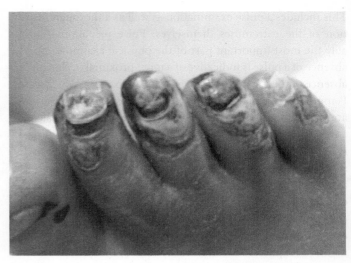

FIGURE 14–17. Patient with severe multilevel occlusive disease and gangrenous toes.

claudication associated with erectile dysfunction is known as the Leriche's syndrome and is consistent with aorto-iliac disease. The impotence is the result of inadequate blood flow through the hypogastric artery.

Ischemic rest pain is easily differentiated from claudication. Rest pain is a constant pain described as a severe aching or burning in the foot. The pain usually localizes to the metatarsal heads but may be worse in the location of a gangrenous toe or ischemic ulcer. This pain often intensifies at night and may be relieved by dependency (ie, hanging the foot over the side of the bed). Rest pain is of far greater consequence that is claudication. Whereas the latter may remain a benign condition, rest pain heralds the onset of gangrene and demands immediate attention.

Tissue loss and gangrene is the most severe form of ischemia (Fig. 14–17). Patients with tissue loss often present with multilevel occlusive disease. Arterial ischemic ulcers are often localized in the distal toes, heel, or sole and dorsum of the foot. Gangrene usually appears as a focal black or dark blue spot over a toe. If not treated, it may spread to other toes, foot, and, in severe cases, the entire leg. There are two type of gangrene: (1) wet (associated with infection) and (2) dry (noninfected). Other causes of leg ulcers are diabetic neuropathy, venous disease, and infection.

Symptoms of spinal stenosis, sciatica, osteoarthritis, or causalgia may be indistinguishable from those of vasculogenic claudication, hence the term "pseudoclaudication," and may have to be ruled out as differential diagnoses. Diabetic neuropathy may be confused with rest pain; however, the pain associated with diabetic neuropathy is not relieved by changes in position and patients often lack the associated physical findings seen in patients with PVD.

Physical Examination

The lower extremities should be carefully evaluated. Physical exam should include palpation, auscultation, and inspection.

TABLE 14–1 • Sign and Symptoms of Acute Arterial Disease
1. Pain
2. Poikilothermia (cold extremity)
3. Pallor (pale or white)
4. Pulselessness
5. Paresthesias (numbness, tingling sensation)
6. Paralysis (rigor)

This includes a pulse examination as well as a thorough inspection of the extremities themselves. Pulse palpation is probably the most important part of the physical examination. The absence of a pulse is indicative of a more proximal occlusion (eg, absence of the CFA pulse indicates aortoiliac occlusive disease). Femoral, popliteal, dorsalis pedis, and posterior tibial arteries are palpated and graded according to the following scale: 0 is a nonpalpable pulse, 1+ is a diminished, but palpable pulse, 2+ is a normal pulse, 3+ is a bounding pulse, and 4+ is an excessively bounding pulse (sometimes seen in patients with arterial aneurysm). A Doppler signal may be used to augment the pulse evaluation but is generally of little value since any flow will produce a signal and only in the presence of a completely occluded artery will the signal be completed absent. In order to perform an accurate pulse examination, both the patient and the examiner need to be in a comfortable and relaxed position. Special attention needs to be paid to any muscle fasciculation, which can often be mistaken for a palpable pulse. If the presence of a palpable pulse is uncertain, the pulse may be counted out to a separate examiner who is palpating the radial or femoral pulse or pulsations on electrocardiogram (ECG) or other monitor can be observed. In the upper extremity, pulses should be examined at the subclavian artery (above the middle of the clavicle); the axillary artery should be palpated in the groove between the biceps and triceps muscle, the brachial artery pulse can be palpated at the antecubital fossa, and the ulnar and radial arteries should be palpated at the wrist on the medial and lateral aspects, respectively.

Palpation is also helpful in assessing the temperature of the extremity. The examiner should use the back of the same hand to assess the temperature of each extremity being examined to compare any difference between them.

Auscultation with a stethoscope is performed to assess for the presence of a bruit. A bruit indicates the presence of a hemodynamically significant stenosis (note that the absence of a bruit does not exclude the presence of significant arterial occlusive disease). Auscultation should be performed at the abdomen, groin to detect any significant aortoiliac disease, at popliteal fossa to detect and Pop A disease. Auscultation over the iliac and femoral arteries should be performed to assess bruits, which may be suggestive of stenoses. In the presence of such a stenosis, a combination procedure with stenting of the iliacs and a peripheral bypass may be warranted.

Inspection of the lower extremity may reveal signs of acute or chronic arterial insufficiency. The patient's foot and toes should be carefully examined. Special attention should be noted in between the toes for any broken skin.

In addition to absent pedal pulses, patients with chronic arterial insufficiency may also present with trophic changes such as muscle atrophy, hair loss, thicken toe nails, ulcerations, or gangrene.

In acute lower extremity ischemia patients may present with skin mottling, cyanosis, pallor or muscle weakness.[19,20]

Inspection of the upper extremity can reveal important information about arterial perfusion. In an acute event the upper extremity may be pallid with diminished motor and sensory functions. In chronic processes you may note ulceration, gangrene, and muscle atrophy in the forearm and wrist.

Upper extremity pulses including the axillary, brachial, radial, and ulnar pulses should be palpated and if there is any question of upper extremity pathology, differential BPs should be checked in the arms. An Allen's test is performed to assess the collateral circulation between the radial and ulnar artery distributions.

The abdomen should be palpated for epigastric or lower quadrant masses. In a thin patient, the aortic pulsation may be prominent and can be mistaken for aneurysmal dilatation. In general, any pulsatile mass in the lower quadrants is an iliac artery aneurysm until proven otherwise. The abdomen may be auscultated for bruits, which are suggestive of renal and/or visceral artery stenoses, although these may be nonspecific findings.

Further examination of the lower extremity includes close inspection of the leg for swelling or lesions. This includes evaluation of the heels and careful evaluation of the skin between the toes. Chronic venous stasis changes or chronic arterial changes are noted, as is the presence of lymphedema, varicosities, and overall skin quality. Finally, venous filling and capillary refill can be used to roughly assess the adequacy of the circulation in the absence of palpable pulses.

In patients with diabetes, it is important to consider the risk of future ulceration. Assessment of the musculoskeletal and neurologic status of the foot is essential in addition to the assessment of the vascular supply. Light-touch sensation is assessed with standardized monofilaments.

TESTING OF THE UPPER AND LOWER EXTREMITIES

Doppler Evaluation[21,22]

Continuous wave (CW) Doppler provides information on motion and flow. CW waveform analysis can provide localized information in patients with incompressible vessel due to wall calcification. CW transducer has two crystals, one constantly transmitting and the other constantly receiving. It is capable of recording all frequency shifts in their path without aliasing (see the following text). Range ambiguity (entire length is evaluated not a specific depth), however, is a limitation as CW Doppler is sensitive to whatever vessels intersect its entire beam. In all Doppler analysis, flow that moves toward the probe is represented as a positive Doppler shift or flow above the baseline. Flow that moves away from the probe is represented as a negative Doppler shift and below the baseline. CW Doppler can be heard audibly, recorded by a chart strip recording, or recorded on film. It is usually a simple analog waveform without the distribution of frequencies that are displayed in the spectral analysis. Zero

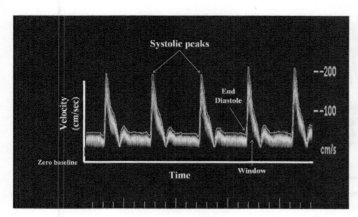

FIGURE 14–18. This image demonstrates the various components of the spectral Doppler waveform.

crossing detectors display an average of the flow velocity (mean frequency not peak frequency).

The magnitude of the Doppler shift is proportional to the angle of incidence, the smaller the angle the higher the Doppler shift (0 degrees will produce the highest Doppler shift) and vise versa (if the angle is 90 degree, there is no Doppler shift because as the cosine of 90 degrees is 0). Doppler shift frequencies are also affected by transducer frequency and the velocity of the red blood cells.

Pulsed Wave Spectral Analysis

Spectral analysis is the method of choice for displaying the Doppler signals. It is a mathematical computation of the reflected pulse that displays individual frequencies and is computed using the fast Fourier transform (FFT) method. It displays all of the Doppler shift frequencies as a bright echo or a shade of gray. It displays time on the horizontal axis and velocity or frequency shift on the vertical axis. In essence, it is a frequency spectrum

of the cardiac cycle. The spectral analysis demonstrates the presence, direction, and the characteristics of the blood flow (Fig. 14–18). In the vascular examination, the spectral waveform analysis has the capabilities of showing the degree of stenosis, site of occlusion, type of vessel, flow disturbances and turbulence, peripheral resistance, and relative flow velocity.

Analysis of Doppler Spectrum Waveform. The Doppler spectrum is a time-velocity waveform that represents changes in blood flow velocities during the cardiac cycle. Time is represented along the horizontal axis, and velocity is depicted along the vertical axis (Fig. 14–19). The intensity or brightness (also referred to as the gray-scale velocity plot) of the spectral line represents the number of red blood cells that are reflecting the ultrasound beam at each velocity. The width of the spectral line represents the range of velocities within a vessel. The width may vary during the normal cardiac cycle, narrowing during systole and widening in diastole. The spectral window is the clear black area between the spectral line and the baseline. Widening of the spectral line (envelope) and filling of the spectral window is called spectral broadening. Spectral broadening is normally seen in the presence of high flow velocity, at the branching of a vessel, or in small-diameter vessels. Spectral broadening can also result from a large Doppler angle, a large sample volume box or gate (>3.5 mm), a sample volume box located close to the vessel wall, or a high Doppler gain setting. Spectral broadening is also inherent in modern multielement ultrasound transducers.

PW Doppler was devised to control the region of active insonation and eliminate the range ambiguity limitation of CW Doppler. Pulsed wave (PW) Doppler systems send ultrasound pulses of a chosen length repetitively to a target at a certain range. Thus, PW Doppler has the advantage of being

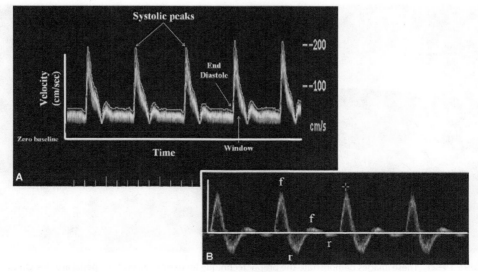

FIGURE 14–19. **(A)** The various components of the spectral Doppler waveform. **(B)** A multiphasic flow waveform (in this case quadriphasic) seen in peripheral vessels in normal resting states. In this case there are both a second forward (f) component and reversed (r) flow component.

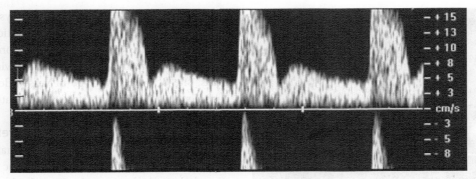

FIGURE 14–20. Aliasing will occur when the velocity exceeds the Nyquist limit. When aliasing occurs, velocities above this limit will be displayed on the tracing opposite to the true direction of blood flow, in this case below the baseline.

"site specific." However, PW Doppler has a major drawback, the "aliasing phenomenon," wherein the Doppler instrument cannot correctly depict higher velocities. Aliasing will occur when the velocity exceeds the Nyquist limit (the Nyquist limit is equal to one half of the pulse repetition frequency). When aliasing occurs, velocities above this limit will be displayed on the tracing opposite to the true direction of blood flow (Fig. 14–20).

Patient Positioning

In general, the optimal position for the vascular evaluation is supine with the extremities at the same level as the heart. The room should be warm (to avoid vasoconstriction). For the lower extremity evaluation, the hip should be externally rotated and the knee slightly bent to allow access to the vessels of interest on the medial aspect of the leg. The leg can be straightened to evaluate the anterior tibial artery as needed. For the upper extremity evaluation, the arms should be at the patient's side and relaxed.

Technique

CW Doppler evaluation of the lower extremities is performed with a 5- to 10-MHz transducer, the frequency to be determined by the depth of the vessel being evaluated. Gel is applied to the area in question. The probe is held at a 45- to 60-degree angle to the skin and fine movements are made to elicit the best possible signal.

In the lower extremity, Doppler waveforms are obtained from the following vessels:

- CFA
- SFA
- Pop A
- PTA
- DPA

If no signals are elicited from the DPA or PTA, waveforms from the peroneal artery can be recorded (Fig. 14–21).

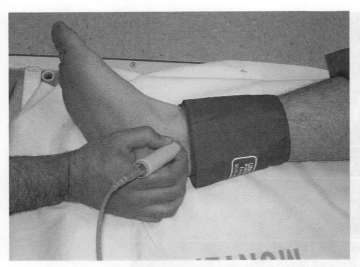
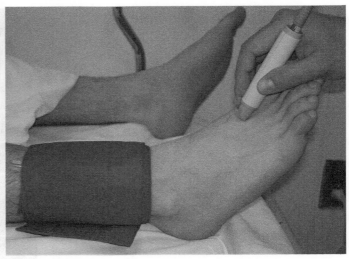

FIGURE 14–21. These images demonstrate the proper technique for examination of the pedal arteries. On the left, the anterior tibial artery is being evaluated in the distal leg as it crosses the extensor crease. On the right, the posterior tibial artery is found medial and immediately distal to the medial malleolus. The Doppler probe is held at a 45- to 60-degree angle to the vessel.

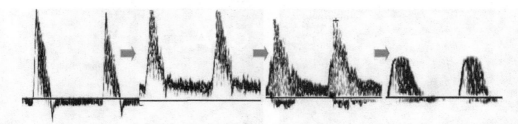

FIGURE 14–22. Spectrum of changes seen in the spectral Doppler waveform with increasing degrees of stenosis (left is normal to right abnormal).

In the upper extremity Doppler waveforms are obtained from the following vessels:

- Subclavian artery
- Axillary artery
- Brachial artery
- Ulnar artery
- Radial artery

Qualitative Interpretation

The Doppler waveform of the arteries in the arms and legs is a graphic representation of the pulsatile blood flow within them. As peripheral arterial occlusive disease progresses the pulsatility diminishes until it is completely lost.

Normal waveforms are multiphasic (generally triphasic or biphasic depending upon vessel elasticity and compliance) at rest and demonstrate a sharp systolic rise, sharp diastolic drop that goes below the baseline (indicative of normal peripheral resistance) and, in some cases, a second forward flow component in diastole (indicative of normal arterial compliance).

As arterial disease progresses, the systolic flow begins to decrease and there is a loss of flow reversal (Fig. 14–22).

Quantitative Interpretation

The two principal mechanisms that control blood volume are cardiac output and peripheral resistance. Cardiac output (mL/s) is the rate of blood flow per minute. Two factors that affect cardiac output are heart rate and stroke volume. Peripheral resistance is controlled by the arterioles and arterial capillaries. These tiny vessels control the volume of blood flow. The arterial resistivity index (RI), also called the resistance index (RI), developed by Leandre Pourcelot, is a measure of pulsatile blood flow that reflects the resistance to blood flow caused by the microvascular bed distal to the site of measurement. The RI is altered by the combination of vascular resistance and vascular compliance. The formula used to calculate RI is (peak systolic velocity – end-diastolic velocity)/peak systolic velocity or

$$RI = (^{v}systole - {^{v}}diastole)/{^{v}}systole$$

This measurement is often used in renal artery imaging. The resistive index is measured using spectral Doppler at the arcuate arteries (at the corticomedullary junction) or interlobar arteries (adjacent to medullary pyramids). The normal range is 0.50-0.70. Elevated values are associated with poorer prognosis in various renal disorders and renal transplant. In children, RI commonly exceeds 0.7, up to 12 months of age and can remain above 0.7 up to 4 years of age.

Pulsatility index (PI) can also be used to evaluate peripheral arterial disease. A decrease in the PI may indicate more proximal disease (Fig. 14–23).

PI = (peak systolic velocity – peak diastolic velocity)/Mean velocity

Normal PI values:

- CFA >5
- Pop A >8
- PTA >14

PI below these values suggests proximal occlusive disease. PI interpretation at the CFA may be affected in the presence of concomitant SFA occlusive disease; therefore the prediction of proximal disease in this setting may be unreliable.

AT in the CFA is used to predict the presence of hemodynamically significant aortoiliac lesions. AT is calculated by measuring the time from the onset of systole to peak systole.

All normal vessel flow profiles should exhibit a rapid rise to from the onset of systole to the peak of systole. Normal AT in

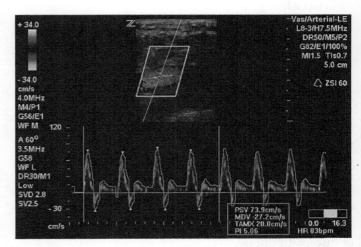

FIGURE 14–23. Calculation of the pulsatility index (PI) using information from four cardiac cycles as marked by the outlined spectra and the yellow calipers. The PI, in the red box, is 5.06 and is within normal limits.

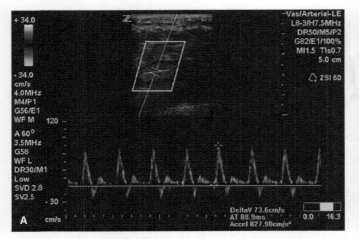
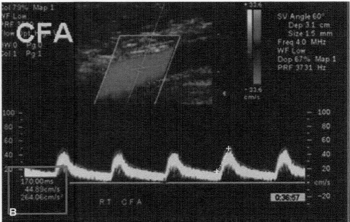

FIGURE 14–24. The acceleration time in (**A**) is 88.9 ms. In (**B**) in a patient with iliac artery occlusion, the acceleration time is 170 ms.

the CFA is <122 ms (Fig. 14–24). AT in the CFA >144 ms suggests an occlusive disease process above that level. As disease progresses the waveforms dampen and the AT increases.

In experienced hands, Doppler waveform analysis is a simple screening test to evaluate for the presence and approximate location of peripheral arterial disease; however, there are limitations and pitfalls to this technique and they are as follows:

1. It requires skill and experience. This is a very technologist-dependent examination that requires skill and training to learn the proper probe positioning, location of the vasculature, and be familiar with the audible signs of the various disease processes and their severity.

2. It sometimes cannot differentiate stenosis from occlusion.

3. It is rendered useless if there is not direct contact with the skin over the vessel (inaccessible vessels secondary to bandage, casts, open wounds).

4. In patients with uncompensated CHF all the waveforms may be damped and the location of the disease may not be detectable.

5. In patients with venous hypertension, the venous signals may be pulsatile and can be confused with arterial signals.

Segmental Pressures[22]

The ankle pressure, and more specifically, the ankle-brachial index (ABI), is the best and most simple method available for screening and assessing the severity of lower extremity peripheral artery disease (PAD). However, ABI results can be inconclusive or the index can be elevated (ie, >1.3) in persons with calcified ankle arteries due to DM, renal failure, or arthritis. In these instances, obtaining toe pressure (TP) measurements, which correlate well with angiographic findings, is advised, providing the patient does not have vasoconstriction with cold toes or vasospastic disease.

Acquiring the ankle pressure. The ABI is the ratio of the systolic blood pressure (SBP) measured at the ankle to that measured at the brachial artery. This index was initially proposed for the noninvasive diagnosis of lower-extremity PAD, but it was later shown that the ABI is an indicator of atherosclerosis at other vascular sites and can serve as a prognostic marker for cardiovascular events and functional impairment, even in the absence of symptoms of PAD.

Before acquiring the ABI, the patient should rest supine in a warm room for at least 10 minutes before testing and not have smoked for at least 1 hour. Place BP cuffs on both arms and ankles. The width of the BP cuff should be at least 20% wider than the diameter of the underlying limb segment. Then apply ultrasound gel over brachial, dorsalis pedis, and posterior tibial arteries. Measure systolic pressures in the arms using a hand-held Doppler over the brachial pulse distal to the cuff at the antecubital fossa. Inflate the cuff 20 mm Hg above last audible pulse and deflate the cuff slowly (2–3 mm Hg/s) and record the pressure at which the pulse becomes audible. Repeat for the contralateral arm. Then measure systolic pressures at the ankles by using the Doppler to locate first the DPA pulse. Inflate the cuff 20 mm Hg above last audible pulse then deflate the cuff slowly and record pressure at which the pulse becomes audible. Repeat the process for the PTA. The ABI value is determined by taking the higher pressure of the two arteries at the ankle and dividing it by the higher of the two brachial systolic pressure measurements. The ABI is a simple ratio and has no unit of measure.

Acquiring the Toe Pressure. The patient should be in a warm comfortable room, supine with arms and legs at heart level. Keep feet warm with a blanket or towel if needed. The patient should rest at least 10 minutes. The goal is for the patient to relax. Place a photocell (see the following text) on the pad of the large toe making sure the pad does not contact the toe cuff. The toe cuff should be wide enough to apply pressure over a large enough area so as to not be a tourniquet and long enough to overlap the bladder. Make sure the Velcro will hold the PPG

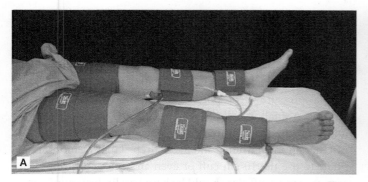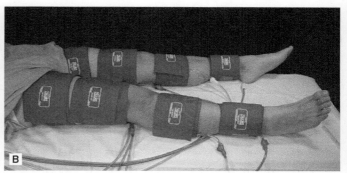

FIGURE 14–25. (A) A patient being evaluated using a three-cuff technique that employs one 20-cm length cuff on the thigh. (B) The four-cuff method, two 12-cm cuffs are used on the thigh. Both techniques employ 10- to 12-cm cuffs around the calf and ankle.

in place but not compress the blood vessels by being too tight. You should see the patient's pulse as a waveform on the chart recorder. Connect the sphygmomanometer to the TP cuff and inflate slowly until the waveform disappears. Note the pressure and continue to inflate until 20–30 mm Hg above that pressure (suprasystolic). Then slowly release the pressure in the cuff at about 2 mm Hg per declination until the waveform reappears. This is the systolic pressure.

The toe-brachial index (TBI) is calculated by dividing the TP by the highest brachial pressure. There is a wide variation of normal TBI values in the literature, but a TBI of less than 0.60 can be considered abnormal. The normal TBI is generally considered to be anything between 0.65 and 0.7 or above.

Segmental pressures are an extension of the ABI and are an indirect noninvasive test that indicates the level and degree of arterial disease and can evaluate disease progression. This test can be performed using a three (thigh, calf ankle) or a four-cuff method (high thigh, above knee, below knee, and ankle), on the lower extremity (Fig. 14–25). The three-cuff method may not differentiate between iliac/common femoral and superficial femoral lesions. The patient should be in the supine position to eliminate the effect of gravity (hydrostatic pressure) and erroneous BP measurements. The head should be slightly elevated. The patient should rest 15–20 minutes to permit stabilization of the pressures. The hip should be externally rotated and the knee slightly bent to facilitate proper Doppler probe placement. The room should be kept warm to avoid the complications of vasoconstriction. Pressures are obtained while the patient is at rest using a CW Doppler probe in the range of 5–10 MHz. A sphygmomanometer is used to measure pressure with a Doppler probe placed at the posterior tibial or dorsalis pedis artery to record the pressure as each individual cuff is activated. The pressure obtained is the pressure underneath the cuff that has been inflated. The cuff at each site is inflated until the systolic pressure sound disappears. The pressure in the cuff is then slowly released (2–3 mm Hg/s) until the sound or the Doppler waveform returns. This measurement is recorded. Bilateral brachial pressures are used as the standard and should be within 20 mm Hg of each other. If there is a greater difference in the

bilateral brachial measurements, this would indicate upper extremity arterial disease. The highest value of the normal two pressures is used as the standard.[22]

In the upper extremity, with a cuff on the upper arm and forearm, the pressures are obtained by first placing the probe at the antecubital fossa to obtain the brachial artery pressure. The probe is placed at the wrist at the medial side to obtain the ulnar artery pressure and on the lateral side to obtain the radial artery pressure. The cuff should be inflated 20–30 mm Hg suprasystolic and deflated slowly (2–3 mm Hg/s) until the signal comes back and the pressure is recorded. Digit pressures can be obtained by placing a small digital cuff over the base of the finger and then using a PPG sensor to detect the return of flow.

Interpretation

In the upper extremity, the study is normal if there is a pressure gradient of less than 20 mm Hg between the right and left brachial pressures or between the upper arm and forearm ipsilaterally. The normal finger to brachial index is >0.80. Pressures gradient of 20 mm Hg or greater between brachial pressures suggest a more proximal obstruction (innominate, subclavian, axillary, or brachial artery) in the arm with the lower pressure. Stenosis of the subclavian artery proximally can sometimes result in reversed vertebral artery flow and the "subclavian steal syndrome" (discussed in detail in Chapter 12). A pressure gradient of 20 mm Hg or greater between the upper arm and forearm suggests an obstruction in the segment between the cuffs. A gradient of >15–20 mm Hg between radial and ulnar artery suggest obstruction in the vessel with the lower pressure. Any finger to brachial index of <0.80 suggests the possibility of hemodynamically significant disease on that side.

In the lower extremity, when using a four-cuff technique, the normal upper thigh pressure is 20–30 mm Hg greater than the brachial pressure. This is because the narrow size of the bladder artifactually elevates the thigh pressure. With the four-cuff technique, the thigh pressure should be equal to or a little higher than the brachial artery pressure.

A pressure gradient of 20 mm Hg or less is considered to be within normal limits. The normal ABI and TBI are >1.0 and

Segmental Pressure Examination

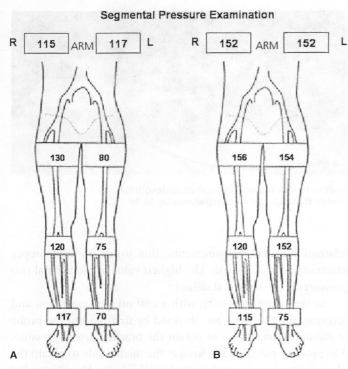

FIGURE 14–26. Segmental blood pressure measurement test. **(A)** Segmental leg pressures in a normal right extremity (ankle brachial index [ABI]: 117/117 = 1.00) and one with a significant left iliac artery stenosis or occlusion (ABI: 70/117 = 0.60). Horizontal and vertical pressure gradients exist at the thigh. **(B)** Segmental leg pressures in a patient with a right superficial femoral artery stenosis and a distal left tibial artery occlusion.

>0.70, respectively. The study is abnormal if there is a pressure gradient of 20 mm Hg or greater between adjacent segments ipsilaterally or if there is a horizontal (right vs left) difference of 20 mm Hg or greater at the same level (Fig. 14–26). In the four-cuff technique an upper thigh pressure 20 mm Hg lower than the brachial pressure indicates inflow disease (aortoiliac or common femoral artery).

Limitations and pitfall associated with this technique are:

- It cannot distinguish stenosis from occlusion.
- It does not provide information regarding specific location for disease but only provides an approximate location.
- In patients with calcified vessels pressures may be erroneously elevated due to medial wall calcification (especially true in diabetic and end stage renal disease patients).
- Patient with surgical incisions may not able to tolerate the pressures.
- Extensive bandages or casts may preclude the ability to wrap the cuffs.
- Inability to elicit a signal distal to the cuff will not allow for the acquisition of a pressure.

Cuff artifact. Limb and digital BP cuffs can vary in width and length, and improper size of the cuff may result in falsely low or high pressures. Pressure artifacts occur when the cuff size

is not appropriate for the girth of the leg or digit. Recommended size is 20% wider than the diameter of the limb. The length of the bladder should be twice its width. Pressure artifacts occur when cuff sizes are not appropriate for very large girth limbs or unusually small limbs. Cuff pressures will vary from intra-arterial pressure in proportion to limb girth such that if the cuff is too small, it will result in erroneously high pressures. If it is too wide, the measurement will be erroneously too low. For instance, in small women and in children, it may be more appropriate to use the 10-cm cuff or even an 8-mm cuff to measure arm pressure. Cuff size should be based on limb circumference.

Standard cuff sizes are listed as follows:

Arm = 12 × 23 cm

Ankle, calf = 10 × 23 cm

Metatarsal = 9 × 20 cm

Digit = 2–2.5 × 5 cm

Thigh = 16–23 cm wide (usually contoured)

Accurate pressure measurements can be obtained only when the head of pressure generated by the bladder can reach the artery in question. When the bladder fails to encircle the limb, the bladder of the cuff must be placed over the artery. In addition, the bladder must compress soft tissue, not bony structures. Therefore, the below-knee cuff should be placed just distal to the tibial tubercle. Failure to adhere to the guidelines will produce falsely elevated pressure readings.

Ranges of disease are as follows:

Normal: systolic ankle pressure is equal to or greater than brachial systolic pressure (a ratio ≥1.0)

Claudication: ABI between 0.6 and 0.9 indicates claudication (sometimes requires exercise testing)

Severe occlusive disease: ABI of less than 0.5 indicates severe occlusive disease (usually does not require exercise testing).

Pressure gradient of more than 20 mm Hg between cuff levels indicates a hemodynamically significant lesion.

TBI can be interpreted as follows:

- 0.64 +/– 0.20 limbs normal
- 0.52 =/– 0.20 claudication in limbs
- 0.23 =/– 0.19 limbs with ulcers or ischemic rest pain

A toe systolic pressure greater than 30 mm Hg may be an indicator that there is healing potential in a foot with ulcers. A normal TBI differs from a normal ABI because the normal BP in the big toe (hallux) is expected to be less than at the ankle or the arm. The normal range for a TBI is considered to be an index >0.65. It the TBI is below 0.65. There is reduced blood flow to the small vessels in the big toe.

Exercise testing is an important adjunct to the segmental pressure evaluation as it can help differentiate patients with true claudication from those with other differential diagnoses (pseudoclaudication). Exercise helps to unmask occlusive disease that is not apparent at rest. It is beneficial in patients with normal or borderline ABIs at rest who present with claudication type symptoms. By monitoring the ankle systolic pressure pre and post exercise, we are able to determine the severity of the arterial occlusive disease process. The magnitude of the immediate pressure drop post exercise and the time for recovery to resting pressure are proportional to the severity of arterial disease.

Technique

After the segmental pressure evaluation identifies the appropriate patient for exercise testing, cuffs are placed at the bilateral ankle and bilateral upper arm. Resting pressures are recorded at the brachial, dorsalis pedis, and posterior tibial arteries bilaterally (if symptomatically) or on the symptomatic side only. The highest ankle pressure and the higher of the brachial artery pressures are used to calculate ABIs. The patient is asked to walk on the treadmill at 2 mph at a 12% incline for 5 minutes or until symptoms force the patient to stop. Immediately post exercise and at 2, 5, and 10 minutes thereafter, the ankle and brachial pressure is recorded until the pressures return to the resting values.

After exercise pressures should increase slightly or remain equal in comparison with the resting pressures. Any pressure drop is considered abnormal. In patients whose pressures return to resting values within 2–6 minutes, single-level disease is suspected. Pressures that return to resting value after 10 minutes are more likely due to multilevel occlusive disease.

Contraindications to the exercise test are shortness of breath, recent history of myocardial infarction, elevated BP >200 mm Hg systolic and >100 mm Hg diastolic, inability or unwillingness to exercise, and patients with symptoms or other findings at rest (ulceration, rest pain).

In patients who are unable to exercise or are disabled, reactive hyperemia testing is an option. The patient is tested in the supine position. After acquisition of the resting pressures, a thigh cuff is inflated to suprasystolic pressure for 3–5 minutes. The thigh cuff is then deflated, and an ankle pressure is recorded immediately after cuff deflation.

In normal patients a drop in ankle pressure of up to 30% may be noticed. Any drop in pressure of up to 50% of the resting ankle pressure may be seen in patients with single-level disease. A >50% ankle pressure drop may be noticed in patients with multilevel disease.

Although it may be useful in some patients, the exercise test is preferred. Reactive hyperemia may be limited in patients who cannot tolerate the pressure exerted by the thigh pressure cuff. In addition, although the exam may uncover an occult stenosis, it may not be clear if the stenosis is in fact the cause of the patient's symptoms as the pressure drop was not brought on by exercise.

Plethysmography[21,22]

Plethysmography provides subjective information about the overall perfusion to the limb. It is not affected by medial calcinosis and is often better tolerated than segmental pressures. It is generally a measurement of volume changes in the extremities for measuring blood flow. It has been used in the past for venous flow studies and venous reflux studies and is now used primarily for arterial studies. Limitations include constant movement (voluntary or involuntary) that may affect the contour of the waveforms, inability to differentiate between stenosis and occlusion, decreasing accuracy in the presence of multilevel disease, excessive bandages, casts, and open wounds, and changes in the pulse waveform contour (may assume an obstructive contour) that can occur in cold rooms.

There are several types of plethysmography.

Air plethysmography in the form of the pulse volume recorder uses air flow to measure volume changes in a limb. It is performed using pneumatic cuffs inflated to a low pressure (~65 mm Hg) that measure the relative changes in pressure in a limb. These instruments provide a good arterial pulse contour waveform.[22] The normal pulse contour has a rapid systolic upstroke, with a prominent dicrotic notch and a down slope that bows toward the baseline in diastole. As disease progresses, changes in the waveform are noted. In mild disease, the rapid systolic upstroke is present and a down slope that bows toward the baseline in diastole is seen; however, the dicrotic notch is absent. Moderate disease yields a rounded systolic peak, loss of the dicrotic notch, and the down slope bows away from the baseline. In patients with severe disease, there is reduced pulsatility in the waveform with a flattened systolic peak and a delayed rise time (Fig. 14–27).

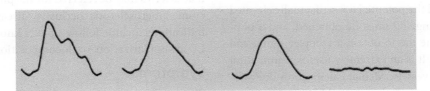

FIGURE 14–27. From left to right are the changes seen in the pulse volume waveforms with increasing levels of disease. Far left is normal. Loss of the dichroitic notch is the first evidence of disease and is seen in the second waveform. The third waveform reveals blunting of the waveform peak on the far right in severe disease there is severe diminution of the pulse volume waveform.

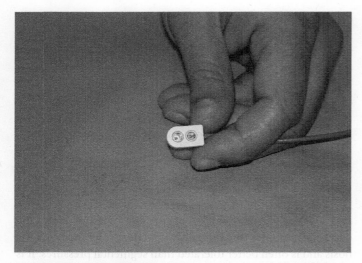

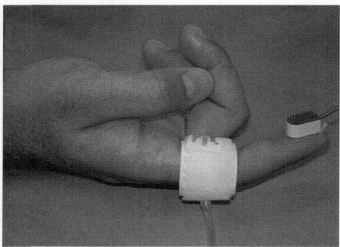

FIGURE 14–28. On the top is the face of the photocell with light-emitting diode and phototransistor. Below is the technique used for acquisition of a digital pressure. The signal from the diode photocell is monitored as the cuff is inflated.

Photoplethysmography (PPG) is performed using a small photocell placed on the extremity, which contains an infrared light (light-emitting diode and a phototransistor) (Fig. 14–28). This photocell identifies subcutaneous flow and produces a pulse contour that can be recorded.[21] This technique is frequently used in vascular examinations to detect blood flow when it becomes difficult with conventional techniques. This may be true in diabetics with medial wall calcification (diabetics and end-stage renal disease patients) and the potential for artifactually elevated leg pressures. In this setting, TP must be obtained, and a photocell can be placed on the toe to obtain a Doppler signal and take a pressure recording. It is an extremely useful examination in patients with calcified vessels. Medial calcification does not extend into the digital arteries making possible to measure systolic TPs. In the upper extremity, evaluation of the digit perfusion helps differentiate fixed arterial disease from vasospastic disorder (cold exposure or stress related).[21]

DUPLEX IMAGING

The clinical role of duplex scanning in the vascular patient has expanded from its earliest applications as the noninvasive exam of choice for the evaluation of atherosclerotic disease of the carotid artery to evaluation of virtually the entire vascular system.

Patients with lower extremity arterial occlusive disease typically undergo a combination of invasive and noninvasive tests prior to lower extremity revascularization. While the patient's symptoms and the results of these tests are used to decide when surgery is needed, the operation is usually planned on the basis of diagnostic arteriography alone. Arteriography accurately defines the location of stenotic and occluded arterial segments and is considered the gold standard for selecting the location of a graft's proximal and distal anastomoses. However, arteriography is invasive and poses the risks of contrast-induced renal dysfunction, puncture site complications, catheter and guidewire-induced vessel wall injury, and allergic reactions. In addition, both standard and digital angiographic techniques occasionally fail to visualize patent low flow distal arterial segments.[23-26]

Duplex ultrasound with color (CDU) can also be used to image the lower extremity and pelvic arteries and is safer and less expensive than arteriography and is also noninvasive. Many studies have shown the clinical utility of CDU for preoperative assessment prior to carotid endarterectomy and for endovascular treatment of short, focal lesions of the aortoiliac and femoropopliteal arteries. We and others have used CDU as the sole imaging technique to evaluate patients prior to lower extremity revascularization.[27-30]

IMAGING THE AORTIC BIFURCATION AND ILIAC ARTERIES

Abdominal scanning requires technical expertise and a thorough understanding of anatomy, physiology, and hemodynamics. Increasing sophistication and refinement of ultrasound technology have allowed for the accurate examination of the deep abdominal and pelvic vasculature, and color flow duplex evaluation of the abdominal aorta and iliac arteries is now performed routinely in most vascular laboratories. Color Doppler vascular ultrasound can routinely interrogate and reliably quantify disease in the aorta and iliac arteries.

Indications

The patient referred for evaluation of the aortic bifurcation and iliac arteries may be referred for the purpose of ruling out aneurysm, atherosclerotic occlusive disease, or dissection. Other indications include follow-up of a known AAA, surveillance of LE revascularization, or documentation of disease progression.

Symptoms

The patient can present with one or a combination of the following symptoms: abdominal, flank or groin pain, a pulsatile abdominal mass, severe disabling buttock or thigh claudication, impotence, manifest signs of lower extremity ischemia, or may be asymptomatic.

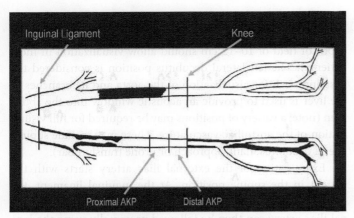

FIGURE 14–30. Diagram that depicts the results of a duplex arterial mapping. On the right, the patient has proximal superficial femoral artery (SFA) disease, with straight line flow through the popliteal artery. Below the knee the patient has an occluded peroneal artery and a short occlusion of the distal posterior tibial artery. The anterior tibial artery is patent and without stenosis throughout its length to the level of the foot. On the left, the patient has an SFA occlusion with reconstitution of the above-knee popliteal artery and three-vessel runoff to the foot.

Blood flow analysis should be performed using both spectral and color Doppler because they are complimentary. Once the color flow image has been optimized, spectral Doppler is used to obtain detailed information of blood flow. A beam angle of 60 degrees or less (45–60) is recommended for interrogation of the blood flow. When used consistently, this helps reduce intra- and interobserver variability. Flow should be sampled at regular intervals 1–2 cm throughout the area of interest and at points of flow disturbance documented by color Doppler. In general, there are three stenosis classifications for aortic and iliac artery stenosis: less than 50%, greater than 50%, or occluded. These are based on a combination of the B-mode examination and flow velocity data. In general, a focal twofold increase in velocity from one segment to another with a change in spectral waveform configuration and poststenotic turbulence suggests the presence of >50% stenosis. A greater than twofold increased velocity with no poststenotic turbulence suggests stenosis less than 50%. If there is disagreement between the B-mode finding and the Doppler data, classification should be made based on the spectral Doppler data. Inability to elicit Doppler or visual evidence of active blood flow under optimal 2D and Doppler settings suggests complete occlusion.

These techniques have allowed the performance of limb salvage procedures in selected patients without the need for diagnostic arteriography. Improvements in vascular ultrasound imaging promise to minimize and/or eliminate the need for routine diagnostic arteriography in many high-risk patients.

LOWER EXTREMITY DUPLEX IMAGING

The most common application of this technique is for the evaluation of the vein bypass graft. It can also be used to identify the exact anatomical location of arterial occlusive disease and to differentiate stenosis from occlusion, for assessment of dialysis access grafts, to assess and define pulsatile masses including aneurysms and pseudoaneurysms and to identify iatrogenic arteriovenous fistulas.[16,17,29,32]

Bypass Graft Imaging[32]

The goal of vein graft surveillance is to identify lesions that may ultimately lead to vein graft occlusion. The rationale for graft surveillance is the progressive nature of atherosclerosis and the tendency of both vein and prosthetic bypass grafts to develop flow-limiting lesions. Duplex ultrasound in conjunction with some form of indirect testing is the recommended surveillance method following lower extremity bypass grafting. At present, frequent surveillance is recommended in the first postoperative year with the initial scan being performed intraoperatively. Studies have shown that grafts followed in a surveillance program have a higher patency rate than those followed only clinically.

Interpretation criteria for identifying stenotic lesions have traditionally focused on identification of focally elevated peak systolic velocities (PSVs) at a site of a stenosis or abnormally low PSVs somewhere within the distal portion of the graft. A PSV of less than 45 cm/s (uniformly throughout the conduit) has been popularized as an indicator of impending graft failure; however, disagreement exists that this value represents an appropriate threshold for all vein grafts. An additional parameter is the use of the mean graft flow velocity (GFV). Mean GFV is calculated by taking an average of 3–4 PSV values in nonstenotic segments of the bypass graft at various levels above and below the knee where applicable. GFV should be greater than 45 cm/s. A GFV of less than 40 cm/s can be present normally in large diameter grafts (>6 mm) or in grafts with limited outflow. Others have advocated the use of flow volume measurements in a predetermined part of the distal graft as a better indicator of impending graft failure, while some have suggested that the significance of change over time, not an absolute velocity or flow value, may be a more sensitive indicator. Most interpretation criteria have been developed for the in situ saphenous vein bypass graft. The same principles can be applied to the reversed vein graft; however, differences in graft diameter and hemodynamics must be considered. There are no established criteria for serial evaluation of prosthetic grafts, and controversy exists in this area. In general, any doubling of velocity from a normal site proximal to the stenosis is consistent with a 50% diameter reduction (a 75% cross-sectional area reduction); however, this assumes a constant diameter.

Exam Preparation and General Considerations. Prior to the evaluation, it is helpful to be familiar with the type of graft being examined. The important elements of this information include the sites of the proximal and distal anastomoses, the type of conduit, and the location of the graft in the leg. Superficial grafts such as in situs or grafts that are tunneled subcutaneously are best evaluated with high-frequency transducers (7.5–10 MHz). Lower-frequency (3–5 MHz) transducers are

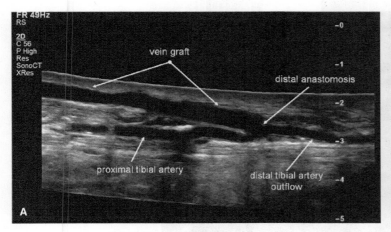
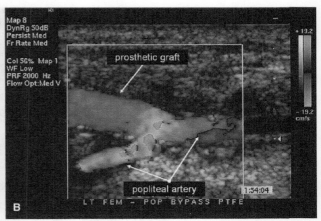

FIGURE 14–31. (A) Gray-scale image of the distal anastomosis of a femoral to posterior tibial artery reversed saphenous vein graft. (B) A color flow image at the distal anastomosis of a femoropopliteal polytetrafluoroethylene (PTFE) prosthetic graft. There is flow beyond the anastomosis moving both retrograde and prograde in the popliteal artery.

best for grafts tunneled anatomically. For grafts anastomosed to the above-knee popliteal or peroneal arteries, it may be necessary to employ a sector or curved array transducer to identify the distal anastomosis and outflow vessel. To avoid the complications of infection, a sterile couplant sheet can be used for imaging in the early postoperative period.

Technical Protocol. The examination starts by identifying the mid portion of the graft in the leg in the transverse orientation. The graft is then followed proximally to its confluence with the inflow vessel where the proximal anastomosis is identified. At this point the transducer is rotated sagittally and the inflow vessel is assessed. The entire length of the graft through the distal anastomosis and outflow artery is then interrogated using both the gray scale image and simultaneously Doppler spectral analysis (Fig. 14–31). Doppler waveforms are obtained using a 60-degree angle and with the sample volume in the center of the vessel and the cursor parallel to the vessel wall. Any angle that varies from the standard should be noted and used on follow-up studies for comparison. The peak systolic and end-diastolic velocity is recorded from waveforms obtained at predetermined sites in the graft, anastomotic sites and inflow and outflow vessels. Data are also recorded at all areas of abnormality as determined by color or spectral Doppler.

Color Flow Doppler. The use of color Doppler is recommended as it provides observation of the graft from a large field of view and significantly reduces the time required to evaluate the graft. The color flow map is used as a guide for the placement of the sample volume, and when proper settings are used, it will easily identify areas of high velocity and turbulent flow. The pulse repetition frequency is lowered until aliasing occurs and then adjusted appropriately to allow good color saturation with the highest velocities seen in the center of the graft. Stenosis is suspected when there are (1) narrowing of the color flow channel;

(2) shift toward the colors representing higher velocities; (3) change in color due to aliasing; (4) prolonged duration of color throughout the cardiac cycle; and (5) color flow bruit (Fig. 14–32).

All abnormal color changes are evaluated by spectral Doppler to determine if an actual velocity increase has occurred keeping in mind that changes in vessel alignment with respect to the scanning lines can cause a color change due to the alteration in Doppler angle. Additionally all sites of flow disturbance are evaluated via the B-mode scan to identify the type of lesion present in the graft conduit. It is imperative to remember that although the B-mode image and color flow information provide important anatomic information and serve as guides to sample volume placement, the severity of the stenotic lesion is categorized only by Doppler spectral waveform analysis.

Causes of Vein Graft Failure. Graft failure can occur by three mechanisms: occlusion by thrombosis, hemodynamic failure, and structural failure (aneurysmal degeneration). The frequency of graft failure is highest within the first 10–14 days (4–10%) post implantation, decreases progressively in the first year, and is approximately 2–4% per year thereafter. Technical errors (suture stenosis, intimal flaps, retained thrombus, graft entrapment, torsion) are the most common cause of failure in the early postoperative period (within 30 days). Late failure can be due to myointimal hyperplasia from preexisting vein graft lesions or atherosclerosis that can develop de novo in vein grafts or disease progression in adjacent native arteries but is most typically seen in the distal runoff bed (Fig. 14–33). It is the period between 30 days and 2 years that occlusive lesions develop, and for this reason, a more aggressive surveillance protocol is employed.

Hemodynamics. Doppler signals will undergo normal changes in the diastolic component of the flow waveform over time. In the early postoperative period, the Doppler waveform may demonstrate continuous forward flow throughout diastole because of a hyperemic response seen after revascularization of a

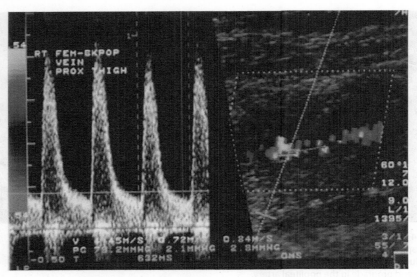

FIGURE 14–32. Color flow image of a stenotic lesion in a vein graft.

severely ischemic limb. Subsequent visits may reveal a change to the more normal peripheral multiphasic type of waveform with reversal of flow in diastole. This of course is dependent on the status of the outflow tract. The PSVs will not change significantly.

If significant decreases (20–30 cm/s) in the peak velocities, as recorded from an index site, are noted, a problem in the graft or adjacent vessels must be suspected. In general, a delayed upstroke (prolonged rise time) infers a problem proximal to the transducer whereas a decrease in diastolic flow suggests a distal lesion. Staccato waveforms, representing to and from motion of blood, are seen proximal to high-grade lesions or occlusion and are usually followed by immediate thrombosis of the graft. This phenomenon can be distinguished form the normal triphasic waveform by its low amplitude and the very short duration of each flow component.

An effective surveillance program must be applicable to all patients, practical in terms of time, effort, and cost, and should provide a means for detecting, grading severity, and assessing

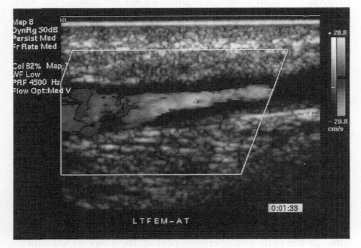

FIGURE 14–33. Color flow image of a patient with a myointimal hyperplastic lesion at the proximal anastomosis of a vein graft as demonstrated by the echo-lucency on the near and far walls of the graft.

progression of lesions. The ultimate goal is detection of the threatened graft before thrombosis occurs.

Lower Extremity Arterial Mapping for Occlusive Disease

Despite surgeons' comfort in the easy-to-interpret format of a conventional arteriogram, compelling reasons exist to research the feasibility of alternatives to this "gold standard" test. Arteriography is expensive, uncomfortable for patients, and encumbered with significant potential complications, including bleeding, hematoma or pseudoaneurysm formation, arterial dissection, embolization, and contrast-induced nephrotoxicity.[23-26] Duplex ultrasonography, on the other hand, is an inexpensive, noninvasive, well-tolerated modality that is capable of accurately distinguishing between normal, stenotic, and occluded vessels.

The rationale for supposing that duplex arterial mapping (DAM) can serve a similar purpose to conventional preoperative arteriography is based on two genres of studies in which both tests are performed in the same patients. The first type of study evaluates whether DAM can accurately evaluate individual arteries and detect 50% or greater stenoses or occlusions when compared to the de facto gold standard of arteriography.[27,28,33-38] A signature study representative of this genre was performed by Moneta et al[39] who compared DAM with arteriography in 150 consecutive patients under consideration for lower extremity revascularization. The authors summarized that for vessels proximal to the crural arteries, duplex technology could adequately visualize 99% of the arteries. The sensitivity for duplex ultrasound in documenting a 50% or greater lesion ranged from 89% in the iliac arteries to a low of 67% within the Pop A. Stenoses could be distinguished from occlusions in almost all cases (98%). In the crural vessels, DAM was able to visualize the anterior tibial, posterior tibial, and peroneal arteries 94%, 96%, and 83% of the time, respectively. The sensitivity of duplex ultrasound for documenting continuous patency of these vessels was 90%, 90%, and 82%, respectively. More recent studies employing newer-generation duplex scanners have yielded improved results especially within the infrapopliteal vasculature where it is now possible to not only document continuous patency of a vessel but also distinguish between greater or less than 50% stenoses.[29]

Knowledge of the presence, degree, and location of arterial stenoses does not necessarily mean that all manner of lower extremity revascularizations can be performed based on duplex examinations alone. However, studies including one performed in our own laboratory have sought to answer the question; "Can duplex scan arterial mapping replace contrast arteriography as the test of choice before infrainguinal revascularization?"[29]

Our study concluded that the need for a femoropopliteal versus an infrapopliteal bypass could be correctly predicted by DAM in 90% of the patients studied. Our study concluded that the need for a femoropopliteal versus an infrapopliteal bypass could be correctly predicted by DAM in 90% of the patients studied. Moreover, both of the anastomotic sites for the bypass were correctly predicted by means of DAM in 90% of the patients who had femoropopliteal bypasses versus only 24% of the patients who underwent infrapopliteal bypasses. We concluded that DAM could reliably predict which patients required femoropopliteal bypasses versus infrapopliteal bypasses.

The following text describes the technique used in our laboratory to perform DAM. In addition, the clinical utility of this modality when compared to conventional arteriography will be explored.

TECHNIQUE FOR DUPLEX ARTERIAL MAPPING

Prior to DAM, patients are advised to perform an overnight fast, wear loose fitting clothing, and expect the examination to last an average of 45 minutes. At the time of the study, the patient is placed supine on a standard examination table. We utilize ATL HDI 3000 and 5000 (Advanced technology Labs, Bothell, Washington) color duplex scanners and start the examination with a broadband L7-4 MHz linear array transducer. First, the CFA on the symptomatic side is insonated. A femoral artery AT greater than 133 cm/s^2 is our criterion to initiate the mapping by scanning the aortoiliac system. A femoral artery AT less than 133 cm/s^2 rules out the presence of significant aortoiliac occlusive disease,[40] and if the patient is free of symptoms or findings (decreased femoral pulse) suggesting aortoiliac disease, we begin by mapping the infrainguinal vasculature only.

For infrainguinal mapping, the leg is externally rotated to facilitate investigation of the thigh and medial calf vessels and returned to its neutral position to evaluate the anterior tibial artery. Different transducers (L12-5 broadband linear or CL 10-5 curved array) are used when necessary to image the more distal vasculature. In this fashion, the common, deep, and

TABLE 14–2 • Stratification of % Arterial Stenosis	
% Stenosis	**Velocity Ratio**
Normal	Triphasic waveform with no spectral broadening
1–19%	Normal waveform with slight spectral broadening and peak velocities increased <30% more than the adjacent proximal segment
20–49%	Spectral broadening with no window under the systolic peak, peak velocity <100% of the proximal adjacent segment
50–99%	Peak velocity 100% more than the adjacent proximal segment and reversed flow component is usually absent; monophasic waveform and reduced velocity beyond the stenosis
Occlusion	No flow in the imaged artery, monophasic preocclusive thump; velocities markedly diminished and waveforms monophasic, tardus parvus flow beyond the occlusion

superficial femoral, above- and below-knee popliteal, anterior, and posterior tibial, peroneal, and dorsalis pedis arteries are all imaged in continuity.

A combination of B-mode and color flow imaging are used to locate the vessels within the appropriate anatomic region and facilitate accurate placement of the sample volume. In the presence of aliasing or narrowing of the color flow channel, a spectral Doppler waveform is obtained and the systolic blood flow velocities are noted proximal to and within the area being interrogated. If the area of interest demonstrates a PSV at least twice as great as that within the adjacent proximal segment, a greater than 50% stenosis is documented. This has been adapted from Jager et al and is detailed in Table 14–2.[38] In the presence of an elevated PSV, but one that is not doubled, a less than 50% stenosis is diagnosed. Finally, the absence of any color flow signal within a vessel confirms the presence of an occlusion. Our technologists also note the presence and degree of calcification within the vasculature and the location of large collateral vessels distal to occlusions.

The significant portions of the examination are recorded on tape for documentation and further surgeon review if desired, and the results are presented on an easy-to-interpret graphical representation of the lower extremity vasculature.

Patients who are going to surgery without arteriography have the skin site overlying the distal anastomosis marked with pen after the surgeon has reviewed the study results and chosen the desired outflow vessel.

Several important technical limitations of DAM must be noted. Examinations may be challenging or impossible to perform in patients with an obese body habitus, severe vascular calcification, or open wounds overlying the course of the named vessels. In addition, the proximal portion of the anterior tibial artery may be difficult or impossible to image as it traverses the interosseous membrane, and the terminal branches of the peroneal artery may not be seen secondary to their small size and deep location within the leg. The degree and extent of mural calcification, exclusive of vessel size, may impact significantly on the pre-bypass decision-making process; however, there is no widely accepted way to measure or grade calcification. There is also no current means to distinguish between the suitability of crural vessels with similar duplex grades of stenoses to harbor the distal anastomosis of a bypass graft. Finally, DAM is a technically demanding study that requires a large amount of experience to perform accurately. During the learning curve, considerable practice, combined with surgeon feedback and comparison of DAM findings to angiography (when performed) is mandatory.

Computed Axial Tomography[41,42]

Computed tomographic (CT) units have an x-ray tube, two scintillation detectors, a line printer, teletyper, and a computer and magnetic disc unit that are used to attain a series of detailed visualizations of the tissues of the body at any depth desired. It is painless, noninvasive, and requires no special preparation; however, there is associated radiation. The body is scanned in two planes simultaneously at various angles. The computer calculates tissue absorption, displays a printout of the numerical values, and produces a visualization of the tissues that demonstrates the densities of the various structures. Tumor masses, infarctions, bone displacement, and accumulations of fluid may be detected.

Angiography, Arteriography, and Digital Subtraction Angiography

Angiography or arteriography is defined as "the roentgenographic visualization of blood vessels following introduction of contrast material and is used as a diagnostic aid."[23,43] It is a radiology procedure where a rapid sequence of films is obtained after injection of contrast material through a catheter that is introduced percutaneously through the femoral or axillary artery. The catheter tip is placed into the selective artery or its branches. Early films show the contrast material in the major arteries followed by subsequent the filling of the smaller arteries. Angiography has the ability to demonstrate intrinsic vascular abnormalities such as atherosclerotic plaques, strictures, occlusions, and malformations. In the extremities, it can also assess the degree of collateral circulation and the patency of the distal vessels. It has long been considered the "gold standard" for vascular examinations and is usually done before surgery or interventional techniques. In some instances, it also solves such diagnostic dilemmas as vasospastic disorders versus occlusive disease of the hands, Buerger's disease, ergotism, temporal arteritis, and periarteritis nodosa. However, angiography is invasive and has some inherent risks with radiation exposure.

Magnetic Resonance Imaging

MRI shows proton density in the body and obtains dynamic studies of certain physiologic functions. Basically, it induces transitions between energy states by causing certain atoms to absorb and transfer energy. This is done by directing a radiofrequency pulse at a substance placed within a large magnetic field. The various measures of time required for material to return to a baseline energy state (relaxation time) can be translated by a complex computer algorithm to a visual image. Magnetic resonance images can be obtained in the transverse, coronal, or sagittal plane. It can penetrate bone without significant attenuation with the underlying tissue clearly imaged. There is no associated radiation.[44]

Treatment for Peripheral Vascular Disease

Treatment programs are tailored to each individual and take into account the needs of the patient and family. The treatment will depend on factors such as the severity of the symptoms, the degree of arterial narrowing or blockage, the impact of the disease on the patient's lifestyle/quality of life, and the patient's overall health. Treatment for patients with PVD may include:

- Controlling risk factors through lifestyle changes and medication
- Endovascular therapy or surgery to reopen arteries of the legs or arms

Controlling Risk Factors and Lifestyle Changes

PVD is a common condition among people who have diabetes and those who smoke. It is critical for diabetics to control their blood sugar levels and for smokers to quit smoking completely. Other essential lifestyle changes are diet and exercise. Diet changes include reducing the amount of cholesterol-containing (fatty) foods and, for overweight people, reducing calories to decrease weight. Exercise helps in weight loss and in building a stronger circulatory system and improving blood flow. Even though PVD may cause pain during exercise, a program of daily walking for short periods may help the patient maintain or regain function. It is also critical for patients with PVD, particularly those with diabetes, to carefully monitor their feet for cuts or wounds and avoid tight-fitting shoes.

Medications

Patients with PVD may benefit from medications to reduce the risk of heart attack and stroke. Among the more commonly prescribed drugs are antiplatelet drugs. These medications make the blood platelets less likely to stick together. Aspirin is the most common, least expensive of these drugs and typically has the fewest potential side effects. Anticoagulants are prescription drugs that prevent blood clots by affecting the proteins in the body's clotting system and require careful monitoring. The drugs include heparin, which is used short term, and warfarin

(Coumadin), which is used long term. Cholesterol-lowering drugs decrease the amount of cholesterol, especially LDL (the "bad" form of cholesterol). These drugs decrease the primary material that make up deposits that narrow or plug arteries and create atherosclerosis. Examples of these drugs are niacin, statins, fibrates, and bile acid sequestrants. Calcium channel blockers help dilate arteries and control high BP. Vitamins such as folate, B_6, and B_{12} help decrease homocystine in the blood. In specific situations, other dietary supplements may be prescribed, such as L-arginine and Omega-3 fatty acids.[45]

Endovascular Therapy and Surgery

Angioplasty and stenting is the mechanical widening of a narrowed or totally obstructed blood vessel and has come to include all manner of vascular interventions typically performed in a minimally invasive or percutaneous method. It is often called percutaneous transluminal angioplasty or PTA for short. PTA is most commonly done to treat narrowing in the leg arteries, especially the common iliac, external iliac, superficial femoral, and popliteal arteries but can also be used to treat narrowings in veins.

This procedure is performed via a puncture of the femoral artery or less commonly the brachial or radial artery. Using various wires, sheaths, and catheters, the interventionalist identifies the narrowed or blocked artery, stretches it open with a balloon, and may or may not place a stent in the area to prevent it from collapsing again. Balloon angioplasty and stenting has generally replaced invasive surgery as the first-line treatment for PVD (Fig. 14–34).[46]

Surgery is the appropriate option for those patients with severe cases of PVD that interfere with daily activities and are not amenable to less invasive forms of intervention. Surgery may include endarterectomy or bypass grafting.

Endarterectomy is a surgical procedure to remove the atheromatous plaque material, or blockage, in the lining of an artery constricted by the buildup of fatty deposits. It is carried out by separating the plaque from the arterial wall. Endarterectomy performed with or without a patch graft. This procedure is more invasive than angioplasty and can be used when a very short segment of an artery is blocked or severely clogged. The surgeon identifies the location of the blockage and then makes an incision over the area. The clogged artery is opened and the diseased segment removed. The artery is closed, or if this will make it too narrow, a small patch of vein or prosthetic graft material is inserted as a cap to maintain a large enough opening for the blood flow.

Surgical bypass treats narrowed arteries by directly creating a detour, or bypass, around a section of the artery that is blocked. Leg artery bypass surgery involves taking a vein from the body or an artificial vein to construct a bypass around a blocked main leg artery. The bypass is, in effect, a secondary system to allow blood to flow to the distal extremity. The vein or graft is sutured in place proximal and distal to the obstruction (Fig. 14–35). It requires at least two incisions: one above and one below the blocked artery. Sometimes, especially when veins are used, longer incisions are necessary.

Inflow operations are performed to restore blood flow in the presence of aortoiliac occlusive disease. Aortobifemoral grafts originate from the aorta and take blood to the femoral arteries at the groins. Aortobifemoral grafting is the most successful type of inflow operation but is also the most invasive. A

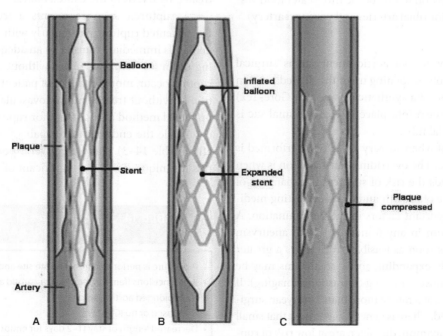

FIGURE 14–34. (A) Collapsed balloon and stent are advanced to the level of stenosis within the vessel. (B) Balloon is inflated and stent is deployed pushing plaque against wall of artery. (C) Plaque is compressed and lumen has been restored.

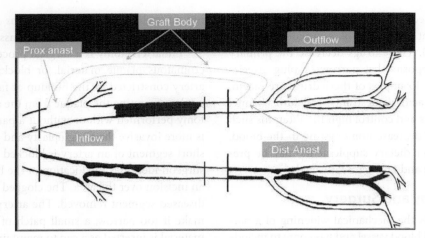

FIGURE 14–35. Bypass graft (dotted orange line) in the left lower extremity. Proximal anastomosis is at the common femoral artery, and the distal anastomosis is at the below-knee popliteal artery.

prosthetic graft is anastomosed to the aorta. The graft has two limbs that are then tunneled under the abdominal muscles to the groins to be anastomosed to the femoral arteries. Axillobifemoral grafts originate from the axillary arteries and take blood to the femoral arteries. This is sometimes the best option in very elderly or very unfit patients as it is a less traumatic alternative to aortobifemoral grafting. Femorofemoral crossover grafts originate from a normal femoral artery in the groin on one leg and take blood to the femoral artery in the groin on the opposite leg.

Outflow operations are performed to restore blood flow to the more distal leg. Femoropopliteal bypass grafts originate from the femoral artery in the groin and take blood to the Pop A either just above or below the knee. Femorodistal or femorocrural bypass grafts originate from the femoral artery at the groin or in the thigh and take blood to one of the three calf blood vessels (anterior and posterior tibial arteries and peroneal artery).[47]

Aortic Aneurysms

The definitive treatment for an aortic aneurysm is surgical repair. This typically involves opening up of the dilated portion of the aorta and insertion of a synthetic (Dacron or Gore-Tex) graft. Once the graft is sewn into place, the aneurysmal sac is closed around the artificial tube.

The determination of when surgery should be performed is complex and case specific. The overriding consideration is when the risk of rupture exceeds the risk of surgery. The diameter of the aneurysm and its rate of growth and other coexisting medical conditions are all important factors in the determination. A rapidly expanding (>5 mm in any 6-month period) aneurysm should be operated on as soon as feasible, since it has a greater chance of rupture. Slowly expanding aortic aneurysms may be followed by routine diagnostic imaging (ultrasound imaging). If the aortic aneurysm grows at a rate of more than 1 cm/year, surgical treatment is considered. There is general agreement that small aneurysms, <4.0 cm in maximum diameter, are at low risk of rupture and should be monitored, whereas an aneurysm 5.4 cm in diameter should be repaired in an otherwise healthy patient.[48]

The endovascular aneurysm repair (EVAR) treatment of AAAs has emerged as a less invasive alternative to open surgical repair.[48] The first endovascular exclusion of an aneurysm was performed by Dr. Parodi and his colleagues in Argentina in 1991. The endovascular treatment of aortic aneurysms involves the placement of an endovascular graft and stent via a percutaneous or open technique (usually through the femoral arteries) into the aneurysmal portion of the aorta. This technique has been reported to have a lower mortality rate compared to open surgical repair and is now being widely used in individuals with comorbid conditions that make them high-risk patients for open surgery. Some centers also report very promising results for the specific method in patients who do not constitute a high surgical risk group. Currently, nearly 80% of all AAAs are treated by EVAR in the United States.

A ruptured AAA represents a true surgical emergency. Documented rupture, particularly with associated hypotension, demands immediate transfer to an adequately equipped operating room for definitive repair without delay. Should aneurysm rupture occur, more than half of patients die before hospitalization or without treatment. Endovascular repair is currently the preferred method of treatment for ruptured AAAs.[48-50]

While the endovascular repair of AAAs offers many benefits (Table 14–3), there are several potential complications of this technique. The most significant of these complications are

---

TABLE 14–3 • Advantages of Endovascular Graft Exclusion of AAAs

- Procedure is performed from remote site and avoids laparotomy.
- Small incisions (femoral, brachial, or carotid artery cutdown for access).
- No prolonged aortic clamping.
- Decreased or no ICU stay.
- Decreased length of stay (1–2 days for endovascular vs 6–8 days for open repair).
- Decreased time to resumption of normal activity level.

TABLE 14-4 • Endoleak Types	
Type 1a, 1b	Endoleak whose origin is at the proximal (1a) or distal (1b) stent attachment site.
Type 2	Endoleak originating from a branch vessel. Possible sources include patent lumbar (posterior to the endovascular graft sonographically), inferior mesenteric (anterolateral to the endovascular graft sonographically), accessory renal or hypogastric arteries or other patent branches of the abdominal aorta. These are best seen in the transverse orientation.
Type 3	Endoleak that originates at the junctions between components of modular devices or from fabric tears within the graft.
Type 4	Transgraft flow or flow that fills the aneurysm sac due to porosity of the graft.
Endotension	Increase in aneurysm size in the absence of endoleak.

endoleak, and graft migration, which have been described for all of the endovascular grafts that have been used to date for endovascular AAA repair.

An endoleak is defined as flow outside of the endovascular graft that perfuses and pressurizes the aneurysm sac. This ongoing pressurization of the aneurysm sac carries with it the persistent risk of aneurysm enlargement and consequently rupture. The presence of an endoleak, therefore, negates the primary goal of the endovascular procedure and results in an aneurysm that remains inadequately treated. Several types of endoleak have been described (Table 14-4). Although, other complications of endovascular AAA repair have been described (Table 14-5), considerable progress in patient selection and surgical technique has reduced the overall rate of these problems.

TABLE 14-5 • Complications Associated With Endovascular Repair of Abdominal Aortic Aneurysms
Aneurysm growth
Embolization
Fabric tears
Graft infection
Graft migration
Hook fracture
Limb thrombosis
Limb separation
Endoleak*

*Common to all endovascular grafts used to date.

Currently, the optimal method for postendovascular graft screening and the most reliable method for detecting endoleak and complications are subject to debate. CT is favored in some centers and color Doppler ultrasound in others[51-56] (Fig. 14-36), although increased use of color duplex ultrasound is suggested for postoperative surveillance after EVAR in the absence of endoleak or aneurysm expansion.[48,56]

Patients undergoing EVAR will probably require routine, lifelong follow-up, and imaging surveillance,[48] and frequent assessment and objective follow-up are critical following EVAR. Color Doppler ultrasound has been used for aortic endovascular graft evaluation and has the advantage of being noninvasive, inexpensive, rapid, safe, nontoxic, easily repeatable, and well tolerated by patients. The combination of color Doppler imaging and Doppler waveform analysis can easily differentiate normal blood flow patterns from abnormal patterns associated with various pathologies. Because color Doppler is relatively inexpensive, easily repeatable, and without known risks, it has played an important role in the postprocedure surveillance follow-up of endovascular interventions.[17,51,54]

The *primary* objectives of the color Doppler examination following endovascular AAA repair will be to:

- Determine whether there is any blood flow in the aneurysm sac (endoleak) and to characterize the type of endoleak, if present
- Measure maximum residual aneurysm sac diameter (assess for enlarging sac size)

In addition, CDU detect other complications associated with the procedure such as iatrogenic injuries and can describe blood flow patterns through the main graft conduit and limbs, including the identification of any kinking, stenosis, or thrombosis that can impair graft function and/or result in end organ ischemia.

Patient Preparation. All patients with endografts potentially can be followed with CDU; however, while there are no real contraindications, there are real challenges. As with all abdominal scanning, the quality of the examination may be degraded in patients with a large body mass index or when abundant bowel gas is present. Patient preparation may be necessary. The patient should fast overnight or for at least 8 hours before the study. This will decrease the amount of intestinal gas and facilitate visualization of the graft and attachment sites. Usually, no other patient preparation is necessary.

Technologist Preparation. To perform a thorough and optimal examination of the endovascular graft, the examiner should be familiar with the various endovascular graft designs. Optimally, the examiner should have information about the specific endograft configuration, including the locations of the proximal and distal attachment sites. In addition, review of the operative report or discussion with the interventionalist or

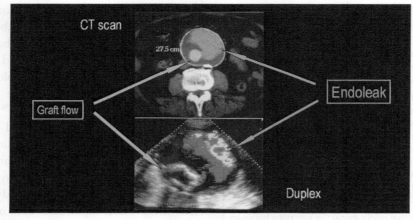

FIGURE 14–36. Top is a CT scan in a patient with an endovascular graft placed to exclude an abdominal aortic aneurysm. Contrast is seen in both the graft and aneurysm sac. Bottom is a color flow image in the same patient that reveals color flow in the graft (blue) and in the aneurysm sac. These findings are diagnostic of endoleak.

surgeon is recommended to determine whether other ancillary procedures were performed.

Ultrasound Examination of Aortic Endografts. The CDU examination of aortic endografts is well described and includes evaluation of the entirety of the endograft with an emphasis on the detection of endoleak and the acquisition of cross-sectional diameter measurements to determine maximum aneurysm size. When an aneurysm sac is excluded from the circulation, it should remain stable or decrease in size over time. Any increase in size suggests that there is preserved blood flow into the aneurysm sac (endoleak) with associated increase in sac pressure, which results in a continued risk for aneurysm rupture. It is also important to determine whether the distal arterial circulation has been preserved by ensuring that there are no kinks or obstructions within the body of the endovascular graft, the graft limb(s), and the inflow and outflow arteries. This can be done using a well-defined protocol.[56]

References

1. Powis RL, Schwartz RA. *Practical Doppler Ultrasound for the Clinician.* Baltimore: Williams & Wilkins; 1991:52.

2. Hallet JW, Brewster DC, Darling RC. *Handbook of Patient Vascular Surgery.* 3rd ed. Boston: Little, Brown; 1995:6.

3. Williams PL, Warwick R, Dyson M, et al., eds. *Gray's Anatomy.* 37th ed. New York: Churchill Livingstone; 1989.

4. Stephens RB, Stillwell DL. *Arteries and Veins of the Human Brain.* Springfield, Charles C Thomas; 1969.

5. McVay CB. *Anson and McVay Surgical Anatomy.* 6th ed. Philadelphia: WB Saunders; 1984.

6. Clemente CD (ed). *Gray's Anatomy of the Human Body.* 30th American ed. Philadelphia: Lea and Febiger; 1985.

7. Zwiebel WJ, Pellerito JS. *Introduction to Vascular Ultrasonography.* 5th ed. Philadelphia: WB Saunders; 2005.

8. Hedrick WR, Hykes DL, Strachman DE. *Ultrasound Physics and Instrumentation.* 3rd ed. St. Louis: Mosby; 1995.

9. Tortora GJ, Grabowski SR. *Principles of Anatomy & Physiology.* 7th ed. New York: Harper Collins; 1993.

10. Hackam DG, Anand SS. Emerging risk factors for atherosclerotic vascular disease. A critical review of the evidence. *JAMA.* 2003;290:932-940.

11. Patterson RF. Basic science in vascular disease. *J Vasc Technol.* 26(1):2002.

12. Maton A, Hopkins J, McLaughlin CW, et al. *Human Biology and Health.* Englewood Cliffs: Prentice Hall; 1993.

13. Tuzcu EM, Kapadia SR, Tutar E, et al. High prevalence of coronary atherosclerosis in asymptomatic teenagers and young adults: evidence from intravascular ultrasound. *Circulation.* 2001;103(22):2705-2710.

14. Fishbein MC, Schoenfield LJ. Heart Attack Photo Illustration Essay on MedicineNet.com.

15. Sales CM, Goldsmith J, Veith FJ. *Handbook of Vascular Surgery.* St. Louis: Quality Medical Publishing; 1994.

16. Kang SS, Labropoulos N, Mansour MA, Baker WH. Percutaneous ultrasound guided thrombin injection: a new method for treating postcatheterization femoral pseudoaneurysms. *J Vasc Surg.* 1998 Dec;28(6):1120-1121.

17. Berdejo GL, Wengerter KR, Marin ML, Suggs WD, Veith FJ. Color flow duplex guided manual occlusion of iatrogenic arteriovenous fistulas. *J Vasc Tech.* 1995;19(2):79-83.

18. Jonathan RB, Hutt, Davies AH. Nonatherosclerotic vascular disease. In: Davies AH, Brophy CM, eds. *Vascular Surgery.* London: Springer; 2006.

19. Hobson RW, Veith FJ, Wilson SE, Veith FJ, eds. Robert W. Hobson (Editor). *Vascular Surgery: Principles and Practice.* Marcel Dekker; October 2003.

20. Hirsch AT, Criqui MH, Treat-Jacobson D, et al. Peripheral Arterial Disease Detection, awareness and treatment in primary care. *JAMA.* 2001 Sep 19;286(11):1317-1324.

21. Gerlock AJ, Giyanani VL, Krebs CA. *Applications of Noninvasive Vascular Techniques.* Philadelphia: WB Saunders; 1988.

22. Needham T. Physiologic testing of lower extremity arterial disease: Segmental pressures, plethysmography and velocity waveforms. In Mansour AM, Labropoulos N, eds. *Vascular Diagnosis.* Philadelphia: Elsevier Saunders; 2005.

23. Hessel SJ, Adams DF, Abrams HL. Complications of angiography. *Radiology.* 1981;138:273-281.

24. Sigstedt B, Lunderquist A. Complications of angiographic examinations. *AJR*. 1978;130:455-460.

25. Formanek G, Frech RS, Amplatz K. Arterial thrombus formation during clinical percutaneous catheterization. *Circulation*. 1990;41:833-839.

26. Lang EK. A survey of the complications of percutaneous retrograde arteriography. *Radiology*. 1963;81:257-263.

27. Larch E, Minar E, Ahmadi R, et al. Value of color duplex sonography for evaluation of tibioperoneal arteries in patients with femoropopliteal obstruction: a prospective comparison with antegrade intraarterial digital subtraction angiography. *J Vasc Surg*. 1997;25:629-636.

28. Karacagil S, Lofberg AM, Granbo A, Lorelius LE, Bergqvist D. Value of duplex scanning in evaluation of crural and foot arteries in limbs with severe lower limb ischaemia—a prospective comparison with angiography. *Eur J Vasc Endovasc Surg*. 1996;12:300-303.

29. Wain R, Berdejo GL, Delvalle WN, et al. Can duplex scan arterial mapping replace contrast arteriography as the test of choice before infrainguinal revascularization. *J Vasc Sur*. 1999;29:100-109.

30. Ascher E, Mazzariol F, Hingorani Salles-Cunha S, Gade P. The use of duplex arterial mapping as an alternative to conventional arteriography for primary and secondary infrapopliteal bypasses. *M J Surg*. 1999;178:162-165.

31. Cramer MM. Color flow duplex examination of the abdominal aorta: atherosclerosis, aneurysm, and dissection. *J Vasc Tech*. 1995;19(5–6).

32. Bandyk DF, Armstrong PA. Duplex Scanning in Vascular Disorders. Surveillance of infrainguonal bypass grafts. In: Zierler RE, ed. Philadelphia: Lippincott, Williams and Wilkins; 2010:341-349.

33. Cossman DV, Ellison JE, Wagner WH, et al. Comparison of contrast arteriography to arterial mapping with color-flow duplex imaging in the lower extremities. *J Vasc Surg*. 1989;10:522-529.

34. Polak JF, Karmel MI, Mannick JA, O'Leary DH, Donaldson MC, Whittemore AD. Determination of the extent of lower-extremity peripheral arterial disease with color assisted duplex sonography: comparison with angiography. *AJR*. 1990;155:1085-1089.

35. Hatsukami TS, Primozich JF, Zierler E, Harley JD, Strandness DE. Color Doppler imaging of infrainguinal arterial occlusive disease. *J Vasc Surg*. 1992;16:527-533.

36. Pemberton M, London NJM. Colour flow duplex imaging of occlusive arterial disease of the lower limb. *Br J Surg*. 1997;84:912-919.

37. Sensier Y, Fishwick G, Owen R, Pemberton M, Bell PRF, London NJM. A comparison between colour duplex ultrasonography and arteriography for imaging infrapopliteal arterial lesions. *Eur J Endovasc Surg*. 1998;15:44-50.

38. Jager KA, Phillips DJ, Martin RL. Noninvasive mapping of lower limb arterial lesions. *Ultrasound Med Biol*. 1985;11:515-521.

39. Moneta GL, Yeager RA, Antonovic R, et al. Accuracy of lower extremity arterial duplex mapping. *J Vasc Surg*. 1992;15:275-284.

40. Kupper CA, Dewhirst N, Burnham SJ. Doppler spectral waveforms for recording peripheral arterial signals: the preferred method. *J Vasc Tecnol*. 1989;13:69-73.

41. Hoff FL, Mueller K, Pearce W. Computed tomography in vascular disease. In: Ascer E, ed. *Haimovici's Vascular Surgery*. 5th ed. Malden: Blackwell Publishing; 2004:chap 6.

42. Mathias Prokop MD, Schaefer-Prokop C. *Spiral and Multislice Computed Tomography of the Body*. Thieme Publishers; 2002.

43. Neiman HL, Lyons J. Fundamentals of angiography. In: Ascer E, ed. *Haimovici's Vascular Surgery*. 5th ed. Malden: Blackwell Publishing; 2004:chap 5.

44. Karmacharya JJ, Velazquez OC, Baum RA, Carpenter JP. Magnetic Resonance Angiography. In: Ascer E, ed. *Haimovici's Vascular Surgery*. 5th ed. Malden: Blackwell Publishing; 2004:chap 7.

45. Stoyioglou A, Jaff MR. Medical treatment of peripheral arterial disease: a comprehensive review. *JVIR*. 2004 Nov;15(11):1197-1207.

46. Lumsden AB, Lin P, eds. *Endovascular Therapy for Peripheral Vascular Disease*. Blackwell Publishing: 2006.

47. Ascer E, ed. *Haimovici's Vascular Surgery*. 5th ed. Malden: Blackwell Publishing; 2004.

48. Chaikof E, Dalman R, Eskandari M, et al. The Society for Vascular Surgery practice guidelines on the care of patients with an abdominal aortic aneurysm. *J Vasc Surg*. 2018;67:1-77.

49. Veith FJ, Gargiulo NJ. Endovascular aortic repair should be the gold standard for ruptured AAAs, and all vascular surgeons should be prepared to perform them. *Perspect Vasc Surg Endovasc Ther*. 2007 Sep;19(3):275-282.

50. Rutherford RB. Randomized EVAR trials and advent of level I evidence: a paradigm shift in management of large abdominal aortic aneurysms? *Semin Vasc Surg*. 2006 Jun;19(2):69-74.

51. Berdejo GL, Lyon RT, Ohki T, et al. Color duplex ultrasound evaluation of transluminally placed endovascular grafts for aneurysm repair. *J Vasc Technol*. 22(4):201-207, 1998.

52. Sato DT, Goff CD, Gregory RT, et al. Endoleak after aortic stent graft repair: Diagnosis by color duplex ultrasound vs. CT scan. *J Vasc Surg*. 1998; 28(4):657-663.

53. Lyon RT, Berdejo GL, Veith FJ. Ultrasound imaging techniques for evaluation of endovascular stented grafts. In: Parodi JC, Veith FJ, Marin ML, eds. *Endovascular Grafting Techniques*. Media: Williams & Wilkins; 1999.

54. Wolf YG, Johnson BL, Hill BB, Rubin GD, Fogarty TJ, Zarins CK. Duplex ultrasonography vs. CT angiography for postoperative evaluation of endovascular abdominal aortic aneurysms repair. *J Vasc Surg*. 2000 Dec;32(6):1142-1148.

55. Zanetti S, DeRango P, Parente B, et al. Role of duplex scan in endoleak detection after endoluminal aortic repair. *Eur J Vasc Endovasc Surg*. 2000;19:531-535.

56. Polak J, Berdejo GL. Ultrasound assessment following endovascular aortic aneurysm repair. In: Zwiebelw and Pellerito J, eds. *Introduction to Vascular Ultrasonography*. 7th ed, Philadelphia: Elsevier Saunders; 2020:chap 25.

Further Readings

Buck DB, van Herwaarden JA, Schermerhorn ML, Moll FL. Endovascular treatment of abdominal aortic aneurysms. *Nat Rev Cardiol*. 2014;11:112-123.

Dua A, Kuy S, Lee CJ, Upchurch GR Jr, Desai SS. Epidemiology of aortic aneurysm repair in the United States from 2000 to 2010. *J Vasc Surg*. 2014;59:1512-1517.

Gunabushanam G, Millet JD, Stilp E, et al. Computer-assisted detection of tardus parvus waveforms on Doppler ultrasound. *Ultrasound*. 2018 May;26(2):81-92.

Illig KA, Donahue D, Duncan A, et al. Reporting standards of the society for vascular surgery for thoracic outlet syndrome. *J Vasc Surg*. 2016;64:23-35. doi: 10.1016/j.jvs.2016.04.039.

Malanga GA, Landes P, Nadler SF. Provocative tests in cervical spine examination: historical basis and scientific analyses. *Pain Physician*. 2003 Apr;6(2):199-205.

Questions

GENERAL INSTRUCTIONS: For each question, select the best answer. Select only one answer for each question, unless otherwise instructed.

1. CW Doppler has how many crystals in the transducer?

   (A) one

   (B) two

   (C) three

   (D) four

2. If flow is toward the transducer, it is represented as a _____ shift.

   (A) positive

   (B) neutral

   (C) variable

   (D) negative

3. Maximum Doppler shift frequency occurs at

   (A) 90 degrees

   (B) 180 degrees

   (C) 0 degrees

   (D) 75 degrees

4. What instrumentation is used for measurement of volume changes in the extremities to demonstrate blood flow?

   (A) CW Doppler

   (B) Color flow Doppler

   (C) plethysmography

   (D) pulse volume recording

5. Which of the following is not true of the spectral analysis?

   (A) mathematical display of the frequency components in the Doppler signal

   (B) computer using the FFT method

   (C) demonstrates the presence, direction, and characteristics of blood flow

   (D) Does not provide measurements of the blood flow

6. Name the components of the spectral analysis labeled on Fig. 14–37.

   (A) _____

   (B) _____

   (C) _____

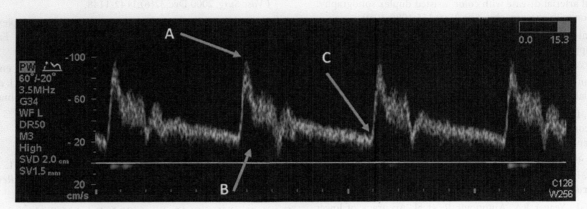

FIGURE 14–37.

7. **Spectral broadening seen on the spectral analysis is most likely due to**

(A) normal arterial waveform

(B) increased bandwidth caused by disturbed flow

(C) decreased bandwidth caused by disturbed flow

(D) increased bandwidth caused by laminar flow

8. **Which statement is *not* true about aliasing?**

(A) Velocities exceed the Nyquist limit.

(B) There is wrap-around of the waveform.

(C) Higher velocities appear on the negative side of the baseline.

(D) Not controlled by the pulse repetition rate.

9. **Fig. 14–38 demonstrates**

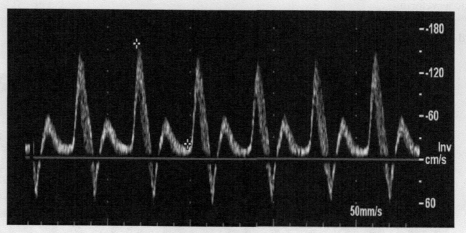

FIGURE 14–38.

(A) aliasing

(B) turbulence

(C) monophasic waveform

(D) triphasic waveform

10. **Fig. 14–39 demonstrates**

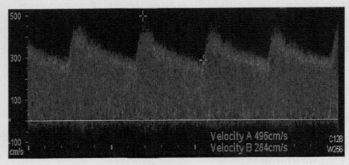

FIGURE 14–39.

(A) spectral broadening

(B) aliasing

(C) monophasic waveform

(D) triphasic waveform

11. **Fig. 14–40 demonstrates**

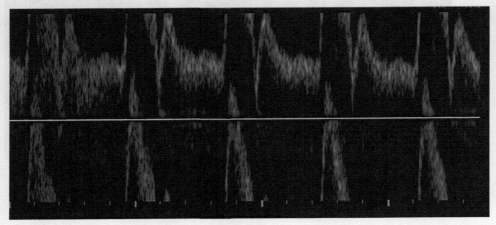

FIGURE 14–40.

(A) dampened waveform

(B) aliasing of the waveform

(C) monophasic waveform

(D) triphasic waveform

12. **Fig. 14–41 demonstrates**

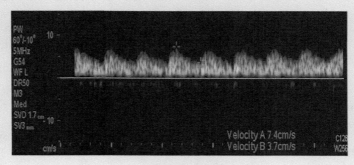

FIGURE 14–41.

(A) spectral broadening

(B) aliasing

(C) turbulence

(D) monophasic waveform

13. **Fig. 14–42 demonstrates**

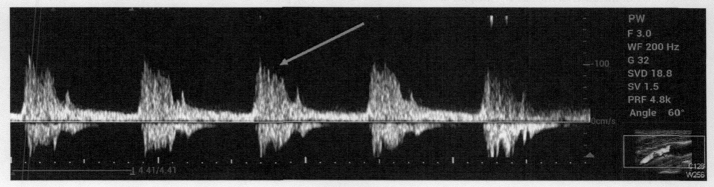

FIGURE 14–42.

(A) to-and-fro flow

(B) aliasing

(C) turbulence

(D) tardus parvus waveform

14. **An interventional procedure where a balloon catheter is placed in a vessel and dilated to eliminate stenotic lesions is called**

(A) digital subtraction angiography

(B) MRI

(C) positron emission tomography

(D) PTA

15. **The physiology of circulation is called**

(A) fluid dynamics

(B) circulatory system

(C) hemodynamics

(D) coronary circulation

16. **Blood movement in concentric layers with the highest velocity in the center of the vessel that creates a parabolic flow profile is**

(A) laminar flow

(B) disorganized flow

(C) boundary layer separation

(D) turbulent flow

17. **What type of plethysmogarphy identifies subcutaneous blood flow?**

    (A) air

    (B) strain gauge

    (C) impedance

    (D) photo

18. **In the poststenotic flow zone, there may be swirling movements and chaotic flow referred to as**

    (A) collateral flow

    (B) turbulent flow

    (C) reversed flow

    (D) laminar flow

19. **Which statement is not true of the Reynolds number?**

    (A) defines the point where flow changes from laminar to disturbed

    (B) is less than 2000 in the normal arterial circulation

    (C) is not included in the basic principles of fluid dynamics

    (D) predicts the stability of a fluid

20. **Laminar flow tends to be disturbed if the Reynolds number exceeds what value?**

    (A) 500

    (B) 700

    (C) 1000

    (D) 1500

    (E) 2000

21. **Disturbed, chaotic flow noted beyond a stenosis/narrowing of a blood vessel is**

    (A) poststenotic turbulence

    (B) velocity jet

    (C) laminar flow

    (D) dampened flow

22. **How is the velocity of blood flow related to the cross-sectional area of the blood vessel?**

    (A) inversely

    (B) directly related

    (C) not related

    (D) variable

23. **BP is**

    (A) volume of blood flowing through the vessel

    (B) average pressure throughout the cardiac cycle

    (C) pulse pressure in circulatory system

    (D) pressure exerted by blood on the wall of a blood vessel

24. **In a resting young adult, the BP is**

    (A) 100 mm Hg during systole and 50 mm Hg during diastole

    (B) 120 mm Hg during systole and 40 mm Hg during diastole

    (C) 150 mm Hg during systole and 70 mm Hg during diastole

    (D) 120 mm Hg during systole and 70 mm Hg during diastole

25. **The expansion and contraction of arteries after each systole of the left ventricle creates a pressure wave termed**

    (A) cycle

    (B) waveform

    (C) pulse

    (D) mean

26. **The resting pulse is**

    (A) between 70 and 80 beats/min

    (B) over 100 beats/min

    (C) under 50 beats/min

    (D) between 25 and 75 beats/min

27. **Each is a predisposing factor for arterial occlusive disease, *except***

    (A) smoking

    (B) diabetes

    (C) hypertension

    (D) bradycardia

28. **What is the most common symptom of lower extremity arterial disease?**

    (A) ulceration

    (B) absence of pulses

    (C) claudication

    (D) cyanosis

29. **Which of the following is not one of the classic six Ps for acute arterial ischemia?**

    (A) pain

    (B) pallor

    (C) pressure

    (D) paresthesias

30. The ABI is used in which examination?

    (A) strain gauge plethysmography

    (B) peripheral angiography

    (C) peripheral venous evaluation

    (D) segmental pressure arterial examination

31. During the segmental arterial pressure examination, the pressure recorded is the pressure

    (A) under the cuff that is inflated and deflated

    (B) at the posterior tibial artery

    (C) below where the cuff is inflated and deflated

    (D) above where the cuff is inflated and deflated

32. In segmental arterial studies, the cuff at each site is inflated until the systolic pressure, sound or Doppler waveform

    (A) appears

    (B) disappears

    (C) remains constant

    (D) none of the above

33. What is used as the standard pressure for segmental arterial studies?

    (A) the lowest posterior tibial artery systolic artery pressure

    (B) the highest common femoral artery systolic artery pressure

    (C) the highest brachial artery systolic artery pressure

    (D) the highest anterior tibial artery systolic artery pressure

34. The bilateral brachial pressures should be within

    (A) 5 mm Hg

    (B) 20 mm Hg

    (C) 25 mm Hg

    (D) 50 mm Hg

35. An ABI of 0.6–0.9 indicates

    (A) normal value

    (B) claudication

    (C) severe occlusive disease

    (D) occlusion

36. An ABI of 0.5 or less indicates

    (A) normal value

    (B) claudication

    (C) severe occlusive disease

    (D) occlusion

37. This is a logical next step in patients with elevated ankle pressures (>200 mm Hg) and suspicion of calcified vessels

    (A) color flow Doppler

    (B) strain gauge plethysmography

    (C) brachial pressures

    (D) toe pressures

38. The normal toe pressure is what?

    (A) equal to the brachial pressure

    (B) equal to the ankle index pressure

    (C) 65% of the brachial pressure

    (D) 75% of the brachial pressure

39. With exercise as flow velocity in a stenosis increases what happens to the pressure across said stenosis?

    (A) increases

    (B) decreases

    (C) remains unchanged

    (D) creates a high variable

40. Composition of the arteries does not include

    (A) intima

    (B) media

    (C) adventitia

    (D) internal capsule

41. As sympathetic stimulation is increased, the smooth muscle of the artery contracts and narrows the vessel lumen. This is called

    (A) vasodilatation

    (B) vascular narrowing

    (C) vasoconstriction

    (D) vasospasm

42. Which artery is present only on right side of the upper extremity?

    (A) brachiocephalic

    (B) subclavian

    (C) thyrocervical

    (D) costocervical

43. Which arterial vessel is a direct continuation of the subclavian?

    (A) vertebral

    (B) common carotid

    (C) axillary

    (D) brachiocephalic

44. The terminal branches of the brachial artery are the
    (A) axillary and subclavian
    (B) palmar and digital
    (C) radial and ulnar
    (D) radial and palmar

45. Which arterial vessel is a continuation of the external iliac artery?
    (A) common femoral
    (B) superficial femoral
    (C) profunda femoral
    (D) popliteal

46. Which vessel lies posterior to the medial aspect of the ankle?
    (A) anterior tibial
    (B) perineal
    (C) posterior tibial
    (D) dorsalis pedis

47. Ischemia is secondary to
    (A) excessive blood flow
    (B) normal blood flow
    (C) decreased blood flow
    (D) none of the above

48. Embolism is
    (A) obstruction of artery by clot or other foreign material
    (B) atherosclerotic plaque formation
    (C) trauma to an artery with resulting occlusion
    (D) dissection of an artery caused by trauma

49. This type of pain is present during exertion and disappears upon cessation of activity?
    (A) rest pain
    (B) claudication pain
    (C) trauma pain
    (D) normal exercise

50. The majority of arterial disease is caused by
    (A) genetic origin
    (B) atherosclerosis
    (C) cardiac disease
    (D) diabetes

51. Blood flow and pressures are not significantly diminished until at least what percentage of the cross-sectional area of the vessel is obliterated?
    (A) 25%
    (B) 50%
    (C) 75%
    (D) 95%

52. Factors that influence a critical stenosis are all, except
    (A) length of the stenosis
    (B) blood viscosity
    (C) peripheral resistance
    (D) all of the above

53. The most common site of atherosclerotic occlusion in the lower extremity is
    (A) common femoral artery bifurcation into superficial and deep femoral artery
    (B) profunda (deep) femoral artery
    (C) distal superficial femoral artery in the adductor canal
    (D) popliteal artery

54. Which artery in the lower extremity passes through the interosseous membrane and courses along the anterolateral aspect of the leg?
    (A) posterior tibial
    (B) anterior tibial
    (C) peroneal
    (D) dorsalis pedis

55. A stenosis or occlusion of the subclavian artery proximal to the vertebral artery can sometimes result in
    (A) subclavian steal syndrome
    (B) thoracic outlet syndrome
    (C) vertebral-basilar occlusive disease
    (D) vertebral artery stenosis

56. Intrinsic compression of the vessels by the clavicle, first rib, and the scalene muscles is characteristic of
    (A) subclavian steal
    (B) thoracic outlet syndrome
    (C) subclavian aneurysms
    (D) Raynaud's disease

57. Provocative maneuvers are used during diagnostic testing for

 (A) Hunter's disease
 (B) Takayasu's disease
 (C) thoracic outlet syndrome
 (D) compartment syndrome

58. A functional vasospastic disorder that affects the small arteries of the extremities is

 (A) Raynaud's disease or syndrome
 (B) Raynaud's phenomenon
 (C) thoracic outlet syndrome
 (D) subclavian steal

59. An obstructive arterial disease that has an underlying systemic or vascular abnormality is

 (A) Raynaud's disease
 (B) Raynaud's phenomenon
 (C) thoracic outlet syndrome
 (D) subclavian steal

60. This entity is a collection of blood contained by surrounding tissue that communicates with an adjacent artery via an extravascular neck or tract

 (A) dissection
 (B) pseudoaneurysm
 (C) arteriovenous malformation
 (D) seroma

61. Which type of aneurysm is associated with an infectious process?

 (A) pseudoaneurysm
 (B) mycotic
 (C) dissecting
 (D) fusiform

62. This condition is usually a result of trauma that causes a sudden tear in the intimal lining of the vessel that produces two lumens?

 (A) pseudoaneurysm
 (B) mycotic aneurysm
 (C) dissection
 (D) saccular aneurysm

63. What modality best provides information regarding the severity of the atherosclerotic process in the evaluation of lower extremity arterial disease?

 (A) color flow Doppler
 (B) spectral waveform analysis

 (C) ABI
 (D) duplex scanning

64. A decrease in peak systolic flow velocity in an arterial bypass graft to less than 40–45 cm/s may indicate

 (A) Pseudoaneurysm in a graft segment
 (B) stenosis of the graft
 (C) occlusion of the graft
 (D) impending graft failure

65. A communication between the artery and the vein is

 (A) pseudoaneurysm
 (B) aneurysm
 (C) AVF
 (D) dissection

66. The Pourcelot index is used to quantify

 (A) arterial flow
 (B) resistance
 (C) turbulence
 (D) volume of flow

67. Tachycardia means

 (A) rapid heart rate
 (B) slow heart rate
 (C) normal heart rate
 (D) irregular heart rate

68. Which of the following is not a noninvasive testing procedure?

 (A) Doppler
 (B) plethysmography
 (C) segmental pressures
 (D) arteriography

69. The ABI is calculated as the

 (A) brachial systolic pressure divided by the ankle systolic pressure
 (B) the ankle systolic pressure divided by the brachial systolic pressure
 (C) brachial diastolic pressure divided by the ankle diastolic pressure
 (D) ankle diastolic pressure divided by the brachial diastolic pressure

70. The units for the ABI are

(A) cm/s

(B) mm Hg

(C) MHz

(D) None of the above

71. What is required before the performance of the vascular noninvasive examination?

(A) evaluation of BP

(B) process screening

(C) patient history

(D) billing procedures

72. The four-cuff segmental pressure evaluation differentiates between

(A) iliac and femoral artery disease

(B) superficial femoral and popliteal artery disease

(C) both A and B

(D) none of the above

73. Normal mean renal artery RI in an adult is

(A) 0.6–0.7

(B) 0.7–0.8

(C) <0.4

(D) none of the above

74. The two major pathways of the cardiovascular system are

(A) arterial and venous

(B) systemic and pulmonary circulation

(C) cerebrovascular and systemic circulation

(D) cerebrovascular, systemic, and pulmonary circulation

75. Which layer of the artery is composed of smooth muscle cells and elastic fibers?

(A) intima

(B) media

(C) adventitia

(D) tunica externa

76. What is the first major branch of the subclavian artery?

(A) thyrocervical

(B) internal mammary

(C) costocervical trunk

(D) vertebral

77. Signs and symptoms of arterial occlusive disease of the lower extremity include

(A) intermittent claudication

(B) dependent rubor

(C) pallor on elevation

(D) all of the above

78. Risk factors that play a part in the development of atherosclerosis of the extremities include

(A) cigarette smoking

(B) hypertension

(C) diabetes

(D) all of the above

79. The Doppler signal in Fig. 14–43 demonstrates

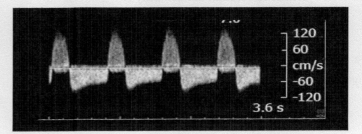

FIGURE 14–43.

(A) triphasic flow

(B) monophasic flow

(C) pseudoaneurysm neck flow

(D) tardus parvus flow

80. With a hemodynamically significant stenosis, one would expect

(A) a focally increased peak-systolic velocity

(B) a decreased peak-systolic velocity and a decreased end-diastolic velocity

(C) no change in the peak-systolic velocity and a decreased end-diastolic velocity

(D) none of the above

81. All of the following can be derived from PW Doppler spectral display, except

(A) presence of flow

(B) direction of flow

(C) characteristics of flow

(D) viscosity of flow

82. Spectral broadening results in the loss of the spectral window below the peak-systolic velocity spectral waveform in systole. Which of the following statements is true?

    (A) A small sample volume placed centrally in the artery should decrease the size of the spectral window.

    (B) The spectral window fills as flow disturbances produce vortices (swirling eddies) with varying flow direction.

    (C) Vortices (rotating flow) will show only forward flow and produce a narrow band of velocities demonstrating a clear spectral window.

    (D) Loss of the spectral window occur only with stenotic lesions of 75% or greater.

83. Appreciable changes in pressure and flow do not occur until the diameter of an artery is reduced by 50% or greater. This degree of narrowing is called

    (A) hemodynamically significant stenosis

    (B) Nyquist limit (50% of the PRF)

    (C) Bernoulli's principle

    (D) Poiseuille's law

84. The principal control mechanisms affecting blood volume changes are

    (A) viscosity and blood vessel diameter

    (B) cardiac output and peripheral resistance

    (C) BP gradients and inertial losses

    (D) energy losses and flow-reducing lesions

85. One advantage of CW versus PW Doppler is

    (A) the ability to differentiate overlying blood vessels

    (B) minimal spectral broadening

    (C) high velocities can be displayed without aliasing

    (D) control of the depth selection of the sample site

86. Factors affecting the Doppler shift frequency include

    (A) Doppler angle

    (B) transducer frequency

    (C) velocity of the red blood cells

    (D) all of the above

87. As hemodynamically significant stenosis becomes more severe, which statement is true?

    (A) Flow volume increases, peak-systolic velocity decreases.

    (B) Flow volume decreases, peak-systolic velocity decreases.

    (C) Flow volume decreases, peak-systolic velocity increases.

    (D) Flow volume increases, peak-systolic velocity increases.

88. The highest peak systolic velocity is found

    (A) at the narrowest portion of the stenotic lesion

    (B) just proximal to the stenotic lesion

    (C) just distal to the stenotic lesion

    (D) both proximal and distal to the stenotic lesion

89. The flow pattern throughout the stenotic lesion will be

    (A) laminar

    (B) retrograde

    (C) disturbed

    (D) none of the above

90. As the radius of an artery decreases there is

    (A) lower resistance to flow

    (B) higher resistance to flow

    (C) no change in the resistance

    (D) variable resistance

91. Which of the following is not used to determine the severity of arterial stenoses?

    (A) peak systolic velocity

    (B) end-diastolic velocity

    (C) systolic velocity ratio

    (D) volume flow

92. With a 50–99% diameter reduction, there will generally be

    (A) spectral broadening with no window under the systolic peak, peak velocity less than 100% of the proximal adjacent segment

    (B) normal waveform with slight spectral broadening

    (C) peak velocity 100% more than the adjacent proximal segment and reversed flow component is usually absent

    (D) none of the above

93. In Fig. 14–44, this image of the iliac artery shows

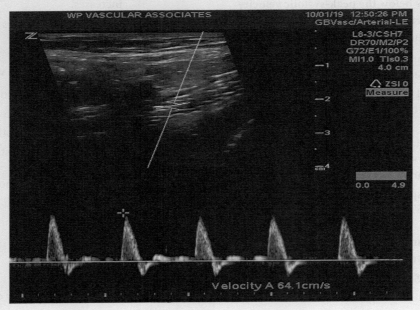

FIGURE 14–44.

(A) iliac artery with stenosis

(B) iliac artery with occlusion

(C) normal flow profile

(D) iliac artery monophasic flow

94. In Fig. 14–45, color flow image and spectral analysis of the external iliac artery shows

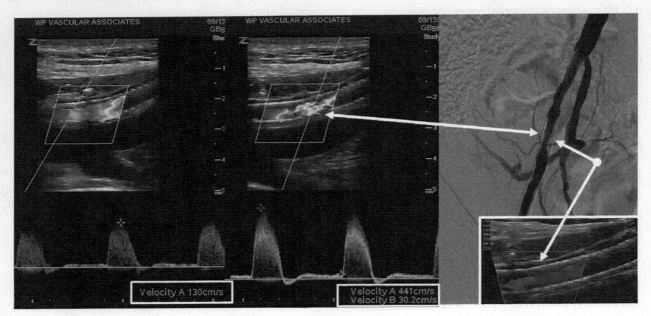

FIGURE 14–45.

(A) normal waveform

(B) site of stenosis

(C) dissection

(D) pseudoaneurysm

95. In Fig. 14–46, the findings are most consistent with

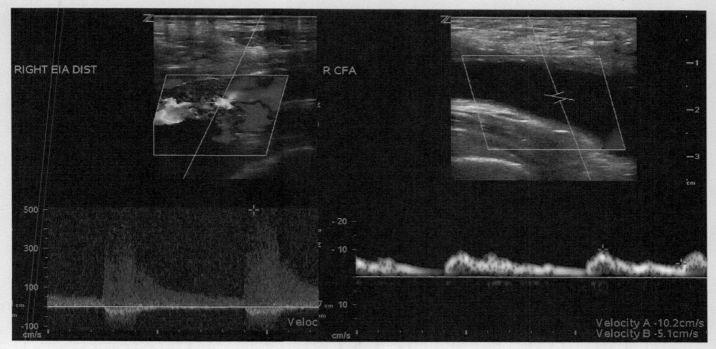

FIGURE 14–46.

(A) plug flow proximal to an occlusion

(B) aliasing secondary to high grade stenosis

(C) aliasing in a mild to moderate stenosis

(D) plug flow distal to an occlusion

96. In Fig. 14–47, physiologic testing of the lower
extremities shows

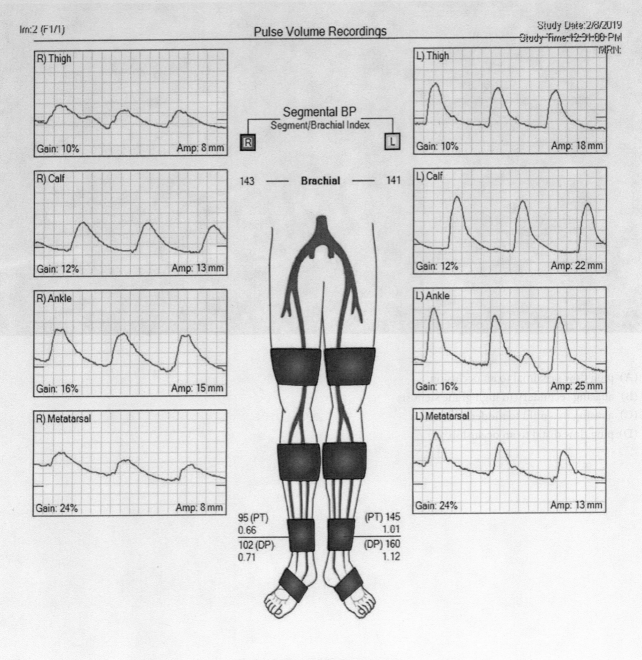

FIGURE 14–47.

(A) severe occlusive disease of the right lower extremity

(B) claudication disease of the left lower extremity

(C) bilateral moderate occlusive disease

(D) moderate right-sided iliac artery disease

97. In Fig. 14–48, the physiologic testing of the lower extremities in this diabetic patient shows

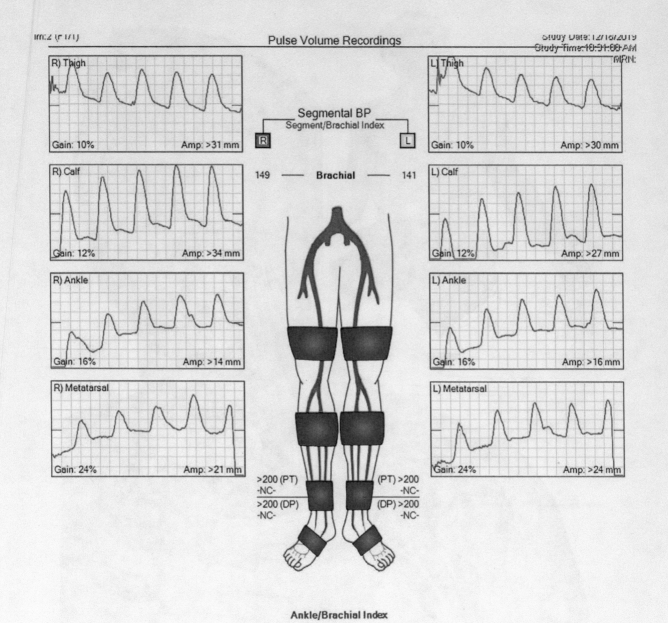

FIGURE 14–48.

(A) normal segmental PVR and pressure study

(B) bilateral arterial disease based on noncompressible vessels

(C) bilateral iliac artery stenosis

(D) normal segmental PVR with elevated ankle pressures likely due to diabetic disease

98. In Fig. 14–49, Adson's maneuver is

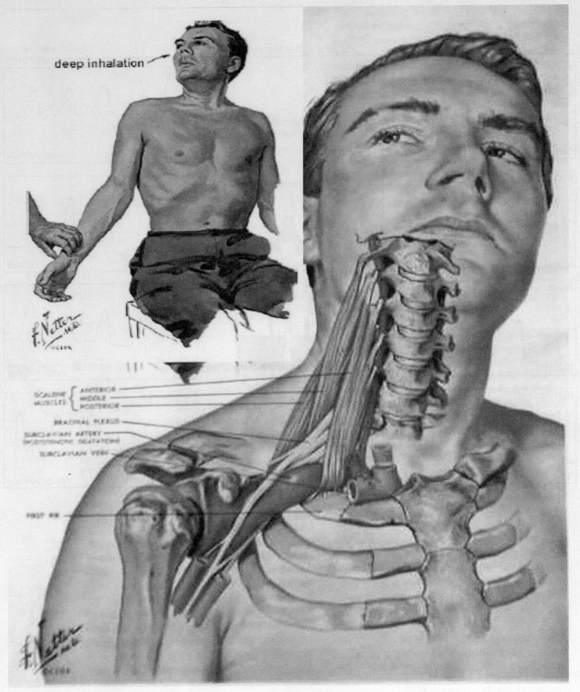

deep inhalation

SCALENE { ANTERIOR
MUSCLES { MIDDLE
          POSTERIOR

BRACHIAL PLEXUS

SUBCLAVIAN ARTERY
(POSTSTENOTIC DILATATION)

SUBCLAVIAN VEIN

FIRST RIB

FIGURE 14–49.

(A) an important and reliable component for thoracic
    outlet compression evaluation

(B) an important and reliable component for Raynaud's
    disease evaluation

(C) an important and reliable component for subclavian
    steal evaluation

(D) no longer widely utilized

99. In Fig. 14–50, the real-time image of the aorta shows

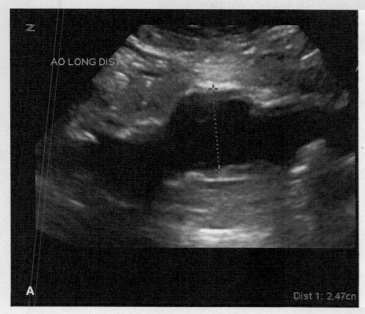 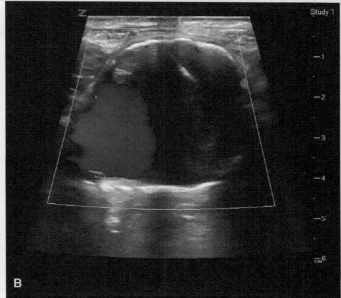

FIGURE 14–50.

(A) long- and short-axis normal aorta
(B) aortic dissection
(C) abdominal aortic aneurysm with calcified wall
(D) abdominal aortic aneurysm with mural thrombus

100. In Fig. 14–51, the ABI on the right is

(A) 0.50
(B) 0.67
(C) 0.33
(D) 0.25

RIGHT

Brachial
Pressure =
160 mmHg

PT = 40 mmHg
DP = 80 mmHg

LEFT

Brachial
Pressure =
120 mmHg

PT = 120 mmHg
DP = 80 mmHg

FIGURE 14–51.

101. Digital BP is generally

(A) within 15–20 mm Hg of the brachial pressure
(B) the same as the brachial pressure
(C) within 10–20 mm Hg of the brachial pressure
(D) within 30–40 mm Hg of the brachial pressure

102. Normal vessel flow profiles should exhibit a
_____ rise time to the onset of systole to the peak
of systole.

(A) very slow
(B) rapid
(C) fluctuating
(D) none of the above

103. Which is not a manifestation of chronic peripheral
arterial occlusive disease

(A) malleolar ulcer
(B) claudication
(C) rest pain
(D) varicose veins

104. A patient with hip and buttock claudication most likely has occlusion of

(A) peroneal artery

(B) iliac arteries

(C) superficial femoral artery

(D) profunda femoris artery

105. Patients with erectile dysfunction (vasculogenic impotence) most likely have occlusion of the _____ as the cause

(A) hypogastric artery

(B) common femoral artery

(C) right renal artery

(D) deep femoral artery

106. A patient with an absent right but normal left common femoral artery pulse may have an occlusion of the

(A) aorta

(B) right deep femoral artery

(C) right common iliac artery

(D) right hypogastric artery

107. Exercise testing helps differentiate patients with true vasculogenic leg pain with ambulation from those with

(A) pseudoclaudication

(B) swelling

(C) ischemic ulcer

(D) rest pain

108. A complete history must include questions around

(A) previous surgical history

(B) risk factors

(C) symptoms

(D) all of the above

109. A thorough physical examination of the patient with suspected arterial occlusive disease includes all the following, except

(A) pulse palpation

(B) palpation for temperature of the extremity

(C) chest x-ray

(D) visual examination of the feet and toes

110. The most common complaint with arterial occlusive disease is

(A) pain

(B) swelling

(C) ulceration

(D) thickened nails

111. A sudden blockage of a main artery is most often seen in patients with

(A) chronic arterial occlusion

(B) acute arterial occlusion

(C) thrombophlebitis

(D) all of the above

112. The most common cause of acute arterial occlusion is

(A) emboli from the heart

(B) trauma

(C) emboli from an abdominal aneurysm

(D) plaque rupture

113. A great toe ulcer is most likely caused by

(A) acute arterial occlusion

(B) thrombophlebitis

(C) chronic arterial occlusion

(D) diabetes

114. A patient with acute arterial occlusion of the lower extremity may present with

(A) skin mottling

(B) cyanosis

(C) pallor

(D) all of the Above

115. Causes for acute arterial occlusion include

(A) embolus

(B) graft thrombosis

(C) trauma

(D) all of the above

116. All of these are common presentations of acute arterial occlusion, except

(A) ulcer

(B) pain

(C) cold extremity

(D) numbness

117. Constant pain in the foot or toes that is relieved by dependency of the extremity is

(A) claudication

(B) rest pain

(C) neuropathy

(D) necrosis

118. The most severe form of chronic arterial occlusive disease is

    (A) calf claudication
    (B) ischemic rest pain
    (C) dependent rubor
    (D) tissue loss and gangrene

119. Patient presenting with rest pain and/or gangrene are most likely to present with

    (A) multilevel occlusive disease
    (B) single-level disease
    (C) tibial disease only
    (D) superficial femoral artery occlusion

120. Arterial ulcers are least likely to occur at the level of the

    (A) toes
    (B) heel
    (C) dorsum of the foot
    (D) medial malleolus

121. Rest pain can be differentiated from diabetic neuropathic pain in that true rest pain is

    (A) often alleviated by dependency
    (B) alleviated by elevation
    (C) alleviated by exercise
    (D) none of the above

122. Which physical findings are often seen in a patient with vasculogenic rest pain

    (A) absent pedal pulses
    (B) dependent rubor
    (C) thickened nails
    (D) all of the above

123. Aortoiliac occlusive disease can result in all, *except*

    (A) a decreased common femoral artery pulse
    (B) calf claudication
    (C) severe thigh and leg swelling
    (D) no symptoms at all

124. A bounding, widened, very prominent popliteal artery pulse can be diagnostic of

    (A) an arterial occlusion
    (B) an aneurysm
    (C) a normal vessel
    (D) a AVF

125. Claudication is

    (A) exercise-related leg pain that is reproduced by the same level of exercise and is relieved by rest
    (B) pain in the distal most aspect of the foot
    (C) pain in the thigh that radiates to the calf and is worst walking uphill
    (D) derived from the Greek word "claudico" meaning to limp

126. Auscultation of the arteries using a stethoscope is performed to detect

    (A) pulse
    (B) pain
    (C) bruit
    (D) thrombosis

127. A weak, pallid upper extremity associated with diminished sensory and motor function of the forearm and hand is most likely consistent with

    (A) acute axillobrachial artery occlusion
    (B) chronic axillary-brachial artery occlusion
    (C) acute axillosubclavian vein thrombosis
    (D) subclavian artery stenosis

128. Upper extremity pulse palpation includes assessment of all, *except*

    (A) palmar artery
    (B) subclavian artery
    (C) brachial artery
    (D) axillary artery

129. A test that is used to assess the collateral circulation to the hand and digits is

    (A) digit to brachial index
    (B) Allen's test
    (C) wrist to brachial index
    (D) ABI

130. A bruit in the epigastric region may be due to

    (A) renal artery stenosis
    (B) renal artery occlusion
    (C) aortic occlusion
    (D) aortic aneurysm

131. **The magnitude of the Doppler shift is**

    (A) inversely related to the angle of incidence

    (B) proportional to the angle of incidence

    (C) no relation to the angle of incidence

    (D) inversely related to the signal to noise ratio

132. **A diameter reduction of 50% corresponds to**

    (A) 25% cross-sectional area reduction

    (B) 50% cross-sectional area reduction

    (C) 75% cross-sectional area reduction

    (D) 95% cross-sectional area reduction

133. **The mathematical computation of the reflected pulse that displays individual frequencies is done using**

    (A) Doppler equation

    (B) Bernoulli's equation

    (C) Poiseuille's equation

    (D) FFT

134. **An endoleak is defined as**

    (A) flow in the endograft limb

    (B) flow outside of the endovascular graft that pressurizes the aneurysm sac

    (C) a pseudoaneurysm of the endograft

    (D) none of the above

135. **The presence of endoleak**

    (A) is of no consequence

    (B) cannot be detected by duplex ultrasound

    (C) carries with it the persistent risk of aneurysm enlargement

    (D) is not a complication of endovascular AAA repair

136. **Advantages of endovascular graft exclusion of AAA include all, *except***

    (A) Decreased length of stay (1–2 days for endovascular vs 6–8 days for open repair).

    (B) Decreased time to resumption of normal activity level.

    (C) Procedure is performed from remote site and avoids laparotomy.

    (D) All of the above.

137. **The primary goal of vein graft surveillance is to**

    (A) identify lesions that may ultimately lead to vein graft occlusion

    (B) measure pressure in the graft

    (C) measure vein graft diameter

    (D) none of the above

138. **What is the recommended modality for vein graft surveillance?**

    (A) pulse palpation along the length of the graft

    (B) segmental pressures

    (C) duplex ultrasound in conjunction with some form of indirect testing

    (D) serial ABIs

139. **More frequent surveillance of vein graft is recommended**

    (A) in the first postoperative year

    (B) in the 12–24 month period

    (C) 2–3 years postoperatively

    (D) after 5 years

140. **All of the following except _____ are useful for vein graft surveillance.**

    (A) flow volume measurements

    (B) mean graft flow velocity

    (C) identification of focally elevated peak systolic velocities

    (D) contrast arteriography

141. **Duplex ultrasound surveillance and criteria for polytetrafluoroethylene (PTFE) grafts**

    (A) is equally effective as for vein grafts

    (B) is not currently well established or widely recommended

    (C) is not possible because of the synthetic material

    (D) none of the above

142. **Superficial vein grafts are best evaluated**

    (A) by manual palpation

    (B) using the ABI

    (C) with high-frequency transducers

    (D) by pulse volume recordings

143. **The pulse volume recorder is a form of**

    (A) PPG

    (B) air plethysmography

    (C) strain gauge plethysmography

    (D) impedance plethysmography

144. Graft failure can occur by mechanisms including all, *except*

   (A) occlusion by thrombosis

   (B) hemodynamic failure

   (C) deep vein thrombosis

   (D) structural failure (aneurysmal degeneration)

145. The frequency of graft failure is highest

   (A) within the first 10–14 days (4–10%) post implantation

   (B) after 1 month to 1 year

   (C) after 1 year

   (D) after 5 years

146. Late failure of vein grafts is most often due to

   (A) suture stenosis

   (B) atherosclerosis that can develop de novo in vein grafts

   (C) intimal flaps that reduce flow

   (D) graft entrapment at flexion sites

147. Late failure of vein graft is most often the result of

   (A) disease progression in adjacent native arteries most typically in the distal runoff bed

   (B) disease progression in adjacent native arteries most typically in the inflow artery

   (C) disease in the conduit itself

   (D) hypercoagulable states

148. In the leg circulation, the most common site of atherosclerosis is the

   (A) popliteal artery

   (B) iliac artery bifurcation

   (C) proximal tibial vessels

   (D) distal superficial femoral artery

149. Which of the following entity is not a risk factor for peripheral artery occlusive disease?

   (A) hypolipidemia

   (B) smoking

   (C) hypertension

   (D) diabetes

150. A pulsatile mass in the groin after catheterization is most likely

   (A) a femoral artery pseudoaneurysm

   (B) a femoral vein false aneurysm

   (C) an AVF

   (D) a femoral artery stenosis

Answers and Explanations

1. **(B)** CW Doppler has two inherent crystals in one transducer: one to receive and one to send continuously.

2. **(A)** *(Study Guide)*

3. **(C)** When the flow is toward the transducer at 0 degrees, the Doppler frequency shift is the greatest (cosine of 0 is 1) and reduced accordingly at other incident angles. A perpendicular or 90-degree angle of insonation results in no detected Doppler shift. Zero degree is not feasible in most clinical applications; we avoid the 90-degree angle and maintain a 30–60-degree for clinical applications.

4. **(C)** Plethysmography is generally a measurement of volume changes in the extremities for measuring blood flow. It has been used in the past for venous flow studies and venous reflux studies and is now used primarily for arterial studies.

5. **(D)** The spectral analysis displays the frequency distribution on a time scale. To process the Doppler signal and calculate all the frequency components, the FFT method is used. The spectral analysis determines the presence, direction, and characteristics of blood flow. The spectral analysis provides the quantification and measurements of the blood flow. This cannot be achieved with color flow imaging alone.

6. Figure
   a. Peak systolic velocity
   b. Window
   c. End diastole

7. **(B)** Spectral broadening means broadening or increase in the bandwidth with filling of the spectral window. This can range from mild to severe and is caused by disturbed flow. Disturbed flow produces increased frequencies and the formation of small eddies that increase the center stream and produce random motion of the blood cells. Spectral broadening is commonly seen with stenosis.

8. **(D)** The Nyquist limit is controlled by the pulse repetition rate. Aliasing is seen with high velocities that exceed the Nyquist limit or 1/2; the pulse repetition rate. It is seen on the spectral analysis waveform display as a wraparound with the higher velocities appearing as a negative reading below the baseline.

9. **(D)** Triphasic waveform that is consistent with a nondiseased, at rest peripheral artery. It demonstrates a rapid systolic rise, prominent flow reversal, and second forward flow component in diastole.

10. **(A)** Spectral broadening is caused by disease and stenosis of the vessel. There is an increase in the frequencies/velocities at any given point in time causing spreading of the bandwidth and loss of the spectral window. These changes are characteristics associated with disturbed flow and stenotic lesions.

11. **(B)** Aliasing will occur when the velocity exceeds the Nyquist limit (the Nyquist limit is equal to one-half of the pulse repetition frequency). When aliasing occurs, velocities above this limit will be displayed on the tracing opposite to the true direction of blood flow.

12. **(D)** Damped monophasic waveform distal to a stenosis. This is because of the slow systolic acceleration and rounding of the systolic peak. The peak systolic velocity will be decreased and the diastolic velocity increased (Table 14–2).

13. **(C)** Turbulence is seen distal to areas of stenosis. In this patient with a 50–69% stenosis of the internal carotid artery, the spectral waveform beyond the lesion shows spectral broadening with complete filling of the spectral window, multiple peaks ("picket fence" sign), and flow above and below the baseline at the same time in the cardiac cycle.

14. **(D)** PTA is the nonoperative dilatation of arterial stenosis using balloon catheters. This procedure has been used to dilate or recanalize arteries or grafts in every anatomic region. It has less risk, shorter recovery time, and is less expensive than surgical revascularization.

15. **(C)** Hemodynamics is the study of the movement of blood and of the forces concerned. This term is commonly used in vascular ultrasound.

16. **(A)** Laminar flow is the normal flow pattern usually seen where blood flow is highest in the center and lowest near the walls creating a parabolic flow profile.

17. **(D)** PPG uses a light sensor that shines light into superficial skin layers, and a photoelectric detector measures the reflected light.

18. **(B)** The poststenotic zone is immediately past an arterial stenosis. The flow becomes disorganized with frank swirling movements.

19. **(C)** The Reynolds number predicts the stability of a fluid and defines the point where flow changes from laminar to turbulent. If the Reynolds number exceeds 2000, laminar flow tends to be disturbed. This is a basic principle in fluid dynamics.

20. **(E)** 2000.

21. **(A)** Poststenotic turbulence is commonly seen immediately distal to an arterial stenosis. In fact, this is usually one of the diagnostic criteria for identification of stenotic lesions. It is described as the flow stream distal to the stenotic lumen spreads out, the laminar flow pattern is lost, and flow becomes disorganized.

22. **(A)** Inversely. The volume flow is proportional to the fourth power of the radius so small changes in the radius can make large changes in the flow. The length of the vessel and the viscosity of blood do not change much in the cardiovascular system, so the changes in blood flow occur primarily as a result of changes in the radius of the vessel and the difference in the pressure energy level.

23. **(D)** BP is the pressure exerted on the wall of a blood vessel by the contained blood, and the difference in the BP within the vascular system provides the immediate driving force that keeps the blood moving. Pulse pressure is the difference between the systolic pressure and the diastolic pressure. The mean pressure is the average BP throughout the cardiac cycle, and blood flow is the volume of blood flowing through a vessel, organ, or circulatory system for a given period of time.

24. **(D)** 120/70 mm Hg. The systolic pressure is the peak BP within a large artery approximately 120 mm Hg. The diastolic pressure is the lowest pressure during the cardiac cycle, approximately 70 mm Hg.

25. **(C)** The pulse is the pressure wave created by the expansion and contraction of the arteries during the cardiac cycle. The pulse pressure is the difference between the systolic pressure and diastolic pressure.

26. **(A)** Pulse rate or number of pulsations per minute varies and is normally 70–80 beats/min.

27. **(D)** The most significant risk factor is the unavoidable family history. Cigarette smoking, diabetes, aging, and hypertension all lead to the development of atherosclerosis. Bradycardia is slowness of the heart rate and pulse rate.

28. **(C)** Claudication is the most common symptom in lower extremity arterial disease. Other symptoms include coldness, cyanosis or color changes, or the absence of pulses. As the ischemia progresses to severe, symptoms will include rest pain, nonhealing ulcers, microemboli, or gangrene of the foot.

29. **(C)** The classic six Ps for acute arterial ischemia are pain, poikilothermia, pallor, paresthesias, paralysis, and pulselessness. If a patient presents with these symptoms, the extremity is examined to assess the severity of the ischemia and to determine the urgency of further tests and treatment.

30. **(D)** The ABI or ankle-brachial pressure is used for peripheral arterial examinations and segmental pressure examinations. Normally, the systolic ankle pressure should be equal to or greater than the systolic pressure. The ratio should be 1.0 or greater.

31. **(A)** The pressure is recorded at the site where the cuff is inflated and deflated, even though the Doppler probe is maintained in place at the posterior tibial artery.

32. **(B)** The cuff at each site is inflated until the systolic pressure, sound, or Doppler waveform disappears. The cuff is slowly released until the sound or Doppler waveform returns. The return of the Doppler sound is then recorded.

33. **(C)** The brachial artery systolic pressure is the standard for segmental arterial studies. The bilateral brachial pressures normally should be within 20 mm Hg of each other. The highest value of the two brachial systolic pressures is used. If the bilateral brachial pressures differ by more than 20 mm Hg, an upper extremity arterial lesion is suspected.

34. **(B)** The brachial systolic pressures should be within 20 mm Hg of each other. If there is a greater difference, an upper arterial lesion is suspected on the side with the lowest value.

35. **(B)** Patients who have intermittent claudication generally have a pressure index in the range of 0.6–0.9 and are required to have exercise testing to evaluate the severity of disease.

36. **(C)** An ankle index of 0.5 or less indicates severe arterial occlusive disease and exercise testing is not required.

37. **(D)** Patients who have calcified vessels may have systolic pressures at the ankle arteries that exceed 200 mm Hg. BP in the toes can be measured using a PPG and is often valuable in assessment of severe peripheral artery disease.

38. **(C)** The normal toe pressure is 60% of the brachial pressures.

39. **(B)** Leg exercise increases blood flow. In the presence of significant arterial disease, the ankle pressure drops after exercise as increased flow across the stenosis results in turbulence and a pressure drop.

40. **(D)** The internal capsule is located in the brain. The composition of the arteries includes: the tunica intima (inner layer), the tunica media (middle layer), and the tunica adventitia (outer layer).

41. **(C)** Vasoconstriction is the decrease in the caliber of the vessels, especially constriction of arterioles, which leads to decreased blood flow to a part.

42. **(A)** The brachiocephalic arises on the right from the aortic arch and gives rise to the right common carotid artery and the right subclavian artery. On the left, there is no brachiocephalic, the left carotid artery arises from the aortic arch.

43. **(C)** The axillary artery is a direct continuation of the subclavian artery. The subclavian descends lateral to the lateral margin of the scalenus anterior to the outer border of the first rib and then becomes the axillary artery.

44. **(C)** Radial and ulnar artery. The brachial artery is a continuation of the axillary artery. It terminates about a centimeter distal to the elbow where it divides and becomes the radial and ulnar arteries.

45. **(A)** Common femoral artery is a continuation of the external iliac artery. It begins at the inguinal ligament midway between the anterior superior iliac spine and the symphysis pubis.

46. **(C)** Posterior tibial artery lies posterior to the medial aspect of the tibia and ankle joint. This artery can be used for segmental pressure measurements along with the distal anterior tibial and dorsalis pedis arteries.

47. **(C)** Ischemia is defined as a deficiency of blood to a part because of the functional constriction or obstruction of a blood vessel. Hallett presents several clinical categories of chronic limb ischemia that are common in dealing with lower extremity arterial disease.

48. **(A)** Embolism is defined as a sudden blocking of an artery by clot or foreign material traveling through the blood stream. There are many origins of embolism, which include air, coronary, infective, pulmonary, and tumors.

49. **(B)** Claudication. This is a classic term used to describe the primary consequence and the most common manifestation of peripheral arterial occlusive disease. It actually means to "limp." It is described as pain during exercise that ceases when the activity is stopped.

50. **(B)** Atherosclerosis is the cause of most arterial diseases today. It is defined by the World Health Organization as a combination of changes in the intima and media of the artery. These changes include focal accumulation of lipids, hemorrhage, fibrous tissue, and calcium deposits.

51. **(C)** The blood flow and pressure are not significantly diminished until at least 75% of the cross-sectional area of the vessel is obliterated. This figure for cross-sectional area can be equated to a 50% reduction in lumen diameter.

52. **(D)** Although the radius is the greatest influence on a critical stenosis other factors also influence the critical stenosis to a lesser extent. They include: length of stenosis, blood viscosity, and peripheral resistance.

53. **(C)** The superficial femoral artery in the adductor canal is the most common site of stenosis or occlusion in the lower extremity and corresponds to claudication in the calf muscle area.

54. **(B)** Anterior tibial artery.

55. **(A)** Subclavian steal syndrome. Occurs more often in the left subclavian artery and is a common atherosclerotic lesion. It is usually discovered because the left brachial BP is significantly lower than the right; however, other clinical symptoms may be present such as arm pain with exercise, dizziness, syncope, visual blurring, or ataxia. Subclavian steal is characterized by reversal of blood flow within the vertebral artery resulting from a hemodynamically significant stenosis or occlusion in the proximal subclavian or innominate artery. The steal is induced because of the decreased pressure in the vessel distal to the stenotic lesion, which leads to retrograde flow in the ipsilateral vertebral artery. Flow on the side of the lesion is recruited from the contralateral vertebral artery and occasionally, the basilar artery.

56. **(B)** Thoracic outlet syndrome is defined as compression of the brachial plexus nerve trunks characterized by pain, paresthesia of fingers, vasomotor symptoms, and weakness of the small muscles of the hand. The subclavian artery leaves the chest by the thoracic outlet. It passes over the first rib, behind the clavicle, and between the anterior and middle scalene muscles. Because of the confines of the thoracic outlet, the subclavian artery, subclavian vein, and brachial plexus are subject to compression. Noninvasive testing for this entity requires special maneuvers, which include exaggerated military position, hyperabduction, and Adson's maneuver. The rationale is to determine any obliteration of the blood flow, which relates to specific positions.

57. **(C)** Multiple maneuvers are used for the evaluation of thoracic outlet syndrome. These positions are used to demonstrate an obliteration of blood flow relating to specific positions. During the maneuvers, the waveforms are recorded by Doppler or PPG to identify any change in blood flow.

58. **(A)** Raynaud's disease is an innocuous vasospastic disorder whereas Raynaud's phenomenon is an underlying systemic or vascular abnormality with vascular occlusion.

59. **(B)** Raynaud's phenomenon is associated with occlusive disease, whereas Raynaud's disease is associated with vasospasm.

60. **(B)** Pseudoaneurysms (false aneurysms) do not have a true arterial wall and are usually the result of vascular injury caused by iatrogenic trauma.

61. **(B)** Mycotic aneurysms are secondary to an infectious process that involves the arterial wall.

62. **(C)** Arterial dissection usually develops secondary to a tear in the intimal layer, which allows blood to enter the wall of the vessel and the creation of two lumens. Characteristically, a moving flap is seen in the lumen of the vessel with real-time imaging.

63. **(C)** ABI quantitates the blood flow. The ABI provides an assessment of the consequence of arterial disease in the extremity and estimates the severity of the disease process. This exam is often used for arterial screening of the lower extremities. Duplex and color flow Doppler provide anatomical detail and hemodynamic information around a stenosis but cannot quantitate the flow.

64. **(D)** A decrease in peak systolic flow velocity to less than 40–45 cm/s may indicate impending graft failure.

65. **(C)** Iatrogenic AVF is an abnormal communication between an artery and a vein.

66. **(B)** The resistive index calculates and quantifies resistance to blood flow. A high-resistance waveform pattern has a

high systolic peak and a low diastolic flow. The resistance can be calculated using the resistive index, systolic frequency (S), minus diastolic frequency (D), divided by the systolic frequency.

67. **(A)** Tachycardia refers to a rapid heartbeat and usually means a heart rate above 100 beats/min.

68. **(D)** Arteriography is an invasive procedures using computerized fluoroscopy for direct visualization of the arterial system after injection of a contrast medium.

69. **(B)** The ABI is the measurement of the SBP at the ankle divided by the highest brachial pressure. It is used to determine the presence and severity of arterial disease.

70. **(D)** There are no units.

71. **(C)** The patient history should always be obtained before the vascular examination. It provides valuable information as to the patient's symptoms and related problems. It also ensures that a complete evaluation of the patient is performed. In some cases, the clinical history may be incorrect or the wrong examination is ordered. By talking to the patient and acquiring history and clinical information, we can make sure our information is correct and the correct exam is being performed. If it is not, we can take the necessary time to talk to the clinician to make sure our information is correct.

72. **(A)** Segmental arterial pressures can be obtained using three or four cuffs. The four-cuff method differentiates between disease above and below the inguinal ligament. This is not possible with the three-cuff method.

73. **(A)** The normal mean renal artery RI for an adult is 0.6 with 0.7.

74. **(B)** The cardiovascular system has two major pathways: the systemic circulation and pulmonary circulation. The path of the blood from the left ventricle through the body is the systemic circulation, and its passage from the right ventricle via the lungs to the left atrium is the pulmonary circulation.

75. **(B)** The tunica media is the fibromuscular middle layer that extends from the internal to external elastic lamina and is circumferential. It is the thickest layer of the arterial and aids in maintaining continuous circulation and appropriate BP by controlling the diameter of the vessel lumen.

76. **(D)** The vertebral artery is the first branch of the subclavian artery. It arises from the posterosuperior aspect of the subclavian artery.

77. **(F)** All of the above. Intermittent claudication is usually the first symptom of arterial disease. As the disease progresses to the point of rest pain, the trophic skin changes, dependent rubor, and pallor on elevation occur. If the level of disease is aortoiliac, it often renders the male impotent because the penile circulation branches from the internal iliac.

78. **(D)** All of the above. Atherosclerosis is a disease process that is influenced by several risk factors: family history, smoking, hypertension, hyperlipidemia, diabetes mellitus, and aging.

79. **(C)** The Doppler signal shows to-and-fro flow seen in a pseudoaneurysm neck.

80. **(A)** A hemodynamically significant lesion is a 50% diameter reduction or greater. As the stenotic segment exceeds 50%, the peak-systolic velocities also increase.

81. **(D)** The spectral analysis demonstrates the presence, direction, and characteristics of the blood flow.

82. **(B)** A clear spectral window indicates laminar flow with little flow disturbance. A small sample volume placed in the central portion of the normal flow stream will produce a crisp, clear window. Flow disturbances, such as vortices and swirling eddies, will decrease the size of the spectral window and should demonstrate flow reversal as well. Spectral broadening can occur with moderate stenotic lesions as well as severe lesions.

83. **(A)** Critical stenosis. The critical stenosis occurs with a diameter reduction of 50% or greater (area reduction of 75% or greater). This is also called a hemodynamically significant lesion.

84. **(B)** The two principal mechanisms that control blood volume are the cardiac output and peripheral resistance. Cardiac output (mL/s) is the rate of blood flow per minute. Two factors that affect cardiac output are heart rate and stroke volume. Peripheral resistance is controlled by the arterioles and arterial capillaries. These tiny vessels control the volume of blood flow.

85. **(C)** The major advantage of CW Doppler is that it can display high velocities without the phenomena of aliasing occurring. Unfortunately, it has no range resolution.

86. **(D)** Doppler shift frequencies are affected by Doppler angle, transducer frequency, and the velocity of the red blood cells. As the Doppler angle decreases between the Doppler beam and the flow stream, there will be an increase in the frequency shift. If the transducer frequency decreases, the frequency shift will decrease. The velocity of the red blood cells will affect the Doppler shift. As the red blood cells move faster, the frequency shift will increase.

87. **(C)** As an arterial stenosis exceeds 60%, the peak systolic velocity will increase and the volume of the flow will decrease.

88. **(A)** The highest velocity is found in the maximal stenotic zone. It is important to profile the stenosis by scanning from the normal vessel through the stenosis to identify the highest velocity and past the stenosis to document the poststenotic turbulence that should be present in all stenotic lesions.

89. **(C)** Disturbed flow is seen throughout the stenotic lesion and just distal to the stenosis in the poststenotic zone. The maximal flow disturbance usually occurs within 1 cm beyond the stenosis.

90. **(B)** As the radius of an artery decreases, the resistance to flow will increase.

91. **(D)** Volume flow is not used in determining the severity of arterial stenosis. There are three stenotic zone velocity measurements commonly used to determine the severity of arterial stenoses: peak systolic velocity, end-diastolic velocity, and the systolic velocity ratio (comparison of peak systole in stenoses to peak systole in the proximal normal segment.

92. **(C)** In a 50–99% diameter reduction of the artery, there will be a loss of reverse flow with forward flow throughout the cardiac cycle, and distal to the stenosis, the waveform will be damped and monophasic (Table 14–2).

93. **(C)** Fig. 14–44. This is a normal multiphasic flow waveform in a patient who is post angioplasty and stent of the external iliac artery. Note the characteristic wire mesh appearance of the intra-arterial stent.

94. **(B)** This color flow image shows in-stent restenosis of the mid to distal external iliac artery. Note the changes in the color flow image at the transition to the site of the stenosis and the associated 3.5-fold elevation in velocity. On the far right is the subsequent arteriogram that confirms and correlates with the color flow duplex findings. The intra-arterial stent is also well seen on the arteriogram. Insert on the arteriogram is the color flow image also showing the reduction in lumen at the site of stenosis.

95. **(B)** Fig. 14–46. The external iliac artery demonstrates aliasing with velocity in excess of 500 cm/s and a loss of the reverse component. There is a color flow bruit seen at the site of the stenosis. In the poststenotic zone, there is a severely dampened monophasic low-velocity waveform consistent with a more proximal high-grade stenosis.

96. **(D)** Fig. 14–47. These findings are consistent with right-sided moderate occlusive arterial disease involving the iliac artery segment. The ABI is 0.7 suggesting one level of disease, and there is calf waveform augmentation suggesting a normal femoral segment. On the left, the ABI and PVR waveforms are within normal limits.

97. **(D)** Fig. 14–48. Normal PVR waveforms at all levels bilaterally. Pressures are likely artifactually elevated due to medial wall calcification in this diabetic patient (this can also be seen in patients with end-stage renal disease).

98. **(A)** Fig. 14–49. The patient is examined in a sitting position with hands resting on thighs. The examiner palpates the radial pulse on the side being tested while the patient actively rotates head to ipsilateral side and the examiner laterally rotates and extends the patient's shoulder. The patient takes a deep breath and is instructed to hold it. The test is positive if radicular symptoms are reported and/or if there is conversion to a diminished or lost radial pulse. This provocative maneuver was once widely utilized; however, it is no longer in vogue as a positive diagnosis of TOS since many people without TOS will show a positive Adson's maneuver and there is minimal evidence of interexaminer reliability.

99. **(C)** Fig. 14–50 shows long- and short-axis imaging of abdominal aortic aneurysms. In Panel A, the long-axis image reveals mural thrombus on the near wall of the aorta. Panel B is a color flow image that shows a lumen where the color is seen; however, most of the aneurysm sac is filled with thrombus.

100. **(A)** The ABI value is determined by taking the higher pressure of the two arteries at the ankle and dividing it by the higher of the two brachial systolic pressure measurements. The ABI is a simple ratio and has no unit of measure.

101. **(D)** The toe-brachial index (TBI) is calculated by dividing the highest toe pressure by the highest brachial pressure. The normal TBI is 0.65–0.7 and above.

102. **(B)** All normal vessel flow profiles should exhibit a rapid rise to from the onset of systole to the peak of systole. Normal AT in the common femoral artery is <122 ms (Fig. 14–19).

103. **(D)** Study guide

104. **(B)** Bilateral thigh, hip, or buttock claudication is consistent with aortoiliac disease.

105. **(A)** Erectile dysfunction is consistent with aortoiliac disease. The impotence is the result of inadequate blood flow through the hypogastric artery.

106. **(C)** The absence of a pulse is indicative of a more proximal occlusion (eg, absence of the common femoral artery pulse indicates aortoiliac occlusive disease). In this case, the presence of a normal pulse at the same level contralaterally excludes significant disease of the aorta. Physical exam should include palpation, auscultation, and inspection. This includes a pulse examination as well as a thorough inspection of the extremities themselves. Pulse palpation is probably the most important part of the physical examination.

107. **(A)** Exercise testing is an important adjunct to the segmental pressure evaluation as it can help differentiate patients with true claudication from those with other differential diagnoses (pseudoclaudication). Exercise helps unmask occlusive disease that is not apparent at rest. It is beneficial in patients with normal or borderline ABIs at rest who present with claudication-type symptoms.

108. **(D)** The value of a history and physical examination should not be underestimated in establishing a correct diagnosis. This part of the patient evaluation also builds the foundation upon which further diagnostic tests and therapeutic interventions may be planned.

109. **(C)** The value of a history and physical examination should not be underestimated in establishing a correct diagnosis. The lower extremities should be carefully evaluated. Physical exam should include palpation, auscultation, and inspection.

110. **(A)** Pain is the most common chief complaint regardless of whether the occlusive disease is acute or chronic. Pain may present as either intermittent claudication or pain at rest.

111. **(B)** Acute arterial occlusion is a sudden and complete blockage of a main arterial supply to the extremity. The most common etiology of an acute occlusion may be embolic or thrombotic (bypass graft or native artery). Most emboli originate in the heart (atrial fibrillation, recent myocardial infarct). Thrombosis of a diseased artery or a bypass graft is common. Another cause for acute occlusion is vascular trauma.

112. **(A)** The most common etiology of an acute occlusion may be embolic or thrombotic (bypass graft or native artery). Most emboli originate in the heart (atrial fibrillation, recent myocardial infarct).

113. **(C)** In chronic arterial insufficiency, you may also note trophic changes such as muscle atrophy, hair loss, thicken toe nails, ulcerations, or gangrene.

114. **(D)** In acute lower extremity ischemia, patients may present with skin mottling, cyanosis, pallor, or muscle weakness.

115. **(D)** Most emboli originate in the heart (atrial fibrillation, recent myocardial infarct) as a cause for acute occlusion; however, other causes of acute occlusion include sudden thrombosis of a diseased artery or a bypass graft as well as vascular trauma.

116. **(A)** The initial presentation is characterized by the presence of the six Ps.

117. **(B)** Rest pain is a constant pain described as a severe aching or burning in the foot. The pain usually localizes to the metatarsal heads but may be worse in the location of a gangrenous toe or ischemic ulcer. This pain often intensifies at night and may be relieved by dependency (ie, hanging the foot over the side of the bed). Rest pain is of far greater consequence than is claudication.

118. **(D)** Tissue loss and gangrene is the most severe form of ischemia.

119. **(A)** Tissue loss and gangrene is the most severe form of ischemia (Fig. 14–15). Patients with tissue loss often present with multilevel arterial occlusive disease.

120. **(D)** Arterial ischemic ulcers are often localized in the distal toes, heel, or sole and dorsum of the foot.

121. **(A)** Diabetic neuropathy may be confused with rest pain; however, the pain associated with diabetic neuropathy is not relieved by changes in position and patients often lack the associated physical findings seen in patients with peripheral vascular disease.

122. **(D)** In addition to absent pedal pulses, patients with chronic arterial insufficiency may also present with trophic changes such as muscle atrophy, hair loss, thicken toe nails, ulcerations, or gangrene.

123. **(C)** Leg swelling is more likely the result of iliocaval vein thrombosis. Aortoiliac arterial occlusive disease may or may not result in symptoms or positive findings.

124. **(B)** Femoral, popliteal, dorsalis pedis, and posterior tibial arteries are palpated and graded according to the following scale: 0 is a nonpalpable pulse, 1+ is a diminished, but palpable pulse, 2+ is a normal pulse, 3+ is a bounding pulse, and 4+ is an excessively bounding pulse (sometimes seen in patients with arterial aneurysm).

125. **(A)** Chronic arterial disease often presents as intermittent claudication. This word is derived from the Latin, claudico, meaning to limp, and is pain that is brought on by exercise and relieved with rest. It is often described as a cramping sensation or a feeling of tiredness or heaviness. It is reproduced by the same level of exercise and is relieved within 2–5 minutes of rest.

126. **(C)** Auscultation with a stethoscope is performed to assess for the presence of a bruit. A bruit indicates the presence of a hemodynamically significant stenosis (note that the absence of a bruit does not exclude the presence of significant arterial occlusive disease).

127. **(A)** In an acute event the upper extremity may be pallid with diminished motor and sensory functions.

128. **(A)** In the upper extremity pulses should be examined at the subclavian artery (above the middle of the clavicle); the axillary artery should be palpated in the groove between the biceps and triceps muscle, the brachial artery pulse can be palpated at the antecubital fossa, the ulnar and radial arteries should be palpated at the wrist on the medial and lateral aspects respectively.

129. **(B)** Allen's test is performed to assess the collateral circulation between the radial and ulnar artery distributions.

130. **(A)** The abdomen may be auscultated for bruits, which are suggestive of renal and/or visceral artery stenoses, although these may be nonspecific findings.

131. **(B)** The magnitude of the Doppler shift is proportional to the angle of incidence; the smaller the angle, the higher the Doppler shift (0 degrees will produce the highest Doppler shift) and vice versa (if the angle is 90 degree, there is no Doppler shift because as the cosine of 90 degrees is 0). Doppler shift frequencies are also affected by transducer frequency and the velocity of the red blood cells.

132. **(C)** In cases of arterial stenosis, specific characteristics are seen. The flow velocity increases upon entering the stenosis because of the decreased cross-sectional area (blood flow and pressures are not significantly affected until at least 50% diameter reduction is seen (equivalent of a 75% reduction in the cross-sectional area).

133. **(D)** Spectral analysis is the method of choice for displaying the Doppler signals. It is a mathematical computation of the reflected pulse that displays individual frequencies and is computed using the FFT method.

134. **(B)** An endoleak is defined as flow outside of the endovascular graft that perfuses and pressurizes the aneurysm sac.

135. **(C)** Endoleak pressurizes the aneurysm sac. This ongoing pressurization of the aneurysm sac carries with it the persistent risk of aneurysm enlargement and potential rupture.

136. **(D)** Table 14–3.

137. **(A)** The goal of vein graft surveillance is to identify lesions that may ultimately lead to vein graft occlusion. The rationale for graft surveillance is the progressive nature of atherosclerosis and the tendency of both vein and prosthetic bypass grafts to develop flow-limiting lesions.

138. **(C)** Duplex ultrasound in conjunction with some form of indirect testing is the recommended surveillance method following lower extremity bypass grafting.

139. **(A)** At present, frequent surveillance is recommended in the first postoperative year with the initial scan being performed intraoperatively. Studies have shown that grafts followed in a surveillance program have a higher patency rate than those followed only clinically.

140. **(D)** Contrast arteriography is invasive; poses the risks of contrast-induced renal dysfunction, puncture site complications, catheter and guidewire-induced vessel wall injury, and allergic reactions; and is not appropriate as a surveillance method.

141. **(B)** There are no established criteria for serial evaluation of prosthetic grafts and controversy exists in this area.

142. **(C)** Superficial grafts such as in situs or grafts that are tunneled subcutaneously are best evaluated with high-frequency transducers (7.5–10 MHz).

143. **(B)** Air plethysmography in the form of the pulse volume recorder uses air flow to measure volume changes in a limb.

144. **(C)** Graft failure can occur by three mechanisms: occlusion by thrombosis, hemodynamic failure, and structural failure (aneurysmal degeneration).

145. **(A)** The frequency of graft failure is highest within the first 10–14 days (4–10%) post implantation, decreases progressively in the first year, and is approximately 2–4% per year thereafter. Technical errors (suture stenosis, intimal flaps, retained thrombus, graft entrapment, torsion) are the most common cause of failure in the early postoperative period (within 30 days).

146. **(B)** Late failure can be due to myointimal hyperplasia from preexisting vein graft lesions or atherosclerosis that can develop de novo in vein grafts or disease progression in adjacent native arteries.

147. **(A)** Late failure can be due to myointimal hyperplasia from preexisting vein graft lesions or atherosclerosis that can develop de novo in vein grafts or disease progression in adjacent native arteries but is most typically seen in the distal runoff bed.

148. **(D)** The superficial femoral artery is a continuation of the common femoral artery. It courses the length of the thigh passing through the adductor canal or Hunter's canal at the distal third of the thigh, where it becomes the above-knee popliteal artery. The most common location of arterial lesions of the leg is the distal superficial femoral artery.

149. *(Study Guide)*

150. These are commonly seen in the groin as complications postcardiac catheterization. A pseudoaneurysm (also known as false aneurysm) is a collection of blood contained by surrounding tissue that communicates with an adjacent artery via an extravascular neck or tract (iatrogenic). It is often the result of injury to the artery, either traumatic or iatrogenic.

15A

Pediatric Neurosonography

Charles S. Odwin and Chandrowti Devi Persaud

Study Guide

INTRODUCTION

Pediatric neurosonology had its beginning in the late 1960s and early 1970s. One of the first applications was the A-mode, or amplitude mode, to determine midline shifts. If, in fact, the midline was shifted, this was an indication of a tumor or pathology. As newer technology and gray-scale imaging emerged, new applications also emerged. The A-mode midline shift examination was quickly replaced with computed tomography (CT). The realization that the open fontanelles in neonates offered a sonographic window to permit ultrasound scanning of the neonatal brain opened new technological advances. Gray-scale imaging became a mainstay in the neonatal department primarily to detect intracranial hemorrhage and monitor enlargement of the ventricles. Ultrasound was also being utilized in neurosurgery to localize lesions and pathology during the surgical procedure. The introduction of color-flow Doppler added diagnostic capabilities for identifying vascular variances and anomalies in the neonate.[1] It was also a time when transcranial Doppler was introduced using the transtemporal window for examination of the adult patients. The advantages of neurosography include more easily available, portability, cost-effectiveness, noninvasiveness, and high sensitivity. Neurosography has been an ongoing expanding specialty for more than 45 years. It now requires the sonographer to have a well-rounded knowledge encompassing anatomy, vascular hemodynamics, positioning, and instrumentation.

INSTRUMENTATION AND TECHNIQUE

Real-time gray-scale imaging using a 5–12 MHz frequency is most commonly used in the evaluation of the neonatal brain. Higher frequencies such as 12 MHz may be used for superficial

structures. Duplex and color-flow Doppler sonography are used to evaluate congenital vascular anomalies, cerebral perfusion, and vascular anatomy.[1]

The anterior fontanelle is used as an acoustic window in the first year of life. It starts to close at 9 months and is completely closed in 13 months.[2] Standard scanning planes and views for evaluations of the brain are coronal, sagittal, and axial.

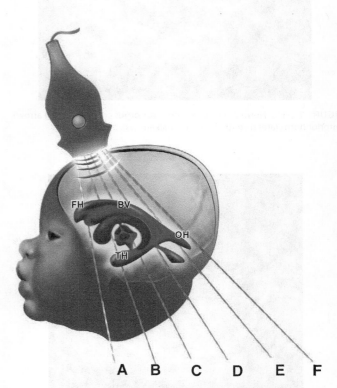

FIGURE 15–1. Schematic of the coronal planes. (**A** to **F**) are scanning planes from anterior to posterior. FH is frontal horn; BV is body of ventricle; TH is temporal horn; OH is occipital horn.

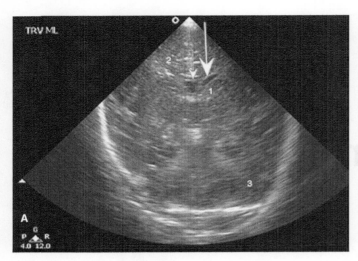

FIGURE 15–1A. Normal coronal sonogram. Cavum septi pellucidi (short arrow); lateral ventricle (long arrow); caudate nucleus (1); frontal lobe (2); temporal lobe (3).

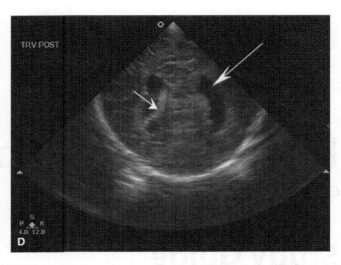

FIGURE 15–1D. Coronal sonogram represents plane D. Choroid plexus (short arrow); trigone of the lateral ventricle (long arrow).

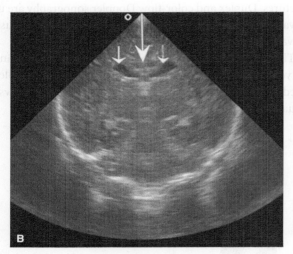

FIGURE 15–1B. Normal coronal sonogram. Corpus callosum (large arrow); anterior horns lateral ventricles (two small arrows).

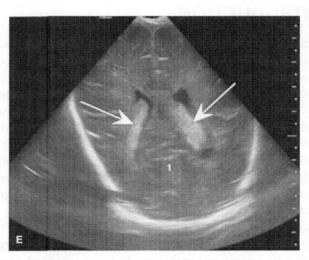

FIGURE 15–1E. Coronal sonogram represents plane E. The two white arrows point to the choroid plexus and the number (1) identifies the cerebellum.

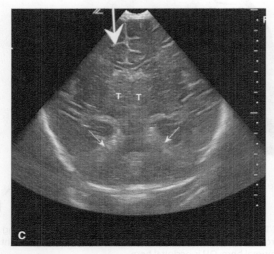

FIGURE 15–1C. Normal coronal sonogram. Cingulate sulcus (large arrow); thalamus (T); tentorium (small arrows).

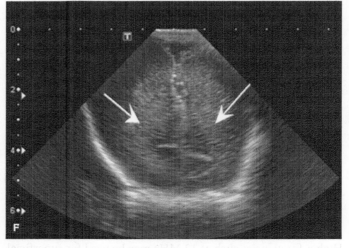

FIGURE 15–1F. Coronal sonogram represents plane F. Area between arrowheads = white matter of the occipital lobe and sulci.

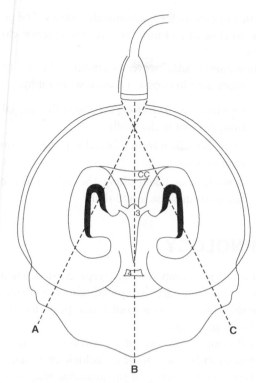

FIGURE 15–2. Schematic of the sagittal planes.

Coronal. These scans are obtained through the frontal fontanelle (Figs. 15–1 A–F). Six standard coronal sonograms taken at the level of:

- frontal horns (anterior to the foramen of Monro)
- foramen of Monro
- posterior aspect of the third ventricle through the thalami
- quadrigeminal cistern
- trigones of the lateral ventricles
- parietal and occipital cortex

Sagittal. These scans are obtained through the frontal fontanelle (Figs. 15–2 A–C). The three standard scans include:

- *Midsagittal plane,* which includes the following anatomical landmarks: cavum septi pellucidi, cavum vergae, corpus callosum, pericallosal artery, cingulate sulcus and gyrus, third ventricle, massa intermedia in the third ventricle, quadrigeminal cistern, and fourth ventricle (Fig. 15–2B).[2]
- *Parasagittal* right planes, which include the following anatomical landmarks: lateral ventricle, choroid plexus, thalamus, and parietal and occipital lobes (Fig. 15–2A).
- *Parasagittal* slightly more lateral than the above on the left, which includes the following anatomical landmarks: the body, occipital and temporal horns of the lateral ventricles, and the glomus (largest) part of the choroid plexus. The frontal, parietal, temporal, and occipital lobes are seen surrounding the lateral ventricle (Fig. 15–2C).

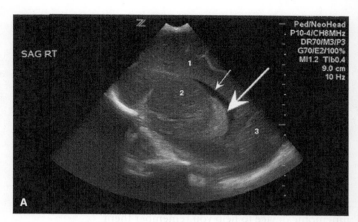

FIGURE 15–2A. Normal parasagittal sonogram. Lateral ventricle (small arrow); choroid plexus (large arrow); parietal lobe (1); thalamus (2); occipital lobe (3).

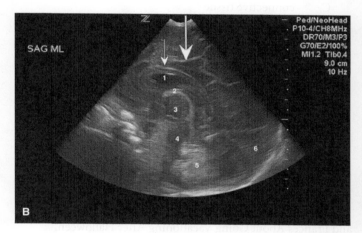

FIGURE 15–2B. Normal sagittal midline sonogram. Corpus callosum (small arrow); cingulate sulcus (large arrow); cavum septi pellucidi (1); choroid plexus (2); third ventricle (3); fourth ventricle (4); cerebellar vermis (5); occipital lobe (6).

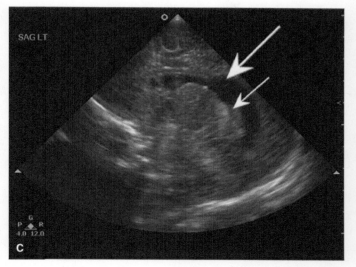

FIGURE 15–2C. Left parasagittal sonogram. Choroid plexus (short arrow); lateral ventricle (long arrow).

Axial. These scans are obtained through the squamosal portion of either temporal bone. To obtain the desired images and anatomical landmarks, the transducer is angled superiorly. The ventricles are seen just above the choroid plexus. The lateral ventricular measurements are obtained in this position or the squamosal fontanelle.

MNEMONICS

Mnemonics are just one of many useful ways to formulate words that will help you remember. How fast you learn, and how much you retain after you learn, may be a big factor in taking examinations. The following are study groups. Formulate your own mnemonic device to help you remember them.

The mnemonic "SCALP" serves as a memory key for the five layers of the scalp listed below:

S   skin
C   connective tissue
A   epicranial aponeurosis
L   loose connective tissue
P   pericranium

The mnemonic "PAD" serves as a memory key for the three layers of membranes called meninges, which cover the brain and spinal cord from inner to outer. The three layers are as follows:

P   pia
A   arachnoid
D   dura

A mnemonic for the 12 cranial nerves is "O,O,O Tell Ted and Frances About Going Vacationing After Halloween."

O   olfactory
O   optic
O   oculomotor
T   trochlear
T   trigeminal
A   abducens
F   facial
A   acoustic
G   glossopharyngeal
V   vagus
A   accessory
H   hypoglossal

The mnemonic "MAPS" serves as a memory key for these fontanelles:

M   mastoid
A   anterior
P   posterior
S   sphenoidal

The time of closure for the fontanelles varies. The posterior is the first to close at 2–3 months, with the anterior closing at 13 months.[2]

The mnemonic "SAC" serves as a memory key for the three scanning planes used in neonatal cranial sonography.

S   sagittal scan taken along the axis of the sagittal suture (longitudinal in the skull)

A   axial scan taken from a lateral approach through the temporal bone.

C   coronal scan taken along the axis of the coronal suture (transverse in the skull)

TERMINOLOGY

Fontanelles are membrane-covered gaps created when more than two cranial bones are juxtaposed, also called soft spots.[2] There are six fontanelles: one frontal, one posterior, two mastoids, and two sphenoidal.

The following definitions of the various anatomic structures associated with sonographic neurologic examinations will enhance your understanding of the anatomic diagrams in the subsequent text.

Arachnoid—The middle layer of meninges covering the brain and spinal cord.

Atrium (Trigone) of the Lateral Ventricles—This is where the anterior, occipital, and temporal horns join.

Brainstem—Part of the brain connected to the forebrain and the spinal cord. It consists of the midbrain, pons, and medulla oblongata.[1]

Caudate Nucleus—Consists of a head, body, and tail. It lies next to the lateral wall of the lateral ventricles.

Cavum Septi Pellucidi—A thin triangular cavity filled with cerebrospinal fluid that lies between the anterior horns of the lateral ventricles.. The cavum septi pellucidi has also been referred to as a fifth ventricle and the cavum vergae as a sixth ventricle.

Central Nervous System—The central nervous system consists of the cerebellum, cerebrum, spinal cord, pons (brainstem), and medulla.

Cerebellum—Portion of the brain that lies posterior to the pons and medulla oblongata below the tentorium.

Cerebral Hemispheres—These are paired brain matter separated from the midline by the falx cerebri.

Cerebrum—The largest part of the brain, which consists of two hemispheres.[1]

Choroid Plexus—Mass of special cells located in all components of the ventricles except for the cerebral aqueduct. They regulate the intraventricular pressure by secreting or absorbing cerebrospinal fluid.[1]

Cistern—Enclosed space serving as a reservoir for cerebrospinal fluid.

Corpus Callosum—Large group of nerve fibers visible superior to the third ventricle that connects the left and right sides of the brain.[1]

Ependyma—The membrane lining the cerebral ventricles.[1]

Epidural—Lies outside the dura mater.

Falx Cerebri (interhemispheric fissure)—A fibrous structure separating the two cerebral hemispheres.

Germinal Matrix—Periventricular tissue including the caudate nucleus. Before 32 weeks gestation, it is fragile and bleeds easily.[1]

Gyri—Convolutions on the surface of the brain caused by infoldings of the cortex.[1]

Massa Intermedia—Also called the interthalamic adhesion, this is the place of fusion between the third ventricle and the medial surface of the thalami.

Meninges—The brain coverings.[1]

Mesencephalon—Midbrain.

Parenchyma—Cortex tissue of the brain.[1]

Pia Mater—The innermost of the three membranes covering the brain and spinal cord.

Pineal Recess—Posterior recess on the third ventricle. There are two posterior recesses: the pineal and the suprapineal recesses.

Prosencephalon—Forebrain.

Rhombencephalon—Hindbrain.

Subdural—Between the dura mater and the arachnoid.

Subependyma—Area immediately beneath the ependyma. In the caudate nucleus, it is the site of hemorrhage from the germinal matrix.

Subarachnoid—Between the arachnoid and the pia mater.

Sulcus—A groove or depression on the surface of the brain, separating the gyri.[1]

Suprapineal recess—One of the two posterior recesses on the third ventricle.

Sylvian Fissure—Lateral cerebri fissure.

Tela Choroidea—Point where the choroid attached to the floor of the lateral ventricles and located behind the foramen of Monro. Most common site of hemorrhage.

Tentorium—V shaped echogenic structure which separates the cerebrum and the cerebellum and is an extension of the falx cerebri.[1]

Thalamus—Two ovoid brain structures situated on either side of the third ventricle superior to the brainstem.[1]

Ventricle—A cavity within the brain containing cerebrospinal fluid.[1]

Vermis Cerebellum—Median part of the cerebellum that lies between the two hemispheres.

ANATOMY

It is essential to know the basic anatomy of the brain. The main parts of the brain are the cerebrum, cerebellum, and the brainstem.

Cerebrum

The cerebrum is divided into two cerebral hemispheres by the longitudinal fissure and connected by the corpus callosum. It is made up of six lobes. The lobes are named according to the skull bones they lie under.

Lobes of the brain and the main functions are the following:

- One frontal lobe—Functions include personality, language, and judgment.
- Two parietal lobes—Functions include senses and muscle control.
- Two temporal lobes—Function is auditory.
- One occipital lobe—Function is vision.

The cerebrum consists of an outer thin gray matter called cerebral cortex and inner white matter. On the surface, there are numerous ridges or convolutions gyri and sulci (grooves). Gyri appear hypoechoic and are marked off by sulci. Sulci appear echogenic. Prominent sulci are pericallosal sulcus, cingulate sulcus and the calcarine sulcus. Deep sulci are called fissures. Fissures appear echogenic and are the longitudinal, transverse, fissure of Rolando (central sulcus), and the Sylvian fissure (lateral sulcus).

Cerebellum

The cerebellum is divided by the vermis into two hemispheres and is separated from the occipital lobe by the transverse fissure superiorly. It has an inner white matter and thin gray outer cortex. On the sonogram, it appears echogenic. Functions include muscle coordination and equilibrium.

Brainstem

Superiorly the brainstem includes diencephalon, midbrain, pons, and the medulla oblongata inferiorly. It lies between the base of the cerebrum and the spinal cord. The diencephalon includes the thalamus and the hypothalamus. The midbrain (mesencephalon) includes the cerebral aqueduct, cerebral peduncle, and the corpora quadrigemina. The brainstem functions mainly for automatic survival, controls the heart beat and breathing, and acts as a relay station for sensory impulses and reflexes.

Basal Ganglia

The basal ganglia is the gray matter that lies deep within the cerebral hemispheres. It includes the caudate nucleus, putamen, and globus pallidus. The caudate nucleus is a common site for intracranial hemorrhage.

There are six ventricles. The first and second are called the right and left lateral ventricles. The lateral ventricles are the largest cerebrospinal filled cavities. Each lateral ventricle is arbitrarily divided into the frontal horn, body, occipital horn, and temporal horn. The third and fourth are below the first and second. Between the frontal horns of the lateral ventricle is the cavum septum pellucidum (CSP) the fifth ventricle; posterior to the CSP is the cavum vergae the sixth ventricle. The third ventricle is bridged by the massa intermedia. There are several foramens, which include the following:

Foramen of Monro—Also termed intraventricular foramen, it divides the frontal horn anteriorly from the body of the ventricle posteriorly and connects the third ventricle with the lateral ventricle.

Aqueduct of Sylvius—Also called the cerebral aqueduct, it connects the third and fourth ventricles.

Foramen of Luschka—The opening in the roof of the fourth ventricle for circulation of the cerebrospinal fluid.

Foramen of Magendie—The opening in the roof of the fourth ventricle for circulation of the cerebrospinal fluid.

The following pages contain illustrations of anatomical structures. Study each illustration carefully, then close your examination book and try to form a eidetic memory of the illustration in your mind. Then draw and label the illustration on a separate sheet of paper without referring to the illustration. Although this process may sound difficult at first, it is a simple method of developing your eidetic memory ability. As sonographers, we see hundreds of sonographic images each day and have probably used eidetic memory without even realizing it. Go ahead and try this with the following illustrations (Figs. 15–3 to 15–9).

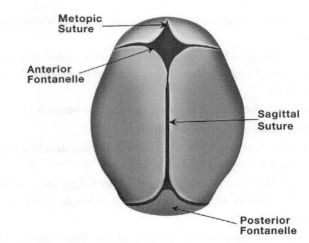

FIGURE 15–4. A diagram of a superior view of the infantile skull.

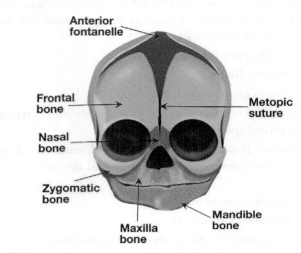

FIGURE 15–5. An anterior view of an infantile skull.

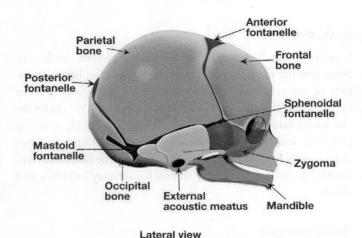

FIGURE 15–3. Diagram of a lateral view of the infantile skull.

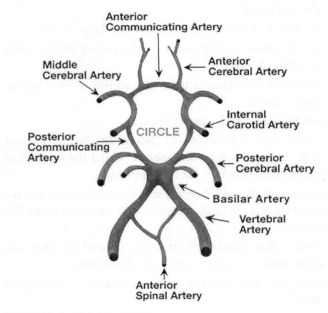

FIGURE 15–6. The circle of Willis.

Ventricular System

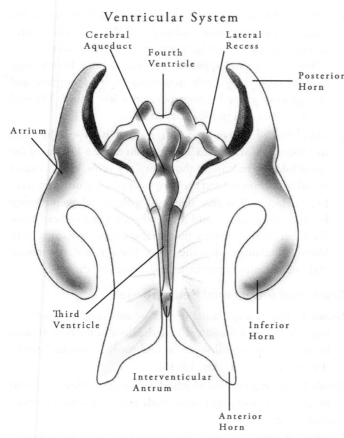

FIGURE 15-7. A diagram of the ventricular system, superior view.

Ventricular System

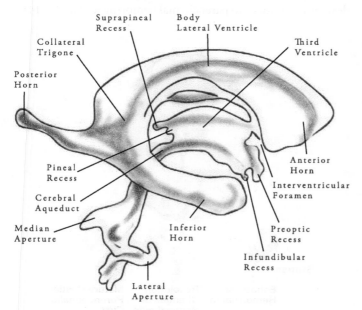

FIGURE 15-8. A diagram of the ventricular system, lateral view.

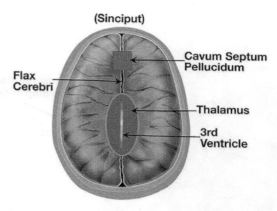

FIGURE 15-9. A diagram of the ventricular system and choroid plexus, lateral view.

DISEASE AND PATHOLOGY

Intracranial Hemorrhage

The most common intracranial pathology in neonates and infants is intracranial hemorrhage.

The most common risk factors are prematurity, gestational age of less than 32 weeks, and low birth weight (<1500 g). Other risk factors include gender (male 2:1), multiple gestations, trauma during delivery, prolonged labor, hyperosmolarity, hypocoagulation, pneumothorax, patent ductus arteriosus, and increased or decreased blood flow. The underlying pathophysiology is hypoxia.[3] Clinical symptoms may include respiratory distress syndrome, hematocrit drop, prematurity (<32 weeks or 1850 g), or problems during delivery. Most bleeds occur within 72 hours after birth. Later complications of hemorrhage include hydrocephalus and porencephalic cyst.[1]

a. *SEH: Subependymal* hemorrhage occurs in the caudate nucleus and can be seen inferior to the floor of the lateral ventricles (Fig. 15–10).[1]

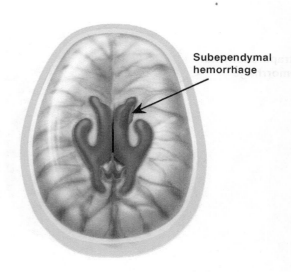

FIGURE 15–10. Subependymal hemorrhage Grade 1.

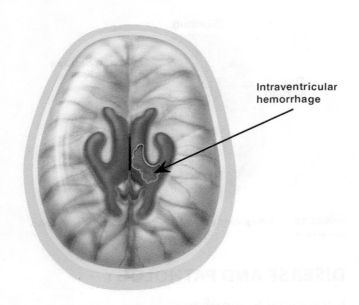

FIGURE 15–11. Intraventricular hemorrhage Grade 2.

b. IVH: *Intraventricular* hemorrhage occurs within the ventricles and can completely fill the ventricles forming a cast (Fig. 15–11).[1]

c. IPA: *Intraparenchymal* hemorrhage occurs within the brain substance, usually near the caudate nucleus and lateral to the ventricles. Dilatation of the lateral ventricles is often associated with parenchymal hemorrhage (Fig. 15–12).[1]

d. CPH: *Choroid* and cerebella hemorrhage occur within the echogenic choroid and cerebellum. They may be difficult to distinguish; however, outline irregularity and increased echogenicity will suggest a hemorrhage.[1]

e. GMH: *Germinal matrix hemorrhage* is the site of many subependymal hemorrhages and is often associated with prematurity.

f. SAH: *Subarachnoid hemorrhage* is located between the arachnoid and pia mater and may be difficult to see on ultrasound unless there is a large amount of blood present.

The sonographic appearance of intracranial hemorrhage changes with time. Early hemorrhages are echogenic and change to decreased echogenicity in a few weeks. The end result is often porencephalic cysts.[1]

g. SDH: *Subdural hemorrhage* is located between the dura mater and the arachnoid. Trauma can cause a tearing of the dural folds or rupture of the medullary veins, which causes blood collection around the periphery of the brain. The cerebral surface will appear flattened with an echogenic space between the cranium and the cerebrum. On a coronal view, fluid can be seen within the interhemispheric fissure, with blood collecting around the brain. The gyri are compressed and become more prominent and closer together.[1]

Grading of Intracranial Hemorrhage[2]

Grade 1. This is a germinal matrix or subependymal hemorrhage. It is seen inferolaterally to the floor of the frontal horn or body of the lateral ventricle and medially to the head of the caudate nucleus (Fig. 15–10).

Grade 2. This is an intraventricular hemorrhage presented with no dilatation and may coexist with germinal matrix hemorrhage (Fig. 15–11).

Grade 3. This type of hemorrhage occur within the brain parenchyma (Fig. 15–12).

Grade 4. This is an intraparenchymal hemorrhage, which may coexist with germinal matrix and intraventricular hemorrhage with or without dilatation and can block the flow of cerebrospinal fluid (Fig. 15–13).

Porencephalic Cyst. This is a cyst arising from the ventricle that develops secondary to parenchymal hemorrhage (Fig. 15–14).

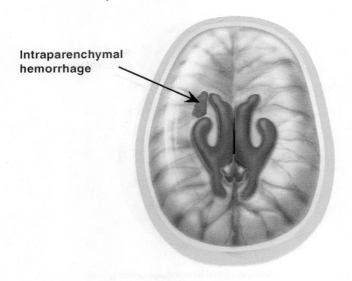

FIGURE 15–12. Intraparenchymal hemorrhage Grade 3.

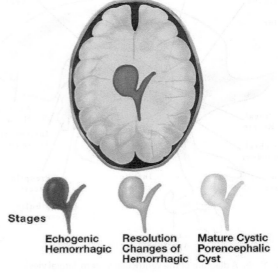

Stages

Echogenic Hemorrhagic   Resolution Changes of Hemorrhagic   Mature Cystic Porencephalic Cyst

FIGURE 15–13. Intraparenchymal hemorrhage Grade 4.

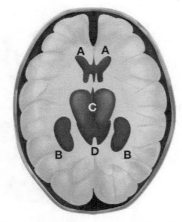

Obstruction with enlargement of the ventricles

A. Anterior horn   **C. Third ventricle**
B. Posterior horn   **D. Fourth ventricle**

FIGURE 15–14. Porencephalic cyst.

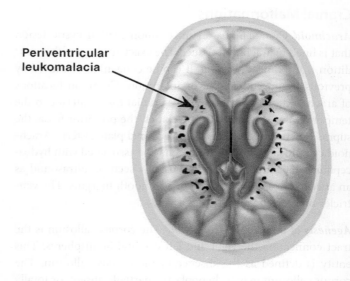

FIGURE 15–15. Periventricular leukomalacia.

Hydrocephalus. Ventricular dilatation is most often secondary to obstruction of the cerebrospinal flow pathways. This is typically associated with enlargement of the head, brain atrophy, and mental deterioration. It is first seen sonographically in the occipital horn, followed by the body and the anterior horn. It can be a minimal, moderate, or marked degree. The third and fourth ventricles are normally barely seen on the scan, so dilatation is easy to visualize.[1] Ultrasound monitors ventricular enlargement and if a shunt placement is required, it can assist in localization. In addition, ultrasound can provide follow-up examinations for the shunt procedure to ensure patency (Fig. 15–14).[1]

Periventricular Leukomalacia. Periventricular leukomalacia (PVL) occurs in neonates who have had asphyxia.[1] It is a region of coagulation necrosis and rarified neutrophile areas that contain swollen axons or macrophages followed by a reaction of microglia cells and astrocytosis. Hemorrhage may accompany the infarction, and the areas of necrosis may liquefy and cavitate.[4] Sonographically, this condition will present with lesions distinctly separate from the caudate nucleus and usually adjacent to the atrium of the lateral ventricles. There will be increased echoes at the external angle of the lateral ventricles, with extensions radiating anterior to the frontal horns. It may be asymmetrical or bilateral. The echo intensity decreases in 2–4 weeks, and cysts or cavities are seen later in the previously echogenic areas (Fig. 15–15).[5]

Intracranial Infections

Encephalitis and Brain Edema. Encephalitis is inflammation of the brain. It is characterized sonographically with an overall increased echogenicity. Brain edema also shows increased echogenicity but has an additional finding; the ventricles become slit like as a result of the brain swelling.[1]

Ventriculitis. Infection of the ventricles is usually associated with encephalitis. It causes dilatation of the ventricles, and they may contain septa and debris. The brain becomes more echogenic, and often there are small cystic areas. The lining of the ventricles appears echogenic on ultrasound, and there may be holes in the borders of the ventricles.[1]

Brain Abscess. Abscesses vary in number and size. They may be lobulated and usually appear as cystic-type lesions with nonhomogeneous echogenic material within. There are usually other signs of ventriculitis and encephalitis.[1]

Intracranial Calcifications. Calcifications in the brain may be seen as a result of infections that occurred during pregnancy. For example, cytomegalovirus inclusion disease or toxoplasmosis. Sonographically, echogenic areas may be seen in the brain with associated shadowing (Fig. 15–16).[1]

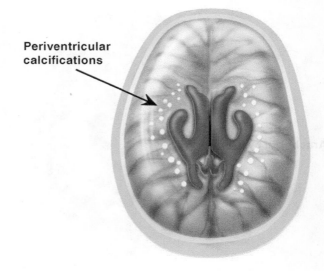

FIGURE 15–16. Intracranial calcifications.

Cranial Malformations

Arachnoid Cyst. This is an uncommon benign cystic lesion that is lined in arachnoid tissue.[1] The exact etiology of this condition is unknown; however, it can be congenital or caused by previous trauma, infection, or infarction. Common locations of arachnoid cysts include middle cranial fossa anterior to the temporal lobe, the cerebral convexities, the posterior fossa, the suprasellar region, and the quadrigeminal plate cistern. Arachnoid cysts located in the midline may be associated with hydrocephalus. The arachnoid cyst is usually seen on ultrasound as an anechoic mass with well-defined smooth margins. The ventricles may also be dilated (Fig. 15–17).[6]

Agenesis of the Corpus Callosum. The corpus callosum is the tract connecting the right and left cerebral hemispheres. This entity is defined as the absence of the corpus callosum. The corpus callosum may be hypoplastic, partially absent, or totally absent. Agenesis of the corpus callosum can be congenital or acquired. Acquired agenesis, for example, can occur as the result of intrauterine insult with anoxia or infarction in the distribution of the anterior cerebral artery. In the congenital type, the posterior portion of the corpus callosum is generally affected, whereas the anterior portion is affected in the acquired type.[6] Patients may be asymptomatic or have seizures, delayed development, hydrocephalus, or cerebral disconnection syndrome.

Real-time ultrasound shows a wide separation of the ventricular frontal horns with an asymmetrical appearance of the lateral ventricles. The third ventricle is high in position, which produces a "rabbit ear" appearance. The normal prominent corpus callosum is not seen on the midline sagittal scan.[6] CT, MRI, and ultrasound may be used to demonstrate this condition.[6]

Holoprosencephaly. This entity is defined as a congenital malformation with partial or complete failure of the primitive

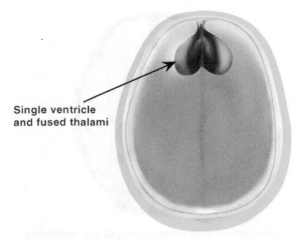

Single ventricle and fused thalami

FIGURE 15–18. Alobar holoprosencephaly.

prosencephalon to form the cerebral hemispheres (telencephalon), and a thalamus and hypothalamus (diencephalon). This leads to a midline cleavage defect with failure to form the cerebral hemispheres and the thalamus. There is a common large ventricle with a horseshoe shape. There are three types of holoprosencephaly:

Alobar (severe form)—A single horseshoe-shaped ventricle with a thin cortical mantle. The thalami are fused, and the third ventricle is absent.[1] This type has severe abnormalities and is not compatible with life (Fig. 15–18).

Semilobar (moderate form)—Anterior horns of the ventricles are present. There is a single occipital horn with partial development of occipital and temporal horns. This form is usually associated with mental retardation.[1]

Lobar (mildest form)[1,6]—A less severe variant than the alobar with considerable cortex present.[1]

Risk factors include maternal diabetes mellitus; toxoplasmosis; trisomies 13, 15, and 18; intrauterine rubella; and Meckel's syndrome. It can be associated with severe facial abnormalities, such as cleft palate, cleft lip, hypotelorism, trigonocephaly, cyclopia, orthocephaly, and cebocephaly.

Real-time ultrasound demonstrates a large central ventricle draping over a bilobed fused thalamus in a horseshoe-shaped appearance. The third ventricle is usually visible in some form with semilobar and lobar types and is small or absent in the alobar type. The falx cerebri and interhemispheric fissure are present to a variable degree in the semilobar and lobar forms, and are usually absent in the alobar forms. The corpus callosum is absent in the alobar form. There is usually some residual brain tissue, depending on the type, with no differentiation of the frontal, temporal, and occipital horns.[6] CT, MRI, and ultrasound demonstrate holoprosencephaly; however, MRI is superior in showing the structural changes caused by holoprosencephaly.

Arnold–Chiari Malformation. This entity is characterized by inferior displacement of the cerebellum and the fourth ventricle

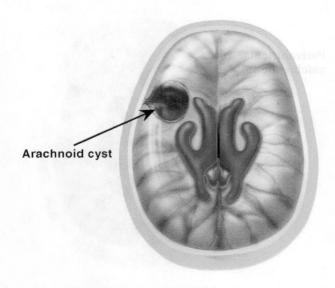

Arachnoid cyst

FIGURE 15–17. Arachnoid cyst.

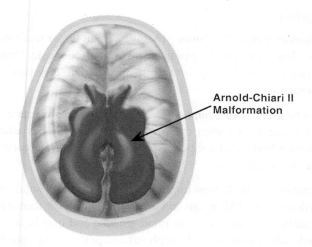

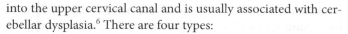

FIGURE 15–19. Arnold–Chiari II malformation.

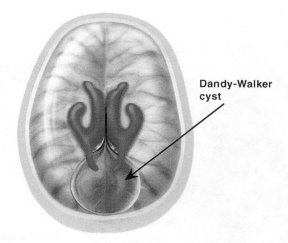

FIGURE 15–20. Dandy–Walker cyst.

into the upper cervical canal and is usually associated with cerebellar dysplasia.[6] There are four types:

Chiari I Malformation—Low-lying cerebellar tonsils below the foramen magnum. Cisterna magna is small or absent. There can be mild elongation and low position of the fourth ventricle. Complications include hydrocephalus and hydromyelia.

Chiari II Malformation—Inferior displacement of the medulla, fourth ventricle, inferior cerebellar tonsils, and vermis, and the presence of a myelocele or meningomyelocele (Fig. 15–19).

Chiari III Malformation—Low occipital and high cervical encephalocele with a bony defect in the infraocciput, posterior rim of the foramen magnum, and posterior arch of the first cervical vertebra. Herniation of the cerebellum, brainstem, fourth ventricle, and upper cervical cord into the defect may occur.

Chiari IV Malformation—Severe cerebellar dysplasia associated with hypoplastic cerebellum, small brainstem, large posterior fossa, and cerebrospinal fluid (CSF) space not causing pressure effects.[6]

Patients may be asymptomatic or have headache, enlargement of the head from hydrocephalus, ataxia, incoordination, signs and symptoms of increased intracranial pressure, and a cervico-occipital soft tissue mass from encephalocele.[6]

Real-time ultrasound shows the cerebellum low in the posterior fossa. The third ventricle may be obscured by the massa intermedia, and the fourth ventricle may be small or absent. The posterior fossa may be small with the cisterna magna not visualized. Hydrocephalus may be present with the lateral ventricles dilated more than the frontal horns. A myelocele or meningomyelocele may be seen at the cervico-occipital junction.[6]

CT, MRI, and ultrasound are used to demonstrate the anomaly. CT and MRI can more effectively demonstrate the bony defects in the occiput, foramen magnum, and C1 and C2 in addition to showing the myelocele or meningomyelocele, fourth ventricle, and brainstem.[6]

Dandy–Walker Malformation or Syndrome. This process is characterized by a cyst in the infratentorial region with absence of the inferior cerebellar vermis and atresia of the foramina of Luschka and Magendie.[7] It is associated with hydrocephalus and presents on ultrasound with a large posterior fossa cyst that communicates with the fourth ventricle and enlargement of the posterior fossa. This condition has been associated with a higher incidence of other anomalies, such as agenesis of the corpus callosum, aqueductal stenosis, porencephalic cyst, encephalocele, holoprosencephaly, and lissencephaly.[7] There will be a small cerebellum and a large posterior fossa (Fig. 15–20).[6]

Hydranencephaly. This is a severe congenital malformation with a complete or almost complete absence of telencephalic structures. The cerebellum, basal portion of the temporal lobes, occipital lobes, and diencephalon are generally preserved. This anomaly is a result of severe intrauterine destructive process, although the exact etiology is uncertain. Neonates may be asymptomatic or have a large head with marked retardation. Transillumination of the skull is increased because of the thinness of the calvarium and increased intracranial fluid. Cerebral activity may be absent on an electroencephalogram.

Sonographically, this anomaly is seen as large bilateral cystic masses in the supratentorial region. Cerebral tissue may be present in the occipital and basal portions of the temporal lobes. The falx cerebri is usually attenuated and deviated (Fig. 15–21).[6]

Congenital Porencephaly. This anomaly is defined as the presence of cystic cavities within the brain matter. These cystic cavities may communicate with the ventricular system, the subarachnoid space, or both.[4]

Microcephaly. This condition is characterized by a decreased head size and reduction of brain mass. It features a typical disproportion in size between the skull and the face. The forehead slopes with a small brain, and the cerebral hemispheres are affected.[5]

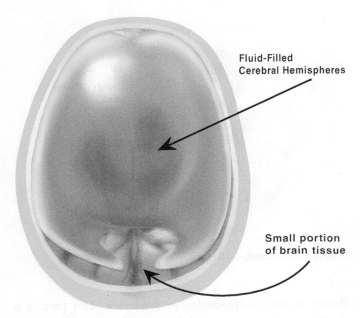

FIGURE 15–21. Hydranencephaly.

Labels in figure: Fluid-Filled Cerebral Hemispheres; Small portion of brain tissue

Cranioschisis. This condition is a splitting of the brain caused by failure of the neural tube to close. The level where the neural tube closes determines which anomalies will be present. Various anomalies include anencephaly, encephalocele, and myelomeningocele.

Vein of Galen Aneurysm and Arteriovenous Malformation. The vein of Galen can become dilated or aneurysmal due to an increased flow from a deep cerebral arteriovenous malformation. The enlarged vein of Galen is seen posterior to the third ventricle and draining posteriorly into the dilated straight sinus and torcular herophili.[7] Sonographically, it appears as a cystic midline space with lateral ventricular dilatation.[2] This condition can be differentiated from other cystic anomalies with color-flow Doppler. Schematic of vein of Galen aneurysm (Fig. 15–22).

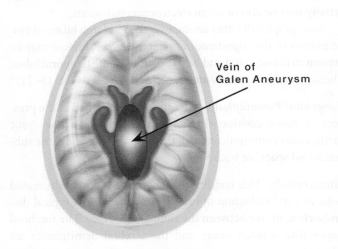

FIGURE 15–22. Vein of Galen aneurysm.

Label in figure: Vein of Galen Aneurysm

Tumors

Choroid Plexus Papilloma. That is a benign tumor that causes the choroid plexus to appear enlarged and echogenic. Hydrocephalus may develop because of obstruction of ventricular foramina.[1]

Corpus Callosum Lymphoma. The lymphoma presents as an echogenic mass within the corpus callosum. It has separated anterior horns that are pointed due to the maldevelopment of the corpus callosum.[1]

Teratoma. This benign tumor has typical irregular, solid mass with areas of calcifications and sometimes with cystic formation. Fetal brain teratoma can be rapid growing and may be associated with obstructive hydrocephalus and polyhydramnious.[1]

Choroid Plexus Cysts

Choroid Plexus cyst (CPC) is associated with fetal aneuploidy, particularly trisomy 18 (Edwards syndrome) at least 50% of the time. Most CPCs disappear spontaneously, usually during the second trimester. Choroid plexus develops in lateral, third and fourth ventricles are responsible for the formation of CSF. Cysts may occur in the choroid plexus during the second trimester with maximal growth and entanglement resulting in entrapment of CSF (Fig. 15–23).

Zika Virus in Pregnancy

Zika virus is spread by daytime-active mosquitoes (Fig. 15–24), its name comes from the Zika Forest of Uganda, where the virus was first isolated in 1947. Not all mosquitoes carry the Zika virus and therefore not every person bitten by infected mosquitoes will get Zika. The infection can be diagnosed by blood or urine test, and currently there is no treatment or cure. Zika virus can be passed from a pregnant woman to her fetus during pregnancy (vertical transmission) can cause birth defect characterized by a small head (microcephaly). This condition can result in intellectual disability and developmental delays after birth (Fig. 15–25).

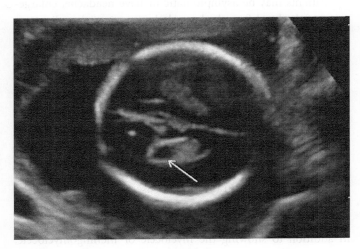

FIGURE 15–23. Arrow points to choroid plexus cyst.

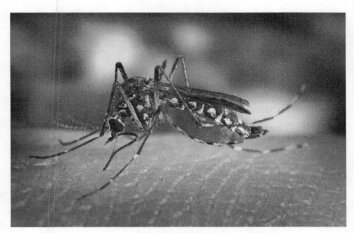

FIGURE 15–24. Dengue aedes mosquito.

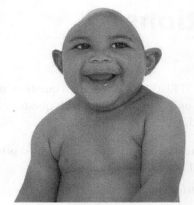

Zika Virus

FIGURE 15–25. Microcephaly due to Zika infection.

References

1. Sanders RC. *Clinical Sonography: A Practical Guide.* 5th ed. Philadelphia, PA: Lippincott Williams & Wilkins; 2016.

2. D'Antoni V, Donaldson OI. A comprehensive review of the anterior fontanelle: embryology, anatomy, and clinical considerations. *Childs Nerv Syst.* 2017 June;33(6):909-994.

3. Fleischer AC, Toy EC, Monteagudo A. *Fleisher's Sonography in Obstetrics & Gynecology: Textbook and Teaching Cases.* 8th ed. New York: McGraw Hill; 2017.

4. Fleischer AC, Manning FA, Jeanty P, et al. *Sonography in Obstetrics & Gynecology Principles and Practice.* 8th ed. New York: McGraw Hill; 2017.

5. Babcock DS, Levine D. *Diagnostic Ultrasound.* 5th ed. St. Louis, MO: Elsevier Mosby; 2018.

6. Meijer G, Steggerda S. *Neonatal Cranial Ultrasonography.* New York: Springer; 2019.

7. Poretti A, Huisman TG. *Neonatal Head and Spine Ultrasonography.* New York: Springer; 2016.

8. Lee JK, Shin OS. Advances in Zika Virus–Host Cell Interaction: Current Knowledge and future perspectives. *Int J Mol Sci.* 2019 March;20(5):1101.

Questions

GENERAL INSTRUCTIONS: For each question, select the best answer. Select only one answer for each question unless otherwise instructed.

1. **Which acoustic windows are used most often in neonatal cranial sonography?**

   (A) anterior and posterior fontanelles

   (B) anterior and sphenoidal fontanelles

   (C) anterior and mastoidal fontanelles

   (D) posterior and sphenoidal fontanelles

2. **On sonography, cytomegalovirus in the neonate is associated with which of the following findings?**

   (A) periventricular calcifications

   (B) small cystic lesions

   (C) encephalocele

   (D) anencephaly

3. **What is another name for the sphenoid fontanelle?**

   (A) lambda

   (B) the anterolateral fontanelle

   (C) the posterolateral fontanelle

   (D) bregma

4. **The anterior fontanelle becomes progressively smaller and, in most cases, closes completely by what age?**

   (A) 6 months

   (B) 2–3 months

   (C) 12 months

   (D) 18 months

5. **What is another name for the mastoidal fontanelle?**

   (A) anterior fontanelle

   (B) posterior fontanelle

   (C) lambda

   (D) posterolateral fontanelle

6. **Which of the following statements about temporal and occipital horns is true?**

   (A) They both diverge laterally as they project from the body of the lateral ventricles.

   (B) They both diverge medially as they project from the body of the lateral ventricles.

   (C) The occipital horn is lateral, and the temporal horns are medial to the body of the lateral ventricles.

   (D) The right temporal horn and the occipital horn are medial, and the left temporal horn is lateral.

7. **The lateral ventricular ratio can be obtained by measuring the distance from the**

   (A) anterior wall to the posterior wall of the lateral ventricle

   (B) midline to medial wall of the lateral ventricle and from the inner wall of the table of the skull

   (C) medial wall to the lateral wall of the lateral ventricle

   (D) midline to the lateral wall of the lateral ventricle and dividing this by the distance from the midline echo to the inner table of the skull

8. **The axial scan is obtained by placing the transducer on the parietal bone just above the**

   (A) styloid process

   (B) coronal suture

   (C) glabella

   (D) external auditory meatus

9. **Which of the following statements regarding the germinal matrix is false?**

   (A) It cannot be visualized as a distinct structure.

   (B) It lies just above the caudate nucleus.

   (C) It disappears between 32 weeks to term.

   (D) It is not a fetal structure.

10. **What is the normal location for the germinal matrix after 24 weeks of gestation?**

    (A) above the caudate nucleus in the subependymal layer of the lateral ventricle

    (B) within the choroid plexus

    (C) inferior to the caudate nucleus

    (D) within the choroid plexus in the trigone

11. **The cisterna magna appears sonographically as**

    (A) echogenic space superior to the cerebellum

    (B) echogenic space inferior to the cerebellum

    (C) echo-free space superior to the cerebellum

    (D) echo-free space inferior to the cerebellum

12. Vascular pulsations are sometimes seen in the Sylvian fissure, which most likely represent the

    (A) anterior cerebral arteries
    (B) posterior cerebral arteries
    (C) basilar artery
    (D) middle cerebral arteries

13. Which of the following statements about the fissure and sulci is true?

    (A) Fissure and sulci both appear echogenic.
    (B) Fissure is echo-free, and the sulci are echogenic.
    (C) Sulci are echo-free, and the fissure is echogenic.
    (D) Fissure and sulci are both echo-free.

14. Where is the CSP located?

    (A) lateral to the corpus callosum
    (B) posterior to the third ventricle
    (C) medial to the thalami
    (D) between the frontal horns of the lateral ventricles

15. The third ventricle is located between the

    (A) CSP
    (B) frontal horns of the lateral ventricles
    (C) thalami
    (D) corpus callosum

16. Increased echogenicity in the brain parenchyma is seen with

    (A) subependymal hemorrhage
    (B) intraventricular hemorrhage
    (C) intraparenchymal hemorrhage
    (D) choroid plexus hemorrhage

17. If dense echogenic material is seen in the ventricle, it is called

    (A) intraventricular hemorrhage
    (B) intraparenchymal hemorrhage
    (C) subarachnoid hemorrhage
    (D) subependymal hemorrhage

18. After an intraparenchymal hemorrhage, the clot retracts and may result in a cystic area communicating with the ventricle. What is this termed?

    (A) holoprosencephaly
    (B) hydranencephaly
    (C) hydrocephalus
    (D) porencephaly

19. Which of the following is *not* a possible contributing factor to intracranial hemorrhage?

    (A) maternal ingestion of aspirin during the final weeks of pregnancy
    (B) extrauterine stress
    (C) intrapartum hypoxia
    (D) pleural effusion

20. A neonate is defined as

    (A) a child during the first 28 days after birth
    (B) a child from 29 days after birth to 1 year
    (C) a fetus of 20 weeks of gestation to a child 28 days after birth
    (D) conception to birth

21. What is the most common site for PVL?

    (A) white matter surrounding the ventricles
    (B) gray matter surrounding the ventricles
    (C) gray matter around the caudate nucleus
    (D) white matter around the cerebellum

22. Disruption of organogenesis in brain development causes specific related brain defects. Such defects do *not* include

    (A) diverticulation
    (B) neural tube closure
    (C) neuronal proliferation
    (D) tuberous sclerosis

23. Which of the following terms is used to describe any hemorrhage within the cranial vault?

    (A) subependymal hemorrhage
    (B) germinal matrix hemorrhage
    (C) intraventricular hemorrhage
    (D) intracranial hemorrhage

24. Which type of intracranial hemorrhage is most common in premature infants?

    (A) subdural hemorrhage
    (B) intraventricular hemorrhage
    (C) intraparenchymal hemorrhage
    (D) subependymal germinal matrix hemorrhage

25. True coronal scans are performed at what angle with the orbitomeatal line?

    (A) 60 degrees

    (B) 90 degrees

    (C) 150 degrees

    (D) They do not have an angle with the orbitomeatal line.

26. Which of the following does *not* designate the term "acoustic window" in cranial sonography?

    (A) a procedure to bypass bone interface

    (B) an opening through which ultrasound can travel with little or no obstruction

    (C) an area in which ultrasound is obstructed

    (D) an area in which ultrasound is not obstructed

27. Which of the following diseases is *not* a common cause of congenital infections of the nervous system?

    (A) rubella

    (B) toxoplasmosis

    (C) gonorrhea

    (D) syphilis

28. Which of the following are *not* sonographic findings of congenital infection of the nervous system?

    (A) microcephaly with enlargement of the ventricles

    (B) a prominent interhemispheric fissure and brain atrophy

    (C) macrocephaly with enlargement of the ventricles

    (D) calcification in the periventricular regions

29. According to the computed tomography grading system for intracranial hemorrhage, which of the following is a Grade 1 hemorrhage?

    (A) subependymal hemorrhage with intraventricular hemorrhage and ventricular dilatation

    (B) subependymal hemorrhage with intraventricular hemorrhage and no ventricular dilatation

    (C) subependymal hemorrhage with intraventricular hemorrhage and intraparenchymal hemorrhage

    (D) isolated subependymal hemorrhage

30. The foramen between the third and fourth ventricles is the

    (A) cerebral aqueduct

    (B) foramen of Monro

    (C) foramen of Magendie

    (D) foramen of Luschka

31. Which of the following is *not* true regarding hydranencephaly?

    (A) Usually, only the brainstem and portion of the occipital lobe remain.

    (B) The falx is usually intact.

    (C) The falx is usually not intact because the head is largely filled with fluid.

    (D) There is a severe loss of cerebral tissue.

32. A Dandy–Walker cyst is usually associated with

    (A) toxoplasmosis

    (B) dysgenesis of the vermis of the cerebellum

    (C) syphilis

    (D) cytomegalovirus

33. The current treatment for hydrocephalus with increased intraventricular pressure is

    (A) Javid's internal shunt

    (B) ventriculoperitoneal (V-P) shunt

    (C) radiation treatment

    (D) ventriculoectomy

34. Which of the following is *not* a sign of hydrocephalus?

    (A) skull bones halo sign on x-ray

    (B) anterior fontanelle sinks

    (C) bulging of the frontal bone of the skull

    (D) decreasing size of ventricles

35. The most common cause of congenital hydrocephalus is

    (A) aqueductal stenosis

    (B) subarachnoid hemorrhage

    (C) interventricular hemorrhage

    (D) intracranial infection

36. Subperiosteal hematomas are also called

    (A) cephalohematomas

    (B) subependymal hemorrhages

    (C) intraventricular hemorrhages

    (D) choroid plexus hemorrhages

37. The cavum pellucidum begins to close at which week of gestation?

    (A) 40 weeks

    (B) 36 weeks

    (C) 12 weeks

    (D) 24 weeks

38. Which of the following best defines the Dandy–Walker syndrome?

   (A) a cyst in the posterior fossa that does not communicate with the fourth ventricle
   (B) a congenital cystic dilatation of the third ventricle
   (C) congenital dilatation of the ventricular system
   (D) a posterior fossa cyst that is continuous with the fourth ventricle

39. Which of the following is a differential diagnosis for hydranencephaly?

   (A) severe hydrocephalus
   (B) Dandy–Walker cyst
   (C) arachnoid cyst
   (D) intracranial teratoma

40. On cranial sonography, the middle cerebral artery is found in the

   (A) region of the Sylvian fissure and above the corpus callosum
   (B) region of the Sylvian fissure and in the circle of Willis
   (C) genu of the corpus callosum and Sylvian fissure
   (D) genu of the corpus callosum and hippocampal sulcus

41. What is the most severe form of hemorrhage?

   (A) germinal matrix hemorrhage
   (B) intraventricular hemorrhage
   (C) subependymal hemorrhage
   (D) intraparenchymal hemorrhage

42. What is another name for the forebrain?

   (A) prosencephalon
   (B) mesencephalon
   (C) rhombencephalon
   (D) myelencephalon

43. Which of the following vessels does *not* form the circle of Willis?

   (A) posterior cerebral arteries
   (B) anterior cerebral arteries
   (C) internal carotid arteries
   (D) external carotid arteries

44. Which of the following is true regarding noncommunicating hydrocephalus?

   (A) It is also called nonobstructive hydrocephalus.
   (B) The cerebrospinal fluid pathways within the brain are blocked.
   (C) Cerebrospinal fluid is blocked within the ventricular system.
   (D) none of the above

45. A Chiari II malformation is defined as

   (A) a congenital abnormality of the brain with elongation of the pons and fourth ventricle and downward displacement of the medulla into the cervical canal
   (B) congenital cystic dilatation of the fourth ventricle caused by atresia of the foramen of Magendie
   (C) congenital formation of a holospheric cerebrum caused by a disorder of the diverticulation of the fetal brain
   (D) none of the above

46. The main arteries supplying the brain are

   (A) one vertebral and one carotid artery
   (B) one basilar artery and two carotid arteries
   (C) two external carotid and two vertebral arteries
   (D) two internal carotid and two vertebral arteries

47. The vertebral artery at the level of the pons is called the

   (A) middle cerebral artery
   (B) basilar artery
   (C) internal carotid artery
   (D) posterior cerebral artery

48. The greatest proportion of the cerebrospinal fluid is produced by

   (A) choroid plexus
   (B) caudate nucleus
   (C) lateral ventricles
   (D) movement of extracellular fluid from blood through the brain and ventricles

49. The sonographic findings of ventriculitis do *not* include

   (A) echogenic ventricular walls
   (B) septated ventricles
   (C) normal-sized ventricles with no debris within
   (D) debris within the ventricles

50. How many cranial bones are there?

   (A) 12
   (B) 10
   (C) 8
   (D) 5

51. Blood between the arachnoid membrane and the pia mater is called

   (A) subarachnoid hematoma
   (B) subdural hematoma
   (C) epidural membrane
   (D) intraparenchymal hematoma

52. The amount of cerebrospinal fluid production in children is

   (A) 140 mL/week
   (B) 140 mL/day
   (C) 532–576 mL/day
   (D) 552–576 mL/week

53. The accumulation of blood between the dura mater and the inner table of the skull is called

   (A) subarachnoid hemorrhage
   (B) subdural hematoma
   (C) epidural hematoma
   (D) intraparenchymal hemorrhage

54. Another name for the temporal horn is the

   (A) anterior horn
   (B) posterior horn
   (C) inferior horn
   (D) lateral horn

55. The largest of all the horns is the

   (A) temporal horn
   (B) occipital horn
   (C) frontal horn
   (D) lateral horn

56. Which of the following are not midline structures?

   (A) third ventricle and fourth ventricle
   (B) cerebral hemispheres
   (C) CSP
   (D) falx cerebri

57. The vein of Galen aneurysm is most likely to be located

   (A) anterior to the third ventricle
   (B) posterior to the foramen of Monro and superior to the third ventricle
   (C) posterior to the foramen of Monro and inferior to the third ventricle
   (D) posterior to the fourth ventricle

58. Which of the following is not a bacterial cause of intracranial infection?

   (A) Haemophilus influenzae
   (B) herpes simplex
   (C) Diplococcus pneumoniae
   (D) bacterial meningitis

59. The central fissure is also called

   (A) Sylvian fissure
   (B) fissure of Rolando
   (C) lateral fissure
   (D) longitudinal fissure

60. Which of the following is the etiology of a porencephalic cyst?

   (A) intracranial infection
   (B) infarction
   (C) intracranial hemorrhage
   (D) trauma

61. Numerous sulci can normally be identified on the premature brain, particularly in the sagittal scan. Identify the condition that would least be likely to obscure the normal sulcal pattern.

   (A) meningoencephalitis
   (B) subdural hematoma
   (C) intracranial infection
   (D) infarction

62. The germinal matrix is largest at which week of gestation?

   (A) 40 weeks (term)
   (B) 24–32 weeks
   (C) 32–40 weeks
   (D) 12–15 weeks

63. **Which of the following is *not* an intracranial tumor?**

    (A) dermoid tumor

    (B) choroid plexus papilloma

    (C) medulloblastoma

    (D) cyclopia

64. **Which of the following *best* describes PVL?**

    (A) ischemic lesions of the neonatal brain characterized by necrosis of periventricular white matter

    (B) a disorder of premature newborns characterized by the increase in vascularity in the periventricular white matter

    (C) a disorder of premature newborns characterized by highly echogenic solid lesions in the parenchyma

    (D) an infection disorder with a decrease in definition of the parenchymal structures

65. **Which of the following is *not* a common infection acquired in utero?**

    (A) herpes simplex

    (B) leukomalacia

    (C) toxoplasmosis

    (D) cytomegalovirus

66. **Which of the following results in the greatest number of neonatal deaths?**

    (A) hypoxia

    (B) erythroblastosis

    (C) trauma at birth

    (D) premature placental separation

67. **Which of the following is *not* a characteristic of lissencephaly?**

    (A) decrease in the size of the Sylvian fissure as the neonatal brain matures

    (B) large ventricles

    (C) less sonographic characteristics because of the inability to differentiate white from gray matter

    (D) large Sylvian fissures

68. **If an infant has a ventriculoperitoneal (V-P) shunt and the fontanelles are bulging, the usual position to assist in drainage is the**

    (A) Trendelenburg position

    (B) lithotomy position

    (C) semi-Fowler's position

    (D) Sims' position

69. **The cerebellum is separated from the occipital lobe of the cerebrum by the**

    (A) interhemispheric fissure

    (B) tentorium

    (C) cerebellar vermis

    (D) parieto-occipital sulcus

70. **The central nervous system consists of the brain and spinal cord. The spinal cord is referred to as the distal continuation of the central nervous system. The terminal portion of the spinal cord is the**

    (A) filum terminale

    (B) conus medullaris

    (C) cauda equina

    (D) pia mater

71. **What region of the lateral ventricular system is the first to dilate in hydrocephalus?**

    (A) the third ventricle

    (B) occipital horns

    (C) frontal horns

    (D) temporal horns

72. **The correct placement for a ventriculoperitoneal (V-P) shunt catheter is**

    (A) frontal horns anterior to the foramen of Monro

    (B) frontal horns posterior to the foramen of Monro

    (C) trigone of the lateral ventricle

    (D) the roof of the third ventricle

73. **Which of the following is least associated with complete agenesis of the corpus callosum?**

    (A) absence of the septum pellucidum

    (B) enlarged septum pellucidum

    (C) wide separation of the lateral ventricle

    (D) displacement of the third ventricle

74. **Which of the following is *not* seen in septo-optic dysplasia?**

    (A) septum pellucidum

    (B) frontal horns

    (C) thalamus

    (D) occipital horns

75. When scanning neonates, excessive pressure should *not* be applied to the anterior fontanelle because it may cause

    (A) increased heart rates
    (B) slowing of the heart
    (C) increased body temperatures
    (D) irregularity of the heart rate

76. When evaluating the intracerebral vessels of an infant's brain, the optimal frequency range for a continuous-wave Doppler transducer is

    (A) 1–3 MHz
    (B) 4–5 MHz
    (C) 1–10 MHz
    (D) 5–10 MHz

77. When using a transcranial approach with the transducer placed 0.5–1.0 cm anterior to the ear and superior to the zygomatic process, the vessel that can be evaluated most accurately in the neonate's brain is the

    (A) middle cerebral artery
    (B) anterior cerebral artery
    (C) posterior cerebral artery
    (D) posterior communicating artery

78. In a normal tracing of a cerebral vessel in a neonate's brain, the maximum systolic velocity is equivalent to the

    (A) peak height
    (B) area under the curve
    (C) slope
    (D) minimum height

79. A Doppler tracing of an anterior cerebral artery in an infant with asphyxia can reveal

    (A) low pulsatility and high diastolic forward flow
    (B) low pulsatility and low diastolic forward flow
    (C) high pulsatility and high diastolic forward flow
    (D) high pulsatility and low diastolic forward flow

80. A Doppler tracing of an anterior cerebral artery in an infant with an intraventricular hemorrhage can reveal

    (A) low pulsatility and low diastolic forward flow
    (B) low pulsatility and high diastolic forward flow
    (C) high pulsatility and high diastolic forward flow
    (D) high pulsatility and low diastolic forward flow

81. The term craniosynostosis denotes

    (A) premature fusion of the cranial sutures
    (B) premature separation of the cranial sutures
    (C) a bluish discoloration of the cranium
    (D) a bluish discoloration of the scalp

82. Hypothermia denotes

    (A) high memory
    (B) low memory
    (C) high temperature
    (D) low temperature

83. When the parietal bones are relatively thin, lateral ventricular measurements can be obtained up to

    (A) 5 years
    (B) 6 months
    (C) 2–3 years
    (D) 6–12 months

84. In cranial sonography, a real-time linear array transducer is limited. Which of the following statements is *not* true of the linear array limitations?

    (A) limited field of view
    (B) inability to visualize the inner lateral table of both sides of the calvarium simultaneously
    (C) able to examine only the central portion of the brain
    (D) producing only a 90-degree pie-shaped image

85. Which of the following sonography planes are *most* comparable with cranial computed tomography?

    (A) axial
    (B) coronal
    (C) sagittal
    (D) occipital

86. The choroid plexus is attached to the floor of the lateral ventricle. Its point of attachment is called

    (A) tela choroidea
    (B) interhemispheric fissure
    (C) pineal body
    (D) caudate nucleus

87. A structure often confused with the third ventricle in the fetus and neonate is the

    (A) cavum septi pellucidi
    (B) choroid plexus
    (C) thalamus
    (D) cavum vergae

88. Between 32 and 40 weeks, the incidence of germinal matrix hemorrhage drops. Approximately what percentage of germinal matrix hemorrhage occurs at 28 weeks of gestation?

    (A) 25%

    (B) 35%

    (C) 40%

    (D) 67%

89. The term *isodense* denotes the following

    (A) same density

    (B) same as sonolucent

    (C) same as echogenic

    (D) same as anechoic

90. Which of the following is associated with an intracranial hemorrhage?

    (A) hyaline membrane disease

    (B) sudden change in blood flow to the region of the germinal matrix

    (C) increase in venous and arterial pressure

    (D) all of the above

91. An infant is defined as a child

    (A) from 29 days after birth to 1 year

    (B) during the first 28 days after birth

    (C) from 1 to 2 years after birth

    (D) from 2 to 6 years after birth

92. Which of the following is *not* an imaginary line from the outer canthus to the external auditory meatus?

    (A) orbitomeatal line

    (B) canthomeatal line

    (C) radiographic baseline

    (D) Reid's baseline

93. Posterior fossa scans are performed at what angle with the orbitomeatal line?

    (A) 150 degrees from the orbitomeatal line and perpendicular to the clivus

    (B) 150 degrees from the canthomeatal line and parallel to the clivus

    (C) 90 degrees perpendicular to the orbitomeatal line and parallel to the clivus

    (D) 120 degrees perpendicular to the canthomeatal line and parallel to the clivus

94. If one sees echogenic material within the occipital horn, it would most likely be correct to assume that there is

    (A) a choroid plexus in the occipital horn

    (B) a choroid plexus in the lateral horn

    (C) an intracranial hemorrhage because no choroid extends into this area

    (D) an intracranial hemorrhage because the tail of the choroid extends into the occipital horn

95. Which of the following does *not* describe hydranencephaly?

    (A) The head is largely filled with fluid.

    (B) The falx is usually intact.

    (C) The loss of cerebral tissue is severe.

    (D) There is a presence of a single midline ventricle.

96. The pericallosal artery is normally seen

    (A) above the corpus callosum

    (B) below the corpus callosum

    (C) in the Sylvian fissure

    (D) between the hippocampal sulcus

97. Approximately how long after ventricular dilatation does the head circumference start to increase?

    (A) 5–7 days

    (B) 3–4 days

    (C) 8 weeks

    (D) 2 weeks

98. If hemorrhage is detected in a newborn on the first examination, studies should be performed

    (A) every 3 days until 2 weeks of age

    (B) every 3 days until 2 months of age

    (C) every 5 days until 3 weeks of age

    (D) every 7 days until 3 weeks of age

99. At which week of gestation is the choroid plexus prominent and may completely fill the lateral ventricle?

    (A) last trimester

    (B) first trimester

    (C) mid trimester

    (D) after birth

100. Hydranencephaly is defined as a

    (A) holospheric cerebrum

    (B) posterior fossa cyst

    (C) congenital cystic dilatation of the fourth ventricle

    (D) head largely filled with fluid and a severe loss of cerebral tissue

101. Which of the following does *not* describe holoprosencephaly?

    (A) formation of a holospheric cerebrum

    (B) disorder of diverticulation of the fetal brain

    (C) cerebral hemispheres and lateral ventricles that develop as one vesicle

    (D) premature fusion of the cranial sutures either complete or partial

102. Which of the following statements about spinal and cranial nerves is true?

    (A) There are 12 pairs of cranial nerves and 12 pairs of spinal nerves.

    (B) There are 12 pairs of cranial nerves and 31 pairs of spinal nerves.

    (C) There are 15 pairs of cranial nerves and 15 pairs of spinal nerves.

    (D) There are 20 pairs of cranial nerves and 20 pairs of spinal nerves.

103. The spinal cord ends at about what vertebral level?

    (A) L2

    (B) L5

    (C) S2

    (D) S5

104. Which foramen connects the third ventricle to the fourth ventricle?

    (A) foramen of Monro

    (B) foramen of Luschka

    (C) foramen of Magendie

    (D) cerebral aqueduct

105. The two anterior recesses on the third ventricle are the

    (A) supraoptic and pineal recess

    (B) pineal and infundibular recess

    (C) infundibular and suprapineal recess

    (D) supraoptic and infundibular

106. Microcephaly is *not* associated with which of the following?

    (A) diverticulosis

    (B) craniosynostosis

    (C) Meckel–Gruber's syndrome

    (D) chromosomal abnormalities

107. The two posterior recesses on the third ventricle are

    (A) preoptic and pineal recesses

    (B) pineal and infundibular recesses

    (C) infundibular and suprapineal recesses

    (D) pineal and suprapineal recesses

108. Another name for massa intermedia is

    (A) interthalamic adhesion

    (B) pineal recess

    (C) preoptic recess

    (D) infundibular recess

109. Which structure is *not* a partition of the dura mater?

    (A) falx cerebelli

    (B) falx cerebri

    (C) tentorium

    (D) cerebellum

110. Bleeding within the cerebral parenchyma is called

    (A) subdural hematoma

    (B) intraparenchymal hemorrhage

    (C) cerebellar hemorrhage

    (D) subarachnoid hematoma

111. Another name for the foramen of Monro is the

    (A) interventricular foramen

    (B) cerebral aqueduct

    (C) foramen of Luschka

    (D) foramen of Magendie

112. Which of the following is *not* part of the brainstem?

    (A) spinal cord

    (B) diencephalon

    (C) midbrain

    (D) pons

113. Midline facial anomalies are often associated with holoprosencephaly. These malformations do *not* include which of the following?

    (A) cebocephaly

    (B) cleft palate

    (C) hypoplasia of the ethmoid bone

    (D) meningomyelocele

114. The meninges covers the brain and spinal cord. Which of the following is *not* one of its layers?

    (A) dura mater

    (B) white matter

    (C) arachnoid membrane

    (D) pia mater

115. Which of the following is *not* an etiology of an arachnoid cyst?

    (A) abnormal mechanism of leptomeningeal formation

    (B) entrapment of subarachnoid space by adhesions

    (C) entrapment of cisternal space by adhesions

    (D) failure of development of the cerebral mantle

116. Which of the following does *not* occur as a result of a vein of Galen aneurysm?

    (A) cardiac failure

    (B) hydrocephalus

    (C) enlarged aorta

    (D) quadrigeminal cyst

117. Which of the following does *not* apply to an arachnoid cyst?

    (A) arachnoid cysts lie between the pia mater and the subarachnoid space.

    (B) arachnoid cysts do not communicate with the ventricles or the arachnoid space.

    (C) arachnoid cysts contain cerebrospinal fluid.

    (D) arachnoid cysts are usually found in the Sylvian fissure, middle fossa, and interhemispheric fissure.

118. Which of the following statements is true about the arachnoid granulations?

    (A) Arachnoid granulations lie in the cingulate sulcus.

    (B) Arachnoid granulations lie in the pericallosal artery where cerebrospinal fluid is reabsorbed by the blood.

    (C) Arachnoid granulations lie in the sagittal sinus and reabsorb cerebrospinal fluid as it circulates.

    (D) Arachnoid granulations lie in the ventricular system and reabsorb cerebrospinal fluid as it circulates.

119. Which of the following is *not* a characteristic of schizencephaly?

    (A) absent corpus callosum

    (B) absent septum pellucidum

    (C) unusually shaped ventricle

    (D) dilated septum pellucidum

120. Eight out of 12 neonates with meningitis usually develop which of the following conditions?

    (A) ventriculitis

    (B) intracranial hemorrhage

    (C) abscess

    (D) encephalomalacia

121. Early scans of a preterm infant brain that has PVL would reveal which of the following findings?

    (A) increased echogenicity at the external angle of the lateral ventricles

    (B) normal echogenicity surrounding the lateral ventricles

    (C) cysts varying from a few small ones to multiple variably sized ones

    (D) markedly decreased vascular pulsations

122. Which of the following arteries is the main nutrient vessel of the subependymal germinal matrix tissue?

    (A) pericallosal artery

    (B) callosal marginal artery

    (C) posterior cerebral artery

    (D) Heubner's artery

123. The most common infections acquired in utero are toxoplasmosis, rubella, cytomegalovirus, and herpes simplex, which is referred to as which of the following terms?

    (A) TORCH

    (B) histogenesis

    (C) cytogenesis

    (D) organogenesis

124. PVL is a result of infarction in the arterial boundary zones also known as which of the following?

    (A) cervical circulation

    (B) watershed circulation regions

    (C) ventriculo-fugal artery region

    (D) ventriculopetal parenchymal artery region

111. **(A)** Intraventricular foramen.

112. **(A)** Spinal cord. The brainstem consists of the diencephalon, the midbrain, the pons, and the medulla oblongata.

113. **(D)** Meningomyelocele is not associated with holoprosencephaly facial anomalies. The facial anomalies that can be associated with holoprosencephaly are cleft palate (fissure), cleft lip (fissure), cyclopia (single orbital fossa), cebocephaly (characterized by a defective nose and closed eyes), and ethmocephaly (characterized by a defect of the ethmoid bone).

114. **(B)** The brain is invested by three membranes termed PAD for pia, arachnoid, and dura mater.

115. **(D)** The causes of an arachnoid cyst are arachnoid lesions, entrapment of subarachnoid or cisternal space, and abnormal leptomeningeal formation.

116. **(D)** A quadrigeminal cyst is not caused by a vein of Galen aneurysm. However, it may be a differential diagnosis because of its location and cystic components. Doppler evaluation should exclude a differential diagnosis.

117. **(A)** Arachnoid cysts lie between the arachnoid membrane and the dura mater and not between the pia mater and the subarachnoid space. Acquired arachnoid cysts are found in cisterns adjacent to the third ventricle, and posterior fossa.

118. **(C)** Arachnoid granulations in the sagittal sinus and reabsorb cerebrospinal fluid as it circulates.

119. **(D)** A dilated septum pellucidum is not a characteristic of schizencephaly. It is characterized by agenesis of the corpus callosum and septum pellucidum in addition to unusually shaped frontal horns of the lateral ventricles.

120. **(A)** Ventriculitis. These neonates initially develop meningitis, edema, and cerebritis. Eight of 12 neonates with meningitis develop ventriculitis. Late complications include subdural effusion, enlarged ventricles, and ventricular septations.

121. **(A)** Increased echogenicity at the external angle of the lateral ventricles. Ischemic lesions may occur at the watershed boundary zones of the periventricular white matter and the centrum semiovale as PVL.

122. **(D)** Heubner's artery. This is the main nutrient vessel of the subependymal germinal tissue, which is destined to give rise to much of the glial cell population of the hemisphere.

123. **(A)** TORCH is the acronym for the most common infections acquired in utero: toxoplasmosis, other (congenital syphilis and viruses), rubella, cytomegalovirus, and herpes simplex virus.

124. **(B)** In the premature infant, the watershed zones are located in the periventricular white matter adjacent to the external margins of the lateral ventricles. The zones lie approximately 3–10 mm from the ventricular wall.

125. **(A)** Grade 4 hemorrhage

126. **(C)** Germinal matrix and intraventricular hemorrhages.

127. **(C)** Unilateral germinal matrix hemorrhage.

128. **(A)** Dandy–Walker cyst.

129. **(B)** Sylvian fissure.

130. **(A)** Cistern magna.

131. **(C)** Enlarged ventricles with an area of porencephaly at the region of the body of the left lateral ventricle.

132. **(B)** Resolving intraparenchymal and intraventricular hemorrhages. The irregularity noted in the choroid plexus region is a sign of intraventricular hemorrhage.

133. **(C)** Hydrocephalus. The abnormal finding is a severe form of post-hemorrhagic hydrocephalus.

134. **(B)** Choroid plexus.

135. **(B)** The abnormal findings in Fig. 15–33 revealed an enlarged lateral ventricle, an enlarged third ventricle, an enlarged fourth ventricle, a dilated foramen of Monro, and a dilated aqueduct of Sylvius.

136. **(D)** Pineal recess. The recess is dilated. The recesses of the third ventricle are as follows: supraoptic, infundibular, pineal, and suprapineal.

137. **(B)** fourth ventricle.

138. **(A)** One of the lateral ventricles. The ventricle is enlarged.

139. **(C)** Temporal horns of the lateral ventricles. Both are enlarged.

140. **(B and C)** A resolving intraventricular hemorrhage and PVL. The lateral ventricles are enlarged, and small cystic areas are seen in the periventricular regions.

141. **(A)** Septal vein.

142. **(B)** Massa intermedia. The massa intermedia or interthalamic adhesion, is visualized best in the presence of ventricular dilatation.

143. **(C)** PVL. This neonate may have had a generalized cerebral edema that led to multiple areas of infarction termed encephalomalacia or porencephaly.

144. **(B)** Multiple irregular-shaped cysts in the glomus part of the choroid plexus. A study done with fetuses that had simple CPCs revealed a normal karyotype and no significant related abnormalities. Babies were delivered with no neurological abnormalities at the time of the neonatal examination. However, a study involving complex CPCs revealed trisomies 18 and 21.

145. **(D)** (B and C.) The abnormality demonstrated is bilateral PVL and intraventricular hemorrhage.

146. **(C)** Frontal horns.

147. **(B)** Septated lateral ventricles. In these sonograms, multiple partitions are seen extending to the lateral walls of the ventricles. This particular case is congenital; however, septated ventricles usually occur in ventriculitis.

148. **(A)** Interhemispheric fissure. The structure is shown in the coronal view.

149. **(C)** Frontal horns of the lateral ventricle. The horns are slightly dilated with a unilateral subependymal hemorrhage.

150. **(D)** Cingulate sulcus.

151. **(A)** Corpus callosum.

152. **(C)** Parieto-occipital sulcus.

153. **(D)** Occipital bone.

154. **(D)** Teratoma.

155. **(B)** Transtemporal and transforaminal windows.

156. **(A)** 0.50–0.57. Blood flow in the brain has a low resistive index.

157. **(D)** Middle cerebral artery is most commonly affected by atherosclerotic disease.

References

1. Meijler G, Sylke J. *Neonatal Cranial Ultrasonography*. 3rd ed. Cham: Springer International publishers; 2019.

2. Norton M, Scoutt LM. *Callen's Ultrasonography in Obstetrics and Gynecology*. 6th ed. New York: Elsevier; 2017.

3. Rumack C, Levine D. *Diagnostic Ultrasound*. 5th ed. New York: Elsevier; 2017.

4. Govaert P, De Vries LS. *An Atlas of the Neonatal Brain Sonography*. 2nd ed. London, England: Mac Keith Press; 2010.

5. Claire FS, Andrew D, *Gray's Surface Anatomy: Ultrasound*. 1st ed. New York: Elsevier; 2018.

6. Hagen-Ansert S. *Textbook of Diagnostic Ultrasound*. 8th ed. New York: Elsevier; 2019.

7. Sutton D. *A Textbook of Radiology and Imaging*. Vol. 2, 7th ed. New York: Williams & Wilkins; 2014.

5. Claire TS, Andrew D. Grays Surface Anatomy. Ultrasound. 1st ed. New York: Elsevier 2018.

6. Hagen-Ansert S. Textbook of Diagnostic Ultrasound. 8th ed. New York: Elsevier, 2019.

7. Sutton D. A Textbook of Radiology and Imaging. Vol. 2. 7th ed. New York: Williams & Williams 2014.

References

1. Abullo O, SvN et. Neonatal Cranial Ultrasonography. 3rd ed. Champaign International publishers 2019.

2. Norton M, Scout LM. Callens Ultrasonography in Obstetrics and Gynecology. 6th ed. New York: Elsevier, 2017.

3. Rumad C, Levine D. Diagnostic Ultrasound. 5th ed. New York: Elsevier, 2012.

4. Govaert P, De Vries LS. An Atlas of the Neonatal Brain Sonography. 2nd ed. London, England: MAC Keith Press, 2010.

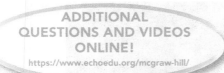
General Applications of Pediatric Sonography

Sumit Pruthi and Elizabeth Snyder

Study Guide

PEDIATRIC ULTRASOUND REVIEW

Introduction

Ultrasonography remains an essential modality in pediatric diagnostic imaging because of its lack of ionizing radiation and ability to perform exams at the bedside without the need for sedation. Although the principles of adult sonography are generalizable, techniques as applied to children are quite different, due to differences in patient size, body composition, and specific entities amenable to sonographic diagnosis in this population. Moreover, specific knowledge of pediatric anatomy, development, and pathology is essential for sonographers performing these exams. This chapter will therefore primarily address anatomy and pathology that is specific in the pediatric population.

In addition to technical factors including choice of transducer and scanning frequency, other factors distinguish pediatric from adult patients. For example, premature or critically ill infants may have difficulty regulating body temperature and children are often unable to cooperate, rendering the examinations particularly challenging in some patients.

NEONATAL BRAIN

The patency of the cranial fontanelles in neonates and infants allows the detailed sonographic evaluation of the brain. Because of its ability to perform exams at the bedside, ultrasound is an important imaging tool for the diagnosis and evaluation of a variety of intracranial pathology in neonates. The exam can be performed as late 12 months of life, when the anterior fontanelle is closed or nearly closed, although in such older patients penetration with the high frequency detailed transducers used in younger infants will not be possible.

Technique

Evaluation of the brain is performed using a 7.5–12 MHz frequency transducer. A 7.5 MHz or higher frequency transducer is typically needed for evaluation of the premature infant, while lower frequency transducers are needed for penetration of the brain in an older infant.[1,2] Linear, higher frequency transducers (eg, 12 MHz or higher) appropriately focused on the near field can be used for the evaluation of superficial structures such as superior sagittal sinus.[1,2]

The anterior fontanelle is the main acoustic window for evaluation of the brain. The posterior and mastoid fontanelles are also used until approximately 6 months of age, when they close.[2] These fontanelles allow for better visualization of posterior structures and the posterior fossa. Images of the brain are obtained in the coronal, sagittal, and axial planes. Video cine clips are very helpful in obtaining a fuller exam.

Anatomy

The exam typically begins by obtaining six standard coronal images through the anterior fontanelle by sweeping slightly from anterior to posterior (Fig. 15–1). Images (from anterior to posterior) are obtained at the level of the following:

- The frontal lobes, just anterior to the frontal horns of the lateral ventricles
- The frontal horns of the lateral ventricles
- The third ventricle
- The body of the lateral ventricle just posterior to the foramina of Monro
- The trigone of the lateral ventricles
- The occipital lobes

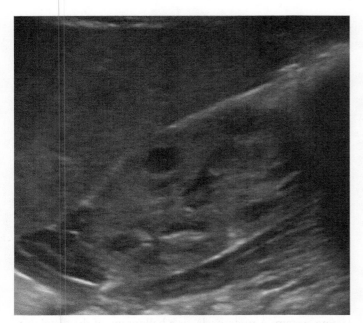

FIGURE 15–12. Normal neonatal adrenal gland. The normal adrenal gland is a triangular structure superior to the upper pole of the kidney.

Congenital Adrenal Hyperplasia

Congenital adrenal hyperplasia is a common cause of ambiguous genitalia in genetically female infants. In these cases, the adrenals are enlarged, losing their lambda two-limb shape, which is substituted by multiple loops, more numerous on the left than on the right. This has been termed "cerebriform appearance" because it appears similar to the gyri in the brain.[39]

Adrenal Hemorrhage

Adrenal hemorrhage in children is most commonly seen in neonates secondary to stress in the perinatal period, although may be also seen in older children or adolescence from blunt abdominal trauma.[39] As in other parts of the body, the appearance of a hematoma in the adrenal gland depends on the age of the hemorrhage. Initially, the hematoma will appear as an echogenic mass without internal vascularity on Doppler imaging. As it evolves, the hematoma may appear as a complex mass, again without internal vascularity. In the chronic setting, the mass may appear calcified, or there may be persistent adrenal calcification without a residual mass.[39] Congenital neuroblastoma is part of the differential diagnosis. Adrenal hemorrhage in neonates can be associated with ipsilateral renal vein thrombosis.

Neuroblastoma

The most common solid adrenal mass in infants and young children is neuroblastoma, a malignant neoplasm of sympathetic neural cells. On ultrasound, neuroblastoma most commonly presents as a heterogeneous solid mass with internal vascularity. There may be foci of internal calcifications which may demonstrate posterior shadowing. Occasionally, neuroblastoma may manifest as a cystic mass, that has imaging overlap with a congenital adrenal cyst or evolving adrenal hemorrhage.[39] Follow-up ultrasound is the best way to differentiate among these diagnoses, as neuroblastoma will typically enlarge and may become more complex, whereas adrenal hemorrhage should slowly resolve over time.[39]

Other Adrenal Masses

Adrenal adenomas, pheochromocytomas and adrenal cortical carcinomas may also rarely present in the pediatric population. On US, adrenal adenomas typically appear as well-circumscribed masses, sometimes with internal vascularity. Pheochromocytomas can appear as an adrenal mass with variable echogenicity and internal vascularity. Adrenal cortical carcinomas are more likely to be larger and heterogeneous, although imaging appearance depends on the size of the mass at the time of diagnosis; these masses may be associated with virilization at presentation, or with syndromic presentation such as Beckwith Wiedemann.[39]

GENITOURINARY TRACT

Ultrasound plays an essential role in the evaluation of the pediatric genitourinary tract and is often the first-line imaging test for the evaluation of the kidneys and bladder.

The kidneys can be imaged both from the coronal approach and the posterior approach. A linear probe is appropriate in neonates and young infants and, when used throughout the study, a posterior approach is not necessary. The coronal approach is superior in imaging of the adrenal gland and of the psoas muscle in the renal fossa. On the other hand, the posterior approach typically brings the kidney closer to the transducer, allowing more detailed renal imaging. In older children, a curvilinear probe is typically used for the coronal approach, while a linear probe should be used for the posterior approach. In some small children, it may be helpful to image the kidneys from a posterior approach, while the child is embraced by their caregiver.[40] Images of the bladder are typically obtained with a linear probe in neonates and infants, and a curvilinear probe in older children, similar to the kidneys. When the bladder is markedly distended, sagittal views including the spine can convey the degree of distension of the bladder. In small children who are not toilet trained, the bladder may be checked multiple times during the exam as it may fill and empty frequently.

Kidneys

Evaluation of kidney length can be compared to normative values based on patient age, height, and/or weight. A 10% difference in size is allowed between the two kidneys. On ultrasound, the renal parenchyma is made up of the outer cortex and triangular, relatively hypoechoic inner medullary pyramids, most prominent and hypoechoic in neonates, and can resemble distended calyces if the scan is technically inadequate. The renal collecting system consists of the calyces, which arise from the apex of the medullary pyramid, and the pelvis, the central portion of the collecting system which connects to the ureter; the calyces are typically nondistended and not individually visible. Longitudinal and transverse views of both kidneys should be performed evaluating for echogenicity, corticomedullary differentiation, and the presence of masses or hydronephrosis. Longitudinal and transverse views are also obtained of the urinary bladder. The bladder volume may be calculated both while full and after voiding, depending on the clinical presentation.

The normal sonographic appearance of the kidneys depends on the child's age. In the neonate or infant, the renal medullary pyramids are large and hypoechoic, and could be mistaken for dilated calyces if the scan is technically inadequate. Cortical echogenicity can be higher than that of older children, and may be slightly higher than or equal to the echogenicity of the liver; in normal kidneys, this enhances the difference between the cortex and the pyramids, or corticomedullary differentiation. The central hyperechoic center seen in adult kidneys is not part of the normal sonographic appearance of the kidneys in young children. Sonographic appearance of the kidneys in older children and adolescents is the same as in adults.

Hydronephrosis

Hydronephrosis, or dilatation of the renal collecting system, may be due to a variety of causes, and is typically evaluated with ultrasound. The severity of hydronephrosis may be evaluated by the degree of pelvocalyceal dilatation, measuring the anterior–posterior diameter of the intrarenal pelvis, and evaluating for any cortical thinning. Society of Fetal Ultrasound (SFU) has designed a grading system for grading neonatal and infant hydronephrosis, whereby Grade 0 denotes no dilatation; Grade 1 (mild) denotes dilatation of the renal pelvis without dilatation of the calyces; Grade 2 (mild) denotes dilatation of the renal pelvis (mild) and calyces (pelvocalyceal pattern is retained); Grade 3 (moderate) denotes moderate dilatation of the renal pelvis and calyces, mild cortical thinning may be seen; and Grade 4 (severe) denotes gross dilatation of the renal pelvis and calyces, and renal atrophy seen as cortical thinning.

Ureteropelvic junction obstruction results from obstruction of the renal pelvis at the level of the origin of the ureter. On ultrasound, findings include dilatation of the affected renal pelvis and calyces, without dilatation of the ureter.

Dilatation of the ureter usually implies reflux, obstruction at the ureterovesical junction, or at the level of the bladder. If there is bladder outlet obstruction as the cause of hydronephrosis, the bladder wall may appear thickened and irregular.

Congenital Anomalies

Congenital anomalies of the kidneys can result in abnormal renal shape or position. A kidney may also be congenitally absent. A pelvic kidney describes a kidney that does not ascend to the upper abdomen and is located in the pelvis. In a horseshoe kidney, the lower poles of the kidneys are fused at the midline, just anterior to the spine. In crossed fused renal ectopia, both kidneys are fused and located on one side of the abdomen.

Renal Duplication

Duplication of the renal collecting system is a common congenital anomaly. Duplication may be complete, with separate upper and lower pole pelves and two separate ureters, or partial. On ultrasound, a duplicated collecting system may be diagnosed when normal renal parenchyma divides the renal pelvis into upper and lower parts. However, if there is no hydronephrosis or dilated ureter, and the renal parenchyma is normal, the duplication is said to be uncomplicated and of no clinical concern.

According to the Weigert-Meyer rule, the lower pole ureter typically inserts into the normal, anatomic location in the bladder. The upper pole ureter, on the other hand, typically inserts inferior to and medial to the site of normal ureteral insertion.[41] Complications arise when the ectopic upper pole ureter becomes obstructed resulting in hydronephrosis of the upper pole collecting system. A ureterocele, or a ballooning of the distal ureter within the bladder wall, may be seen as a cystic appearing outpouching adjacent to the ureterovesical junction. The upper pole ureter may insert outside of the bladder altogether, in the urethra or vagina in girls, in the seminal vesicles in boys. When there is hydroureteronephrosis of the upper pole, it is important to assess the parenchyma for loss of corticomedullary differentiation, as it is often dysplastic. Vesicoureteral reflux may occur in the lower pole ureter, but typically the parenchyma of the lower pole is normal.

Cystic Renal Disease

Cystic renal disease typically refers to genetic conditions, such as autosomal recessive and autosomal dominant polycystic renal disease, or to developmental conditions, most commonly multicystic dysplastic kidneys (MCDKs), and renal cystic dysplasia.

Autosomal recessive polycystic kidney disease typically can present prenatally, in neonates, or in older children, depending on the degree of renal involvement. When presenting in neonates, the kidneys appear markedly enlarged and echogenic because the cysts are small, made up of hyperplastic tubules; with high-resolution linear transducers, some of the tiny cysts can be resolved. If autosomal dominant kidney disease presents in children, it typically does not present until late childhood or adolescence. Because renal cysts are much less common in children than adults, even one cyst typically requires sonographic follow up to evaluate for the development of additional cysts. Occasionally, autosomal dominant disease may present in neonates, and very rarely may resemble autosomal recessive disease.

MCDK is a congenital malformation of the kidney that typically presents as multiple noncommunicating cysts separated by absent or echogenic, dysplastic renal parenchyma. MCDK is thought to be caused by early in utero obstruction, with atresia of the ureteropelvic junction or the pelvis and infundibula.

A MCDK may be followed by ultrasound to ensure involution. MCDKs by definition, have no function. The condition is very rarely bilateral, but when this happens, the child functionally has no kidneys.

Renal cystic dysplasia refers to a spectrum of abnormal renal development or renal damage from in utero obstruction or reflux. Kidneys show decreased or no corticomedullary differentiation, and may have some tiny cysts, often distributed in the periphery. These kidneys have variable function. These findings should be sought in upper poles of duplex kidneys when hydronephrotic, and in the kidneys of patients with posterior urethral valves.

Renal Tumors

Wilms tumor is the most common solid renal tumor in children, which most commonly presents between ages 1 and 5 years.[41] Typically, it appears as a large, solid, heterogenous mass with internal vascularity. The tumor may spread into the renal vein and even extend into the IVC and right atrium. This will appear as echogenic thrombus, which will demonstrate internal Doppler flow. The unaffected kidney must also be examined as 5–10% of children will have bilateral tumors.[41]

Mesoblastic nephroma is a benign solid renal mass which typically presents in the prenatal or neonatal period. Renal cell carcinoma may occur in childhood, but typically occurs later than Wilms tumor, in older children or adolescents.

Pelvis

Ultrasound is the modality of choice for imaging of the pelvic organs in children. In neonates and infants, evaluation can be carried out with the linear transducer. Transperineal scanning can also be performed, most easily in neonates. A curvilinear probe is typically used in older children, the frequency of which depends on the size of the child. Organs are imaged in both the sagittal and transverse planes, and the ovaries are measured in three planes. A full bladder should be used as an acoustic window. Occasionally, a bladder catheter may need to be placed to fill the bladder.

Female Pelvis

The size and sonographic appearance of the uterus and ovaries depend on the developmental stage of the child. In the neonate, the uterus appears relatively prominent with an echogenic endometrial stripe, caused by stimulation from maternal hormones, although its length is 2–3 cm. After 2–3 months of age, the uterus, particularly the fundus, decreases in size and appears flat and rectangular. The uterus will maintain this shape until puberty, measuring usually between 2.5 and 3 cm in length.[42] Similarly, neonatal ovaries may appear prominent and may contain several cysts until 9–12 months of age. Prior to puberty, the ovaries typically measure less than 1 cm^3 in volume. The post-pubertal appearance of the uterus and ovaries is similar to that in adults.

Congenital Anomalies

Hydrocolpos or hydrometrocolpos describes fluid and/or blood distending the vagina and endometrial canal, usually from obstruction. Common causes of obstruction include imperforate hymen, a stenotic or atretic vagina, or a vaginal septum.[42] These are typically found in adolescents after the onset of menses. When found in neonates with large masses, it is usually due to a combination of reflux of urine and/or meconium, as in urogenital sinus or cloacal anomalies. On ultrasound, the distended vagina will appear as a tubular cystic or hypoechoic mass posterior to the bladder. The clue to the diagnosis is identification of the uterine cervix and uterus above the cystic mass, with variable distension of the endometrial canal.

Ambiguous Genitalia

Ultrasound plays an important role in the workup of ambiguous genitalia. The presence of the uterus and vagina can be confirmed. Gonads can be identified in the pelvis, inguinal canals, or in the labia, and ovaries can be distinguished from testes by the presence of multiple small anechoic follicles whereas testes have a homogenous echotexture.

Testes

In the newborn period, the testes appear rounded or oval and demonstrate homogenous echotexture with echogenicity usually less than that of adolescent testes (Fig. 15–13). Until puberty, flow in the testes is slow, usually 5 cm/s or less, and will need high-frequency linear transducers and low-flow settings for identification. On color Doppler, the vessels typically appear as small foci of color signal, versus the branching pattern seen in adolescents.[42] After puberty, the testes remain homogenous but appear slightly more echogenic. They typically measure between 3 and 5 cm in length.

Cryptorchidism is a congenital abnormality in which in the testes do not descend into the scrotum. They may be located anywhere along their embryologic descent from the retroperitoneum to the inguinal canal.

Testicular Torsion

As in adults, testicular torsion results when the testicle twists about the spermatic cord, compromising blood supply. Ultrasound with color and spectral Doppler is the exam of choice

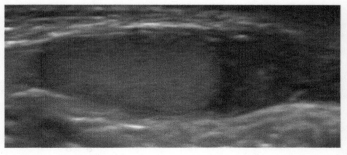

FIGURE 15–13. Normal neonatal testicle.

for the diagnosis. The diagnosis is confirmed with ultrasound by demonstrating decreased or absent flow in the affected testicle, compared to normal flow in the contralateral testicle. Depending on the duration of the torsion, the testicle may appear normal in echotexture, or may appear more hypoechoic or heterogeneous than normal, which usually portends a poorer prognosis.

Torsion of the testicular or epididymal appendages is the most common cause of acute scrotal pain in prepubertal boys.[42,43] In contrast to testicular torsion, in torsion of the testicular appendage, Doppler flow to the affected testicle will be increased compared to the contralateral side. A round, echogenic avascular focus adjacent to the testicle—the torsed appendage—may be seen in some cases.

Neonatal Hips

Developmental dysplasia of the hip (DDH) results when an infant's hip does not form normally; in milder cases, the acetabulum is small and the hip is located, in more severe cases the hip is subluxed or frankly dislocated. Because early intervention is essential in preventing long-term sequelae of this condition, early and accurate diagnosis is essential. Ultrasound is useful as the femoral head is cartilaginous as it has not yet ossified; therefore, it is easily evaluated sonographically. Ultrasound is the diagnostic modality of choice for diagnosis and evaluation of DDH up to 6 months of life before the femoral head starts to ossify. Neonates with abnormal physical exam of the hip or a risk factor for DDH, eg, breech delivery, family history, undergo ultrasound.

A screening hip ultrasound for DDH is performed around 6 weeks of age. Prior to this, hips may appear immature from laxity from maternal hormones, but this may resolve prior to 6 weeks of age. The exam is performed with a linear high-frequency transducer. Both hips are examined. The exam consists of a static and dynamic portion. Static images are obtained in the coronal view at rest and transverse view of the hip while flexed. A transverse view of the hip with stress is also performed to evaluate stability. The exam should be performed with the infant relaxed. The parent can talk to or comfort the child or toys or music can be used for distraction as needed.

To obtain the coronal view, the transducer is placed along the lateral aspect of the patient's hip. The correct view should begin with identifying a straight iliac line and should include the acetabular roof, the triradiate cartilage, and the most inferior portion of the ischium in the same plane (Fig. 15–14). The cartilaginous femoral head appears hypoechoic with small internal echogenic foci. The coronal view can be obtained in physiological neutral position, with approximately 15–20 degrees flexion or in a flexed position.[44] In this view, the morphology of the acetabulum, thickness of fibrofatty pulvinar and the degree of femoral head coverage can be evaluated. The acetabular angle may also be measured. The angle is defined by the acetabular roof and the vertical iliac line, and an angle greater than 60 degrees is normal (Fig. 15–15).

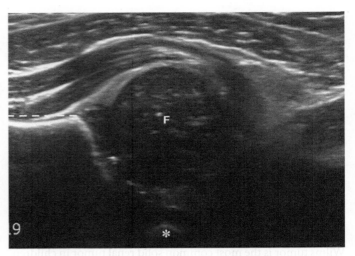

FIGURE 15–14. Normal coronal view of the hip. The cartilaginous femoral head (F) sits within the acetabulum. The iliac line (dashed line) and ischium (*) are also visible in the standard coronal view of the hip.

The transverse view of the hip is obtained both with and without stress. The transducer is turned 90 degrees from the coronal view placed perpendicular to the lateral aspect of the hip, parallel to the femoral shaft while the hip is flexed. Gentle posterior and superior stress is then applied to the hip to evaluate for any change in the position of the femoral head with respect to the posterior acetabulum. If there is a change, then the hip is considered unstable. Application of stress maneuvers is omitted when hips are being examined in a harness or splint device.

Follow-up ultrasound is also used to evaluate infants after a period of observation or treatment. On follow-up studies the patient can be examined outside of harness unless otherwise requested by the orthopedic surgeon.

Hip Effusion

Hip pain or limping in a child can be caused by a variety of pathologic conditions. Because pelvic radiographs may be

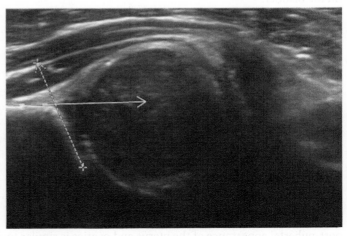

FIGURE 15–15. Normal coronal view of the hip demonstrating the normal alpha angle.

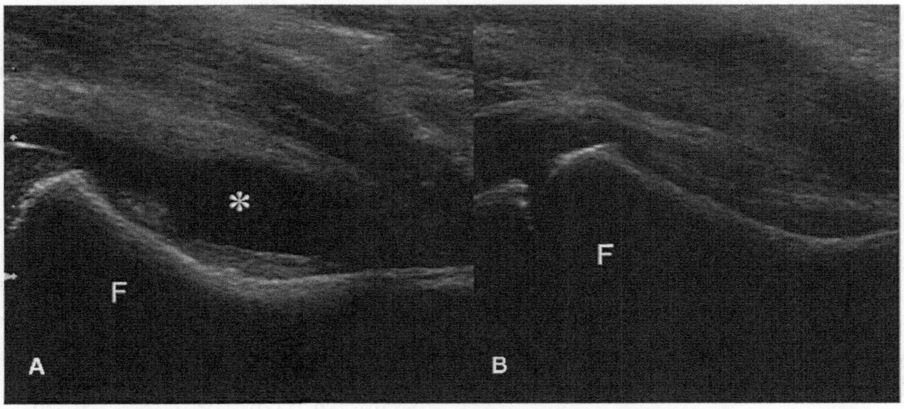

FIGURE 15–16. Sagittal oblique ultrasound images of the hip. **(A)** Image demonstrates a hip joint with an effusion (*). **(B)** The image is a normal hip with no effusion. F—femoral neck.

normal in a child with a hip effusion, ultrasound is often used to determine if an effusion is present.

The exam is performed with a high-frequency linear transducer with the child in the supine position with the hips in neutral position. The hip is scanned from an anterior approach, in a sagittal oblique plane along the long axis of the femoral neck, following the iliopsoas tendon to its insertion at the lesser trochanter. The underlying femoral head and neck are identified by their brightly echogenic linear anterior cortex. The anterior hip joint capsule is identified as a thin echogenic line superficial to the femoral neck cortex and should appear linear or concave in the normal hip. In the case of effusion, the anterior capsule demonstrates a convex margin, and anechoic or hypoechoic fluid is seen deep to the joint capsule anterior to the femoral neck (Fig. 15–16).[45] The asymptomatic hip is typically imaged for comparison.

References

1. Rumack CM, Auckland AK. Neonatal and infant brain imaging. In: Rumack C, Levine D, eds. *Diagnostic Ultrasound*. 5th ed. Philadelphia, PA: Elsevier; 2018, pp. 1511-1572.

2. Gupta P, Sodhi KS, Saxena AK, et al. Neonatal cranial sonography: a concise review for clinicians. *J Pediatr Neurosci*. 2016;11:7-13.

3. Ladino Torres MF, DiPietro MA. Spine ultrasound imaging in the newborn. *Semin Ultrasound CT MRI*. 2014;35:652-661.

4. Wolf S, Schneble F, Tröger J. The conus medullaris: time of ascendence to normal level. *Pediatr Radiol*. 1992;22:590-592.

5. Patterson S. Sonographic assessment of the neonatal spine and the potential for new technologies to aid in diagnoses. *J Diagn Med Sonogr*. 2009;25:4-22.

6. Agarwalla PK, Dunn IF, Scott RM, Smith ER. Tethered cord syndrome. *Neurosurg Clin N Am*. 2007;18:531-547.

7. Lowe LH, Johanek AJ, Moore CW. Sonography of the neonatal spine: Part 2, spinal disorders. *Am J Roentgenol*. 2007;188:739-744.

8. Guimaraes CV. Neuro. In: Donnelly L, ed. *Fundamentals of Pediatric Imaging*. 2nd ed. Philadelphia, PA: Elsevier; 2016, pp. 243-320.

9. Unsinn KM, Geley T, Freund MC, Gassner I. US of the spinal cord in newborns: spectrum of normal findings, variants, congenital anomalies, and acquired diseases. *RadioGraphics*. 2000;20:923-938.

10. Bansal AG, Oudsema R, Masseaux JA, Rosenberg HK. US of pediatric superficial masses of the head and neck. *RadioGraphics*. 2018;38:1239-1263.

11. Weinstock MS, Patel NA, Smith LP. Pediatric cervical lymphadenopathy. *Pediatr Rev*. 2018;39:433-443.

12. Ahuja AT, Ying M, Ho SY, et al. Ultrasound of malignant cervical lymph nodes. *Cancer Imaging*. 2008;8:48-56.

13. Brown RE, Harave S. Diagnostic imaging of benign and malignant neck masses in children—a pictorial review. *Quant Imaging Med Surg*. 2016;6:591-604.

14. Ablin DS, Jain K, Howell L, West DC. Ultrasound and MR imaging of fibromatosis colli (sternomastoid tumor of infancy). *Pediatr Radiol*. 1998;28:230-233.

15. Penny SM. Sonographic diagnosis of fibromatosis colli. *J Diagn Med Sonogr*. 2006;22:399-402.

16. Ahuja AT, Wong KT, King AD, Yuen EHY. Imaging for thyroglossal duct cyst: the bare essentials. *Clin Radiol*. 2005;60:141-148.

17. Wadsworth DT, Siegel MJ. Thyroglossal duct cysts: variability of sonographic findings. *Am J Roentgenol*. 1994;1630:1475-1477.

18. Bhat V, Salins PC, Bhat V. Imaging spectrum of hemangioma and vascular malformations of the head and neck in children and adolescents. *J Clin Imaging Sci*. 2014;4:31.

19. Mulligan PR, Prajapati HJS, Martin LG, Patel TH. Vascular anomalies: classification, imaging characteristics and implications for interventional radiology treatment approaches. *Br J Radiol*. 2014;87:20130392.

20. Behravesh S, Yakes W, Gupta N, et al. Venous malformations: clinical diagnosis and treatment. *Cardiovasc Diagn Ther*. 2016;6:557-569.

21. Joshi P, Vasishta A, Gupta M. Ultrasound of the pediatric chest. *Br J Radiol*. 2019;92:20190058.

22. Nasseri F, Eftekhari F. Clinical and radiologic review of the normal and abnormal thymus: pearls and pitfalls. *RadioGraphics*. 2010;30:413-428.

23. El-Halaby H, Abdel-Hady H, Alsawah G, et al. Sonographic evaluation of diaphragmatic excursion and thickness in healthy infants and children. *J Ultrasound Med*. 2016;35:167-175.

24. Chavhan GB, Babyn PS, Cohen RA, Langer JC. Multimodality imaging of the pediatric diaphragm: anatomy and pathologic conditions. *RadioGraphics*. 2010;30:1797-1817.

25. Gale HI, Gee MS, Westra SJ, Nimkin K. Abdominal ultrasonography of the pediatric gastrointestinal tract. *World J Radiol.* 2016;8:656-667.

26. Hernanz-Schulman M. Infantile hypertrophic pyloric stenosis. *Radiology.* 2003;227:319-331.

27. Edwards EA, Pigg N, Courtier J, et al. Intussusception: past, present and future. *Pediatr Radiol.* 2017;47:1101-1108.

28. Di Serafino M, Mercogliano C, Vallone G. Ultrasound evaluation of the enteric duplication cyst: the gut signature. *J Ultrasound.* 2015;19:131-133.

29. Sangüesa Nebot C, Llorens Salvador R, Carazo Palacios E, et al. Enteric duplication cysts in children: varied presentations, varied imaging findings. *Insights Imaging.* 2018;9:1097-1106.

30. Druten J van, Khashu M, Chan SS, et al. Abdominal ultrasound should become part of standard care for early diagnosis and management of necrotising enterocolitis: a narrative review. *Arch Dis Child Fetal Neonatal Ed.* 2019;104:F551-F559.

31. Epelman M, Daneman A, Navarro OM, et al. Necrotizing enterocolitis: review of state-of-the-art imaging findings with pathologic correlation. *RadioGraphics.* 2007;27:285-305.

32. John SD, Munden MM. The pediatric gastrointestinal tract. In: Rumack C, Levine D, eds. *Diagnostic Ultrasound.* 5th ed. Philadelphia, PA: Elsevier; 2018, pp. 1833-1869.

33. Shimanuki Y, Aihara T, Takano H, et al. Clockwise whirlpool sign at color Doppler US: an objective and definite sign of midgut volvulus. *Radiology.* 1996;199:261-264.

34. Patino MO, Munden MM. Utility of the sonographic whirlpool sign in diagnosing midgut volvulus in patients with atypical clinical presentations. *J Ultrasound Med Off J Am Inst Ultrasound Med.* 2004;23:397-401.

35. Back SJ, Maya CL, Khwaja A. Ultrasound of congenital and inherited disorders of the pediatric hepatobiliary system, pancreas and spleen. *Pediatr Radiol.* 2017;47:1069-1078.

36. Kanegawa K, Akasaka Y, Kitamura E, et al. Sonographic diagnosis of biliary atresia in pediatric patients using the "triangular cord" sign versus gallbladder length and contraction. *Am J Roentgenol.* 2003;181:1387-1390.

37. O'Hara SM. The Pediatric liver and spleen. In: In Rumack C, Levine D, eds. *Diagnostic Ultrasound.* 5th ed. Philadelphia, PA: Elsevier; 2018, pp. 1730-1774.

38. Chung EM, Lattin GE, Cube R, et al. From the archives of the AFIP: pediatric liver masses: radiologic-pathologic correlation. Part 2. Malignant tumors. *RadioGraphics.* 2011;31:483-507.

39. Bittman ME, Lee EY, Restrepo R, Eisenberg RL. Focal adrenal lesions in pediatric patients. *Am J Roentgenol.* 2013;200: W542-W556.

40. Paliwalla M, Park K. A practical guide to urinary tract ultrasound in a child: pearls and pitfalls. *Ultrasound J Br Med Ultrasound Soc.* 2014;22:213-222.

41. Paltiel HJ, Babcock DB. The pediatric urinary tract and adrenal glands. In: Rumack C, Levine D, eds. *Diagnostic Ultrasound.* 5th ed. Philadelphia, PA: Elsevier; 2018, pp. 1775–1832.

42. Simpson WL, Chaudhry H, Rosenberg HK. Pediatric pelvic sonography. In: Rumack C, Levine D, eds. *Diagnostic Ultrasound.* 5th ed. Philadelphia, PA: Elsevier; 2018, pp. 1870-1919.

43. Rakha E, Puls F, Saidul I, Furness P. Torsion of the testicular appendix: importance of associated acute inflammation. *J Clin Pathol.* 2006;59:831-834.

44. AIUM-ACR-SPR-SRU practice parameter for the performance of an ultrasound examination for detection and assessment of developmental dysplasia of the hip. *J Ultrasound Med.* 2018;37:E1-E5.

45. Grissom LE, Harcke HT. The pediatric hip and other musculoskeletal ultrasound applications. In: Rumack C, Levine D, eds. *Diagnostic Ultrasound.* 5th ed. Philadelphia, PA: Elsevier; 2018, pp. 1920-1941.

Questions

1. Until what age can head ultrasound be typically performed?

   (A) 3 months
   (B) 6 months
   (C) 12 months
   (D) 18 months

2. Which of the following brain structures is imaged through the mastoid fontanelle?

   (A) cerebellar hemispheres
   (B) corpus callosum
   (C) lateral ventricles
   (D) third ventricle

3. What is the standard number of images obtained in the coronal plane through the anterior fontanelle in the evaluation of the neonatal brain?

   (A) four
   (B) five
   (C) six
   (D) seven

4. An ultrasound probe is placed approximately 1 cm posterior to the helix of the ear. What fontanelle is most likely being imaged?

   (A) anterior
   (B) mastoidal
   (C) occipital
   (D) posterior

5. In what plane are images of the brain obtained from the mastoid fontanelle?

   (A) axial
   (B) coronal
   (C) parasagittal
   (D) sagittal

6. Until what age can ultrasound of the brain be typically performed?

   (A) 4 months
   (B) 6 months
   (C) 12 months
   (D) 18 months

7. Which of the following structures is normally seen in a midline sagittal image of the brain?

   (A) body of the lateral ventricles
   (B) cerebellar hemispheres
   (C) corpus callosum
   (D) sylvian fissure

8. Which of the following is a fluid-filled structure between the frontal horns of the lateral ventricles?

   (A) cavum septum pellucidum
   (B) corpus callosum
   (C) foramen magnum
   (D) fourth ventricle

9. An echogenic mass is seen at the caudothalamic groove in a premature infant. What is the most likely diagnosis?

   (A) choroid plexus cyst
   (B) GMH
   (C) normal choroid plexus
   (D) tumor

10. Ultrasound in a premature infant demonstrates hemorrhage at the caudothalamic groove as well as in the lateral ventricle. The ventricles are normal in size. What is the grade of GMH in this infant?

    (A) Grade I
    (B) Grade II
    (C) Grade III
    (D) Grade IV

11. Which of the following is a sonographic finding in diffuse cerebral edema?

    (A) enlargement of the lateral ventricles
    (B) increased gray-white matter differentiation
    (C) increased separation between the frontal horns of the lateral ventricles
    (D) slit-like lateral ventricles

12. **Which of the following is a sonographic finding of alobar holoprosencephaly?**

    (A) fused thalami

    (B) normal corpus callosum

    (C) normal lateral ventricles

    (D) normal third ventricles

13. **Sonographic findings of the Chiari II malformation include which of the following?**

    (A) absent cerebellar vermis

    (B) cystic dilatation of the posterior fossa

    (C) fused thalami

    (D) small posterior fossa with downward displacement of the cerebellar tonsils

14. **Which of the following is true regarding the appearance of intracranial hemorrhage on ultrasound?**

    (A) It always appears cystic.

    (B) It always appears echogenic.

    (C) It always appears hypoechoic.

    (D) Its appearance depends on the age of hemorrhage.

15. **At what level does the conus medullaris normally terminate?**

    (A) T12–L1

    (B) L1–L2

    (C) L3–L4

    (D) L4–L5

16. **Until what age can spinal cord ultrasound be typically performed?**

    (A) 1–3 months

    (B) 4–6 months

    (C) 6–8 months

    (D) 10–12 months

17. **The echogenic line along the surface of the spinal canal is which of the following?**

    (A) arachnoid-dura mater complex

    (B) central echo complex

    (C) cauda equina

    (D) pia mater

18. **Which of the following spinal structures is evaluated with M-mode imaging?**

    (A) arachnoid mater

    (B) cauda equina

    (C) craniocervical junction

    (D) vertebral bodies

19. **Which of the following is associated with a tethered spinal cord?**

    (A) limited motion of nerve roots on M-mode and cine images

    (B) spinal cord located in the center of the spinal canal

    (C) termination of the conus at the T10 level

    (D) thin appearance of nerve roots of the cauda equina

20. **Myelomeningocele is associated with which brain malformation?**

    (A) Chiari I

    (B) Chiari II

    (C) Chiari II

    (D) Dandy–Walker malformation

21. **Patients with dorsal dermal sinuses are most at risk for which of the following?**

    (A) meningitis

    (B) paralysis

    (C) stroke

    (D) urinary tract infections

22. **What is the most common clinical presentation of fibromatosis colli?**

    (A) a 2-week-old infant presenting with a unilateral neck mass

    (B) a 1-year-old presenting with a supraclavicular mass

    (C) a 2-week-old presenting with bilateral neck masses

    (D) a 1-year-old presenting with a painful submandibular mass

23. **Which muscle is affected in fibromatosis colli?**

    (A) latissimus dorsi

    (B) serratus anterior

    (C) sternocleidomastoid

    (D) trapezius

24. **Which of the following is true about thyroglossal duct cysts?**

    (A) Real-time sonography may aid in the diagnosis.

    (B) They always appear anechoic.

    (C) They may have internal vascular flow on Doppler imaging.

    (D) They may be solid lesions.

25. **An infant presented with a reddish palpable mass in the neck. Ultrasound imaging demonstrates an echogenic mass with increased vascularity and a high-density of vessels within the mass. What is the most likely diagnosis?**

    (A) dermoid cyst

    (B) epidermoid cyst

    (C) infantile hemangioma

    (D) LM

26. **Phleboliths are typical of which vascular lesion?**

    (A) arteriovenous malformation

    (B) infantile hemangioma

    (C) LM

    (D) VM

27. **Which of the following is true regarding LMs?**

    (A) They always appear anechoic.

    (B) They never contain fluid-fluid levels.

    (C) They may contain phleboliths.

    (D) They may present as rapidly expanding masses.

28. **What is the typical echogenicity of the thymus?**

    (A) equal to or slightly less echogenic than the liver

    (B) equal to or slightly more echogenic than the liver

    (C) significantly less echogenic than the liver

    (D) significantly more echogenic than the liver

29. **How many layers of bowel are typically seen on ultrasound?**

    (A) two

    (B) three

    (C) five

    (D) six

30. **In HPS, how long does the pyloric channel measure?**

    (A) less than 2 mm

    (B) less than 10 mm

    (C) less than 14 mm

    (D) less than 20 mm

31. **Which of the following techniques are used for the evaluation of HPS?**

    (A) high-frequency linear transducer and M-mode imaging

    (B) high-frequency linear transducer and cine imaging

    (C) low-frequency curved transducer and M-mode imaging

    (D) low-frequency curved transducer and cine imaging

32. **Which of the following makes the diagnosis of small bowel–small bowel intussusception more likely than an ileocolic intussusception?**

    (A) internal echogenic fat

    (B) size less than 1.8 cm

    (C) size greater than 2.5 cm

    (D) target sign

33. **What does the term pneumatosis describe?**

    (A) air in the bowel wall

    (B) air in the bowel lumen

    (C) air in the portal venous system

    (D) free air in the peritoneum

34. **What is the upper limit of normal for the diameter of the normal appendix?**

    (A) 4 mm

    (B) 5 mm

    (C) 6 mm

    (D) 7 mm

35. **What is the most common cause of hepatic metastases in children?**

    (A) breast cancer

    (B) lymphoma

    (C) neuroblastoma

    (D) Wilms' tumor

36. **Which of the following is the most useful sonographic finding of biliary atresia?**

    (A) absent gallbladder

    (B) contracted gallbladder

    (C) echogenic liver

    (D) triangular cord sign

37. The adrenal glands are located immediately superior to which organ?

(A) bladder

(B) kidneys

(C) liver

(D) pancreas

38. Which of the following describes a normal appearance of a neonatal adrenal gland?

(A) cerebriform

(B) cystic

(C) globular

(D) triangular with internal echogenic line

39. Which of the following ultrasound findings suggests a diagnosis other than an adrenal hemorrhage?

(A) complex cystic mass with calcification

(B) complex cystic mass with internal vascularity

(C) complex cystic mass without internal vascularity

(D) echogenic mass without internal vascularity

40. A 2-week-old infant is found to have a cystic mass in the right adrenal gland. What is the best way to distinguish between adrenal hemorrhage or cystic neuroblastoma in this patient?

(A) age of patient

(B) CT scan

(C) follow-up ultrasound

(D) MRI

41. A triangular hypoechoic area is seen in the spleen in a 4-year-old child with sickle cell anemia. What is the most likely diagnosis?

(A) abscess

(B) calcification

(C) hemangioma

(D) infarct

42. Which of the following is true regarding the sonographic appearance of neonatal kidneys?

(A) The cortex appears more echogenic than in older children.

(B) The cortex appears more hypoechoic than in older children.

(C) The cortical surface appears smoother than in older children.

(D) There is typically no corticomedullary differentiation.

43. According to the Weigert–Meyer rule, in a duplicated kidney where does the upper pole ureter insert?

(A) anatomically

(B) inferior and lateral to the normal ureteral insertion

(C) inferior and medial to the normal ureteral insertion

(D) superior and lateral to the normal ureteral insertion

44. A neonate undergoes abdominal ultrasound for distension and the kidneys appear markedly enlarged and echogenic with loss of corticomedullary differentiation. What is the most likely diagnosis?

(A) autosomal dominant polycystic kidney disease

(B) autosomal recessive polycystic kidney disease

(C) MCDK

(D) nephrogenic rests

45. Which of the following is true regarding the sonographic appearance of testicles in the neonate?

(A) Doppler flow appears similar to adults.

(B) They may appear spherical or ovoid.

(C) They typically appear more hyperechoic than adolescent testes.

(D) They typically measure between 3 and 5 cm in length.

46. An 8-year-old male presents with sudden onset of right testicular pain. Sonographic evaluation demonstrates a hypervascular right testicle with an echogenic avascular pretesticular focus. What is the most likely diagnosis?

(A) epididymitis

(B) rhabdomyosarcoma

(C) testicular torsion

(D) torsion of the testicular appendage

47. How may neonatal ovaries be differentiated from testes in an infant with ambiguous genitalia?

(A) homogeneous echotexture

(B) location in the inguinal canal

(C) location in the pelvis

(D) presence of small internal anechoic foci

48. An infant is examined for hip dysplasia. What is a normal alpha angle?

(A) anything greater than 40 degrees

(B) anything less than 40 degrees

(C) anything greater than 60 degrees

(D) anything less than 60 degrees

49. A newborn infant has a history of breech presentation. At what age should a screening ultrasound for hip dysplasia be performed?

    (A) 1 week
    (B) 2 weeks
    (C) 6 weeks
    (D) 8 weeks

50. In the evaluation of hip joint effusion, along what axis is the hip scanned?

    (A) along the long axis of the femoral neck
    (B) along the short axis of the femoral neck
    (C) along the long axis of the greater trochanter
    (D) along the short axis of the greater trochanter

51. What type of probe is used for the evaluation of a hip effusion in a child?

    (A) high-frequency curvilinear probe
    (B) low-frequency curvilinear probe
    (C) high-frequency linear probe
    (D) low-frequency linear probe

52. Which of the following findings suggests a hip joint effusion?

    (A) concave configuration of the anterior joint capsule
    (B) convex configuration of the anterior joint capsule
    (C) linear configuration of the anterior joint capsule
    (D) symmetric appearance of both hips

23. In the following image, the structure indicated by the arrow is a distended gastrocnemius/semimembranosus bursa. Which of the following best describes this finding?

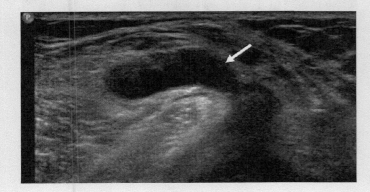

(A) popliteal bursitis

(B) noncommunicating with the posterior knee joint

(C) Baker's cyst

(D) knee-joint effusion

24. A joint is visualized on ultrasound as

(A) a synovium-filled space between two cortical surfaces

(B) a cartilaginous space between two cortical surfaces

(C) a synovium filled space between two cartilaginous surfaces

(D) a cartilaginous space between two cartilaginous surfaces

25. A joint effusion may be indicated on ultrasound by the presence of

(A) low-level echoes

(B) septations

(C) solid material

(D) displacement of the capsule by fluid

26. Ultrasound for joint effusions would definitely be the preferred imaging modality in patients with which of the following findings?

(A) adjacent fracture

(B) joint prosthesis

(C) rheumatoid arthritis

(D) adjacent ganglion cyst

27. Ganglion cysts are *not* likely to form in relation to

(A) joint capsules

(B) tendon sheaths

(C) muscles

(D) joint effusions

28. Which of the following statements is true regarding ganglion cysts?

(A) They are most commonly located along the volar aspect of the ankle.

(B) They are most commonly spongy at palpation.

(C) They are best treated with percutaneous drainage.

(D) They are often related to prior trauma.

29. Ultrasound can be useful in treatment as well as diagnosis of musculoskeletal disorder. What is this due to?

(A) the ability of ultrasound to be able to capture quicker images of needle placement than CT or MRI

(B) the ability of ultrasound to be able to discern the gap between the tendon and its sheath avoiding rupture of the sheath

(C) the ability of ultrasound to better distinguish soft tissue from bony structures than CT or MRI

(D) the ability of ultrasound to distinguish the needle better than CT or MRI

Questions 30–31: Match the structures indicated in the following image with the terms in Column B.

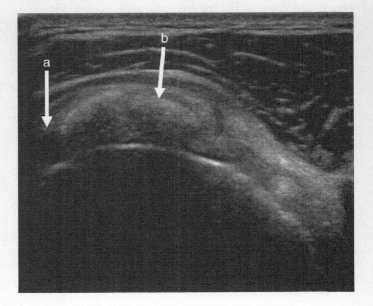

COLUMN A   COLUMN B

30. _____   (A) Calcification

31. _____   (B) Posterior portion of the supraspinatus tendon

Questions 32–34: Match the structures indicated in the following image with the terms in Column B.

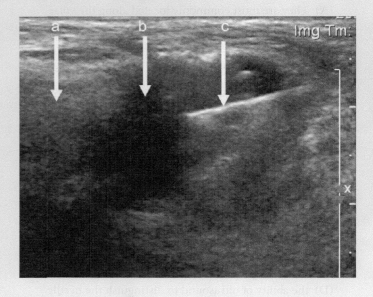

COLUMN A	COLUMN B
32. _____	(A) Neuroma
33. _____	(B) Needle
34. _____	(C) Interdigital webspace

35. Why use the color hue (chroma map) on neuroma studies?

(A) improved visualization

(B) improved specular reflection

(C) reduction in anisotropic effect

(D) reduction of speckle

Questions 36–39: Match the structures indicated in the following image with the terms in Column B.

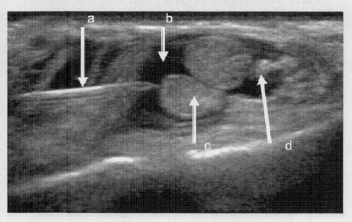

COLUMN A	COLUMN B
36. _____	(A) Peroneal tendons of ankle
37. _____	(B) Needle
38. _____	(C) Tendon vinculum
39. _____	(D) Distended tendon sheath postinjection

40. The needle used in ultrasound-guided therapeutic injections appears

(A) echogenic with posterior acoustic enhancement

(B) echogenic with posterior reverberation artifact

(C) hypoechoic with posterior acoustic enhancement

(D) hypoechoic with posterior reverberation artifact

41. The following image represents a procedure described in the body of the text. What sort of procedure is it?

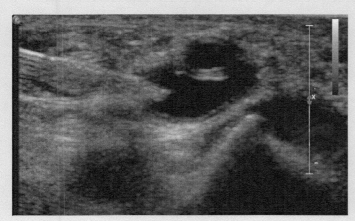

(A) ultrasound-guided biopsy
(B) x-ray-guided injection
(C) diagnostic ultrasound
(D) ultrasound-guided aspiration/injection

Questions 42–44: Match the structures indicated in the following image with the terms in Column B.

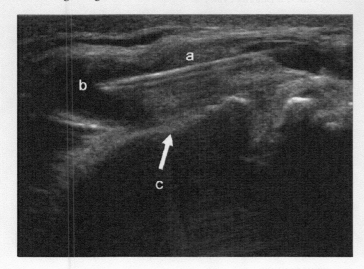

COLUMN A	COLUMN B
42. _____	(A) Cyst
43. _____	(B) Needle
44. _____	(C) Bone

45. The following image is an example of which of the following types of sonography?

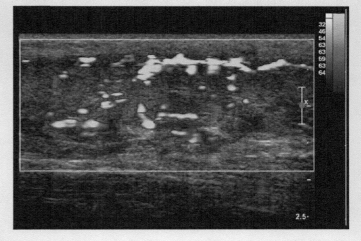

(A) Pulse-wave (PW) Doppler
(B) continuous-wave (CW) Doppler
(C) 2D color Doppler
(D) color power Doppler

Answers and Explanations

1. **(C)** MRI has been the preferred method of evaluating abnormalities of the musculoskeletal system. However, sonography is recognized as advantageous due to its ability to image in real time while watching manipulation of the affected anatomy.

2. **(D)** Sonography is unable to delineate information beyond the cortical surface of bony structures due to the acoustic impedance mismatch from the adjacent soft tissue.

3. **(A)** PDI is a technique used to display the detection of blood flow without displaying direction or having dependence on angle of insonation.

4. **(B)** PDI has been utilized to assess vascularity associated with low-flow states seen in the musculoskeletal system when assessing degree of injury and its response to treatment.

5. **(C)** Tendons typically demonstrate a surrounding layer of echogenic tissue. However, this is not always representative of a synovial sheath but is sometimes the adherent connective tissue (paratendon).

6. **(C)** The anisotropic effect is an artifact of sonographic imaging when the beam is less than perpendicular to the tissue and a hypoechoic region is identified suggesting an abnormality.

7. **(A)** Multiple factors determine tendon thickness, but the best method for assessing normal versus abnormal thickness for a particular patient is to compare the affected tendon to the unaffected contralateral tendon.

8. **(B)** Calcification within any region of the body is demonstrated sonographically as having an echogenic interface with a discrete shadow posteriorly.

9. **(A)** With diffuse inflammation of the tendon, there is sonographic evidence of diffuse inflammation.

10. **(A)** Complete tendon ruptures often result in the formation of an adjacent hematoma and muscle retraction.

11. **(B)** Cartilage.

12. **(C)** Supraspinatus tendon.

13. **(D)** Pre-bursal.

14. **(A)** Subcorticoid subdeltoid bursa.

15. **(B)** Presence of fluid within the biceps sheath has a 95% positive predictive value.

16. **(B)** The sonographic appearance of echogenic striations within hypoechoic bands of is classic for the echogenic perimysium and the hypoechoic muscle fiber bulk.

17. **(C)** The "dirty shadow" appearance is a result of the gas formation within the infected collection of fluid.

18. **(A)** The appearance of an intramuscular hematoma will change over time. With appropriate response to treatment, the resolving injury may often return to a near normal appearance.

19. **(D)** If a hematoma does not resolve entirely, it will often result in a calcification along the periphery.

20. **(D)** Normal bursae are typically too small to identify definitively with sonography. Visualization of this anatomy often suggests pathology immediately.

21. **(A)** The normal bursa is 2 mm thick or less.

22. **(D)** Acute bursitis is most often anechoic in nature due to the recent injury. The appearance of complicated fluid is suggestive of an inflammatory response. This can further be evaluated using PDI to confirm hyperemia.

23. **(C)** If a fluid collection connects with the joint space, it is not considered simply bursitis. Fluid collection along the gastrocnemius muscle communicating with the knee joint is called a Baker's cyst.

24. **(A)** Cartilage should be seen below the echogenic joint margin and a small hypoechoic space between the bony structures of the joint.

25. **(D)** Any sonographic evidence of internal echoes within a joint effusion suggests inflammation or infection of the effusion. Additional imaging modalities may be preferred to further characterize the findings.

26. **(B)** Ultrasound may be utilized effectively on essentially any patient and may be preferred for those patients with prosthesis due to the artifacts seen on CT and MRI.

27. **(D)** Ganglion cysts are often connected the joint capsule but are not a result of a joint effusion.

28. **(D)** Ganglion cysts typically occur on the dorsal aspect of the wrist and ankle and are often presumed to be related to prior trauma.

29. **(D)** Real-time imaging during the insertion of the needle allows for more rapid. Sequential imaging of the advancement of the needle tip during the procedure simultaneously.

30. **(B)** Posterior portion of the supraspinatus tendon.

31. **(A)** Calcification.

32. **(B)** Needle.

33. **(C)** Interdigital webspace.

34. **(A)** Neuroma.

35. **(A)** Use of a chroma map assists in differentiating adjacent tissues of similar acoustic properties. This allows the subtle differences in the neuroma characteristics to stand out.

36. **(C)** Tendon vinculum.

37. **(A)** Peroneal tendons of the ankle.

38. **(D)** Distended tendon sheath post injection.

39. **(B)** Needle.

40. **(B)** When the beam crosses the interface of the metal needle shaft, there is strong reflection (echogenic), but the small space between the walls of the lumen often results in the reverberation artifact due to delayed signal return from the far wall of the needle lumen.

41. **(D)** There is a cystic mass present with needle guidance directed toward the mass. Due to the cystic nature of this abnormality, aspiration of its contents would be likely.

42. **(B)** Needle.

43. **(A)** Cyst.

44. **(C)** Bone.

45. **(D)** Color power Doppler provides information obtained by the amplitude of moving blood cells. This method of imaging does not indicate velocity and is not dependent on angle to demonstrate flow making it much more sensitive to low-flow states as seen in the musculoskeletal system.